AF758128

Principles of Specialty Nursing
Under the Auspices of the *European Specialist Nurses Organisations (ESNO)*

Series Editor

Françoise Charnay-Sonnek
ESNO
European Specialist Nurses Organisations
Brussels, Belgium

The role of the specialist nurse in Europe is still not clearly defined. Despite the fact that there have been formal training programs – e.g. for nurse anaesthetists, operating room nurses, intensive care and mental health nurses – for years now, the practices, status, duration and content of training can vary greatly from country to country. Some other specialist roles, e.g. for Diabetes, Dialysis, Urology and Oncology, have successfully been established in Europe with the help of professional transnational collaborations. Moreover, advances in medical technologies and more sophisticated treatment will not only require specialist nurses in order to ensure quality and safety of care, but will also call upon them to assume new roles in their professional field to compensate for physician shortages. Most of the available literature on specialty nursing practice currently comes from the USA, Canada, and Australia, and accordingly reflects evidence-based nursing in these countries. Therefore, there was and is a need to establish European evidence-based practice on the basis of different clinical experiences. This series, which encompasses books for each specialty, will shape evidence-based practice in Europe, while also integrating lessons learned from other continents. Moreover, it will contribute to clarifying the status of the specialist nurse as an advanced practice nurse.

More information about this series at http://www.springer.com/series/13892

José Carlos Santos • John R. Cutcliffe
Editors

European Psychiatric/Mental Health Nursing in the 21st Century

A Person-Centred Evidence-Based Approach

Springer

Editors
José Carlos Santos
Escola Superior de Enfermagem de Coimbra
Nursing School of Coimbra
Coimbra
Portugal

John R. Cutcliffe
Cutcliffe Consulting
Kingston
Canada

School of Nursing
Coimbra
Portugal

ISSN 2366-875X ISSN 2366-8768
Principles of Specialty Nursing
ISBN 978-3-319-31771-7 ISBN 978-3-319-31772-4 (eBook)
https://doi.org/10.1007/978-3-319-31772-4

Library of Congress Control Number: 2017964372

© Springer International Publishing Switzerland 2018
This work is subject to copyright. All rights are reserved by the Publisher, whether the whole or part of the material is concerned, specifically the rights of translation, reprinting, reuse of illustrations, recitation, broadcasting, reproduction on microfilms or in any other physical way, and transmission or information storage and retrieval, electronic adaptation, computer software, or by similar or dissimilar methodology now known or hereafter developed.
The use of general descriptive names, registered names, trademarks, service marks, etc. in this publication does not imply, even in the absence of a specific statement, that such names are exempt from the relevant protective laws and regulations and therefore free for general use.
The publisher, the authors and the editors are safe to assume that the advice and information in this book are believed to be true and accurate at the date of publication. Neither the publisher nor the authors or the editors give a warranty, express or implied, with respect to the material contained herein or for any errors or omissions that may have been made. The publisher remains neutral with regard to jurisdictional claims in published maps and institutional affiliations.

Printed on acid-free paper

This Springer imprint is published by Springer Nature
The registered company is Springer International Publishing AG
The registered company address is: Gewerbestrasse 11, 6330 Cham, Switzerland

Foreword I

According to various national mental health-care policies and position statements regarding contemporary mental health care, the person who uses such services (i.e., client, service user) is no longer a passive recipient. The service user is no longer "reduced" to being little more than a disease or malfunctioning brain. And the care context should no longer be one dominated by doctors/nurses, wherein the care is focused on diagnosis, symptomatology, and associated pharmacological responses. The National Survivor User Network (accessed 30 January 2017), for instance, highlights how the mental health service user involves the:

active participation of a person with lived experience of mental distress in shaping their personal health plan, based on their knowledge of what works best for him.

These policy statements, which show a large degree of convergence and consistency across international borders, indicate that mental health service users can no longer be considered as "third parties," disconnected from their own treatment and the health system. In contemporary European mental health care, the service user has to be considered as a "partner," the cocreator/codesigner of the care pathway, and, importantly, an expert by experience. And so for someone who is a passionate advocate for service users, it is so very heartening and reassuring to read a Psychiatric/Mental Health nursing textbook that encapsulates the values and practices inherent to these policies and position statements. It is uplifting to read a book in which the role(s) and the involvement of the service user are addressed throughout and, simultaneously, reflect innovation and evidence-based practice in Psychiatric/Mental Health nursing.

Furthermore, one of the defining characteristics of person-centered P/MH nursing is the desire to form partnerships with service users, work with (alongside) rather than work "on" such individuals. P/MH nurses wishing to practice with such a person-centered or humanistic focus regard the service users as experts (and owners) of their own experiences and their own care. Indeed, in such relationships, both parties are recognized as human beings having the same values and the same rights in the promotion of their interests. An informed service user will then be able to choose among the various treatment options and will feel as if he/she is an actor of its treatment. Similarly, an informed P/MH nurse would consider the whole of the service user's situation and challenges, taking intrapersonal, interpersonal, familial, professional/occupational, and social/environmental factors/experiences into account when responding to the service user's needs and tailoring and planning the care in line with their needs. This holistic and integrated approach allows for a greater care consolidation and has a beneficial influence on outcomes like recovery, user's satisfaction, and security of care. And so upon reading the book, I took great comfort and solace from how the editors had integrated these key concepts and used them as the underpinning for the individual chapters.

Upon reading the book, I was also struck by a further key underpinning for this book, namely, that of evidence-based or evidence-informed practice. I was also delighted to see how the editors have linked evidence-informed P/MH nursing practice with the service user involvement. Evidence indicates that mental health service user involvement in treatment/policy making can and does have a positive impact. It enables a greater understanding of the service user's whole situation, experiences, background, and "environment" and thus enables services to be shaped to the user's need. This increases the quality of the care and the cost-effectiveness. But, as one of the authors rightly writes, this approach can be only sustainable if users are primarily considered as citizens; this concept of citizenship is central to relation and participation in society. This is the first P/MH nursing textbook that I have read that brings these three key concepts together into one philosophical underpinning for the book and, importantly, demonstrates that they are not mutually incompatible, far from it.

The book also highlights how European and occidental mental health care per se still has a way to go before it can claim to have endorsed and operationalized personcentered, holistic, evidence-informed, and service user-informed mental health care. To get there, this requires of course that mental health-care professional's behavior and culture change fundamentally. For service users and those championing service user involvement, the care model should be based on the client's needs by asking this question: "What matters to you?" Communication styles and patterns have to become more transparent and explicit at the individual, team, and organization level. Education of P/MH nurses, psychiatrists, psychologists, and other mental health professionals should include a holistic vision of the care as well as the multiprofessional care model in order to remove the barriers between different professions and specialties. Adopting this configuration of mental health care remains challenging and contains unanswered questions; however, it represents the mental health-care system of the future, and this book completely reflects this trend.

As a result, I endorse and recommend this book without hesitation or pause.

For any mental health practitioner, especially P/MH nurses, who wish to adopt a progressive, emancipatory approach to practice, this book is a must read.

Brussels, Belgium Françoise Charnay-Sonnek

Foreword II

Back in 1984, at the tender age of 18, I took a job as a nursing assistant in an acute male psychiatric ward of a mental hospital outside Bristol in the UK. I only worked there for a few months—before disappearing off to explore India—but the experience remains clearly etched in my mind. I particularly remember one young man—let's call him Rob—who was admitted shortly after I started, highly agitated, restless and manic. I'd never seen anyone so unwell. Yet four months and a few interesting incidents later, Rob walked out of that hospital with a smile, a wave and his head held high, his mind mended. Since I too was young and had no formal nursing qualifications, I spent a lot of time on the ward with Rob and so was able to witness his journey to recovery on an almost daily basis. At the end of my time working there, I thought I would be unlikely to find such a rewarding job ever again, and so that has proved in many ways. Working with numbers and policies and forms is not nearly as interesting as directly working to help people get better from mental health problems.

I begin with this little account because it speaks to two pivotal issues underlying the mental health nursing profession (and this book): the value of mental health and our individual as well as collective need to nurture, protect and—where indicated—restore it and the potential for and power of recovery from mental health problems, both in its clinical and personal sense. I don't know what happened to Rob after that hospital admission, but at discharge his mental health state was evidently stabilized and his functional capacities were restored to the extent that he was able to go back to his course of study.

Our mental health and well-being is a precious but fragile asset, shaped by a myriad of different factors that may be either protective or harmful. It is therefore appropriate and reassuring that due place and recognition is given in this new textbook to the underlying determinants of mental health and the explicit adoption of a biopsychosocial approach to its understanding. Improved knowledge and awareness about the many possible factors that may lead to someone becoming ill and coming into contact with mental health services would seem to be a vital prerequisite for a more nuanced and holistic response to a person's needs. The pursuit of a person-centred approach to mental health nursing is indeed a recurring and deservedly central theme of this book and one that resonates strongly with broader (inter)national agendas to strengthen health systems and workforce development policies.

In this volume, attention is also given to the needs of particular subpopulations, including refugees and migrants. Europe is witnessing a huge inward movement of people, many of them scarred by conflict, civil unrest, or persecution, which not only increases the numbers of people who could benefit from decent, responsive mental health services but also poses new challenges for mental health nurses and other frontline workers, including issues of cultural sensitivity and language. These and other issues are nicely picked up in a section devoted to the competencies required of nurses working in mental health.

A further important challenge and need concerns how to foster effective collaboration or joint working arrangements with other professional groups. There is more than enough evidence to support the value of collaborative care in its true sense, but all kinds of real-world barriers seem to get in the way of its proper implementation, including weak clinical governance, vertical budgeting arrangements and ill-defined roles and responsibilities. So a further competency need extends to working well with other health professionals as well as working well with users of services! In support of this strategic need, the WHO Regional Office for Europe has had the pleasure of hosting a number of knowledge exchange meetings between lead representatives of staff groups active in mental health in the region—including Horatio.

A final critical area of strategic need relates to the inclusion of service users in the processes and decisions that affect their lives. This is a foundational principle of the WHO *European Mental Health Action Plan 2013–2020* and one given renewed emphasis in a recent (2017) *Report of the Special Rapporteur to the UN on the right of everyone to the enjoyment of the highest attainable standard of physical and mental health*. Issues around the engagement, involvement and participation of service users are explored in Chap. 3 of this book, including issues of informed consent, shared decision-making and legal capacity. This has also been a major area of developmental work for WHO over the last decade, culminating in the release of a comprehensive set of *QualityRights* training and guidance materials for assessing and improving standards of care and human rights protection across different mental health-care settings and in ways that are fully in line with the *UN Convention on the Rights of Persons with Disabilities*. It is incumbent on mental health nurses to be not only cognizant but also respectful of the human rights of those whom they are caring for.

I congratulate the editors and authors for putting together this new book and share the hopes and expectations they have for the translation of a person-centred, evidence-based and rights-oriented approach to mental health promotion, protection and restitution into everyday nursing practice.

Dan Chisholm
Programme Manager for Mental Health
Division of NCDs and Promoting Health through the Life-Course
WHO Regional Office for Europe, Copenhagen, Denmark

Preface

Why Another Psychiatric/Mental Health Nursing Textbook?

That is a good place to start.

In our long careers in psychiatric/mental health nursing, neither of the editors has ever found one textbook that featured the key emphases and elements that we wanted and needed to see. Sure, some textbooks included some of these desired emphases and elements; those published during the last ten years or so may have included material on evidence-based practice. Others have something of a humanistic or person-centred focus. One or two have eschewed the dominant bio-psychiatry, pharmacologically-skewed, and containment driven (i.e. defensive practice) dominant discourse of most Occidental, contemporary mental health care. And a few have made some effort to reflect a European emphasis—to a greater or lesser extent and with mixed results. But no P/MH textbook has brought these emphases together—up until now. For those involved in leading the writing, editing and production of this book, this publication represents the first genuinely European, Person-centred, evidence-based, P/MH nursing textbook that questions the hegemony of bio-psychiatry, places the human connection and therapeutic relationship as central and sees service users as our partners in care.

The initial idea for the book belongs with Jose, and with apologies to Tolkien, 'the tale grew in the telling' once this became a collaborative, co-edited text with the addition of John. One of our early and easy design decisions was to compile a list of contributors that genuinely represented and reflected as many European nations as possible rather than having the more typical, 'Anglo-Saxon'-heavy author composition. For a genuinely European P/MH nursing textbook, the Editors felt it should include contributions emanating from lesser known European authors and often unrepresented European nations. Further, the editors felt that the book could have more utility and applicability if we invited a few contributions from non-European scholars, arguably broadening its appeal and widening the audience that might see something meaningful and experience a 'phenomenological ah ha!'

As with most journeys, our path from conceptualisation to realisation was neither linear nor lacking turbulence. And at the risk of sounding trite, maybe there was something worthwhile and enabling in such struggles? The destination 'tastes' even sweeter for the challenges encountered *en route*. And so the project that began in earnest in 2016 comes to fruition in 2018. Maybe as the textbook evolved during its production, it may also be the case that the editors (and authors?) are changed as a result of their experiences.

In closing, if the contributions from the authors, representing around 20 different countries, are anything to go by, there remains an international appetite for the form(s) of P/MH nursing and mental health care featured and focused on in this book, both in the mental health care providers and the services users—the recipients and consumers of such care. This is heartening. While the published evidence seems to suggest that the passion for interpersonally focused P/MH nursing care may have passed its zenith, the same body of work continues to highlight that desire that service users have to receive and engage in such care. And so to see these key ideas embraced and embedded throughout this book gave the editors hope for the future. After all, as Peplau (1995, p.x), the so-called Founding Mother of P/MH nurse, stated:

> Despite our current emphasis on medical diagnoses, sophisticated technology, economic cutbacks and "quick fixes", what patients need most in the midst of this health care maze is sensitive and caring individuals who are willing to enter into interpersonal relationships that foster hope and prevent hopelessness.

Coimbra, Portugal
Kingston, Canada
November 2017

José Carlos Santos
John R. Cutcliffe

Acknowledgements

The editors have a number of people and organisations that they need to offer their profound thanks to, and without whom this book could not have been produced.

Firstly, to each of the publishers that gracefully provided permission to contributors to reproduce part or all of their previously published works, we extend our appreciation and thanks. Where such reproductions have occurred, we include acknowledgments and thanks at the end of these individual chapters. However, the editors would like to offer our thanks again here to the publishing houses: Taylor Francis, Elsevier and Wiley.

Secondly, it is perhaps tautological to point out that without the outstanding work and contributions of our authors, this book would not exist. To each contributor, whether a sole or co-author—the editors are proud to be associated with each of you and want each of you to know that your contributions have elevated the overall academic quality and clinical utility of this book. Thank you.

Thirdly, to the foreword writers, Françoise and Dan; we greatly appreciate your Forewords and the endorsement of the book, and both of which offer some thoughtful and interesting insights and comments.

Fourthly, to the publishing team, Nathalie and Madona, and everyone else at Springer; we know the effort and energy you put into this book. We hope and trust that you are happy with the finished product and what a way to start a book series. Thank you.

Fifthly, to our families, Joao Santos and Rita Santos, and to Maryla, Natalia and Charlotte—we could not have done this without your unfailing support, love and encouragement. This one is for you!

And lastly to all the clients, family members and significant others that we have encountered in our respective mental health care careers; we are honoured to have shared in your journey and hope that, in some small way, we made a difference for the better.

Contents

Part I Principles and Approaches

1 **Introduction: Remembering the Person: The Need for a Twenty-First-Century, Person-Centred European Psychiatric/Mental Health Nursing Textbook** 3
John R. Cutcliffe and José Carlos Santos

2 **Oxymoronic or Synergistic: Deconstructing the Psychiatric and/or Mental Health Nurse** 13
John R. Cutcliffe, Chris Stevenson, and Richard Lakeman

3 **Service User Involvement and Perspectives** 29
Marta Ferraz

4 **Taxonomies: Towards a Shared Nomenclature and Language**. 37
Carlos Alberto da Cruz Sequeira and Francisco Miguel Correia Sampaio

5 **Theories of the Interpersonal Relationships, Transitions and Humanistic Theories: Contribution to Frameworks of Psychiatric/Mental Health Nursing in Europe**. 49
José Carlos Carvalho and Raul Alberto Cordeiro

6 **An Introduction to the Art and Science of Cognitive Behavioural Psychotherapy** 59
John Swan and Graham Sloan

7 **Psychodynamic and Psychoanalytical Theory, Approaches and Clinical Relevance: Applying the Psychoanalytic Principles and Practices to Mental Health Nursing**. 75
J. Lopes and John R. Cutcliffe

8 **The Biopsychosocial Approach: Towards Holistic, Person-Centred Psychiatric/Mental Health Nursing Practice** 89
José Carlos Santos, Marie Bashaw, Will Mattcham, John R. Cutcliffe, and Kelly Graziani Giacchero Vedana

9 **Trauma-Informed Care: Progressive Mental Health Care for the Twenty-First Century** 103
John R. Cutcliffe, Rodger Travale, and Tyler Green

10 **Competences for Clinical Supervision in Psychiatric/Mental Health Nursing** 123
John R. Cutcliffe and Graham Sloan

11 **European and Worldwide Mental Health Epidemiology and Trends** 141
Evanthia Sakellari

12 **Mental Health Nurses and Responding to Suffering in the Twenty-first Century Occidental World: Accompanying People on Their Search for Meaning** 151
John R. Cutcliffe, Jan Kare Hummelvol, Arild Granerud, and Bengt Erikson

Part II Settings and Contexts

13 **Acute Inpatient Psychiatric/Mental Health Nursing: Lessons Learned and Current Developments** 169
Roland van de Sande

14 **Community Psychiatric/Mental Health Nursing: Contexts and Challenges—The Case of Nurse Prescribing and Recovery-Focused Interventions** 183
Steve Hemingway and Neil Brimblecombe

15 **Unearthing the Theoretical Underpinnings of "Green Care" in Mental Health and Substance Misuse Care: History, Theoretical Origins, and Contemporary Clinical Examples** 195
John R. Cutcliffe and Rodger Travale

16 **Nursing People in Prisons, Forensics and Correctional Facilities** 211
Tommy Dickinson, Amrita Mullan, Kirsty Lippiatt, and Julie Ann Owen

17 **eHealth, Telematics and Telehealth** 223
Nina Kilkku

18 **Public Health and Ecological Approaches: The Example of eHealth for Adolescent Mental Health Support** 235
Anttila Minna, Kurki Marjo, and Välimäki Maritta

Part III Psychiatric/Mental Health Nursing Competencies and Ways of Working

19 **Forming and Maintaining Interpersonal Relationships** 247
Manuel José Lopes

20 Psychiatric/Mental Health Nursing Core Competencies: Communication Skills 259
Cândida Loureiro, Helena Quaresma, and José Carlos Santos

21 Group Work in Psychiatric/Mental Health Nursing: The Case for Psychoeducation as a Means to Therapeutic Ends 269
Evelyn Gordon and Maeve Kenny

22 A Family-Focused, Recovery Approach When Working with Families When a Parent Has a History of Mental Health Problems: From Theory to Practice 283
Darryl Maybery and Andrea Reupert

23 Psychiatric/Mental Health Nursing and Mental Health Promotion: An Eight Steps Path 293
José Carlos Rodrigues Gomes

24 Therapeutic Milieu: Utilizing the Environment to Promote Mental Wellness 309
Tyler D. Green

25 Psychiatric/Mental Health Nursing Nonphysical Competencies for Managing Violence and Aggression: De-escalation and Defusion 319
Hulya Bilgin and Zeynep Ozaslan

Part IV Human Experiences of Mental Health Problems and Psychiatric/ Mental Health Nursing Responses

26 Problems Affecting a Person's Mood 337
German López-Cortacans, Carme Ferré-Grau, and José Carlos Santos

27 The Person Experiencing Anxiety 353
Columba McLaughlin

28 Integrated Care – 'Schizophrenia': A Challenge for Psychiatric/Mental Health Nursing 371
David González-Pando and Fernando Alonso-Pérez

29 Human Experiences of and Psychiatric/Mental Health Nurses' Responses to Problems Related to Dementias and Cognitive Impairment 385
Helena Quaresma, Cândida Loureiro, and José Carlos Santos

30 Problems Related to Substance and Alcohol Misuse 395
Fatma Yasemin Kutlu and Gul Dikec

Part V Specific Challenges

31 **Problems Related to Eating, Nutrition, and Body Image** 425
Christopher Modica

32 **Suicide and Self-Harm** 441
José Carlos Santos

33 **A Systematic Perspective of Violence and Aggression in Mental Health Care: Toward a More Comprehensive Understanding and Conceptualization** 453
John R. Cutcliffe and Sanaz Riahi

34 **The Withdrawn or Recalcitrant Client** 479
Richard Lakeman

35 **Confronting Goffman: How Can Mental Health Nurses Effectively Challenge Stigma? A Critical View of the Literature** 493
L. Bates and T. Stickley

Part VI Special Populations

36 **Psychiatric/Mental Health Nursing Care of Children and Adolescents** 507
António Jorge Soares Antunes Nabais, Lucília Rosa Mateus Nunes, John R. Cutcliffe, and José Carlos Santos

37 **Psychiatric/Mental Health Nursing Care of the Older Adult: Mental Health in Old Age** 521
Bengt Eriksson and Arild Granerud

38 **Psychiatric/Mental Health Nurses Care of the Client Who Presents with Both Mental Health and Substance Misuse Problems** 533
John R. Cutcliffe, Rodger Travale, and T. Green

39 **Non-European and European Migrants in Acute Adult Inpatient Mental Healthcare: Dissociation and Identity** 549
Yasmine Souiah-Benchorab, Stephen Adshead, and Jean-Manuel Morvillers

40 **Working with Individuals Who Are Homeless** 561
Cheryl Forchuk

41 **Mental Health Problems and Risks in Refugees During Migration Processes and Experiences: Literature Overview and Interventions** 571
Cossu Giulia, Maura Galletta, and Carta Mauro Giovanni

About the Editors

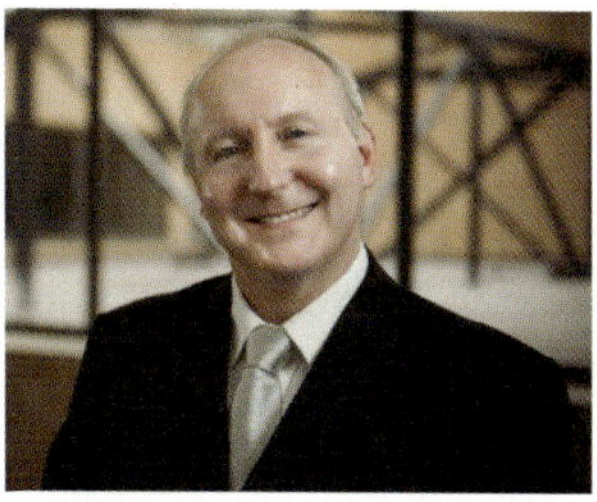

Dr. John R. Cutcliffe is the owner/operator of Cutcliffe Consulting, a health care/higher education/corrections consulting firm that operates in the USA, Canada, and Europe. He is an esteemed academic, having held three Endowed Research Chairs; he also practices as a psychotherapist. He also holds Adjunct Professor positions at the University of Ottawa, Canada; the University of Coimbra, Portugal; and the University of Malta, Malta. Most recently, John held the 'Blanke Endowed Research Chair in Nursing Research'/Director for the Center for Nursing Research at Wright State University, Ohio, USA. His two previous Endowed Professorial Research chairs were the 'David G. Braithwaite Research Chair' at the University of Texas and the 'Acadia Professorship in Psychiatric and Mental Health Nursing' at the University of Maine, both in the USA.

John's clinical background is in nursing, having completed his psychiatric nurse and then his general nurse education in the United Kingdom. John's research interests focus on hope, suicide, and clinical supervision, and he was recognised by the federal government of Canada and cited as one of the top 20 'Research Leaders of Tomorrow' for his research focusing on hope and suicidology.

He has published extensively—over 120 peer-reviewed papers, 35 chapters, over 50 professional/editorial/non-peer-reviewed papers, 11 books, and over 90 abstracts/conference proceedings. As of June 2017, his work has been cited more than 5647 times (according to Google Scholar), his 'H' Index is 39; his I-10 index is 100. His work on suicide and care of the suicidal person has been translated into German, Japanese, Dutch, Spanish, Mandarin Chinese, Portuguese, Korean, Turkish, and Italian. He has over $5,000,000 dollars of extra-mural research funding as Primary/Co-Investigator and his research findings, particularly those pertaining to suicide and hope, are now found in best practice guidelines in several parts of the world. John has a track record of successful doctoral student supervision, operationalized through his primary and Adjunct appointments. As a result, he has a track record of providing doctoral supervision via distance to his internationally located students. He has served as the national Canadian Representative for the International Association of Suicide Prevention and the Director of the International Society of

Psychiatric Nurses: Education and Research division: he is the Associate Editor for the highest ranked Psychiatric/Mental Health Nursing Journal as well as serving on the boards of eight other health or education focused journals. And in 2012 he was invited by the Director of Medicine at Yale University to join the first international advisory board on Clinical Supervision.

He retains his interest in clinical work, particularly in psychotherapy and advancing a more human-focused approach to Psychiatric/Mental Health nursing—in psychiatric facilities, corrections facilities, and substance misuse facilities; care of the suicidal person, inspiring hope, clinical supervision, and dealing with violence and aggression.

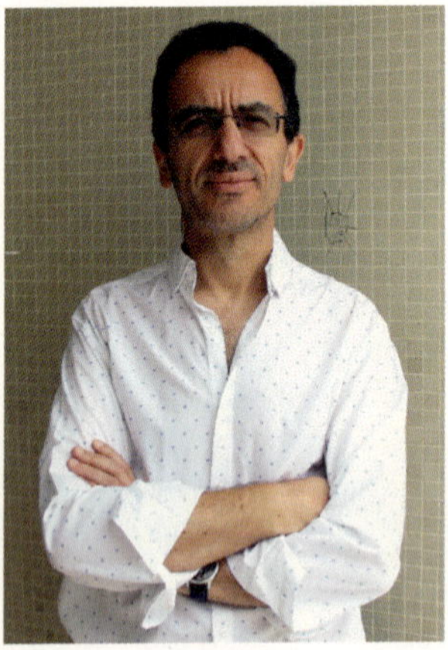

José Carlos Santos is a Coordinating Professor at the Nursing School of Coimbra. He has a background in nursing and experience in general and psychiatric hospitals. He completed his nursing degree (1986), mental health specialisation (1997), and master's degree (2000) in Coimbra, and his doctoral degree (2006) at the University of Porto.

He is a researcher of the Health Sciences Research Unit: Nursing (UICISA:E), Nursing School of Coimbra. He coordinates the 'Prevention of suicidal behaviours' project, which has three main areas: adolescents—prevention of suicidal behaviours in schools; families—prevention of suicidal behaviours with the families; and professionals—guidelines and tools to prevent suicidal behaviours. He is also a researcher at the Portuguese Observatory on Health Systems.

José is a professor of Mental Health/Psychiatric Nursing in doctoral and master's programmes, and in an undergraduate nursing degree. He is currently the coordinator of the master's degree in Mental Health and Psychiatric Nursing at the Nursing School of Coimbra.

He is a renowned specialist in suicidal behaviours. He was President of the Portuguese Society of Suicidology (2011–2013) and Rapporteur for the Portuguese Suicide Prevention Plan (2013–2020). He supervises both national and international master's dissertations and doctoral theses in this field. He also works in the Suicide Research and Prevention Unit at the Coimbra University Hospital.

José is a member of several health-related organisations where he occupies a position of responsibility.

He has published extensively in this field. He is the author or coauthor of 5 books, 13 chapters, over 30 peer-reviewed papers, and over 60 abstracts/conference proceedings in Portuguese and English. He is a board member or referee of several journals.

His interests focus on suicidal behaviours and their impact on the family, society, and professionals, liaison psychiatry, and mental health/psychiatric nursing in general.

Contributors

Stephen Adshead School of Health and Human Sciences, University of Essex (Southend on Sea), Colchester, UK

Fernando Alonso-Pérez University of Oviedo, Oviedo, Spain

Marie Bashaw Assistant Professor of Nursing, Wright State University, Ohio, USA

L. Bates Substance Misuse Nurse, Dudley and Walsall Mental Health Partnership NHS Trust, Dudley, UK

Hulya Bilgin Florence Nightingale Nursing Faculty, Psychiatric and Mental Health Nursing, Istanbul University, Istanbul, Turkey

Neil Brimblecombe South London and Maudsley NHS Foundation Trust, London, UK

José Carlos Carvalho Escola Superior de Enfermagem do Porto (Nursing College of Porto), Porto, Portugal

Raul Alberto Cordeiro Polytechnic Institute of Portalegre, Portalegre, Portugal

Carlos Alberto da Cruz Sequeira Nursing School of Porto, Porto, Portugal

Scientific Pedagogical Unit, "Nursing: Discipline & Profession", Nursing School of Porto, Porto, Portugal

Research Group "NursID: Innovation & Development in Nursing" Center for Health Technology and Services Research (CINTESIS), Porto, Portugal

Portuguese Society of Mental Health Nursing, Porto, Portugal

John R. Cutcliffe Cutcliffe Consulting, Kingston, Canada

School of Nursing, Coimbra, Portugal

Tommy Dickinson The University of Manchester, Manchester, UK

Gul Dikec Nursing Department, Health Science Faculty, Istinye University, Istanbul, Turkey

Bengt Eriksson Inland Norway University of Applied Science, Faculty of Public Health, Hedmark University College, Elverum, Norway

Marta Ferraz Coordinator of the Advisory Commission for User and Caregiver Participation, National Mental Health Programme, DGS, Director of the Oeiras Psychosocial Rehabilitation Unit, ARIA, Mira, Portugal

Carme Ferré-Grau Department of Nursing, Rovira i Virgili University, Tarragona, Spain

Cheryl Forchuk Western University, London, ON, Canada

Maura Galletta Department of Medical Science and Public Health, University of Cagliari, Cagliari, Italy

Kelly Graziani Giacchero Vedana Ribeirão Preto College of Nursing - PAHO/WHO Collaborating Centre for Nursing Research Development, University of São Paulo, Butantã, Brazil

Carta Mauro Giovanni Department of Medical Science and Public Health, University of Cagliari, Cagliari, Italy

Cossu Giulia Department of Medical Science and Public Health, University of Cagliari, Cagliari, Italy

José Carlos Rodrigues Gomes Health Research Unit, School of health Sciences, Polytechnic Institute of Leiria, Leiria, Portugal

David González-Pando University of Oviedo, Oviedo, Spain

Amrita Goomany Sheffield Health & Social Care NHS Foundation Trust, Sheffield, UK

Evelyn Gordon School of Nursing and Human Sciences, Dublin City University, Dublin, Ireland

Arild Granerud Inland Norway University of Applied Science, Faculty of Public Health, Hedmark University College, Elverum, Norway

Tyler Green Clinical Instructor and Psychiatric Nurse Practitioner, Wright State University Ohio, New York, NY, USA

Tyler D. Green College of Nursing and Health, Wright State University, Dayton, OH, USA

T. Green Owner/Operator Cutcliffe Consulting, University of Coimbra, Dayton, Portugal

Steve Hemingway University of Huddersfield, Huddersfield, UK

Jan Kare Hummelvol Inland Norway University of Applied Science, Faculty of Public Health, Hedmark University College, Elverum, Norway

Maeve Kenny Principal Clinical Psychologist, St Vincent's Hospital, Fairview, Dublin, Ireland

Nina Kilkku School of Health Care, Tampere University of Applied Sciences, Pirkanmaa, Finland

Fatma Yasemin Kutlu Mental Health and Psychiatric Nursing Department, Florence Nightingale Nursing Faculty, Istanbul University, İstanbul, Turkey

Richard Lakeman Adolescent Mental Health Nurse Navigator/Clinical Nurse Consultant, Cairns and Hinterland Health Service District, Queensland Health, Brisbane, Australia

School of Health & Human Science, Southern Cross University, Lismore, NSW, Australia

Kirsty Lippiatt King's College London, London, UK

J. Lopes RN Mental Health Specialist, Psychoanalitic Psychotherapist, School of Health Care, Polithecnical Institute of Setúbal, Setúbal, Portugal

Manuel José Lopes São João de Deus School of Nursing, University of Évora, Évora, Portugal

German López-Cortacans Primary Care Center, Catalan Institute of Health, Barcelona, Spain

Cândida Loureiro Nursing School of Coimbra, Coimbra, Portugal

Välimäki Maritta Department of Nursing Science, University of Turku, Turku, Finland

School of Nursing, Hong Kong Polytechnic University, Hung Hom, Hong Kong

Kurki Marjo Department of Child Psychiatry, University of Turku, Turku, Finland

Will Mattcham Assistant Professor of Nursing, Cleveland State University, Ohio, USA

Darryl Mayberry Department of Rural Health and Professor Rural Mental Health Research, Director School of Rural Health - Monash University, Moe, VIC, Australia

Columba McLaughlin Ulster University, Coleraine, UK

Anttila Minna Department of Nursing Science, University of Turku, Turku, Finland

Christopher Modica Wright State University, Dayton, OH, USA

Jean-Manuel Morvillers EPS Maison Blanche, Paris, France

Université Paris 13, Sorbonne Paris Cité, Chaire Recherche Sciences Infirmières, Laboratoire Educations et Pratiques de Santé (LEPS), (EA 3412), UFR SMBH, Bobigny, France

Amrita Mullan Sheffield Health & Social Care NHS Foundation Trust, Sheffield, UK

António Jorge Soares Antunes Nabais Centro Hospitalar Lisboa Central, Hospital D. Estefânia, Lisboa, Portugal

Lucília Rosa Mateus Nunes Nursing Department, Escola Superior de Saúde—Instituto Politécnico de Setúbal, Setúbal, Portugal

Julie Ann Owen King's College London, London, UK

Zeynep Ozaslan Nursing Department, Health Sciences Faculty, Kocaeli University, Kocaeli, Turkey

Helena Quaresma Nursing School of Coimbra, Coimbra, Portugal

Andrea Reupert Faculty of Education, Krongold, Monash University, Clayton, VIC, Australia

Sanaz Riahi Clinical Information and Adolescent Services, Ontario Shores Mental Health, Whitby, ON, Canada

Evanthia Sakellari Department of Public Health and Community Health, Athens University of Applied Sciences, Athens, Greece

Department of Nursing Science, University of Turku, Turku, Finland

Francisco Miguel Correia Sampaio Nursing School of Porto, Porto, Portugal

Research Group "NursID: Innovation & Development in Nursing" Center for Health Technology and Services Research (CINTESIS), Porto, Portugal

Psychiatry Department, Hospital de Braga, Braga, Portugal

Roland van de Sande Institute of Nursing Studies, Utrecht University of Applied Sciences, Utrecht, The Netherlands

Parnassia Psychiatric Institute, The Hague, The Netherlands

José Carlos Santos Escola Superior de Enfermagem de Coimbra, Nursing School of Coimbra, Coimbra, Portugal

Graham Sloan Consultant Nurse in Psychological Therapies, Psychological services, NHS Ayrshire and Arran, Ayr, Scotland, UK

Psychological Therapies Training Coordinator, NHS Education for Scotland, NHS Ayrshire and Arran, Ayr, Scotland, UK

Yasmine Souiah-Benchorab EPS Maison Blanche, Paris, France

Chris Stevenson Formerly Head of School of Nursing and Professor, Dublin City University, Dublin, Ireland

T. Stickley Associate Professor, School of Nursing, Midwifery and Physiotherapy, University of Nottingham, Nottingham, UK

John Swan Division of Neurosciences and Medical Education Institute, College of Medicine, Dentistry and Nursing, University of Dundee, Dundee, UK

Rodger Travale Healthcare Manager, Chiron Health Services, Prince George Regional Correctional Centre, British Columbia, Canada

Part I

Principles and Approaches

1 Introduction: Remembering the Person: The Need for a Twenty-First-Century, Person-Centred European Psychiatric/Mental Health Nursing Textbook

John R. Cutcliffe and José Carlos Santos

1.1 The Need for a Contemporary European Psychiatric/Mental Health Textbook

Anyone who has paid even only cursory attention to the global news over the last decade or so should be well aware that Europe has endured, and in many ways is still enduring, significant upheaval, major socio-economic and geopolitical changes/challenges.[1] These challenges and developments can have a direct and indirect impact on mental health-care policy (Santos and Cutcliffe 2013), on mental health service user outcomes and experiences (Simou and Koutsogeorgou 2014) and on psychiatric/mental health nursing practice, education and research (WHO 2012). According to the World Health Organisation—European Regional Office (2017)— mental health problems account for almost 20% of the burden of disease in the WHO European Region and now affect one in four people in Europe at some time in their life. Additionally, according to the findings of several significant studies (see, e.g. European College of Neuropsychopharmacology 2011), results reveal that (so-called) mental disorders have become Europe's largest health challenge in the twenty-first century. To further

[1] See, for example, major economic meltdown; Syrian refugee crisis, rise of anti-establishment and the nouveau right, Britain's decision to Brexit.

J.R. Cutcliffe (✉)
Cutcliffe Consulting, Kingston, Canada

School of Nursing, Coimbra, Portugal
e-mail: jcutcliffe@outlook.com

J.C. Santos
Escola Superior de Enfermagem de Coimbra, Nursing School of Coimbra, Coimbra, Portugal
e-mail: jcsantos@esenfc.pt

© Springer International Publishing Switzerland 2018

J.C. Santos, J.R. Cutcliffe (eds.), *European Psychiatric/Mental Health Nursing in the 21st Century*, Principles of Specialty Nursing,
https://doi.org/10.1007/978-3-319-31772-4_1

compound and complicate the situation, the clinical focus and indeed very nature of mental health problems and resultant responses to mental health-care needs have been annexed by those who would seek to locate the discourse firmly within biological psychiatry.[2] For instance, the relevant literature draws attention to:

- The creeping encroachment of the medicalisation of everyday life (see Szasz, 2007; Cutcliffe and Lakeman In Press; Whittaker 2010, 2012; Lakeman and Cutcliffe 2009, 2016)
- The continuing acceptance and pushing (some use the term 'marketing') of the biological hypothesis of mental health even in the face of an absence of convincing or compelling scientific evidence (Deacon 2013; Lakeman and Cutcliffe 2016)
- The exponential expansion of so-called psychiatric diagnoses in the various iterations of the DSM, both in terms of scope and sheer number,[3] despite the fact that such diagnoses represent a consensus of opinion within certain American Psychological Association members and are, in no way, scientific constructs (see also Phillips et al. 2012)

Furthermore, P/MH nurses and all mental health-care practitioners are now firmly embedded in and have to operate within the epoch of evidence-based practice (see, e.g. Buccheri et al. 2010). While the editors are more comfortable with and prefer to use the term 'evidence-informed',[4] we nevertheless wholeheartedly embrace the concept of evidence-informed care and practice and, accordingly, all contributing authors to this book we asked to write their chapters in this context. For some people, there is a trend to delegitimise independent facts and create a climate of epistemological relativism,[5] resulting in situations where opposing parties rely on their own facts. For the editors of this book, we deliberately eschew 'Alt' news and other non-peer-reviewed sources of information. All authors and contributors to this book were required to use sources of information that, where possible and appropriate,[6] were subject to the common scientific academic practices of falsifiability, verifiability, empirical tests, peer review and independent verification/reproducibility. As a case in point, the editors draw attention to the thorny issue of biological psychiatry and the paucity of evidence.

[2] And with this the almost automatic response to mental health problems being the prescription of pharmaceuticals.

[3] According to Spitzer et al. (1978), the DSM I had about a dozen separate diagnoses, whereas now this number has grown to 265 in DSM V (Ghaemi 2013).

[4] Given that even the most modest estimates suggest that the amount of practice that can accurately claim to be evidence based is about 40%—with other studies suggesting even lower numbers, it is something of an overreach to adopt the term 'evidence-based practice'.

[5] Indeed the Orwellian term 'alternate facts' has been advanced recently by a senior advisor to Donald Trump (i.e. Kellyanne Conway). See http://www.cbsnews.com/news/kellyanne-conway-alternative-facts-internet-memes/.

[6] Not all research paradigms or methods see reproducibility as possible or necessary to establish credibility, truth value or validity of findings; readers are referred to the vast literature available on qualitative research methodology and the various underpinning philosophical views.

As Cutcliffe and Lakeman (In Press) highlighted in a paper that was accepted for publication in *Skeptic* (http://www.skeptic.com/):

> Senior Lecturer at Harvard Medical School and the former Editor in Chief of *The New England Journal of Medicine*) Marcia Angell draws together the findings and arguments of Kirsch (a psychologist), Whittaker (a journalist) and Carlat (a psychiatrist) pertaining to the biological causation hypothesis. She asserts, "but the main problem with the theory is that after decades of trying to prove it, researchers have still come up empty-handed. All three authors document the failure of scientists to find good evidence in its favor. Neurotransmitter function seems to be normal in people with mental illness before treatment." Angell highlights how Carlat refers to the chemical imbalance theory as a "myth", and how Kirsch concludes "It now seems beyond question that the traditional account of depression as a chemical imbalance in the brain is simply wrong.

Accordingly, if operating judiciously within the evidence-informed approach, then P/MH nurses ought to be aware of the biological hypothesis but treat it with a healthy degree of scepticism—given the lack of evidence supporting (for a recent review, please see Cutcliffe and Lakeman In Press; Lakeman and Cutcliffe 2016). At the same time, accepting and operating within the boundaries of a genuinely scientific discipline requires P/MH nurses to retain an open mind to the possibility that the biological hypothesis may indeed turn out to be accurate; one does not close down the possibility of having to accept this hypothesis in the face of new and compelling evidence. Thus, throughout the book, the reader will find that the editors eschew certain terms, preface some terms with the expression 'so-called' and/or place such terms in 'scare, shudder or sneer' quotation marks as a way to illustrate their unconfirmed nature.

1.2 A Different Psychiatric/Mental Nursing Textbook

When one acknowledges and accepts the actuality of the mental health challenges facing Europe, the need for a P/MH nursing textbook that both acknowledges the existence of and is contextualised by these challenges, becomes clear. There is a need for P/MH nursing textbook that includes contemporary material on recently discovered key aetiological findings and resultant policy/practice shifts, for instance, the overwhelming and compelling evidence that links childhood trauma with the development of mental health problems in adult life (see Chap. 9 on Trauma-Informed Care). There is a need for a textbook that reflects the more contemporary global shift in drug/substance misuse policy—not least the massive and significant shift from a criminal justice-driven response to a treatment-driven response to substance misuse (see Chaps. 30 and 39). Furthermore, there is a need for a P/MH nursing textbook that adopts and promotes a person or client-centred approach as essential and one that adopts a more critical stance on biopsychiatry and pharmacological responses as the mainstay of our care responses and interventions. That is not to say that such views have no place in our practice (or in this book for that matter). But it is to say that there are already plentiful examples of textbooks that adopt and embrace the biological view of psychiatry and see pharmacological intervention as the mainstay of mental health care. Yet what are noticeably absent or at least spartan in this body of literature are P/MH nursing textbooks that emphasise the interpersonal use of self and that identify, illustrate and expand the multiple ways that P/MH nurses might offer help and care for/with clients without relying predominantly on psychotropic drugs, defensive practices and/or containment measures.

Consequently, this book has been designed, written and edited with a deliberate focus on interpersonally focused ways of working as a P/MH nurse. *It was designed and constructed with a specific intent to identify, explain and explore the various (multiple) ways that P/MH nurses might enact the full and wide range of skills and interventions that they have available to them, rather than limiting, curtailing and kerbing their therapeutic potential.* The book was conceived as a deliberate counterpoint to the many P/MH nursing textbooks (in the view of the editors at least) that emphasise defensive practices, containment measures, risk aversion, risk preoccupation and litigation avoidance: to paraphrase P/MH nursing textbooks that emphasise the *Psychiatric or Yang* at the expense of the *Mental Health or Yin* (Cutcliffe 2000). And the book was conceptualised as a conduit for reinforcing the critical (for the editors at least) shift in policy that sees mental health service users as partners in their own care and that sees such individuals as experts by experience and very often, according to the epidemiological evidence, as individuals trying to come to terms with and find ways to cope with their own traumatic past. For the editors of this book, one of the defining characteristics of person-centred P/MH nursing is the desire to form partnerships with service users, work with (alongside) rather than work 'on' such individuals.[7] Such P/MH nurses see the service users themselves as experts (and owners) of their own experiences and their own care. We wholeheartedly endorse and support the views expressed by the National Survivor User Network (2017), namely, that mental health service user involvement is the *active participation of a person with lived experience of mental distress in shaping their personal health plan, based on their knowledge of what works best for them* (emphasis added). The editors concur with the stated view:

> Service user involvement is about making sure that mental health services, organisations and policies are led and shaped by the people best placed to know what works: people who use mental health services. They are experts by experience.

And that:

> Service-user leadership is fundamental to designing, delivering and checking services that support people to fulfil their potential. Only by transforming services in the way that the people who use them want us to can better outcomes be achieved at a time of real budget constraint.

A further design decision for this textbook involved the editors wanting to acknowledge the existence of certain unresolved issues and debates that are relevant

[7] As this suggests a power differential between service user and P/MH nurse people with mental health problems

to P/MH nurses and nursing, and moreover, the editors wished to ensure that the book included chapters on some issues that, while significant and important, hitherto have remained under-examined and under-discussed. Such issues include:

1. Expose/explore multiple meanings, inconsistencies, contradictions and hidden agendas in the texts 'psychiatric/mental health' nursing.
2. Address the lack of a consistent nomenclature in mental health care.
3. And by no means least, consider the very nature of our responses to people experiencing mental health problems and challenges.

1.3 The Structure of the Book

The book is composed of six sections: (1) Principles and Approaches, (2) Settings and Contexts, (3) Psychiatric/Mental Health Nursing Competencies and Ways of Working, (4) Human Experiences of Mental Health Problems and Psychiatric/ Mental Health Nursing Responses, (5) Specific Challenges and (6) Special Populations.

The first section focuses on cross-cutting and/or overarching principles that have relevance and application to all areas of mental health care and on principle, interpersonal theoretical approaches. The second section focuses on the wide range of different settings and contexts that mental health is delivered and in which P/MH nurses operate. The editors further wished to include chapters in the book on historically atypical and/or nontraditional settings where P/MH nurses now work. While various models or approaches to mental health-care delivery are (and have been historically) evident across Europe,[8] significant quantities of mental health care in Europe traditionally involved large asylums and institutionalised care (see WHO—ROE 2017). Indeed, reflecting the fundamental shift away from such care delivery approaches, the WHO—ROE (2017) states:

> The commitment to deinstitutionalization and the development of community-based mental health services has continued, although progress is uneven across the Region. The consensus is that care and treatment should be provided in local settings, since large mental hospitals often lead to neglect and institutionalization. Thus, a focus on the expanding role of primary care, working in partnership with multidisciplinary mental health staff in community-based facilities, has become central. (WHO—ROE 2017)

Accordingly, the editors wanted to ensure that a twenty-first-century P/MH nursing textbook includes chapters that accurately reflect the variety of 'new', contemporary and/or nontraditional settings and contexts in which European mental health care is delivered. Accordingly, in addition to focusing on inpatient and community care settings, the editors also commissioned chapters on mental health care in

[8] Not least the examples of the exciting service delivery developments associated with *Psychiatrica Democratica* in Italy (Crossley 2006) and mirrored in Spain (Ferre Navarete and Palanca 2005).

correctional facilities, therapeutic communities and care delivered via eHealth and telehealth.

The third section focuses on the range, breadth and variety of skills available to and used by (some) twenty-first-century P/MH nurses, and these are considerable. P/MH nurses now work as individual therapists (or counsellors) and family therapists. They work to de-escalate and defuse potentially violent and aggressive situations. P/MH nurses co-ordinate and facilitate a variety of groups. They engage in primary mental health promotion and even ecological mental health promotion activities. P/MH nurses also work indirectly with clients via mediums such as the 'therapeutic milieu' and the unit environment. Accordingly, in addition to P/MH nursing skills that are used frequently (e.g. communication skills, interpersonal relationship formation skills), the editors wanted to include other chapters that focus on the skills that, if the literature is accurate, appear to be given less emphasis in some curricula and some other P/MH nursing textbooks.

The fourth section focuses on a range of commonly experienced mental health challenges; indeed, the challenges in this section reflect those mental health challenges described as contributing the most to the 'Global Burden of Disease Study' (see Whiteford et al. 2013). For the editors, it seemed logical to focus on the more commonly encountered and experienced mental health problems rather than the less common, more esoteric.

Lastly, the final two sections of the book focus on specific clinical challenges facing P/MH nurses and populations that present additional complexity and difficulties. While suicide and self-harm are not isolated to clients with mental health problems, it is very well documented that the risk of suicide and self-harm are significantly higher in this population and the same argument can be advanced regarding exposure to and risk of violence/aggression. Similarly, people who are reluctant to engage with health-care professionals (for a variety of reasons) or indeed can be recalcitrant with all are likely to be encountered by P/MH nurses in mental health-care systems. And even a cursory examination of the relevant policy literature will highlight how mental health care remains bedevilled by stigmatised attitudes and ignorance. Though cautious about singling out certain populations (as in so doing one invariably inadvertently excludes other populations), the editors decided that the merits of including these populations outweigh the drawbacks. As a result, the editors wanted to see the challenges presented by children, adolescents and young people, especially given the empirical links between traumatic childhood experiences and mental health challenges. The well-documented 'ageing' population and resultant massive growth in older adults (more people living longer, baby boomer birth rate much higher than 'Millennials' and 'Gen-Xers') means that this population, and the mental health challenges they present, could not be omitted. A further population which, according to the literature (see Chap. 39), has been underserved and yet presents with significant mental health problems is those people who experience simultaneous mental health problems *and* substance misuse problems. Despite the large numbers of people who were former inpatients in mental health facilities and many who are currently experiencing mental health challenges, the homeless population receives scant attention in P/MH nursing literature. And the final population that warrants special attention, especially given the significant increase in migration and (mass) refugee movements from war-torn countries, are indeed migrants and refugees.

1.4 Closing Remarks

This book is a tool for better P/MH nursing practices and innovative approaches. According to the European Mental Health Action Plan (WHO—ROE 2017), which highlights a number of objectives for mental health care in Europe (see Box 1.1), the plan is guided by three main aims:

a). Improve the mental well-being of the population and reduce the burden of mental disorders, with a special focus on vulnerable groups, exposure to determinants and risk behaviours.
b). Respect the rights of people with mental health problems and offer equitable opportunities to attain the highest quality of life, addressing stigma and discrimination.
c). Establish accessible, safe and effective services that meet people's mental, physical and social needs and the expectations of people with mental health problems and their families.

(WHO 2012, p. 3)

Box 1.1 Objectives for Mental Health Care in Europe

- Everyone has an equal opportunity to realise mental well-being throughout their lifespan, particularly those who are most vulnerable or at risk.
- People with mental health problems are citizens whose human rights are fully valued, respected and promoted.
- Mental health services are accessible, competent and affordable, available in the community according to need.
- People are entitled to respectful, safe and effective treatment.
- Health systems provide good physical and mental health care for all.
- Mental health systems work in well-coordinated partnership with other sectors.
- Mental health governance and delivery are driven by good information and knowledge (WHO 2012).

These three issues are interdependent, indivisible and mutually enforcing and imply the need for interventions not only within traditional mental health institutions but also within the community. The issues highlight how the focus of P/MH nursing practice ought to be aligned with vulnerable groups, by advocating for the rights of such groups, but also the need to work with 'healthy' people, by empowering their citizenship. These aspects are perhaps beyond traditional and historical views of clinical practice, but they should be included if P/MH nurses are to embrace the full scope of their practice, the full width and depth of populations with whom they can work with therapeutically and the full breadth of locations and settings in which mental health care can be delivered.

In closing, the editors will not belabour how the main objectives for mental health care in Europe (Box 1.1) are very similar to the focus, philosophy and emphasis in practice stressed and given prominence throughout this book. Perhaps then, for P/MH nurses and other mental health practitioners who are striving or even aspiring to enact these WHO—ROE aims, this book is a valuable resource.

References

Buccheri R, Trygstad L, Buffum MD, Gerlock AA (2010) Developing an evidence-based practice for psychiatric nursing. J Psychosoc Nurs 48(5):3–5

Crossley N (2006) Contesting psychiatry: social movements in mental health. Routledge, London

Cutcliffe JR (2000) Fit for purpose? Promoting the human side of mental health nursing. Br J Nurs 9(10):632–637

Cutcliffe JR, Lakeman R (In Press) 21st century snake oil: the pseudoscience of contemporary psychiatry. Skeptic

Deacon BJ (2013) The biomedical model of mental disorder: a critical analysis of its validity, utility, and effects on psychotherapy research. Clin Psychol Rev 33:846–861

European College of Neuropsychopharmacology (2011) The size and burden of mental disorders in Europe. https://www.sciencedaily.com/releases/2011/09/110905074609.htm

Ferre Navarete F, Palanca I (2005) Mental health care in Madrid. Eur Psychiatry 20(2):279–284

Ghaemi SN (2013) Requim for DSM Psychiatric Times. http://www.psychiatrictimes.com/authors/s-nassir-ghaemi-md-mph

Lakeman R, Cutcliffe JR (2009) Misplaced epistemological certainty and pharmaco-centrism in mental health nursing. J Psychiatr Ment Health Nurs 16:199–205

Lakeman R, Cutcliffe JR (2016) Diagnostic sedition: re-considering the ascension and hegemony of contemporary psychiatric diagnosis. Issues Ment Health Nurs 37:125–130

National Survivor User Network (2017) Service user involvement in the delivery of mental health services. http://www.together-uk.org/wp-content/uploads/downloads/2014/06/Service-User-Involvement-briefing.pdf. Accessed 30 Jan 2017

Phillips J, Frances A, Cerullo M et al (2012) The six most essential questions in psychiatric diagnosis: a pluralogue part 2: issues of conservatism and pragmatism in psychiatric diagnosis. Philos Ethics Humanit Med 7:8. https://www.ncbi.nlm.nih.gov/pmc/articles/PMC3390269/

Santos JC, Cutcliffe JR (2013) The recent global socioeconomic crisis and its effects on mental health in Portugal. Ment Health Nurs 33(6):33–35

Simou E, Koutsogeorgou E (2014) Effects of the economic crisis on health and healthcare in Greece in the literature from 2009 to 2013: a systematic review. Health Policy 115(2-3):111–119

Spitzer RL et al (1978) Research diagnostic criteria: rationale and reliability. Arch Gen Psychiatry 35:773

Szasz, T (2007) The Medicalization of Everyday Life: Selected Essays. Syracuse University Press, Syracuse.

Whiteford HA, Degenhardt L, Rehm J, Baxter AJ, Ferrari AJ, Erskine HE et al (2013) Global burden of disease attributable to mental and substance use disorders: findings from the global burden of disease study 2010. Lancet 382(9904):1575–1586

Whittaker B (2010) Mad in America: bad science, bad medicine, and the enduring mistreatment of the mentally ill. Basic Books, New York

Whittaker B (2012) Anatomy of an epidemic: magic bullets, psychiatric drugs, and the astonishing rise of mental illness in America. Broadway Paperbacks, New York

World Health Organisation—European Regional Office (2017) Mental health. http://www.euro.who.int/en/health-topics/noncommunicable-diseases/mental-health. Accessed 15 Jan 2017.
World Health Organisation—Regional Office for Europe (2017) European mental health action plan. http://www.euro.who.int/__data/assets/pdf_file/0004/194107/63wd11e_MentalHealth-3.pdf. Accessed 30 Jan 2017.
World Health Organization (2012) Risks to mental health: an overview of vulnerabilities and risk factors: Background paper by WHO Secretariat for the development of a comprehensive mental health action plan. http://www.who.int/mental_health/mhgap/risks_to_mental_health_EN_27_08_12.pdf

Oxymoronic or Synergistic: Deconstructing the Psychiatric and/or Mental Health Nurse

2

John R. Cutcliffe, Chris Stevenson, and Richard Lakeman

2.1 Introduction

With apologies to William Shakespeare and his classic work 'Romeo and Juliet', in answer to his question: 'What's in a name? That which we call a rose by any other name would smell as sweet', we would respectfully disagree with the Bard and suggest: a great deal. At the most fundamental (literal) level, names are simply a collection of letters and/or symbols that identify a person or entity. However, the value and power of names have long been recognized and expressed throughout human history. Etymologists point out how people's names were far from mere cosmetic or audible aesthetics; they symbolized and communicated specific meanings and messages. Similarly, philosophers engage in (for some semantic, for others substantive) discussions about names, characterizing them as, amongst others, descriptors and linguistic mechanisms for reference. As a result, whether for referential, descriptive purposes or symbolic, communication purposes, names it seems matter.

Accordingly, the authors of this chapter seek to radicalize a debate which has taken place intermittently concerning the name, existence, nature, function and place of so-called psychiatric/mental health nursing. We do so because even a

J.R. Cutcliffe (✉)
Cutcliffe Consulting, Kingston, Canada

School of Nursing, Coimbra, Portugal
e-mail: jcutcliffe@outlook.com

C. Stevenson
Formerly Head of School of Nursing and Professor, Dublin City University, Dublin, Ireland

R. Lakeman
Adolescent Mental Health Nurse Navigator/Clinical Nurse Consultant,
Cairns and Hinterland Health Service District, Queensland Health, Brisbane, Australia

© Springer International Publishing Switzerland 2018

J.C. Santos, J.R. Cutcliffe (eds.), *European Psychiatric/Mental Health Nursing in the 21st Century*, Principles of Specialty Nursing,
https://doi.org/10.1007/978-3-319-31772-4_2

cursory examination of the names and terms used internationally to signify a nurse who specializes in working with people with mental health problems will illustrate the absence of a shared nomenclature. Nurses who claim to engage in the same form and type of nursing care do not share the same title (signifier). Secondly, we do so because such transposition of names can be regarded as an *epistemological sleight of hand*, whereby some allege an isomorphic relationship between 'psychiatric' and 'mental health' without ever having substantiated these phenomena as immediately transposable/transplantable. And thirdly, we do so because there is a body of evidence (both discursive and to a lesser extent empirical) which lends support to the view that there may very well be two distinct phenomena: 'psychiatric' nurses and 'mental health' nurses—who are not necessarily interchangeable.

Accordingly, this chapter will, respectively, (1) apply a historical analysis identifying and problematizing how 'psychiatric' and/or 'mental health' nursing has metamorphosed according to service geography and deconstruct the very terms themselves; (2) be informed by the work of de Saussure (1916/1983) and Derrida (1978) in an attempt to expose/explore multiple meanings, inconsistencies, contradictions, hidden agendas and multiple meanings in the texts 'psychiatric, mental health and psychiatric/mental health' nursing; (3) highlight the possible existence of psychiatric and mental health nurses as separate but complimentary nurses; and (4) promote a much needed expanded debate about these terms and the implications arising out of their use/acceptance.

2.2 Has Psychiatric/Mental Health Nursing Ever Really Existed?

2.2.1 Geography as Destiny

Historically, what nurses who work with psychologically distressed people were called (i.e. what 'signifiers' such nurses had) has to a large extent depended on where they have worked (Rogers and Pilgrim 2001), various public and/or mental health policy positions (see Ramshorn and Pearlmutter 1982) and the vagaries of passing fashion (Nolan 1993). In the United States, for example, Ramshorn and Pearlmutter (1982) point out that:

> '*psychiatric nursing* (emphasis added) as a clinical speciality arose during this (medical-therapeutic model 1945–1960) period'.

Whereas the so-called community mental health movement in the United States of America (USA), with an alleged emphasis on shifting from a psychiatry/medical model to a community-located, mental health model did not occur until after 1960. These authors continue to illustrate however how while the policy espoused a 'mental health' focus and a corresponding shift in practice, in reality, no such fundamental changes in practice could be demonstrated; these practices were still drawing on a traditional medical model. On a related note, Hedlund and Jeffrey (1993) assert that the term *psychiatric nursing* (emphasis added) arose in the United States because these nurses wished to distinguish and/or differentiate themselves from their general hospital counterparts. These authors continue:

> 'the addition of mental health to psychiatric nursing…dates back to the early 1990s… This (community mental health) movement led nurse educators to believe that psychiatric nurses had an important community health role to play'.

Interestingly, so while the 'signifier' of 'mental health' nursing was added to reflect the change in geographical location where the care occurred and to reflect the shift in mental health policy, the evidence indicates that little significantly altered in terms of practice delivery. In this sense 'psychiatric' or 'mental health' nurse has been a signifier of where one works in much the same way that 'domiciliary, community or public health' nurses qualified their titles. Indeed Peplau (1989) suggested that it might be useful to think of nurses who practice *in* psychiatric settings as *psychiatric nurses* (emphasis added).

Similar shifts in the 'signifier' can be located in the UK historical and policy literature. Nolan (1993), for example, points out that the attendants of the asylum became 'mental nurses' in the mental hospitals of the United Kingdom. The titling (signifier) changed as 'mental hospitals' were rebranded 'psychiatric hospitals' and services expanded to become 'mental health' services. An examination of various reports, for example, the 1968 UK government report 'Psychiatric Nursing Today and Tomorrow', clearly use the term *psychiatric nursing*, as did the 'Salmon Report' (Nolan 1993). Indeed while there is some small degree of variance in the terms used pre-1982 in the UK, the common signifier is *psychiatric nurse(ing)*. Two key phenomena appear to be closely linked to the shift from 'psychiatric' to 'mental health' signifiers during the 1980s: a policy shift towards community care and the so-called 1982 syllabus. As with the United States, community (mental) health care was supposed to promote a 'person-centred' approach and an emphasis on (mental) health promotion (Nolan 1993); according to Rogers and Pilgrim (2001), it held out the promise of a humanitarian alternative to long-term institutionalized care. It also contributed to a shift in signifier for those nurses who worked in the community alongside people with mental health problems: 'community mental health' nurse. Perhaps evidence of this can be found in the UK Department of Health's Mental Health Nursing Review, commissioned in 1992 and resulting in the document 'Working in Partnership' (Department of Health 1994). Clarke (1999, p. 9) makes this point most clearly when he states that:

> 'one recommendation of the *Mental Health Nursing Review Team* (original emphasis) (1994) was that all psychiatric nurses – whether in the community or located in the hospital – be awarded the title 'mental health nurse'.

Similarly, the 1982 syllabus was written specifically to emphasize interpersonal skills and interpersonal ways of working, to distance such nurses from the 'asylum or institution' (both in terms of where the education/preparation occurred and in terms of the imagery/associations and views of such institutions that were pervasive in the general population). Just as the name (signifier) of 'asylum attendants' had shifted to 'nurses' during the 1920s (Nolan 1993), the issue of names (signifiers) was once more of central importance to this population of nurses during the 1980s which saw an increase in the use of the terms 'therapist' and 'mental health'. Again, while the use of these terms was not consistent and often the terms 'Psychiatric' and 'Mental Health' were used interchangeably, even a cursory review of the extant literature will show a dramatic increase in the use of the term 'Mental health' nurse during and subsequent to this period.

The analysis above is clearly not the full story as, at least for nurses themselves, the title is imbued with symbolism, and in the case of 'mental health nursing', at least it may signify aspirations for a particular kind of praxis (Chambers 2006). In the text entitled 'The Mental Health Nurse', various nursing leaders of the time in their chapters used the terms, 'mental health' or 'psychiatric nurse', interchangeably. This professional ambivalence about the title seems to be resolving if the titles of contemporary nursing textbooks are any indicator. While occasionally nursing texts prior to 1990 included the term 'mental health' in the title (e.g. Morgan and Moreno 1973), more often the term 'psychiatric nursing' was used (e.g. Stuart and Sundeen 1987). This gave way to various combinations: psychiatric-mental health nursing (e.g. Glod 1998), psychiatric mental health nursing (no hyphen) (e.g. Fortinash and Holoday-Worret 1996) or psychiatric and mental health nursing (e.g. Barker 2003). While this change has been by no means a linear process, in certain parts of the world (e.g. the UK, Australia), one is far more likely today to have the 'psychiatric' omitted altogether (e.g. Fontaine 2009; Norman and Ryrie 2004). Consider, for example, the very title of this journal or that the Royal College of Nursing (recovered 2011) stated at their most recent congress that:

> '*Community mental health nurses (CMHNs), formerly community psychiatric nurses,* (emphasis added) have been instrumental in the transition of mental health services from an institutional setting to a community setting'.

However, in other parts of the world (e.g. Canada, the United States), the term 'mental health' nurse is rarely used. Indeed, Nolan and Hopper (2000) in referring to nursing in the 1960s use the term 'mental health' nursing which would have been unthought of and unthinkable in that era. Norman and Howell (2000, p. 560) consign 'psychiatric' nursing to the past when they use the phrase 'Psychiatric nursing (now Mental Health nursing)'. Notwithstanding that these texts reflect different styles, somewhat different emphases, and particular geographic outlooks, a 'Shelf Browser' would be hard pressed to discern any substantive differences that might somehow signify a different philosophy or practice associated with 'mental health', 'psychiatric' nursing or any combination thereof. We extend this position in the following section.

2.2.2 Deconstructing Psychiatric and/or Mental Health Nursing

In our deconstructive approach to the 'psychiatric' and/or 'mental health' nurse, we are informed by the work of de Saussure (1916/1983), who was interested in semiotics—the science of signs—and the problem of how they are representative of the world. We were also influenced by and drew upon aspects of the work of Derrida (1978) who used the term deconstruction in a specific way as the work of exposing, multiple meanings, inconsistencies, contradictions, hidden agendas and multiple meanings in texts. Text in this context is not just written words but includes conversation, art, non-verbal communication and practices—essentially anything that can be 'read' for meaning. Saussure divided a sign into a signifier (the written or spoken word) and the signified (the concept or meaning of the word). Taken together, they refer to something in the world. Saussure pointed out that there is no necessary relationship between the signifier and the signified, for example, between the word schizophrenic and the concept of psychotic illness (or, as we shall argue later, between the words 'Psychiatric nurse', 'Mental Health nurse' or 'Psychiatric/ Mental Health nurse' and the concepts of P/MH nursing) as one could just as easily conjoin the concept of psychotic illness with the word 'fantasia'. In addition, there is no necessary relationship between the sign (the signifier + signified) and its referent in the world. For example, the sign (as word and concept) could be replaced with other words and concepts. Accordingly, using the label 'PN', 'MHN' or 'PMHN' is a way to distinguish people in practice and implies a set of skills that can then be *presumed* in each person so labelled, although we confront that assumption later in the paper.

2.3 The 'Psychiatric' Nurse

Psychiatry is allied to the biomedical model, and its quest is therefore, at least in part, for the 'magic bullet' to cure so-called mental illness. However, despite many promises, medication to treat the underlying bio-dysfunction of so-called mental illness has had, at best, equivocal results (Antonuccio et al. 2002; Breggin 1994, 2000; Cutcliffe and Lakeman 2010; Kirsch et al. 2002, 2008; Lehman 2004; Moncrieff et al. 1998; Storosum et al. 2001). Despite the questionable track record of psychiatry, 'Psychiatric nurses' have attached themselves to the biomedical version of distress, and this may represent, at least in part, a political agenda in relation to supporting the case for arguing that nursing is a profession. For example, the relatively recent emergence of 'Psychiatric Nurse Practitioner' has shifted their practice closer to the traditional role of psychiatrists (Bailey 1996) and moreover describes this practice shift as 'Advanced Psychiatric Nursing'. This alliance offers a 'geographic location', that is, the dysfunctional brain, that defines practices in the same way that previously nurses have been described and directed by their physical location, as argued above. Indeed, in this instance, the signifier 'Psychiatric nurse' does have a relationship with its signified—the concept of the 'Psychiatric nurse' who is assisting in the execution of a bio-psychiatric approach. Together (as a sign) they point to specific practices, for example, monitoring symptoms, ensuring medication compliance, tracking response to medication, observing to prevent risk to self and others, and engaging in control and restraint, each of which are practices which are easily detected. However, in a paper reviewing what 'Psychiatric Nurses' do on a day-to-day basis, Cowman et al. (2001) found that there was more scope to the role than suggested by the sign. Notwithstanding the possible lack of conceptual clarity in some of the described activities in Cowman et al. (2001), these authors found that 'Psychiatric Nurses' typically assessed patient needs and planned care, engaged in caring interactions, engaged in pharmaceutical interventions, were involved in education (teaching and learning), documented information, and co-ordinated services of nurses and other professionals. Furthermore they communicated with other professionals and other grades of staff and managed the administration/organization of the clinical area. Cowman et al. (2001) looked at 'psychiatric nursing' across a range of clinical environments and so may have inadvertently described the activity of psychiatric *and* mental health nurses, leaving the signifier, signified and sign 'psychiatric nursing' intact.

2.4 The 'Mental Health' Nurse

If the text 'psychiatric nurse' deconstructs itself, is the text 'mental health nurse' any better placed? One issue immediately arises in relation to the multiple meanings of the word 'mental' ranging from 'cerebral, mind, psychological, rational, and intellectual' to 'mad', although the range is rarely acknowledged. Such multiple meanings are problematic in relation to the articulation between 'mental', 'health' and 'nursing'. Accordingly, one should ask: What is mental health? Is it 'psychological health or mad health'? Many global health organizations have consistently defined mental health as more than the absence of illness (see, e.g. World Federation for Mental Health 2004), and for some, it is now de rigueur to speak of holistic health promotion (i.e. no health without mental health). 'Mental health' nurses sometimes deal with these matters by claiming a holistic approach and an emphasis on mental health promotion (Jane-Llopis et al. 2005; Parham 2008; Wand 2011), but problems arise: (1) Firstly, if the scientific and mental health-care community is unable to advance a definitive view of mental health per se, does this not undermine any attempts to promote mental health (Cutcliffe and McKenna 2011)? This issue is further bedevilled by the multiple and not necessarily convergent definitions of 'mental health'. If 'mental health' nurses are not conceptually clear on what exactly it is that they are supposed to be promoting, how can they then be sure that they are promoting it? (2) Holism is expansive and so requires a position of knowing all (Clarke 2006; Forster and Stevenson 1996; Russell 1946). In effect, valuing breadth while trying to define the specialty of 'mental health nursing' means that deconstruction happens. (3) The traces of the 'psychiatric' linger in 'mental health' nursing practice despite claims to being more holistic. For example, some nurses now described as 'mental health' nurses are adept at reinventing the 'psychiatric' in their new arenas of practice. Holmes (2006) makes a similar point when he refers to the United Kingdom Chief Nursing Officer's (2005) call for 'mental health' nurses to prioritize moving clients towards more healthy lifestyles when the predominant discourse in education and service ideologies is biomedical. This awkward conflation of 'mental health' nursing with 'psychiatric nursing' is also evident in the Scottish (Scottish Executive 2006) and English (Dept. of Health 2006) reviews of mental health nursing which emphasize both the importance of recovery *and* the value of nurses acquiring prescribing privileges.

The political agenda concerning the development of 'mental health nurses' has been touched upon above in relation to the move from the asylums to more community-based care and with it the idea that a more proactive, mental health promotion approach was possible. Here was a discipline in need of redefinition, and the conjoining of 'mental', 'health' and 'nursing' was an attempted solution. Three studies serve to demonstrate the arbitrariness of the signifier/signified 'mental health' nurse as multiple meanings of it are generated. Porter (1993) has argued that post-institutional 'mental health nursing' is splitting into different specialties. Kudless and White (2007) point out the 'community mental health' nurses function in a range of behavioural health-care settings, and those different roles require different skills and competencies. Norman and Howell (2000, p. 560) noted that different camps have polarized the debate about the nature of 'mental health nursing', with one camp promoting the uniqueness of 'mental health nursing' and the other seeing it as a function that is shaped by a multidisciplinary mental health service and (that) it can be fulfilled by anyone. In summary, a deconstruction of 'mental health' nursing reveals how tenuous the relationship between the term and the actual practice is. The everyday activity of many 'mental health' nurses typically has little to do with mental health, and the term 'mental health' remains undefined; it is ambiguous and amorphous, perhaps a misnomer but perhaps serves as an aspiration.

2.5 Reinventing the Already Punctured Wheel: The 'Psychiatric/Mental Health' Nurse

'Psychiatric/mental health' nursing is an inherently conflicted combination. Barker (2008: Foreword) states:

> 'The concept of psychiatric/mental health nursing is quite a mouthful, and one that is not easily digested'

And we would argue, indigestible. We disagree with the largely unexamined prescription for practice—namely, the conflation of 'psychiatric' with 'mental health' nurse. How can a 'psychiatric/mental health' nurse practice when the philosophy of one part (bio-psychiatry) is in conflict with another (holistic, person-centred care)? There are many examples of how this philosophical conflict might impact on practice: the person who refuses (or insists on) taking psychotropic medication; the person who insists that they are not psychotic; and the person who situates her/his problems in family dynamics. Cutcliffe (2008) has advanced a similar argument. In response to the rhetorical questions:

1. What is 'psychiatric' and/or 'mental health' nursing?
2. What do nurses do in enacting P/MH nursing?

Cutcliffe (2008) alluded to fundamental differences between two broad groups of P/MH nurses, and these groups can be categorized as those describing themselves as 'psychiatric' nurses and others as 'mental health' nurses. For Cutcliffe (2008) 'psychiatric' nurses can be described as a largely subservient discipline and an extension of psychiatry's social control mechanism(s), for the policing, containment and correction of already marginalized people. 'Psychiatric' nurses carry out a number of defensive, custodial, uncritical and often iatrogenic practices and treatments, which are based on a false epistemology and misrepresentation of what are, by and large, 'human problems of being' and represent these as so-called mental illnesses (Cutcliffe 2008), whereas those describing themselves as 'mental health' nurses can be described as a specialty branch of the discipline of nursing and a specialty craft if you will that operates primarily by working alongside people with mental health problems, helps such individuals and their families find ways of coping with the 'here and now' (and past), assists in discovering and ascribing individual meaning to the person's experiences, and explores opportunities for recovery, reclamation and personal growth—all through the medium of the therapeutic relationship (Cutcliffe 2008).

Given the, for some, contentious nature of these positions, it behoves the authors to offer explanation and substantiation. As alluded to above, the extant literature is unequivocal in identifying that 'psychiatric nurses', by and large, locate the causation and aetiology of mental health problems as having a biological origins; these views are in turn based on biomedical, Descartes' principles of mind-body dualism and reductionism (Descartes et al. 1988; Beresford 2010). Similarly, this particular aetiological construct then leads logically to 'standard' or common medical model interventions, not least pharmacological responses, and thus their embracing of nurse prescribing (see, e.g. Bailey 1996; Gournay 2000a, b; Jones and Gray 2008a, b). They utilize the term 'mental illness' and refer to this as an illness like any other. For 'psychiatric nurses', 'mental illness' then is seen to reside in the individual; hence the frequency of terms/expressions such as people *having a mental illness* and *people with schizophrenia* (see Hannigan and Cutcliffe 2002) and the literature shows that this group of nurses adopt (and/or are comfortable with) a range of care practices that are in keeping with these views. Pharmacological interventions are seen as de rigueur and indeed the mainstay of 'psychiatric nursing' practice; Jones and Gray (2008b), for example, *refer to antipsychotic drugs as the cornerstone of treatment for people with schizophrenia* (emphasis added). This group of nurses regards mental illnesses as 'disorders' that need fixing and that sometimes the person with the disorder may not know what is in his/her own best interests. For this group of nurses, this not only necessitates but morally sanctions the use of a range of containment and/or control practices (see, e.g. Vuckovich and Artinian's excellent 2005 study). Whether this is the forced administration of medication, the use of physical restraint and seclusion rooms, forcibly 'assisting' the person to undertake electroconvulsive therapy, locking doors, restricting the person's freedom of movement, removing personal items or placing the person 'under' close observations—all such activities are undertaken, allegedly, 'for the patient's own good—or/and for the safety of others' (Cutcliffe 2008).

In contrast, 'Mental health' nurses, by and large, acknowledge the current uncertainty and ambiguity concerning the aetiology of mental health problems and leave room for the view that these are 'human problems or living, being or existence', an unavoidable (and maybe necessary) part of the human experience or condition. They emphasize and hold sacrosanct the interpersonal nature of 'mental health' nursing believing that they themselves are the most useful therapeutic 'tool' at their disposal (Peplau 1952; Barker 1999). Though 'mental health' nurses can be seen to embrace a range of theoretical approaches to interpersonal work (and/or therapy), there is consensus on the view that such talking therapies exist, at least to some extent, to help the person experiencing mental health problems, cope with (and find meaning in) their experiences, not necessarily cure or fix (see Wilhemina recovered 2011). The pioneering and seminal contributor to the recovery movement in the United States, Dr. Pat Deegan (recovered 2011) makes this point most clearly when she states:

> 'Recovery does not refer to an end product or result. It does not mean that one is "cured" nor does not mean that one is simply stabilized or maintained in the community. Recovery often involves a transformation of the self wherein one both accepts ones limitation and discovers a new world of possibility. This is the paradox of recovery i.e., that in accepting what we cannot do or be, we begin to discover who we can be and what we can do'.

For Cutcliffe (2008) 'mental health' nurses are uncomfortable with adopting psychotropic pharmacological interventions as the mainstay (or cornerstone) of mental health care, especially in the light of the documented, questionable efficacy of and well-documented iatrogenic harm caused by many of these agents (Moncrieff et al. 1998; Healy 2003, 2005; Moncrieff et al. 2005; Moncrieff and Kirsch 2006; Lakeman and Cutcliffe 2009; Cutcliffe and Lakeman 2010).

In summary, as identified above, a deconstructionist 'view' might conclude that there is an unspoken agenda embedded in the confluence of the signifier 'psychiatric/mental health nursing'. With the well-documented shifts in policy from institutionalized care, including the closure of large psychiatric institutions, to community-based care, with the increased recognition of consumer-led and/or consumer-informed care and more recently with a shift in mental health policy that embraces a 'recovery-focused' approach, 'psychiatric nurses' had to reinvent/realign themselves to be congruent with these shifts in policy. In this context, the conjoining of 'psychiatric/mental health nursing' might be seen as a rhetorical device aimed at convincing the external world of the discipline's development. When examined, however, the device is exposed as unsustainable because of the problematic connection and the conflict between a psychiatric model which implies control and coercion (Barker and Stevenson 2000) and one which is allegedly oriented more to the whole person in context.

2.6 'Janus'-Like or Irreconcilable: Our Ongoing Attempts to Square the Circle

Having engaged in the deconstruction of 'psychiatric' and/or 'mental health' nursing, the authors of this paper liken the awkward and ill-thought-out attempt to conflate 'psychiatric' *and* 'mental health' nursing under the same homogenous title as akin to attempts to square the proverbial circle, which was, despite a considerable intellectual effort by geometers, discovered/proved to be impossible. Even a cursory examination of the relevant theoretical, discursive and empirical literature will show that many authors/scholars continue to use these 'signs' interchangeably. Others may wish to advance the position that 'psychiatric' and 'mental health' nurses are metaphorically, merely two different sides of the same coin or the faces of the two-faced Roman God—Janus. In such a case, the authors cannot ignore the symbolism here whereby one of Janus' faces is looking into the past and the other facing into the future. However, our deconstruction illustrates that there are currently too many irreconcilable philosophical views, theoretical positions/underpinnings and practice examples which illustrate that such a conflation does not reflect the realities of clinical practice. Moreover, rather than being esoteric musings, it is worth examining how this unfitting conflation impacts on mental health care. In order to do so, we return to the issue of signs/signifier.

Consider the expectations that 'signs' have of/for mental health service users/consumers. The client who uses or wishes to use mental health services has certain (implicit and/or explicit) expectations—which are at least in part based on the 'signifier'—just as clients who use other health-care services do. For instance, when one chooses to visit the 'dentist' (sign), one has certain expectations that the dentist will examine and/or treat one's teeth (and gums to a lesser extent—though a periodontist may disagree). One would be shocked and disappointed if the dentist ignored one's teeth and focused on one's finger nails, neurological status or the alignment of your spine. Similarly, when a woman visits the ob-gyn clinic, she has a clear expectation of where the clinical practice/examination will focus. If the physician focuses only on hair loss or checks her long-distance vision, one would expect that the woman would be reluctant to use that ob-gyn physician again.

Accordingly, it is worth examining the literature to see if there is any record/evidence of what mental health service users/consumers expect to receive when the 'signifier' is 'mental health' services. The first key finding is that while services use the signifier 'mental health', what service users actually mostly encounter is a service dominated by the 'medical model'; they actually encounter 'psychiatric care' (with its focus on diagnosis, symptomatology and associated pharmacological response) and that this is a repeated *bone of contention* for service users (see, e.g. Gordon et al. 1979; Elbeck and Fecteau 1990; Beech and Norman 1995; Shephard et al. 1995; Cutcliffe et al. 1997; Murray 1997; Mental Health Foundation 2000; Forrest et al. 2000; Rose 2002; Walcraft 2003; Coffey et al. 2004; Boardman 2005). The second key finding reported in this literature is the overzealous reliance on medication, the desire for 'talking therapies in place of (or in addition to) medication and the (extensive) level of dissatisfaction with this over-use of medication (and its associated iatrogenic effects.) The third key finding goes to the value that service users place on interpersonal relationships with their mental health clinicians particularly if such relationships are 'natural, warm and human' rather than distant, cold and professional, if they are founded on respecting the persons' dignity, treating him/her with due respect and providing emotional support (see Cutcliffe 2008).

Not only do these findings clearly resonate with early policy positions emanating from the mental health service user recovery movement (see Deegan recovered 2011), but very similar findings continue to appear in more recent service user service evaluations and surveys. Findings reported in the Mental Health Foundation report (2000; Rose 2002) indicate an overwhelmingly predominant theme running through service users' 'most helpful' supports was the role and value of relationships with other people, in all their different forms, and, in many cases, the specific relationships with mental health professionals. Similarly, Bowcroft (recovered 2011) reporting on the first official survey of the United Kingdom National Health Service Mental Health inpatients revealed high levels of dissatisfaction with services. According to Bowcroft (2011), two particular areas of concern were highlighted (again): the failure to focus on patients' needs and the dangers posed to vulnerable individuals by potentially violent fellow patients. Bowcroft (recovered 2011) continues to report that almost half (48%) said the potential side-effects of prescribed medicines were not explained to their satisfaction, and only 41% said they were given enough time to discuss their condition with nurses. Disturbingly similar findings have been repeatedly reported and highlighted by MIND (see, e.g. MIND recovered 2011). MIND surveys and reports indicate that (a) 98% of respondents visiting their GP for mental health problems were prescribed medication, despite the fact that less than one in five had specifically asked for it/them; (b) over half (54%) of the respondents felt they had not been given enough choice; and (c) of those who had tried alternative treatments, over one in three had to take the initiative and ask for it—and often pay for it—themselves.

This body of literature then illustrates that while there is some sense of satisfaction with some aspects of the 'psychiatric' services, there is more corresponding discontent and dissatisfaction with the lack of 'mental health'-focused services. This is despite the extant policy literature being replete with rhetorical hyperbole regarding recovery (see, e.g. the US President's New Freedom Commission on Mental Health 2003). Furthermore, there is also some evidence to suggest that 'psychiatric' services are often a *wolf in sheep's clothing*; that is to say, service user are *sold a bill of goods* that they should expect to receive 'mental health care' and then what they actually receive is 'psychiatric care'. One final inference that can be drawn from the key findings in this body of work is that the current documented and widespread dissatisfaction of many service users with 'mental health' services is, at least in part, attributable to expectations based on the 'signs'—which ultimately bear little or no resemblance to the signifier. One wonders if there is a sense of service users feeling 'duped' or 'conned' that there was an element of dishonesty or, more accurately, disingenuousness in the portrayal of so-called mental health services.

Conclusions

Our deconstruction of the limited literature indicates that what nurses who work with psychologically distressed people are called has to a large extent depended on where they have worked (Rogers and Pilgrim 2001), various public and/or mental health policy positions (see Ramshorn and Pearlmutter 1982) and the vagaries of passing fashion (Nolan 1993). Accordingly, while it may presently be 'in vogue' to refer to the conflated term, 'psychiatric/mental health nursing', our deconstructionist view is that there is, at least in part, an unspoken agenda embedded in the confluence of the signifiers 'psychiatric/mental health nursing'. There are currently too many irreconcilable philosophical views, theoretical positions/underpinnings and clinical practices to enable nurses to practice simultaneously as both a 'psychiatric' and 'mental health' nurse. In this context, the conjoining of 'psychiatric/mental health nursing' might be seen as a rhetorical device aimed at convincing the external world of the discipline's development and communicating to service users the type of care they can expect to receive. Unfortunately, compelling evidence within the service user evaluation literature indicates that it is disingenuous to camouflage 'psychiatric' services as 'mental health' services, and as signifiers, signified and signs, 'psychiatric and/or mental health nursing' are sustained by political agendas which do not necessarily prioritize the needs of the person in distress or dovetail with the contemporary mental health policy literature.

There are real implications for practice designated as 'psychiatric and/or mental health nursing'. Being less restricted in the flow of practice, by abandoning the existing grammar (Wittgenstein 1953) of 'psychiatric and/or mental health nursing', and, in place, having separate but parallel 'psychiatric' and 'mental health' services (and nurses) would offer opportunities for a different more individualized recovery-oriented approach to those in emotional trouble. However, this is difficult to envisage in the established knowledge/power nexus of 'psychiatric/mental health' services with vested professional interests. Furthermore, clearly demarked and honest 'signs' for both 'mental health' care and 'psychiatric care' would not only be a more *honest* approach but it would also be in keeping with the service user literature that highlights the expectation that there are two signs (and thus two services): psychiatric *and* mental health services.

Acknowledgement This chapter has been reproduced, with kind permission from the publisher. Wiley, from the journal article referenced: Cutcliffe, J.R., Stevenson, C. & Lakeman, R. (2013) Oxymoronic or synergistic: deconstructing the psychiatric and/or mental health nurse *International Journal of Mental Health Nursing* 22, 125–134.

References

Antonuccio DO, Burns DD, Danton WG (2002) Antidepressants: a triumph of marketing over science?. Prev Treat 5(1). Article 25. http://www.journals.apa.org/prevention/volume5/pre0050025c.html. Retrieved 2008

Bailey KP (1996) Preparing for prescriptive practice: advanced psychiatric nursing and pharmacotherapy. J Psychosoc Nurs 34:16–20

Barker P (2008) Foreword. In: Morrissey J, Keogh B, Doyle L (eds) Psychiatric/mental health nursing: an irish perspective. Gill and Macmillan, Dublin

Barker P (1999) The philosophy and practice of psychiatric nursing. Churchill Livingstone, Edinburgh

Barker P (ed) (2003) Psychiatric and mental health nursing. Arnold, London

Barker PJ, Stevenson C (eds) (2000) The construction of power and authority in psychiatry. Butterworth Heineman, Oxford

Beech P, Norman IJ (1995) Patients' perceptions of the quality of psychiatric nursing care: findings from a small-scale descriptive study. J Clin Nurs 4:117–123

Beresford MJ (2010) Medical reductionism: lessons from the great philosophers. QJM Int J Med 103(9):721–724

Bowcroft G (recovered 2011) Most mental health patients do not feel safe, survey reveals The Guardian Newspaper. http://www.guardian.co.uk/society/2009/sep/24/mental-health-patients-feel-unsafe
Boardman J (2005) New services for old – an overview of mental health policy in beyond the water towers: the unfinished revolution in mental health services 1985–2005. The Sainsbury Centre for Mental Health, London
Breggin P (1994) Toxic psychiatry – drugs and electroconvulsive therapy: the truth and the better alternatives. Harper Collins, London
Breggin PR (2000) Reclaiming our children. Peresus Books, Cambridge
Chambers M (2006) The case for 'mental health' nurses. In: Cutcliffe JR, Ward MF (eds) Key debated in psychiatric/mental health nursing. Churchill Livingstone Elsevier, London, pp 33–45
Clarke L (1999) Challenging ideas in psychiatric nursing. Routledge, London
Clarke L (2006) So what exactly is a nurse? J Psychiatr Ment Health Nurs 13:388–394
Coffey M, Higgon J, Kinnear J (2004) 'Therapy as well as tablets': an exploratory study of service users' views of community mental health nurses (CMHNs) responses to hearing voices. J Psychiatr Ment Health Nurs 11:435–444
Cowman S, Farrelly M, Gilheany P (2001) An examination of the role and function of psychiatric nurses in clinical practice in Ireland. J Adv Nurs 34(6):745–753
Cutcliffe JR (2008) Has the die been cast? rediscovering the essence of psychiatric/mental health nursing. Br J Nurs 17(2):88–92
Cutcliffe JR, Lakeman R (2010) Challenging normative orthodoxies in depression: Huxley's Utopia or Dante's Inferno? Arch Psychiatr Nurs 24(2):114–124
Cutcliffe JR, Dukintis J, Carberry J, Tilley C, Turner S, Anderson-Moll D, Cooper W (1997) User's views of their continuing care community psychiatric services. Int J Psychiatr Nurs Res 3(3):382–394
Cutcliffe JR, McKenna HP (2011) What does it mean to engage in mental health promotion: Does one size fit all? Int J Nurs Stud 48, 915–917.
Deegan P (recovered 2011) Recovery and the conspiracy of hope. Presented at "There's a person in here": the sixth annual mental health services conference of Australia and New Zealand, Brisbane, Australia, 16 September 1996. http://www.patdeegan.com/pat-deegan/lectures/conspiracy-of-hope
Department of Health (1994) Working in partnership: a collaborative approach to care. HMSO, London
Derrida J (1978) Writing and difference. Routledge, London
Dept of Health (2006) From values to action: The Chief Nursing Officer's Review of mental health nursing London HMSO
Descartes R, Cottingham J, Stoothoff R, Kenney A, Murdock D (1988) The philosophical writing of descartes in three volumes. Cambridge University Press, Cambridge
Elbeck M, Fecteau G (1990) Improving the validity of measures of patient satisfaction with psychiatric care and treatment. Hosp Community Psychiatry 41(9):998–1001
Fontaine KL (ed) (2009) Mental Health Nursing. Pearson/Prentice Hall, Upper Saddle River
Forrest S, Risk I, Masters H, Brown N (2000) Mental health service user involvement in nurse education: exploring the issues. J Psychiatr Ment Health Nurs 7:51–57
Fortinash KM, Holoday-Worret PA (eds) (1996) Psychiatric mental health nursing. Mosby, St Louis
Forster S, Stevenson C (1996) Holistic thinking: personhood and the biopsychosocial model. In: Cooper N, Stevenson C, Hale G (eds) Integrating perspectives on health. Open University Press, Buckingham
Glod CA (ed) (1998) Contemporary psychiatric-mental health nursing. F.A. Davis, Philadelphia
Gordon D, Alexander DA, Dieztan J (1979) The psychiatric patient: a voice to be heard. Br J Psychiatry 135:115–121
Gournay K (2000a) Commentaries and reflections on mental health nursing in the UK at the dawn of the new millennium: commentary 2. J Ment Health 9(6):621–623
Gournay K (2000b) Role of the community psychiatric nurse in the management of schizophrenia. Adv Psychiatr Treat 6:243–249

Hannigan B, Cutcliffe JR (2002) Challenging contemporary mental health policy: time to assuage the coercion? J Adv Nurs 35(5):477–484
Healy D (2003) Lines of evidence on the risk of suicide with selective serotonin reuptake inhibitors. Psychother Psychos 72:71–76
Healy D (2005) Psychiatric drugs explained, 4th edn. Elsevier, Edinburgh
Hedlund NL, Jeffrey FB (1993) Overview of psychiatric nursing. In: Rawlins RP, Williams SR, Beck CK (eds) Mental health – psychiatric nursing: a holistic life-cycle approach, 3rd edn. Mosby, St. Louis, pp 2–16
Holmes C (2006) The slow death of psychiatric nursing: what next? J Psychiatr Ment Health Nurs 13:401–415
Jane-Llopis E, Barry M, Hosman C, Patel C (2005) Mental health promotion works: a review. Promot Educ Suppl 2:9–25
Jones M, Gray R (2008a) Partial agonists and suicide: the role of the mental health nurse. J Psychiatr Ment Health Nurs 15(3):253–259
Jones M, Gray R (2008b) Time to wake up and smell the coffee: antipsychotic medication and schizophrenia. J Psychiatr Ment Health Nurs 15(4):344–348
Kirsch I, Moore TJ, Scoboria A, Nicholls SS (2002) The emperor's new drugs: an analysis of antidepressant medication data submitted to the U.S. Food and Drug Administration. Prev Treat 5. Article 23. Available: http://www.journals.apa.org/prevention/volume5/pre0050023a.html. Retrieved 2008
Kirsch I, Deacon BJ, Huedo-Medina TB, Scoboria A, Moore TJ, Johnson BT (2008) Initial severity and antidepressant benefits: a meta-analysis of data submitted to the food and drug administration. PLoS Med 5(2):e45. https://doi.org/10.1371/journal.pmed.0050045
Kudless MW, White JH (2007) Competencies and roles of community mental health nurses. J Psychosoc Nurs 45(5):36–44
Lakeman R, Cutcliffe JR (2009) Misplaced epistemological certainty and pharmaco-centrism in mental health nursing. J Psychiatr Ment Health Nurs 16:199–205
Lehman P (2004) Coming off psychiatric drugs: successful withdrawal from neuroleptics, antidepressants, lithium, carbamazepine and tranquilizers. Peter Lehman Publishing, Shrewsbury
Mental Health Foundation (2000) Strategies for Living: a summary report of user-led research into peoples' strategies for living with mental distress. The Mental Health Foundation, London
MIND (recovered 2011) Mind says mental health patients survey findings are just "the tip of the iceberg". http://www.mind.org.uk/news/2048_mind_says_mental_health_patients_survey_findings_are_just_the_tip_of_the_iceberg
Moncrieff J, Kirsch I (2006) Efficacy of antidepressants in adults. Br Med J 331:155–157
Moncrieff J, Wessely S, Hardy R (1998) Meta-analysis of trials comparing antidepressants with active placebos. Br J Psychiatry 172:227–231
Moncrieff J, Hopker S, Thomas P (2005) Psychiatry and the pharmaceutical industry: who pays the piper? Psychiatr Bull 29:84–85
Morgan AJ, Moreno JW (1973) The practice of mental health nursing: a community approach. Lippincott, Philadelphia
Murray L (1997) How can clients and carers become allies? Nurs Times 93:40–42
Nolan P (1993) A history of mental nursing. Stanley Thornes, Cheltenham
Nolan P, Hopper B (2000) Revisiting mental health nursing in the 1960s. J Ment Health 9(6):563–573
Norman I, Howell V (2000) Mental health nursing in the UK at the dawn of the new millennium. J Ment Health 9(6):559–561
Norman I, Ryrie I (eds) (2004) The art and science of mental health nursing: a textbook of principles and practice. Open University Press, Maidenhead
Parham J (2008) Keeping promotion and prevention on the agenda in mental health: issues and challenges. Aust e-J Adv Ment Health 7:1–5
Peplau HE (1952) Interpersonal relations in nursing, 2nd edn. Macmillan, London
Peplau H (1989) Psychiatric nursing: role of nurses and psychiatric nurses. In: O'Toole AW, Welt SR (eds) Interpersonal theory in nursing practice. Springer Publishing Co., New York, pp 120–133

Porter S (1993) The determinants of psychiatric nursing practice: a comparison of sociological perspectives. J Adv Nurs 18:1559–1566

President's New Freedom Commission on Mental Health (2003) Achieving the promise: transforming mental health care in America, Final report. http://www.mentalhealthcommission.gov/reports/FinalReport/FullReport.htm.

Ramshorn MT, Pearlmutter D (1982) Social, cultural and historical aspects of mental health care. In: Haber J, Leach AM, Schudy SM (eds) Comprehensive psychiatric nursing, 2nd edn. McGraw-Hill Book Company, New York, pp 5–15

Rogers A, Pilgrim D (2001) Mental health policy in Britain: a critical introduction, 2nd edn. Basingstoke, Macmillan

Rose D (2002) Users' voices: the perspectives of mental health service users on community and hospital care. The Sainsbury Centre for Mental Health, London

Royal College of Nursing (Royal College of Nursing Congress 2011) [Cited 30 Aug 2016] Available from: URL: http://www.rcn.uk/newsevents/congress/congress_2011

Russell B (1946) History of western philosophy. George Allen and Unwin, London

de Saussure F (1916/1983) Course in general linguistics (trans. Roy Harris). London, Duckworth

Scottish Executive (2006) National review of mental health nursing in Scotland: rights, relationships and recovery: the report of the national review of mental health nursing in Scotland. Scottish Executive, Edinburgh

Shephard G, Murray A, Muijen M (1995) Perspectives on schizophrenia: a survey of user family carer and professional views regarding effective health care. J Psychiatr Ment Health Nurs 4:403–422

Storosum JG, Van Zwieten BJ, Van den Brink W, Gersons BPP, Broekmans AW (2001) Suicide risk in placebo-controlled studies of major depression. Am J Psychiatry 158:1271–1275

Stuart GW, Sundeen SJ (1987) Principles and practice of psychiatric nursing. C.V. Mosby, St Louis

Vuckovich PK, Artinian BM (2005) Justifying coercion. Nurs Ethics 12(4):370–380

Walcraft J (2003) The mental health service user movement in England. The Sainsbury Centre for Mental Health, London

Wand T (2011) Real mental health promotion requires a reorientation of nursing education, practice and research. J Psychiatr Ment Health Nurs 18:131–138

Wilhelminia GTD (recovered 2011) Mental health nurses' knowledge and views on talking therapies in clinical practice. Thesis submitted to the Victoria University of Wellington 2008. http://researcharchive.vuw.ac.nz/bitstream/handle/10063/675/thesis.pdf?sequence=2

Wittgenstein L (1953) Philosophical investigations (trans. G.E.M. Anscombe). Blackwell, Oxford

World Federation for Mental Health (2004) The relationship between physical and mental health: co-occuring disorders.. http://www.wfmh.org. Accessed Feb 2011

3 Service User Involvement and Perspectives

Marta Ferraz

3.1 Introduction

> You can't consider the brain in isolation from the social world and experiences people Have…. (Bental 2003)

Over recent decades, the involvement of users in health care, namely, in mental health care, has become the tenet of health and mental health plans in most countries that have developed community-based services. Mental health reforms have put a greater emphasis on care within the community and similarly on the participation of users in the services and supports that are developed (Thornicroft and Tansella 2006; WHO 2013, 2015; Millar et al. 2016). And while the authors of this chapter are fully supportive of this policy development, questions of clarity and clinical application still remain. For instance, perhaps it should be asked: what exactly are we talking about when we refer to user involvement? Why should users be involved? And what facilitates or hinders the process of involving users?

Mental health service user involvement, in general, aims to ensure that mental health services, provider institutions, and policies are oriented and molded by those best placed to identify what works—the persons that use mental health services or, in other words, the experts by experience. Scientific and practical evidence has demonstrated the following:

(a) That significant and effective involvement of the persons that use, or have used in the past, has become an indispensable part of, health and social, care

M. Ferraz
Coordinator of the Advisory Commission for User and Caregiver Participation, National Mental Health Programme, DGS, Director of the Oeiras Psychosocial Rehabilitation Unit, ARIA, Mira, Portugal
e-mail: martasofiaferraz@gmail.com

© Springer International Publishing Switzerland 2018

J.C. Santos, J.R. Cutcliffe (eds.), *European Psychiatric/Mental Health Nursing in the 21st Century*, Principles of Specialty Nursing,
https://doi.org/10.1007/978-3-319-31772-4_3

provision in mental health. When capacity is built so that people are able to participate actively in the planning, implementation, and evaluation of services, such services experience significant improvements, and those service users involved also see their skills and self-esteem enhanced (Linhorst 2006; Weinstein 2010).

At its most basic level, mental health service user involvement is characterized (or defined) as the active participation of a person with lived experience of mental health problems, in the design of his/her care plan, valuing his/her knowledge/experience of so-called mental illness. Nonetheless, both the relevant literature and wider policy papers on this subject tend to use the term "user involvement" in a much wider scope than these early definitions. Thus, the term has come to mean the active inclusion of users' perspectives in the design, commission, delivery, and evaluation of services, as well as in the development of mental health policy at local and national levels (WHO 2013; Millar et al. 2016; Tait and Lester 2005).

3.2 Potential Outcomes

Empirical literature in the area of mental health service user involvement tends to indicate and include positive results at various levels (Thornicroft and Tansella 2006). At an individual level, mental health service user involvement has been found to:

- Improve health and treatment outcomes, as well as staff and patient relationships, namely, in what comes to trust.
- Increase satisfaction with care, sense of dignity and self-worth.
- Reduce complaints.
- Empower the client, leading to greater responsibility for care.
- Result in safer care.

On an organizational level, mental health service user involvement can increase the chance that policies and services are informed, relevant, appropriate, and targeted to the clients. It enables a greater understanding of the links between health, lifestyle, and the circumstances in which people lead their lives. Ultimately, it seems to improve public perception and confidence in the services provided, besides, delivering better service outcomes thus making them more cost-effective. With respect to community, mental health service user involvement leads to improved policies that address inequalities in health. Services become more equitable and inclusive, helping to address social exclusion and responding better to the needs of the community served. At this level, once again, mental health service user involvement reduces complaints and increases trust (Millar et al. 2016; Linhorst 2006; Tait and Lester 2005).

Although the benefits have become growingly apparent and recognized, the desired user involvement across the mental health sector has been inconsistent if not demagogic (Bee et al. 2015; Lewis 2014; Thornicroft and Tansella 2006). A simple principle that has proved difficult to put into practice, as it cannot be reduced to:

- Giving permission/consent, being engaged or empowered by others
- Participation in client satisfaction surveys
- Participating in other persons' terms (e.g., providers, commissioners, and/or regulators)
- One time attendance or involvement with the responsibility of representing the views of all service users
- Over-dependence on the same, few persons to represent the "user community" without reference and/or connection to the latter

Genuine user involvement must entail the assurance that people with lived experience are given the opportunity to assert their perspective and be heard in their own right. In other words, user involvement is about giving people the choice and opportunity of being active participants in their own lives, not passive bystanders (Roe and Davidson 2005).

3.3 Attributes

Millar et al. (2016) have identified five defining attributes of service user involvement within of mental health and social care contexts: person-centered approach, informed decision making, advocacy, obtaining service user views and feedback, and collaborative work. Bearing in mind the principles underlying modern mental health reforms, none of the characteristics should be a surprise or even unattainable. In fact, if reforms are put in place according the orientations of WHO (2013, 2015), all of these attributes should be present thus making user involvement an integral part of current mental health policies, plans, and service provision.

A person-centered approach in community-based mental health calls for taking into account the personal and social circumstances of an individual, as well as clinical issues, not only in care planning but also in the development of policies, plans, and services/programs. In truth, the principle should extend beyond treatment and care services to the wider support network of the person in mental distress and those that might interact, even if only occasionally, with him/her. Person centeredness calls for erecting a relationship where empathy and respectful listening, treating service users with dignity, respecting them as individuals, and building trust are paramount. Besides identifying individual needs and challenges, a person-centered approach should build on the strengths, resiliencies, and aspirations of the service user, acknowledging the person's views and experiences (Bee et al. 2015; Linhorst 2006; Millar et al. 2016; Tait and Lester 2005; Roe and Davidson 2005; Slade and Davidson 2011).

Another defining attribute of user involvement is informed decision making. So that decisions may be made with responsibility, people must be informed about what they're deciding about and what choices they have. People can only take responsibility if they are given appropriate information, in an adequate language and accessible way. This perspective of informed decision making regards not only treatment and care at an individual level but pertains to involvement in decisions about services at a collective level too (Mancini 2008; Tait and Lester 2005; Weinstein 2010).

Various authors have highlighted the importance of advocacy as an aspect of service user involvement (Millar et al. 2016). In this sense, advocacy encompasses users advocating for themselves/each other in a variety of ways that go beyond having access to an independent advocate or preparing advanced directives. It may entail having access and talking to policymakers and the media, involvement in peer support groups; participating in research; having a role in the planning, development, and evaluation of services; providing training; and even writing papers for publication in the field, thus challenging stigma and discrimination (Weinstein 2010).

Service users' priorities have been identified as being very different from those of mental health professionals and caregivers (Lewis 2014; Linhorst 2006; Millar et al. 2016; Thornicroft and Tansella 2006). Therefore, obtaining their views and feedback is an important part of user involvement but cannot be limited to consultation if it is to be effective. There is a need to invest in service user leadership, through empowerment and delegation of responsibility in all aspects of mental health and social care service provision. This might mean creating mechanisms for promoting users' participation and empowering them, for example, mutual help groups and user boards to design and/or evaluate programs, and even hiring them to manage/provide services.

Another final aspect that needs to be in place for successful service user involvement is joint decision making regarding policies, service design, delivery, and evaluation. Again, considering and valuing the user's expertise as someone with unique personal knowledge of what it's like to live and cope with having a mental illness (Slade and Davidson 2011) and providing mechanisms that make working in partnership possible are crucial for meaningful involvement. Examples of partnerships that have been useful at a service level are hiring peer support workers. In this instance, people with lived experience are hired as part of the support team their role being that of providing support by example (modeling), being an example of success, and facilitating disclosure and sharing with other users who might relate easier to someone that has undergone a similar experience—a peer. Viewing the service user as a partner with invaluable, complementary experiential knowledge, rather than as competing with empirical professional knowledge, has great potential at an individual level but also, and equally important, at organizational and community/societal levels. At the latter, it can influence government; parliament; civil service and professionals groups through lobbying, briefings, and reports; and also the media and other informal mechanisms, providing evidence and direct contact with examples of success (Millar et al. 2016; Lewis 2014; Roe and Davidson 2005).

3.4 Challenges

User involvement is only sustainable if people are viewed primarily as citizens and are able to set the agenda instead of just following it. The concept of citizenship is central to relating and participating, in other words being involved, in society. If users are only viewed in a consultative role, the exercise of choice and need articulation are compromised. This is further aggravated by stigma and discrimination known to be present in the mental health setting, most times resulting in social exclusion. All together these factors impose structural constrains to the "practice of citizenship" and participation. Bearing this in mind, at a macro level, governments, policies, and providers must emphasize user rights, information, access, and choice, redressing involvement as an enriching and empowering process in itself for service users. At all levels, it means not only implicating them in decision making but mobilizing service users to participate effectively, as well as implanting mechanisms to engage users and avoid tokenistic forms of involvement (Lewis 2014; Kemp 2010; WHO 2015).

Tait and Lester (2005) have identified several barriers that seem to contribute to the existing gap between user involvement in theory and practice. The scarce information available to service users about the nature of mental health problems, side effects of medication, alternative forms of treatment, and mental health law in general make effective involvement difficult. Involvement can be costly, including transport and time, and make it unreasonable for most service users, and services themselves, as these expenses are not usually contemplated in annual budgets. Concerns about representativeness rise invariably when service user involvement is promoted. As do the discrepancies between manifested support of user involvement and actual sharing and transferring of power. Fortunately, despite the hiatus between rhetoric and practice reality, the evidence of positive practice has increased over time. Aspects that may be critical to success are suggested by Gosling (in Weinstein 2010) including starting from an established common platform of shared values and beliefs; clearly and honestly stating everyone's power; speaking about equity, not equality; possibility of challenging the status quo; respecting the terms and considering the benefits of and for those involved; no retaliation; and option of engaging and disengaging along the way.

Service user involvement is intended to promote high-quality health and personal social services that are safer and more accessible. In order to be meaningful, it cannot be "a one-off intervention" or an isolate program (Tait and Lester 2005; Bee et al. 2015), it must become part of the own fabric of mental health services affecting every aspect of mental health and social care provision.

3.5 General Recommendations

Recovery is a concept that has also emerged in the last decade and become part of the principles of modern mental health and social care service provision (WHO 2013, 2015). A goal of mental health service provision (Roe and Davidson 2005), recovery as a paradigm gives emphasis to choice, and responsibility in the process of regaining a valued role, as defined by the person in recovery, in life (Mancini 2008; Slade and Davidson 2011). Due to their characteristics, user involvement can lead to recovery, and recovery can fuel involvement; thus, we close this chapter with some recommendations for user involvement and recovery viewing the concepts as a two-way street (Weinstein 2010):

- Focus on people strengths and their identity as person, not on their symptoms and identity as a user/patient.
- Keep hope and optimism up, as people need to feel recognized and valued by their potential and skills.
- Keep people informed, give them the opportunity and encouragement to choose.
- Allow for individual uniqueness—cultural background, spirituality, and, even, sexuality can give strength and direction to participation and personal recovery.
- Address issues that might impede involvement and recovery, such as lack of meaningful relationships, activities, and housing.
- Implant measures to avoid exclusion, discrimination, and stereotyping—participation requires acceptance.
- Adapt language.
- Work in a collaborative fashion, review evidence together, and make decisions in partnership.
- Avoid bureaucratic "by the book" thinking—effective involvement and recovery approaches require creativity.
- Recruit staff that have the capacity to be humble, to respect humanity, and to foster hope.

3.6 Final Words

User involvement can only be truly effective if people recognize in each other complementary knowledge and skills. Collaboration means working together, viewing and valuing distinct know-hows, and building from the skills and strengths of each individual. This chapter was written in partnership, a reflection of the work we have been doing and modeling for some years now—working collaboratively we can have excellent results and the satisfaction of respecting others and being respected in dignity as human beings.

References

Bee P, Price O, Baker J, Lovell K (2015) Systematic synthesis of barriers and facilitators to user-led care planning. Br J Psychiatry 207(2):104–114. https://doi.org/10.1192/bjp.bp.114.152447

Bental R, HG Publishing (2003) "What was that you said again?" - a new look at psychosis, The Human Givens Institute, Chalvington. Retrieved from: http://www.hgi.org.uk/archive/newlook-psychosis.htm#.VyZqQmODBSU on 20 April 2016

Gosling J (2010) The ethos of involvement as the route to recovery. In: Weinstein J (ed) Mental health, service user involvement and recovery. Jessica Kingsley, Philadelphia, pp 201–215

Kemp P (2010) Introduction to mental health service user involvement. In: Weinstein J (ed) Mental health, service user involvement and recovery. Jessica Kingsley, Philadelphia, pp 15–29

Lewis L (2014) User involvement in mental health services: a case of power over discourse. Sociol Res Online 19(1.) Retrieved from: http://www.socresonline.org.uk.html

Linhorst D (2006) Empowering people with severe mental illness: a practical guide. Oxford University Press, New York, NY

Mancini AD (2008) Self-determination theory: a framework for the recovery paradigm. Adv Psychiatr Treat 14(5):358–365. https://doi.org/10.1192/apt.bp.107.004036

Millar S, Chambers M, Giles M (2016) Service user involvement in mental health care: an evolutionary concept analysis. Health Expect 19(2):209–221

Roe D, Davidson L (2005) Destinations and detours of the users' movement. J Ment Health 14(5):429–433. https://doi.org/10.1080/08893670500270734

Slade M, Davidson L (2011) Recovery as an integrative paradigm in mental health. In: Thornicroft G, Szmukler G, Mueser KT, Drake RE (eds) Oxford textbook of community mental health. Oxford University Press, London, pp 26–33

Tait L, Lester H (2005) Encouraging user involvement in mental health services. Adv Psychiatr Treat 11(3):168–175. https://doi.org/10.1192/apt.11.3.168

Thornicroft G, Tansella M (2006) Growing recognition of the importance of service user involvement in mental health service planning and evaluation. Epidemiol Psichiatr Soc 14(1):1–3

World Health Organization (2013) Mental health action plan 2013–2020. WHO, Geneva

World Health Organization (2015) The European mental health action plan 2013–2020. WHO - Regional Office for Europe, Denmark

Weinstein J (2010) Conclusion: the way forward for service user involvement and recovery. In: Weinstein J (ed) Mental health, service user involvement and recovery. Jessica Kingsley, Philadelphia, pp 201–215

4 Taxonomies: Towards a Shared Nomenclature and Language

Carlos Alberto da Cruz Sequeira and Francisco Miguel Correia Sampaio

4.1 Introduction

This chapter will focus on the main nursing taxonomies, with special focus on their relation to mental health, and emphasize their usefulness to care conception, care documentation and clinical practice. Thus, four main classifications will be analysed: the International Classification for Nursing Practice (ICNP®), from the International Council of Nurses (ICN 2010), this being the only nursing taxonomy included in the World Health Organisation (WHO) Family of International Classifications, since 2008; the Nursing Interventions Classification (NIC); and the Nursing Outcomes Classification (NOC), as well as the International Nursing Diagnoses, approved by NANDA International, Inc. (NANDA-I). These connections (Johnson et al. 2011) show significant relevance to the nursing process, since

C.A. da Cruz Sequeira (✉)
Nursing School of Porto, Porto, Portugal

Scientific Pedagogical Unit, "Nursing: Discipline & Profession,", Nursing School of Porto, Porto, Portugal

Research Group "NursID: Innovation & Development in Nursing" Center for Health Technology and Services Research (CINTESIS), Porto, Portugal

Portuguese Society of Mental Health Nursing, Porto, Portugal
e-mail: carlossequeira@esenf.pt

F.M.C. Sampaio
Nursing School of Porto, Porto, Portugal

Research Group "NursID: Innovation & Development in Nursing"
Center for Health Technology and Services Research (CINTESIS), Porto, Portugal

Psychiatry Department, Hospital de Braga, Braga, Portugal

© Springer International Publishing Switzerland 2018

J.C. Santos, J.R. Cutcliffe (eds.), *European Psychiatric/Mental Health Nursing in the 21st Century*, Principles of Specialty Nursing,
https://doi.org/10.1007/978-3-319-31772-4_4

they allow the understanding of the set of outcomes related to a specific nursing diagnosis (and also to identify the indicators enabling these outcomes evaluation). They also enable the identification of the suggested nursing interventions to respond to the specific nursing diagnosis.

As a result of the long-term experience in teaching and clinical practice and consistent with a reflexive approach, the authors of this chapter aim to call readers' attention to the importance of these classifications, their potentialities, limitations and challenges to their use. Thus, the main goals of this chapter are:

- To describe the main nursing taxonomies
- To analyse advantages and disadvantages related to its use
- To relate taxonomies with the nursing discipline, particularly with clinical practice in mental health
- To identify the main challenges and opportunities concerning its use

4.2 Overview of Taxonomies in Nursing

Taxonomy can be defined as the science of principles and methods of the several elements encompassing a scientific area (Infopédia 2014). Throughout the years and in the several different health domains, taxonomies have been considered increasingly important. Nowadays and especially in developed countries, nursing is increasingly based on evidence derived from research (and other forms of evidence), and thus taxonomies are required to help classify nursing knowledge (Hughes 2008).

This information highlights the importance of using taxonomies to classify and hierarchize any science domain knowledge. The question is then to determine if nursing will be able to exist as an evidence-based, scientific discipline without the development of taxonomies. It is not difficult to imagine what the implications might be to nursing if each professional used an individual language in the care conception, potentially describing the same situations in different perspectives. There would be impediments to the continuity of care. Electronic documentation of care would be nontransferable. It is likely that present and future nursing is and will likely be significantly dependent on the development of taxonomies, enabling nurses to:

- Describe nursing care.
- Adopt a common language between nurses.
- Electronically document nursing care.
- Draw on relevant information obtained from other clinical practice contexts.
- Compare nursing care between different clinical practice contexts.
- Identify people's nursing care needs, meaning nursing diagnosis.
- Prescribe nursing interventions.
- Provide information to managers and policy decision-makers concerning nursing care needs.

- Inform the population and other health professionals on the specific nurses' intervention areas.
- Contribute to the development of research databases.
- Promote consolidation of a professional nursing identity, while an autonomous discipline.
- Extract indicators sensitive to nursing care (epidemiological, of structure, process and outcome).

Regardless of the specific context, nurses' professional practice is based on two domains: (1) the collaborative domain, in which another health professional prescribes the intervention but the nurse is responsible for its execution (e.g. to assist a surgery, to prepare a patient for a medical examination, etc.), and (2) the autonomous domain, in which the nurse is responsible for identifying the person's needs; for naming this need through one or more nursing diagnoses; for prescribing nursing interventions with referential integrity, capable of achieving health gains; and for assessing outcomes (Ordem dos Enfermeiros 1996). According to this approach, taxonomies need to "speak to", at least in part, nursing assessment, interventions and outcomes, since these three axes represent the nursing practice core. Thus, it is essential to understand the importance of applying taxonomies to the nursing profession and discipline. Clark and Lang (1992, p. 109) summarize this issue stating as they do:

> If we cannot name it, we cannot control it, practice it, teach it, finance it, or put it into public policy.

There are several research studies that emphasize the existence of a higher diagnostic accuracy when nurses are found to have an educational background based on standardized language (Levin et al. 2004; Müller-Staub et al. 2007; Paans et al. 2012), as well as higher consistency regarding nursing care documentation (Paans et al. 2010).

4.3 Nursing Taxonomies and Structure

The International Classification for Nursing Practice® (ICNP®) is a third generation classification that, based on the Version 2 (ICN 2010) analysis, and aims to be a logical transition towards a fourth generation classification, meaning a classification that combines diagnosis, interventions and nursing outcomes. In order to achieve this objective, ICNP® catalogues have to be developed since they can fill a practical need in building health information systems by describing nursing care (ICN 2008). The ICNP® classification is organized into seven axes: focus, judgement, means, action, time, location and client:

- Nursing diagnosis = label for "Focus" axis + label for the "Judgement" axis; the use of terms from other axes or the use of more terms from the "Focus" axis and/or "Judgement" is optional.

- Example: impaired cognition, low self-esteem, risk for delusion, etc.
- Nursing intervention = label for "Action" axis and this must include at least one "Focus"; terms from any other axes and from the "Action" can be included.
- Example: teaching memory technique, demonstrating relaxation technique, etc.

The main issue deriving from the ICNP® underlying methods is the variety of diagnostic and intervention alternatives, meaning that if this process lacks clear regulation, it is very likely to result in multiple diagnosis and interventions, similar to what occurred in the Portuguese context (Paiva et al. 2014). As an example, with the focus "cognition", multiple combinations are possible: reduced cognition, impaired cognition, altered cognition, etc.

Both NANDA-I and the ICNP® include nursing diagnosis; however the first sets the defining characteristics and factors related to this subject (Johnson et al. 2011). This will enable a better contextualization of the nursing diagnosis, potentially providing a more accurate identification. Nevertheless, and contrary to the ICNP®, this is a hermetic classification that does not consider the combination of terms to determine nursing diagnosis, thus considered a constrainable option. Some examples found are situational low self-esteem, ineffective impulse control, risk for chronic low self-esteem, etc.

Both ICNP® and NANDA-I identify two types of nursing diagnoses (effective diagnostic and potential diagnoses). The Nursing Interventions Classification (NIC) (Bulechek et al. 2012) lists the interventions, specifies their definition and describes the related performed activities. Currently, the implemented nursing information systems in some health services, which include the description of the specific activities for each intervention, enable a better characterization of some nursing interventions. This will help to add information to some complex interventions, while others might not need further clarification. For example, the concept "cognitive restructuring" does not solely define the nursing activities necessary for optimal nursing performance. Cognitive restructuring may involve activities related to the beliefs and cognitive errors or dysfunctional thoughts. Thus, evaluating the effectiveness of interventions can be difficult, if the specific activities are not clearly documented.

In some cases, these interventions are performed by different nurses, responsible for prescribing, implementing and evaluating, so it is important to rely on documented procedures integrating the different activities. As an example, the intervention "promoting emotional support" does not specify the activities described in the NIC classification, which can involve different activities, such as sharing emotions, help people recognize emotions, provide safety feelings, etc. Thus, assessing the interventions' effectiveness can be difficult if there is no evidence on the specific related activities. Since these processes involve different nurses, the interventions' documentation may very likely involve different activities.

It is important to raise a discussion on the true meaning of "nursing interventions" and define "good practices". This discussion should necessarily address interventions such as the "environmental safety management" or "communication management". The NIC is a classification that encompasses nursing interventions, best practices and proposed goals related to a diagnosis, for example, cognitive restructuring (intervention), presence (good practice) and self-esteem enhancement (outcome).

Finally, we will attempt to analyse the NOC taxonomy (Moorhead et al. 2012). Nursing diagnoses (and relevant data) and interventions have been the main research focus in nursing with little attention given to the outcomes. However, through the results evaluation, it is possible to identify indicators expressing the importance of nursing interventions. In the particular case of the NOC, the nursing results presented consist of a set of indicators that should be submitted to an evaluation in order to determine if the outcome was effectively achieved or not. A Likert scale, from 1 to 5, is used to assess each indicator. Thus, the NOC provides outcomes for a set of indicators extracted from validated standardized instruments, allowing a specific evaluation for the nursing practice.

4.4 Advantages and Disadvantages in the Use of Taxonomies

4.4.1 In Nursing Care

The main advantage of using taxonomies is the possibility of nursing care being based on a common language among nurses, enabling documentation of assessment, interventions and nursing outcomes through health information systems. Nursing can benefit from the use of taxonomies, since they enable the development of patterns for nursing care planning. This may be achieved, in the view of the authors, for example, by developing the ICNP® catalogues (nursing data subsets) for specific focus or nursing diagnosis, enabling to fill a practical need in building health information systems with all the advantages in adopting a standardized nursing language.

Regarding the nursing process, which is currently in its third iteration (Pesut and Herman 1998), it is worth considering what impact taxonomies may have and how they may be "woven into" the nursing process per se. Recent knowledge development activities in classification systems (Pesut and Herman 1998) appear to include an emphasis on including and specifying outcomes, testing/measuring of meeting these outcomes (or not). In this context, the concept of nursing care has been increasingly linked to outcomes, and this blending of nursing process and taxonomies was operationalized in the clinical reasoning model "outcome-present state-test" (OPT) (Pesut and Herman 1999). In this model, the patterns and relations between nursing diagnoses and outcomes are linked, and their connections are explained; a key issue will emerge enabling the dynamic of the ongoing system. The keystone issue represents the core of the system dynamic and provides a leverage point for intervention that shifts the patient system from a present problem-oriented state to a specified desired-outcome state (Kuiper et al. 2016) (e.g. see Fig. 4.1). Efforts are made to try and identify the "central" or key nursing diagnosis as the thinking goes that if this central issue or need can be resolved, then this will also help resolve other related nursing diagnoses and problems (Pesut and Herman 1999). In the view of the authors,

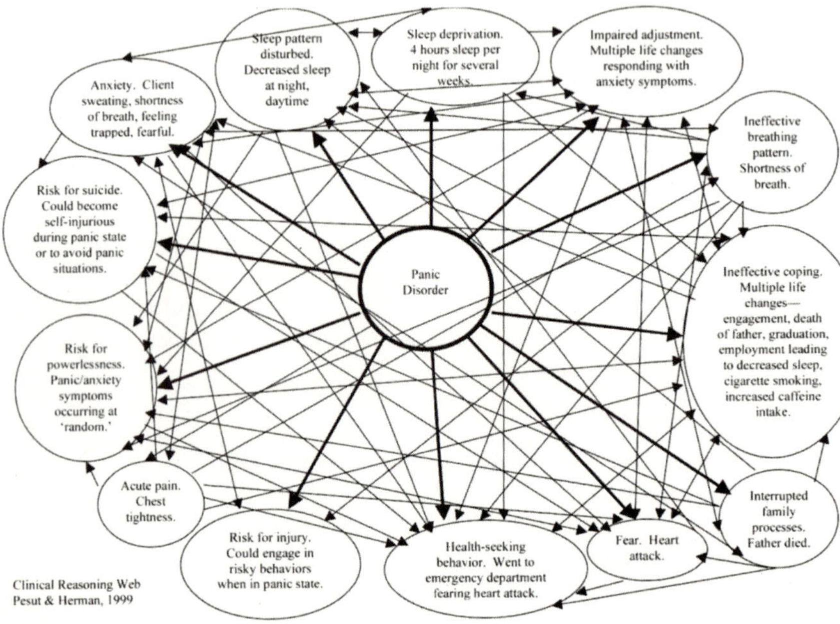

Fig. 4.1 Sample of one student's clinical reasoning web. Source: Kuiper et al. (2016)

this is very important and relevant in a mental health context, since there are some potential diagnoses that influence others (e.g. a cognition diagnosis includes other diagnoses at memory level, thought, language, attention, etc.). Accordingly, it is important to establish guidelines to determine in which situations the nurse's attention should be focused on the major diagnosis or in the minor diagnoses.

For the authors of this chapter, it is important to identify problems (nursing diagnosis) and then apply clinical reasoning that allows to understand the relationship between them and identify the "keystone" issue. Thus, it is possible to place the focus of care (intervention) on the main nursing diagnosis as a way to give a more meaningful response to the problem. The nursing taxonomies are essential in this process, since the clinical reasoning model OPT (Pesut and Herman 1999) presents itself as a conceptual framework for operationalizing their use. Thus, "present state" can be defined as a nursing diagnosis and "outcome state" as outcomes sensitive to nursing care (Pesut and Herman 1999; Sequeira, 2006). The nursing interventions are the actions enabling the person's transition (Meleis 2010) from a problematic condition to more desirable "outcome states".

P/MH nurses are encouraged to consider the following steps when considering patterns of the language used in the nursing process (Sequeira, 2006):

1. *Initial assessment*—data/evidence—how to describe these data?
2. *Diagnosis hypotheses*—which data support them?—are new data needed?
3. *Interview*—complete data for each diagnosis based on evidence (for each diagnosis, evidence-based data research is necessary).

4. *Identify the nursing diagnosis or diagnoses*—should identification consider only real diagnoses or should also focus on the potential diagnoses?
5. To agree with the person on the *care goals*.
6. *Negotiate interventions* with the person—more evidence is needed on identifying more effective interventions to a diagnosis response.
7. *Prescribing interventions*—to establish an action plan with a sequence and frequency of implementation for each intervention based on each single case.
8. *Perform interventions*—the existence of quality standards is essential to ensure greater interventions' effectiveness.
9. *Evaluate interventions' outcomes*.
10. *Complete the interventions* if the desired outcomes are achieved, or *reframe* the entire plan.

In terms of disadvantages, the different taxonomies do not clearly identify the nursing process. This means that, if one wishes to utilize the model described in the previous paragraph, then it may not be possible to list and describe relevant data to the identification of those diagnoses, establish a relationship between data and diagnosis and identify the specific outcomes to each nursing diagnosis and assure that a particular outcome is in fact addressed to a specific nursing diagnosis. Thus, an argument can be made that if one wishes to use this model, then it is necessary to create a taxonomy that enables P/MH nurses to describe and ensure data completeness in relation to nursing diagnoses and guarantee that nursing interventions have a referential integrity to a specific diagnosis.

4.4.2 In Nursing Care Documentation

Care documentation utilized by P/MH nurses is a further reason for the use of taxonomies. McCormick and Jones (1998) state http://www.nursingworld.org/MainMenuCategories/ANAMarketplace/ANAPeriodicals/OJIN/TableofContents/Vol31998/No2Sept1998/Isonetax onomyneeded.aspx:

> …market forces, or competition, necessitates accountability, and documentation is required to substantiate accountability for processes and outcomes of care. Data on outcomes related to quality and costs will provide information to the public, and ultimately enable consumers and payers to determine health care-related value, and make tradeoffs in level of quality desired for a given cost.

Despite the growing trend, in many parts of Europe, to move towards the wholesale adoption and implementation of electronic health records, it is also evident that these information technologies require the inclusion of a standardized language. It has been argued that this is the most effective way to generate data, the analysis of which ought logically to be able to help improve the quality of care provision (McCormick and Jones 1998). Moreover, for the authors of this chapter, electronic health records should contribute to best nursing practice quality and enhance its visibility. Indeed and considering the importance of information systems to policy decision-making and resources allocation (Clark 1998), nursing care documentation that relies on a shared taxonomy could help information systems promote and highlight the impact of the nursing discipline in health systems (Doyle 2006).

The replacement of paper documentation and records, by electronic health records, has already garnered worldwide support (Coffey et al. 2015; Wang et al. 2013). In Portugal, the majority of health institutions have already implemented this system. The electronic data recording is also under regulation concerning access and personal data protection (Paiva et al. 2014). Thus, data should be used in a responsible way (including addressing relevant ethical issues such as the reliability of care documentation). This could have a major contribution to improve the quality and safety of the user, help to increase the efficiency and effectiveness of the provision of care and enable autonomy and control of the nursing practice, enhancing it as a profession as well as a science. However, without a standardized language resource, it is not possible to identify, aggregate, analyse and compare the specific type of data related to nursing care (Jones et al. 2010).

4.5 Taxonomies in Psychiatric/Mental Health Nursing

In the specific context of the P/MH nursing, it seems clear that there is still a long way to go before evidence can be obtained which shows that the existing taxonomies can impact and improve current clinical practice. Despite the work already developed in this area, the desired quality achievement of nursing taxonomies in P/MH nursing is still a major challenge. There is already a set of interventions described in Nursing Interventions Classification (NIC), which are of reference, for the context of psychiatry. However, these interventions still need to be culturally validated in many countries, since this classification was based on the American reality.

The development of studies that evaluate the effective value of interventions, like relocation stress reduction (5350), cognitive restructuring (4700) and reminiscence therapy (4860), will be very useful for awareness on the health gains associated with its implementation. In the specific case of the Nursing Interventions Classification (NIC), there is a domain almost entirely composed by interventions in the field of mental health and psychiatric nursing. Thus, the "domain three" in this classification is identified as "behavioural domain" and includes six dimensions: "behavioural therapy", "cognitive therapy", "communication enhancement", "coping assistance", "patient education" and "psychological comfort promotion" (Bulechek et al. 2012). Some of the intervention examples that can be found in these dimensions are "cognitive restructuring", "behaviour modification" and "counselling".

However, the NIC does not provide information on the procedures of these interventions. Their creation and validation will be an asset for the documentation in health information systems. With the existence of the procedures, it will be also easier for the nurses to use them in the clinical practice, teaching them and evaluating them. At this level, a focus group study carried out by Sampaio et al. (2014) enabled the identification of some nursing interventions described in the NIC and that can be considered of psychotherapeutic domain. In Table 4.1, these nursing psychotherapeutic interventions are described.

Table 4.1 Nursing psychotherapeutic interventions

Brief psychodynamic interventions	Cognitive interventions	Behavioural interventions	Humanistic interventions
Life story	Decision-making support (5250)	Self-modification assistance (4470)	Counselling (5240)
–	Anger control assistance (4640)	Smoking cessation assistance (4490)	Motivational interview
–	Mood management (5330)	Eating disorders management (1030)	–
–	Grief work facilitation (5290)	Family process maintenance (7130)	–
–	Crisis intervention (6160)	Socialization enhancement (5100)	–
–	Self-awareness enhancement (5390)	Role enhancement (5370)	–
–	Self-esteem enhancement (5400)	Behaviour modification (4360)	–
–	Body image enhancement (5220)	Suicide prevention (6340)	–
–	Coping enhancement (5230)	Family integrity promotion (7100)	–
–	Hope inspiration (5310)	Simple relaxation therapy (6040)	–
–	Anxiety reduction (5820)	Assertiveness training (4340)	–
–	Relocation stress reduction (5350)	Impulse control training (4370)	–
–	Cognitive restructuring (4700)	–	–
–	Reminiscence therapy (4860)	–	–

The "domain three" included in the NOC, entitled "psychosocial health", also includes four dimensions with a significant relation to the mental health and psychiatric nursing context. These dimensions are described as "psychological well-being", "psychosocial adaptation", "self-control" and "social interaction" (Moorhead et al. 2012). As an example, some nursing outcomes can be found in these referred dimensions: "self-esteem", "social interaction skills" and "will to live". The identification of psychotherapeutic interventions, based on the NIC, and the NOC indicators are extremely useful resources for the nursing practice in the context of psychiatry. However, it is still necessary for nurses and investigators to be made aware of the necessity of more investigation work on the interventions procedures, the interventions effectiveness and the psychometric proprieties of the NOC indicators.

Conclusions

For the authors of this chapter, it is of the utmost importance that P/MH nurses search for and ultimately reach consensus on the most relevant taxonomies to their everyday work. It can also be argued that they eventually work on specific taxonomies enabling a better characterization of people's needs and the activities developed by P/MH nurses. According to ICNP® /NANDA International, Inc.

(NANDA-I), there are areas which it is not possible to achieve a diagnosis, as the ones related to certain changes in thinking or types of violence. The Nursing School of Porto is working on an ongoing research project, on the development of archetypes/clinical data models. This project aims at providing inputs to improve nurses' clinical decision-making, supported on national parameter records and in the opinion of experts for each intervention area. The creation of clinical data models can be an important support to nurses concerning the scientific evidence related to care plans. Thus, it will be possible to develop clinical data models, meaning a set of data, diagnosis, interventions and outcomes, addressing anxiety, stress, agitation, delusion, etc. The existence of these clinical data models will also be essential to enhance clinical practices, as they can be replicated and eventually improved in other contexts/countries, facilitating consensus building (Sequeira 2014).

References

Bulechek GM, Butcher HK, Dochterman JM, Wagner C (2012) Nursing interventions classification (NIC), 6th edn. Elsevier, St. Louis, MO

Clark J (1998) The international classification for nursing practice project. Online J Issues Nurs 3(2). Retrieved from: www.nursingworld.org/MainMenuCategories/ANAMarketplace/ANAPeriodicals/OJIN/TableofContents/Vol31998/No2Sept1998/TheInternationalClassificationForNursingPracticeProject.aspx

Clark J, Lang N (1992) Nursing's next advance: an internal classification for nursing practice. Int Nurs Rev 39(4):109–111

Coffey C, Wurster LAM, Groner J, Hoffman J, Hendren V, Nuss K, Covert J (2015) A comparison of paper documentation to electronic documentation for trauma resuscitations at a level I pediatric trauma center. J Emerg Nurs 41(1):52–56. https://doi.org/10.1016/j.jen.2014.04.010

Infopédia (2014) Dicionário da Língua Portuguesa. [em linha]. Porto: Porto Editora, 2003–2017. [consult. 2016–06-02]. Disponível na Internet: https://www.infopedia.pt/dicionarios/lingua-portuguesa/taxonomia

Doyle M (2006) Promoting standardized nursing language using an electronic medical record system. AORN J 83(6):1335–1342. https://doi.org/10.1016/S0001-2092(06)60147-6

Hughes RG (2008) Patient safety and quality: an evidence-based handbook for nurses. [em linha]. Rockville: AHRQ Publication No. 08–0043 [consult. 2016–06-02]. Disponível na internet: https://archive.ahrq.gov/professionals/clinicians-providers/resources/nursing/resources/nurseshdbk/nurseshdbk.pdf

International Council of Nurses (2008) Guidelines for ICNP® catalogue development. Geneva: Author

International Council of Nurses (2010) ICNP® version 2 – international classification for nursing practice. Geneva: Author

Johnson M, Moorhead S, Bulechek G, Butcher H, Maas M, Swanson E (2011) NOC and NIC linkages to NANDA-I and clinical conditions: supporting critical reasoning and quality care, 3rd edn. Mosby, Maryland Heights, MO

Jones D, Lunney M, Keenan G, Moorhead S (2010) Ann Rev Nurs Res 28:253–294. https://doi.org/10.1891/0739-6686.28.253

Kuiper R, Pesut DJ, Arms TE (2016) Clinical reasoning and care coordination in advanced practice nursing. Springer Publishing Company, New York, NY

Levin RF, Lunney M, Krainovich-Miller B (2004) Improving diagnostic accuracy using an evidence-based nursing model. Int J Nurs Terminol Classif 15(4):114–122. https://doi.org/10.1111/j.1744-618X.2004.tb00008.x

McCormick KA, Jones CB (1998) Is one taxonomy needed for health care vocabularies and classifications?. Online J Issues Nurs 3(2). Retrieved from: www.nursingworld.org/MainMenuCategories/ANAMarketplace/ANAPeriodicals/OJIN/TableofContents/Vol31998/No2Sept1998/Isonetaxonomyneeded.aspx

Meleis AI (2010) Transitions theory: middle range and situation specific theories in nursing research and practice. Springer Publishing Company, New York. NY

Moorhead S, Johnson M, Maas ML, Swanson E (2012) Nursing outcomes classification (NOC), 5th edn. Elsevier, St. Louis, MO

Müller-Staub M, Needham I, Odenbreit M, Lavin MA, Van Achterberg T (2007) Improved quality of nursing documentation: results of a nursing diagnoses, interventions, and outcomes implementation study. Inter J Nurs Terminol Classif 18(1):5–17. https://doi.org/10.1111/j.1744-618X.2007.00043.x

Ordem dos enfermeiros (1996). Regulamento do exercício profissional do Enfermeiro (REPE) – Decreto de lei n° 161/96, de 4 de Setembro. Ordem dos Enfermeiros, Lisboa

Paans W, Sermeus W, Nieweg RMB, van der Schans CP (2010) Prevalence of accurate nursing documentation in patient records. J Adv Nurs 66(11):2481–2489. https://doi.org/10.1111/j.1365-2648.2010.05433.x

Paans W, Sermeus W, Nieweg RMB, Krijnen WP, van der Schans CP (2012) Do knowledge, knowledge sources and reasoning skills affect the accuracy of nursing diagnoses? A randomised study. BMC Nurs 11:11. https://doi.org/10.1186/1472-6955-11-11

Paiva A, Cardoso A, Sequeira C, Morais EJ, Bastos F, Pereira F et al (2014) Análise da parametrização nacional do Sistema de Apoio à Prática de Enfermagem - SAPE®. Escola Superior de Enfermagem do Porto, Porto. Retrieved from: http://www.esenf.pt/fotos/editor2/i_d/publicacoes/apn-978-989-98443-5-3.pdf

Pesut DJ, Herman J (1998) OPT: transformation of nursing process for contemporary practice. Nurs Outlook 46(1):29–36. https://doi.org/10.1016/S0029-6554(98)90022-7

Pesut D, Herman JA (1999) Clinical reasoning: the art and science of critical and creative thinking. Cengage Learning, Boston

Sampaio FMC, Sequeira C, Lluch Canut T (2014) Intervenciones NIC del dominio conductual: Un estudio de focus group de intervenciones psicoterapéuticas de enfermería. In Asociación Española de Nomenclatura, Taxonomia y Diagnósticos de Enfermería (AENTDE) (Eds.), X Simposium AENTDE "Lenguaje enfermero: identidad, utilidad y calidad" (pp 718–721). Seville: author

Sequeira C (2006) Introdução à prática clínica: Do diagnóstico à intervenção em enfermagem de saúde mental e psiquiátrica. Coimbra: Quarteto. Disponível em:https://www.researchgate.net/publication/275518330_Introducao_a_Pratica_Clinica_-_do_diagnostico_a_intervencao_em_saude_mental

Sequeira C (2014) Editorial: Consensos em saúde mental - diagnósticos, intervenções e resultados. Revista Portuguesa de Enfermagem de Saúde Mental 11:6–8

Wang N, Yu P, Hailey D (2013) Description and comparison of documentation of nursing assessment between paper-based and electronic systems in Australian aged care homes. Int J Med Inform 82(9):789–797. https://doi.org/10.1016/j.ijmedinf.2013.05.002

Theories of the Interpersonal Relationships, Transitions and Humanistic Theories: Contribution to Frameworks of Psychiatric/Mental Health Nursing in Europe

5

José Carlos Carvalho and Raul Alberto Cordeiro

5.1 Introduction

Since the 1980s, a discernible shift in European mental health policies has resulted in a significant shift towards community-centred or community-based mental health care (Samele et al. 2013). Simultaneously, most European countries have increasingly been disposing of traditional psychiatric hospitals. This deinstitutionalisation process has resulted in a significant reduction in the number of beds in the existing psychiatric hospitals, and yet this diminution of inpatient services has occurred in lieu of a structural change that includes the creation of psychiatry departments in general hospitals and community-based services. A further important shift in European mental health care, which for some is concomitant with the movement away from deinstitutionalisation, is that of embracing client-centred care, a focus on interpersonal ways of working, and working within a humanistic conceptual framework (Caldas de Almeida and Killaspy 2011). It is within this context that the authors of this chapter draw attention to three major theoretical trends and resultant theoretical frameworks, which have been utilised in psychiatric/mental health nursing care: interpersonal relation-based theories, humanistic-based theories and transition-based theories.

J.C. Carvalho (✉)
Escola Superior de Enfermagem do Porto (Nursing College of Porto), Porto, Portugal
e-mail: zecarlos@esenf.pt

R.A. Cordeiro
Polytechnic Institute of Portalegre, Portalegre, Portugal

© Springer International Publishing Switzerland 2018

J.C. Santos, J.R. Cutcliffe (eds.), *European Psychiatric/Mental Health Nursing in the 21st Century*, Principles of Specialty Nursing,
https://doi.org/10.1007/978-3-319-31772-4_5

5.2 Rediscovering Peplau

Researchers, educators and clinicians have long recognised the profound influence of the mid-twentieth century focus on interpersonal relations on nurses and nursing (Lego 1999). However, in the present time, both in nursing and other health science fields, neuroanatomy, neurobiology/neurophysiology and the pervasive influence of big pharmaceutical companies, have replaced interpersonal theories as the key to the understanding of human behaviours (Lakeman and Cutcliffe 2009, 2016; Cutcliffe and Lakeman 2010). Consequently, even a cursory examination of contemporary mental health-focused literature, policy and theory will show a noticeable and, for the authors of this chapter, an exaggerated 'biological concern' in the personal and interpersonal evaluation of mental health and the experience of being a mental health service user. Given the very well-documented and widespread discontent that the majority of mental health service users have repeatedly reported concerning the overuse of drugs and absence of interpersonal, 'talk therapy' (Cutcliffe et al. 2015), the authors join the chorus of like-minded P/MH nurses in encouraging P/MH nurses to revisit, reconsider the original concepts of the interpersonal relationships in P/MH nursing (Peplau 1991) and rediscover their transforming power as an important ingredient of effective P/MH nursing.

5.3 Theories of Interpersonal Relationships in Psychiatric/ Mental Health Nursing

For those Europeans who embrace and accept interpersonal focused P/MH nursing, Hildegard Peplau is thought of and regarded as the 'Mother' of P/MH nursing (Howk et al. 1998). In general, the interpersonal relations theories, like Peplau's (1991), highlight the importance of and subsequently emphasize the development of interpersonal relations between the nurse and the client; for Peplau, this relationship is an opportunity for mutual learning and growth. Peplau (1991) placed as many demands for reflection and change on the nurse as on the patient. The nurse had to know herself/himself as well as the patient (D'Antonio et al. 2014). For Peplau, nursing, in its essence, is an interpersonal process; the nurse–patient relationship was the centre of P/MH nursing practice. Peplau (1991) identified four sequential phases in the interpersonal relationship: orientation, identification, exploitation and resolution. And while there is movement through these stages, Peplau makes room for some multidirectional movement with the stages, at times, overlapping one another. In addition to the four phases or stages, Peplau also describes a number of different professional rules that the P/MH adopts: stranger, educator, resource, counsellor, leader or substitute. A further critically important conceptualisation (if not philosophical stance) is Peplau's conceptualisation of the patient (or client) as a partner in the nursing process (Alligood and Tomey 2010).

These key conceptual and theoretical elements are for the authors of this chapter, appropriate and culturally sensitive to the European culture, and in line with World

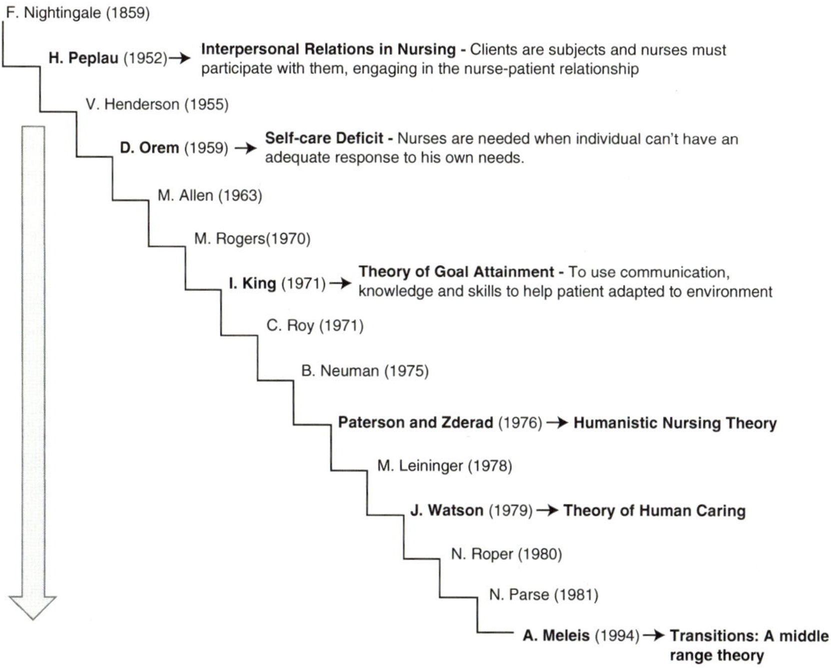

Fig. 5.1 Evolution of Nursing Theories

Health Organisation Regional Office for Europe (WHO: ROE). Wherein, respect to the future of European mental health care, the WHO: REO stipulates that:

> The mental health programme will base all its work on the following principles; all its activities will be: driven by the needs and experiences of people, communities and society; based on the best evidence, including both scientific evaluation and local experience; and sensitive to local cultures and resources, and respectful of diversity. (WHO-ROE 2005, p. 141)

On the other hand, some strategic mental health policy changes, as for example, focussing only on the treatment of so-called severe mental illnesses and the need to offer care solely centred on an economic cost-benefit calculation, has compromised the application of Peplau's framework (Jones 1996). For a brief history of nursing theories, see Fig. 5.1.

5.4 Humanistic Theories and Person-Centred Approaches

The person-centred approach was initially developed and advanced in the USA during the 1940s and is commonly associated with 'humanistic' models and thinking.

> It has its roots in humanistic psychology and the primarily European concepts of phenomenology and existentialism. (Trahar 2004, p. 8)

Viewed through a humanistic lens, the human being, independently of the circumstances which surround him, possesses the innate capacity of assuming the control of his/her own life and of promoting his/her own development by means of the exclusively humane capacities of choice, creativity and self-fulfilment. The key of the learning process in the humanistic vision is *becoming a person*, which emphasises learning as a personal process, particularly learning from the individual's life experiences (Rogers 2004).

Among the main theorists of the humanistic perspective, Abraham Maslow (1908–1970), who for some is considered the spiritual father of the humanist movement, developed the motivation theory centred in the self-fulfilment concept. A further key contributor to this humanistic perspective is Carl Rogers (1902–1987), who advanced the key argument concerning the innate capacity for each person to further develop his/her capacities and potentials. Rogers (2004) offered important conceptualisations and arguments convinced that the human being is conscientious of his/her own experiences and is capable of evaluating and correcting them. Rogers extended his humanistic, person-centred perspective to the treatment of emotionally disturbed people. Rogers brings into psychotherapy a different perspective of the person and, consequently, a diverse perspective of the person who seeks for assistance and the therapist/client relation—a non-directive approach of the therapeutic relation. In contrast with the idea that reduces humans to an existence fatally determined by factors that are both outer (social or cultural pressures for instance) and inner (unconscious impulses or inherited characteristics) and hinder his/her free will capacities, Rogers (2004) sees the human being as inherently gifted with liberty and power of choice, a humanist perspective of the therapeutic relation and the care.

For some, at least, these important elements of humanistic thinking have a major influence in contemporary mental health care. Josephine Paterson and Loretta Zderad, for instance, regard nursing as an interaction involving the development of experiences lived by the nurse and the patient. Focus is the dialogical intersubjective relationship experienced by human beings for the use of their potentials in order to be better; a truly ecological relation. They start from the appreciation of singularity of the unique being rich in diverse experiences and exchanges, which develop from community life and individual experiences. Paterson and Zderad (1988) defend the importance of considering humanistic nursing as an end worth fighting for or an attitude which strengthens individual endurance needed to reach a difficult target, or, more essentially, as an important value which enriches the nursing practice (see Fig. 5.2).

The humanistic perspective tends to highlight life experience of the formal therapeutic actors as a source of knowledge that is relevant to care practice (O'Connor 1993; Kleiman 2001; McCamant 2006). Paterson and Zderad characterise their theory as a *metatheory*, in the sense that it describes the nursing process in abstract terms (McCamant 2006). The meaning of humanistic nursing is founded in *the phenomenon of nursing as it is experienced in the everyday world* (Paterson and Zderad 1976, p. 23). The process of humanistic nursing is described as 'incarnate men (patient and nurse) meeting (being and becoming) in a goal-directed (nurturing well-being and more-being), intersubjective transaction (being with and doing with) occurring in time and space (as measured and as lived by patient and nurse) in a

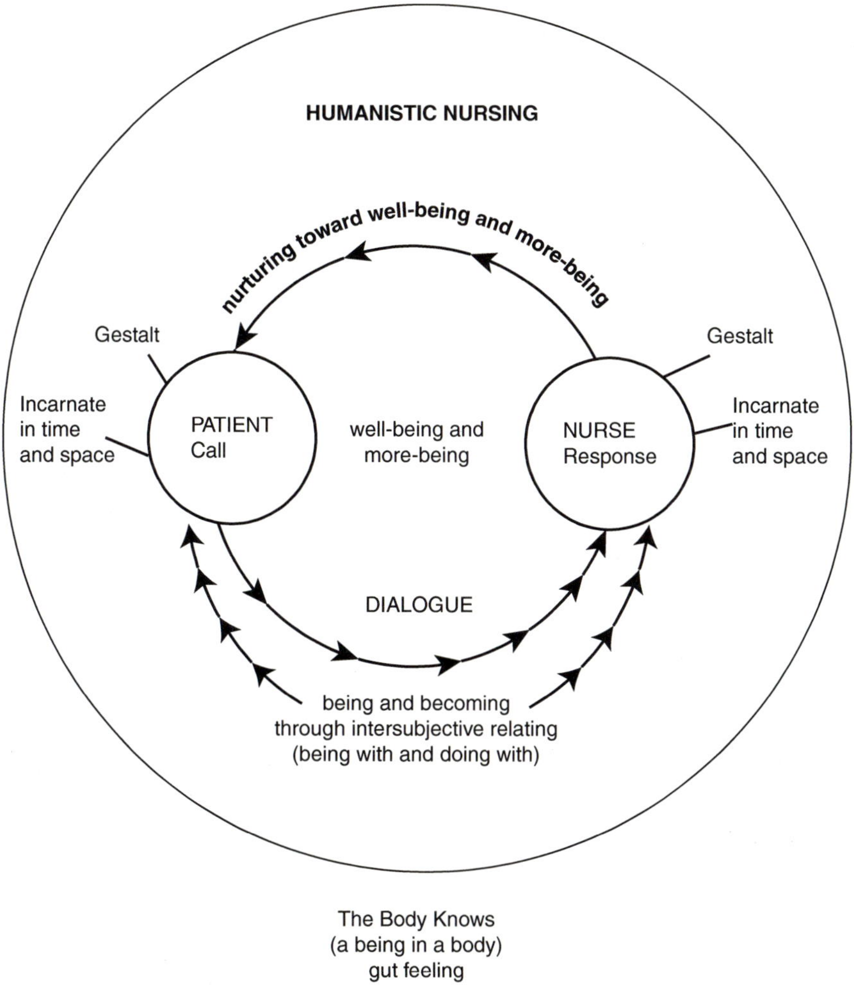

Fig. 5.2 Conceptual framework of humanistic nursing theory (Parker and smith 2005)

world of men and things' (p. 23). In other words, the nurse–patient relationship is characterised by interactions designed to promote well-being and existential growth in the context of the lived world. The nurse cares for the patient by presence or being with the patient and other nursing actions or activities.

Humanistic theories developed, at least in part, as a tacit rejection of and response to the orthodox, psychoanalytical thought of the time: namely, that a person's destiny was determined in the early life. Humanistic theories emphasise a person's capacity for self-actualisation, growth, development—at all stages of life. Humanists believe that the person contains within himself the potential for healthy and creative growth.

Paterson and Zderad's Humanistic Nursing Theory draws upon both Humanism and Existentialism (Paterson and Zderad 1988).

Humanism attempts to take a broader perspective than a reductionalist approach of the individual's potential and tries to understand each individual from the context of their own personal experiences.

Existentialism is a philosophical approach to understanding life. It's the belief that thinking begins with the human—the feeling, acting, living individual. Existentialism emphasises the individual's free-choice, self-determination and self-responsibility.

Nursing dialogue is when a nurse and patient come together. The nurse presents her/his self as a helper ready to assist the patient. The nurse is open to understanding how the patient feels with the intention of improvement. Openness is an essential quality for humanistic nursing dialogue. Humanistic-based nursing involves more than a technically competent relationship between the nurse and client. Instead, it determines that nursing is a responsible quest, a transactional relation whose meaning demands concepts founded in the existential conscience of a nurse as herself and the other (Paterson and Zderad 1988).

According to Paterson and Zderad (2008, p. 3),

> Humanistic nursing embraces more than a benevolent technically competent subject-object one-way relationship guided by a nurse in behalf of another. Rather it dictates that nursing is a responsible searching, transactional relationship whose meaningfulness demands conceptualization founded on a nurse's existential awareness of self and of the other.

It envisages the possibility of looking with a different perspective to the one who needs help and to the one who is willing to help; the one who provides care is someone with a certain type of care available and the one taken care of is someone with certain needs (Wu and Volker 2012), presenting the nursing care as a living and communicative encounter. Humanistic and person-centred nursing encounters require the nurse to be open to every experience, and he/she needs to go beyond 'doing with'. It involves a human being helping another in an inter-human and intersubjective transaction, with the aim of increasing responsible choices, not only in the absence of sickness but in the human possibility of well-being and better-being.

5.5 The Perspective of Transitions in Psychiatric/Mental Health Nursing

Transition (from the Latin *transitiōne)* means *act or effect of passing from one state, period, matter or place to another* and is a contemporary concept which is woven into the theory of crisis (Teixeira et al. 2010; Page 1998; Jacobson 1980; Meleis and Trangenstein 1994). Transition process can include disturbance of balance, a disturbance of a stable condition, which immediately demands new patterns of behaviour and to which a response arouses, usually, through mechanisms and usual reactions available to each person to deal with problems. The transition is defined as the passage from one phase of life, condition or state to another (Meleis and Trangenstein 1994; Meleis 2010). The transition involves how people respond to change with the passage of time (Kralik et al. 2005). The transition refers to the complex interactions between client/environment. According to Chick and Meleis (1986), the transitions are categorized as within the nursing field when the health/disease or responses to the transition are manifested in the domain of behavioural health.

Examination of the relevant literature suggests that for P/MH nursing (at least), the goal of care provision has morphed beyond addressing pathological issues to the response of the individual to the health and life processes, as well as the transition processes that happen throughout the life cycle. In a world that is in permanently changing, the human being experiences transitional periods and is frequently put to the test regarding his/her capabilities to deal with those changes. Humanistic P/MH nursing then requires consideration of the person's experiences, as well as the person's responses to health challenges and consequences of the transitions (Meleis and Trangenstein 1994).

There are several different theoretical and clinical (practical) reasons for considering transitions, and how people react to, cope with and are affected by them, as a matter of P/MH nursing. Nurses spend a great part of their time caring for people who are experiencing one or more changes in their lives which may well have impact and or effect on health (family, social, personal and life cycle transitions). Some authors (Meleis et al. 2000; Schumacher 1995; Schumacher et al. 1998; Nolan et al. 1995) have led the introduction of this issue into the discourse about nursing. Meleis et al. (2000, p. 13) highlights the necessity of considering transitions because:

> Nurses (…) tend to be the carers who prepare clients for transitions which approach and facilitate the learning process of new competences related to the experiences of health and sickness. (Meleis et al. 2000, p. 13)

According to Meleis (2010), this middle-range theory arose from the analysis of the 'transition' concept as a core concept in nursing and aims to provide a structure which allows the description, understanding, interpreting and/or explaining nursing specific phenomena, which reflect and emerge from the practice. These theories aspire to offer a systematic construct of the mission, nature and objectives of nursing (Meleis 2010).

Meleis and her collaborators point out:

> Changes in health status may provide opportunities for enhanced well-being and expose individuals to increased illness risks, as well as trigger a process of transition. (Meleis et al. 2000, p. 52)

The Middle-Range Transition Theory (Meleis et al. 2000) includes three main concepts: the nature of transitions (types, patterns and properties), the conditions (facilitators and inhibitors) and the response patterns, perceived as indicators of the process (to feel connected, interact, being located, trust and coping) and result (fluid and flexible identities; mastery) and 'nursing therapeutics' (see Fig. 5.3).

The transitions are complex and multidimensional phenomena in which it is possible to identify five features (awareness, involvement, change and difference, transition period and critical points and events), which normally are related among each other (Meleis et al. 2000). The awareness is related to the *perception, knowledge and recognition of a transition experience*, considered a key feature of the entire process, and the individual, to be in transition, needs to be aware of the changes in

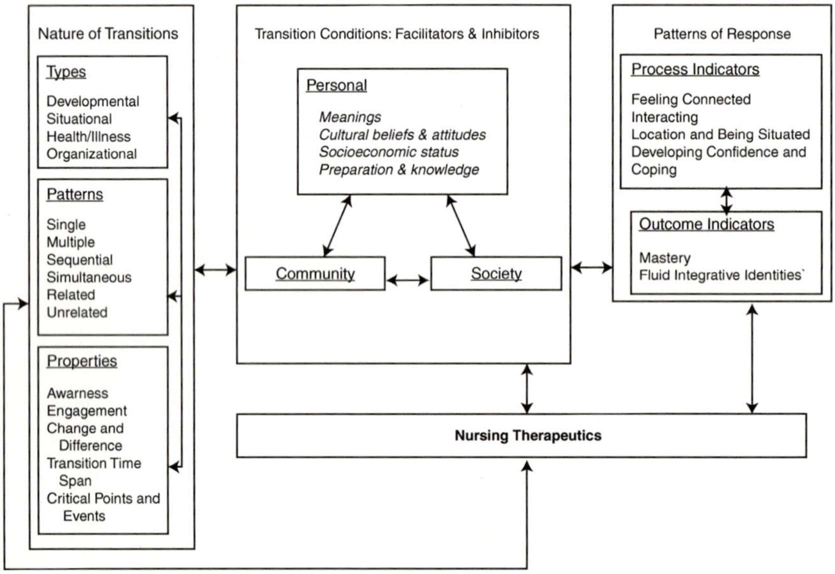

Fig. 5.3 Transitions middle-range theory Meleis et al. (2000)

course. Involvement is understood as the degree to which the person appears to be implicated with the processes inherent to the transition. The awareness level influences the level of involvement, since the level of involvement of someone who is aware of the changes that took place, will obviously be different from the one who does not identify them (Meleis et al. 2000; Meleis and Trangenstein 1994). Transitions are the *result of changes and result in changes* (Meleis et al. 2000), so change and difference are considered essential properties of transition. The existence of changes (physical, social, personal, emotional and environmental) is another property of transitions, some related with the ongoing transition process, others not. All transitions feature changes through time. Any process starts with the first signs of change and goes through a period of instability with advances and withdrawals till a potential end, where the individual acquires a new concept of stability. Transition time is, thus, variable and many times indefinite, which requires a continuous evaluation of the results though time, alert nonetheless to the fact that this evolution is not blindly considered linear, as it might be difficult or even impossible to define time barriers (Meleis et al. 2000).

In a first approach to the person who has been diagnosed with so-called mental illness, it is important that the nurse evaluates the insight, recognised as the capacity to gain an accurate and deep understanding of someone or something. In case the client does not possess an insight, he/she could never experience a transition. Nevertheless, the transition theory could be utilised in the approach to the family member who is providing care, in which the nurse evaluates the different fields associated to a transition. Besides this, and in line with the humanistic theory, it is important that the nurse seeks to find an interpersonal relation of proximity and trust with the client himself/herself.

Conclusion

In this chapter, we aimed at highlighting the main concepts of three theoretical foundations of P/MH nursing; we seek for anchors that connect them to the cultural and scientific specifications of Europe. P/MH nursing has adopted, in the formation of its theoretical references, concepts which do not completely adapt to the history of the professionals and psychiatric institutions in Europe, neither to the specialist professionals training. It is our belief that theoretical basis of broaden social, cultural and clinical should be more adapted to the European reality. People are different, culture are different, history are different, mental health problems and challenges are different, P/MH nursing history is different, so must be different today's approach to so-called mental illness. Although today we have a cross-cultural overview of world, our habitat remains special and foundation of our ecological balance, especially in an imbalance table between us and the world, in the context of mental health. A theoretical foundation for the framework in mental health nursing in Europe should always consider its history and cultural diversity, its history in the care of the mental illness and the history of its education in general nursing and particularly in specialised P/MH nursing. We do not point out a theoretical orientation. That would be too bold. But we say clearly: P/MH nursing in Europe needs to have a humanist look of the person, see it at all stages of their life cycle with all the inherent transitions discovering and constantly rediscovering the advantages of developing interpersonal relations as a therapeutic interaction field. This is the humanist framework for P/MH nursing in Europe.

References

Alligood M, Tomey A (2010) Nursing theorists and their work, 7th edn. Elsevier, Mosby

Caldas de Almeida JM, Killaspy H (2011) Long-term mental health care for people with severe mental disorders. European Commission. (Last accessed on 2016 Oct 30). Available from: http://ec.europa.eu/health/mental_health/docs/healthcare_mental_disorders_en.pdf

Chick N, Meleis AI (1986) Transition a nursing concern. In: Chinn PL (ed) Nursing research - methodology, issues and implementation. Aspen, Rockville, pp 237–257

Cutcliffe JR, Lakeman R (2010) Challenging normative orthodoxies in depression: Huxley's Utopia or Dante's Inferno? Arch Psychiatr Nurs 24(2):114–124

Cutcliffe JR, Santos JC, Kozel B, Taylor P, Lees D (2015) Raiders of the lost art: a review of published evaluations of inpatient mental health care experiences emanating from the United Kingdom, Portugal, Canada, Switzerland, Germany and Australia. Int J Men Health Nurs 24(5):375–385

D'Antonio P, Beeber L, Sills G, Naegle M (2014) The future in the past: Hildegard Peplau and interpersonal relations in nursing. Nurs Inq 21(4):311–317

Howk C, Brophy GH, Carey ET, Noll J, Rasmussen L, Searcy B, Stark NL (1998) Hildegard E. Peplau: psychodynamic nursing. In: Tomey AM, Alligood MR (eds) Nursing theorists and their work, 4th edn. Mosby, St. Louis, pp 335–350

Jacobson GF (1980) Crisis theory. New Dir Ment Health Serv 1980:1–10. https://doi.org/10.1002/yd.23319800603

Jones A (1996) The value of Peplau's theory for mental health nursing. Br J Nurs 5(14):877–881

Kleiman S (2001) Josephine Paterson and Loretta Zderad: humanistic nursing theory with clinical applications. In: Parker ME (ed) Nursing theories and nursing practice. F.A. Davis, Philadelphia, pp 151–168

Kralik D, Visentin K, Van Loon A (2005) Transition: a literature review. J Adv Nurs 55(3):320–329
Lakeman R, Cutcliffe JR (2009) Misplaced epistemological certainty and pharmaco-centrism in mental health nursing. J Psychiatr Ment Health Nurs 16:199–205
Lakeman R, Cutcliffe JR (2016) Diagnostic sedition: re-considering the ascension and hegemony of contemporary psychiatric diagnosis. Issues Ment Health Nurs 37:125–130
Lego S (1999) The one-to-one nurse-patient relationship. Perspect Psychiatr Care 35:4–23
McCamant KL (2006) Humanistic nursing, interpersonal relations theory, and the empathy-altruism hypothesis. Nurs Sci Q 19:334–338
Meleis AI (2010) Transitions theory: middle-range and situations specifics theories in nursing research and practice. Springer Publishing Company, New York
Meleis AI, Sawyer L, Im E, Messias D, Schumacher K (2000) Experiencing transitions: an emerging middle-range theory. Adv Nurs Sci 23(1):12–28
Meleis A, Trangenstein P (1994) Facilitating transitions: redefinition of the nursing mission. Nurs Outlook 42(6):255–259
Nolan M, Ready J, Grant G (1995) Developing a typology of family care: implications for nurses and other service providers. J Adv Nurs 21:256–265
O'Connor N (1993) Paterson and Zderad: humanistic nursing theory. Sage, Newbury Park
Page LJ (1998) The crisis in mental health theory. Int J Men Health 27(1):33–61
Parker ME, Smith MC (2005) Nursing theories and nursing practice. FA Davis, p. 128
Paterson JG, Zderad LT (1988) Humanistic nursing. National League for Nursing, New York
Paterson JG, Zderad LT (1976) Humanistic nursing. John Wiley & Sons, New York
Paterson J, Zderad LT (2008) Humanistic nursing. Project Gutenberg eBook. Available from: http://www.gutenberg.org/files/25020/25020-8.txt
Peplau HE (1991) Interpersonal relations in nursing: offering a conceptual frame of reference for psychodynamic nursing. G.P. Putnam's Sons, New York
Rogers C (2004) On becoming a person. Constable and Robinson Ltd., London
Schumacher KL (1995) Family caregiver role acquisition: role-making through situated interaction. Sch Inq Nurs Pract 9:211–271
Samele C, Frew, S., Urquia N (2013) Mental health systems in the European Union Member States, Status of Mental Health in Populations and benefits to be expected from investments into mental health. A report prepared on behalf of the Institute of Mental Health, Nottingham for the EU Executive Agency for Health and Consumers. (Last accessed on 2016 Oct 30). Available from: http://www.ec.europa.eu/health/mental_health/docs/europopp_full_en.pdf
Schumacher KL, Stewart BJ, Archbold PG (1998) Conceptualization and measurement of doing family caregiving well. Image J Nurs Sch 30:63–69
Teixeira J, Meireles J, Carvalho JC (2010) A teoria das transições em saúde mental (The theory of transitions in mental health). Revista Portuguesa de Enfermagem de Saúde Mental (Port J Ment Health Nurs) 4:45–52
Trahar S (2004) Models of counseling. Guidance and counseling in education. Unit handbook
WHO European Office (2005) Mental health action plan for Europe: facing the challenges, building solutions. WHO European Ministerial Conference on Mental Health, Helsinki. (EUR/04/5047810/7)
Wu HL, Volker DL (2012) Humanistic nursing theory: application to hospice and palliative care. J Adv Nurs 68(2):471–479

An Introduction to the Art and Science of Cognitive Behavioural Psychotherapy

6

John Swan and Graham Sloan

6.1 Introduction

Psychiatric/mental health nurses, especially those who wish to operate as psychotherapeutic agents, often draw on a range of theoretical approaches and interventions. One such approach, and the particular interventions and practices subsumed within it, which can be found with conspicuous regularity in many P/MH nursing settings, is that of cognitive behavioural therapy. As a result, this chapter will provide a succinct overview of the evidence base for CBT. Its key methods, competencies and the therapeutic skills associated with CBT will be examined, as will some of the developmental journey towards how psychiatric/mental health nurses may better utilise CBT within their everyday practice. First, we will begin with an overview of its key features, evidence base, methods and therapeutic skills for CBT.

6.2 What is Cognitive Behavioural Therapy (CBT)?

Cognitive behavioural therapy (CBT) is a psychological (cognitive) and behavioural approach to change based on scientific principles and interventions that empirical research has proven to be effective for a multitude of clinical conditions and presenting problems (Roth and Fonaghy 1996). CBT has two key influences, behaviour therapy as developed

J. Swan
Division of Neurosciences and Medical Education Institute,
College of Medicine, Dentistry and Nursing, University of Dundee,
Dundee, UK

G. Sloan (✉)
Consultant Nurse in Psychological Therapies, Psychological Services,
NHS Ayrshire and Arran, Ayr, Scotland, UK

Psychological Therapies Training Coordinator, NHS Education for Scotland,
NHS Ayrshire and Arran, Ayr, Scotland, UK
e-mail: graham.Sloan@aapct.scot.nhs.uk

© Springer International Publishing Switzerland 2018

J.C. Santos, J.R. Cutcliffe (eds.), *European Psychiatric/Mental Health Nursing in the 21st Century*, Principles of Specialty Nursing,
https://doi.org/10.1007/978-3-319-31772-4_6

by Wolpe and others in the 1950s and 1960s and cognitive therapy, founded by Aaron Beck in the late 1950s, early 1960s. Beck proposed a model of therapy which focused on conscious mental processes. Prior to these developments, there had been an emphasis on 'unconscious' processes. Beck, while recognising that unconscious processes do exist, created a model that aimed at facilitating clients to become more aware of their conscious experience of meaning-making. Beck's model is based on the rationale that an individual's emotions and behaviour are largely determined by the way in which they interpret the world (Westbrook et al. 2007). The model focuses on the role and content of cognitions in emotional disorders. Thus, the '**C**' of CBT represents 'cognition' and refers to how people think and create meaning about situations, symptoms and things that happen in their lives, and how they develop beliefs about themselves, others and the world.

> 'Men are disturbed not by things, but by the view which they take of them.'

The cognitive component uses techniques to help people become more aware of how they reason and the kinds of thinking that contribute to the meaning they attach to events, people and relationships. There are three levels of cognition: automatic thoughts, underlying assumptions and schema (core beliefs). Automatic thoughts and images are the specific moment-to-moment experiences that pass through our minds; they are situation specific. For example, 'this chapter will be rejected by the editors'. Underlying assumptions or intermediate beliefs are cross-situational and can be thought of as rules or principles of living. These can usually be expressed in a conditional 'if…then…' format. For example, 'if this chapter is rejected, then I will never get over it'. Underlying assumptions can also be expressed as should or must statements—'everything I do should be perfect', 'I must agree to all requests received'. Core beliefs are global and absolutistic beliefs which are developed as a result of life experiences and are thought to be influenced by our relationships with significant others. These can be expressed in the form of 'CBT is the best therapy', 'men are lazy', 'I am useless' and 'the world is dangerous'.

In CBT, it is important to gain some understanding of the influence of an individual's experiences on his or her belief system. Beliefs and schema are thought to be formed as a result of experiences and exposure to events, people or relationships. CBT emphasises the importance of critical incidents which, when congruent with the content of existing beliefs, can serve to trigger them. These, in turn result in information being processed in a particular biased manner. The anxious person, for example, who understands themselves to be vulnerable, and anxiety to be overbearing, will see themselves as weak and unable to cope and events as threatening, too risky or indeed life threatening (Table 6.1).

In his cognitive model of depression, Beck proposed the presence of a negative cognitive triad, composed of negative views about self, world (others) and the future (Beck et al. 1979): *I can't do anything right, people expect so much from me, things will never change, and I'll never be able to write interesting material.* A number of processing errors or thinking distortions have been identified, which include all-or-nothing thinking, overgeneralisation, discounting the positive and jumping to conclusions. Importantly, we are all susceptible to such processing errors, but it is the pervasive negative bias that distinguishes depressed individuals from nondepressed individuals. See Table 6.2 for some examples.

Table 6.1 Three levels of cognition

Automatic thoughts
'The editors won't find this chapter interesting'
Underlying assumptions
'We should be able to write really interesting material'
Core schema
'We're useless'

Table 6.2 Thinking errors (Willson and Branch 2006)

All or nothing—student who gets 98% for exam—'I didn't do well enough, I'm useless'
Overgeneralisation—a single event is perceived as a never-ending pattern of defeat—student fails one exam—'I never do well in exams or assignments'; 'nothing ever goes right'
Discounting the positive—rejecting positive experiences by insisting they don't count. Getting 98% in a recent assignment is deemed a 'fluke', 'easy marker' or 'examiner error'
Jumping to conclusions—the student who fails an exam might think 'that's it now, I'll get kicked off the course' or 'the tutors will think so badly of me'

The **B** of CBT stands for a behavioural approach and is derived from two basic ideas. First, we generally do things to keep us safe, avoid bad things or to earn reward/reinforcement. Second, we need to feel safe enough in order to gradually change unhelpful behaviours. So with a combination of the previous cognitions and behavioural principles, the depressed person will try and keep themselves safe. They will avoid those situations, people and relations which trigger feelings they find difficult to tolerate. So with behavioural activation (Martell et al. 2010), it is important to establish interests, activities particular to the person we are working with, be guided by their pace of working and support the person towards achieving their goals.

6.3 Empirical Foundations of CBT

Cognitive therapy for depression came along in the late 1970s early 1980s with the publication of Beck's seminal text. Following on from its use with people experiencing depression (Beck et al. 1979), CBT has become more widespread and has been subjected to both outcome (see, e.g. Schreiber et al. 2015) and process-focused research (see, e.g. Price et al. 2016). Findings from empirical research inform that it is a valuable and effective therapy for a broad range of psychological difficulties (Roth and Fonaghy 1996). According to the evidence-based clinical practice guideline (DoH 2001), and the more recent Matrix (NHS Education for Scotland 2014), CBT has a strong evidence base in helping people with:

- Depressive disorders
- Panic disorder and/or agoraphobia
- Social phobia
- Simple phobia
- Generalised anxiety disorder
- Health anxiety

- Post-traumatic stress disorder
- Obsessive-compulsive disorder
- Eating disorders (bulimia)

CBT is acknowledged as being an effective psychological treatment for people with psychosis (SIGN 1998; NICE 2009). It is also a useful therapy for assisting with the psychological issues associated with physical health conditions such as irritable bowel syndrome, chronic fatigue syndrome, chronic pain, cancer and diabetes (White 2001; SIGN 2010).

6.4 CBT: Key Methods

CBT is a focused, structured, educational and usually time-limited psychological therapy which has as a key aim, reducing the distress experienced by the person you are assisting. Another important therapy aim is teaching the person skills which they will be able to put into practice to help assist them in the future.
The key methods of CBT which are applied to achieve these aims include:

- The therapeutic relationship
- Assessment strategies
- Case conceptualisation
- Structure
- Cognitive techniques
- Behavioural interventions

6.5 Therapeutic Relationships

Box 6.1 The therapeutic relationship—reflective space
What do we mean by the therapeutic relationship?
How collaborative is your style/approach with clients?
What are the benefits?
What are the difficulties in working collaboratively with your client?

Emphasised the importance of a collaborative therapy relationship in which clients are able to progress and work towards their recovery through exploration of empirically generated evidence rather than therapist persuasion or coercion. This is consistent with attachment theory (Bowlby 1969) and self-efficacy. Bowlby (1969) argued that an effective therapy relationship can provide a secure base from which a client is able to explore. In this respect the relationship is helpful because it provides a safe, sheltered space in which clients can take a deep breath, consider their problems in context, engage in an explorative, guided discovery with another person, gain perspective, make mistakes, re-experience old wounds and problematic issues in a safe and secure environment, recover the strength to re-confront life and try new behaviours. In all, the relationship provides a supportive structure (Sloan 1999) within which clients' generative, self-healing capacities can optimally operate.

6.6 Assessment Strategies

In CBT, the assessment approach sometimes referred to as functional analysis is concerned with reaching an understanding of the client's thinking, feeling and behaviours that contribute to the difficulties they experience. Essentially, functional analysis is the foundation of assessment practice within CBT and includes the key areas depicted in Table 6.3.

To assist in this process, a variety of methods can be incorporated and include clinical interview, case history, information from others, questionnaires and rating scales, diaries and on occasion role play.

6.7 Case Formulation

In CBT the case formulation is a hypothesis about the client's areas of difficulty. The case formulation pulls together the information from the assessment of the client's difficulties and relates this to the cognitive model and theoretical literature relevant to these. There are a range of templates for case formulation, Fig. 6.1 is only one example. The case formulation is shared and collaboratively negotiated with the client as it instils a clear rationale for treatment.

Table 6.3 Key areas of assessment

1. Five Ws
What are the main problems?
Where does the problem occur?
When does it occur?
Why (feared consequence or belief)?
With whom?
2. FIND
Frequency, intensity, number and duration
3. ABC analyses
Antecedents, behaviour, consequences
4. Development of the problem
5. Goals and expectations of therapy
6. Medication and substance use
7. Assets and strengths
8. Impact of problems on client's life
9. Mental health status
10. Medical history
11. Ethico-legal
12. Personal history
13. Family history
14. Developmental history

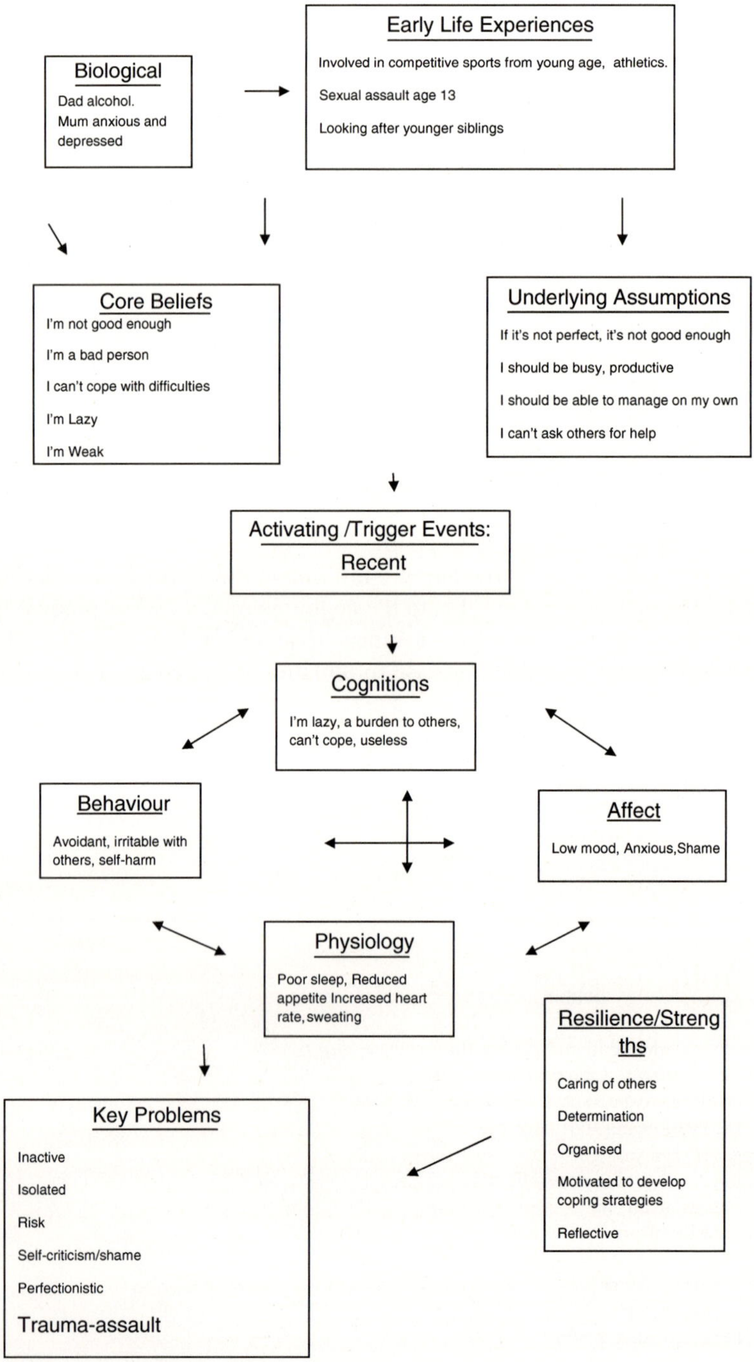

Fig. 6.1 Example of case formulation

Table 6.4 Structure of therapy session

Checking in and review patient's emotional state
Set the agenda: feedback from last session, reviewing homework, current issues for session
Agreeing homework
Summarising session (patient and therapist)
Elicit feedback, both positive and negative feedback, about session

6.8 CBT: Structure of Therapy

A typical course of treatment of CBT might consist of somewhere between 12 and 20 sessions (Simmons and Griffiths 2009). In more complex cases this may be extended. Ideally, sessions will take place usually weekly or fortnightly providing adequate time for practice, experimentation, reflection and maintaining momentum. Individual sessions normally last somewhere between 45 and 60 min. The initial sessions (1–4) focus on engagement, assessment, socialisation to CBT format and case formulation. During the next stage (sessions 5–16), the emphasis is on interventions that will assist with the problem areas identified from the formulation. Throughout the course of treatment, there will be regular reviews, where time will be taken to repeat psychometric measures comparing these with baseline measures, elicit subjective feedback from the client on changes and progress with their personal goals. Towards the end of treatment, sessions can be less frequent and focus on relapse prevention leading onto 'booster sessions' and follow-up appointments (sessions 17–20) (Table 6.4).

At the commencement of every therapy session, the therapist will elicit the client's current emotional state and how they've been managing between sessions which can be prompted by asking: 'How have things been since the last session?' If there is a sense of importance to what is being shared, the therapist can enquire: 'It sounds like this is really important for you, is this something we should make time for and discuss more fully today?'

Agenda setting must be collaborative and the items must have meaning for the client. The client is encouraged to contribute items so that the agenda is client-driven—it is their therapy. Therapist can ask: 'what's your best hope for today's session?' or 'how will you know that today's session has been worthwhile?' Once agenda items have been agreed, the order and priority can be negotiated.

Throughout the session, frequent summaries of key learning points are made. Towards the end of the session, a summary sought from the client can be helpful. This facilitates insight into the level of understanding and any areas where uncertainty and confusion remain. During CBT, we also encourage our clients to keep notes or on occasion audio record the therapy sessions and maintain a therapy folder.

Box 6.2 Agenda setting—reflective space

How often would you set an agenda with your client?
When you do, does it help or hinder?
What sort of feedback do you receive from your clients?
Does this feedback help or hinder the therapeutic alliance?

6.9 Feedback

The therapist elicits the client's feedback to determine their understanding of and response to the session. Sessions may provoke distressing cognitions and related emotions and also trigger unpleasant memories or traumatic images which may not otherwise be revealed. Consequently, failing to elicit such feedback may leave the client with misunderstandings, negative interpretations or additional distress. At the beginning of each session the therapist should elicit feedback concerning the previous therapy session: 'Since we met have you had any thoughts about the last session?' And towards the end of the current therapy session, the therapist can ask specifically for any negative reactions to therapist, content and formulation, check whether anything you said or did has upset the patient, ask if anything was not clear, ask what was helpful or unhelpful, enquire how the patient is feeling and invite other questions or comments.

It is essential that the therapist responds to this feedback in an open, non-judgemental and nondefensive manner. The therapist can view such feedback as a gift that will help to develop the therapeutic relationship and influence positive change for the client.

6.10 CBT: The Place of Homework

Box 6.3 Homework—reflective space

What experience do you have in using homework when working with clients?

How do they respond?

How do you manage any resistance to homework?

How does homework contribute to recovery?

Homework assignments create a link between sessions ensuring that the client continues to work on problems in the hundreds of hours between therapy sessions (Kazantis et al. 2005). Such homework tasks enable the collection of data to add to exploration of a topic, the testing out of predictions (Bennett-Levy et al. 2004), experimenting with new behaviours and cognitions, place significance and emphasise on the client's active involvement in the change process and encourage self-monitoring, self-evaluation and self-reinforcement.

Again this process must be a collaborative enterprise, both client and therapist collaboratively identifying, negotiating and clarifying an assigned task relevant to the session targets. It is essential that the therapist elicits the client's understanding of the rationale for all homework agreed and ensuring that the client understands its parameters. Homework should be specific with details clearly explained and written down where appropriate and as necessary. When negotiating a homework task, it is important to elicit any anticipated difficulties, doubts and predictions of outcome. And during the subsequent therapy session, any outcome of the homework, progress, difficulties and conclusions requires discussion, reflection and if required adjustment.

Table 6.5 Cognitive methods

Identifying, evaluating and modifying negative automatic thoughts
Identifying, evaluating and modifying underlying assumptions or rules for living
Identifying, evaluating and modifying core beliefs
Evaluating worries
Information and logical errors
Putting things in perspective
Schema-focused therapy
Examining and challenging cognitive distortions
Challenging self-critical thoughts

Table 6.6 Lists various behavioural methods

Exposure-based treatment strategies
Reinforcement
Modelling and role play
Activity scheduling
Behavioural experiments
Relaxation

6.11 CBT: Cognitive and Behavioural Models

As explained previously, cognitions can be understood to exist at three levels, automatic thoughts, underlying assumptions and core beliefs. Consequently, a range of methods that aim to target each of these levels is required. Tables 6.5 and 6.6 list some of these methods.

6.12 Competent CBT

The practice of all psychological therapies calls for both art and science. The practice of CBT is no different. The practice of CBT has its roots in the scientific tradition, and the 'success' and popularity of CBT owe much to the fact that the therapy has been subjected to thousands of research trials which have demonstrated patient acceptability, good levels of effectiveness and efficacy. Thanks to this scientific endeavour, the CBT community of practitioners feels it has a handle on 'what works for whom' (Roth and Fonaghy 1996), and there is a fair degree of confidence that CBT has a wide utility. However, it is important to inject a note of caution to balance the all-encompassing positive reputation that CBT has accrued. The note of caution is this: there are limits to the effectiveness of all psychotherapies, and in our training programme, we share with our students the secret of being a good therapist or mental health worker (MHW).

The secret of being a good therapist is having the 'right' patient working with you. The Safran and Segal suitability criteria attempt to go some way towards ensuring client engagement. Another 'secret' we share is that when you put the unique individual human dimension into the theory around psychopathology and the

Table 6.7 Safran and Segal suitability criteria

1. Accessibility of automatic thoughts
2. Awareness and differentiation of emotions
3. Acceptance of personal responsibility for change
4. Compatibility with cognitive rationale
5. Alliance potential in-session
6. Alliance potential out-of-session
7. Chronicity of problems
8. Security operations
9. Focality
10. General optimism about therapy

competent practice of CBT, you come hard up against the limitations of an empirical or scientific approach to therapy (Table 6.7).

Individuals rarely come to mental health services or psychological therapy services with one clinical disorder or one discrete problem of living as a consequence of being unwell. Individuals rarely present in the manner that the textbooks say they might. Most commonly people present with complex mixes of clinical disorder; most people who are depressed also present with features of anxiety disorders and vice versa. A significant proportion of people who present to mental health services have experienced the presenting problems of living over reasonably long to very long periods of time. This element of chronicity is predictive of reduced benefits from psychological input. Other factors which influence outcome and vary from patient to patient no matter which disorder they present with are motivation and readiness for change, the nature of their interpersonal networks and the socio-economic circumstances they find themselves in.

In the face of these (and other) challenges to working effectively with people, it is hard to maintain adherence to evidence-based practice, and all MHWs can fall victim to 'creative eclecticism' (trying any old thing in desperation) or what has been termed more kindly as 'therapist drift' (Waller 2009; Waller et al. 2012).

One route to reconciling the tension between the need for science and the need for 'artful' approaches to helping people change is to be found in the development of CBT training programmes using an evidence-based approach to defining a framework of which elements of CBT practice and theory are most effective in given clinical presentations. This framework places significant importance on the art of applying these treatment approaches to individuals but defines, as far as possible, these nebulous artful skills into a set of operationalised and measurable competences. Those dimensions which are the science and art of being a competent and effective MH practitioner are put on the same footing, and it is clear that it is the blending of core competences (the science bit) and metacompetences (the art bit) which needs to be addressed in training, development and supervision.

As trainers, clinicians and supervisors in CBT, we welcome the recent introduction of a competence framework for CBT (Roth and Pilling 2007, 2008). Roth and Pilling, with expert input from the CBT community, set out a framework which identified five specific aspects of competence which trainers, practitioners and supervisors should seek to blend to enhance outcomes for patients:

1. *Generic therapeutic competences*: These are competences foundational to the delivery of any psychological therapy or package of care and include the ability to engage and assess patients, knowledge of mental health theory and practice, developing and maintaining working alliances and clinical supervision.
2. *Foundational or basic CBT competences*: A set of knowledge and skill which includes awareness and skill of core CBT principles, working collaboratively, forming and sharing formulations which use the cognitive behavioural model of the maintenance cycle of problems of living.
3. *Specific CBT techniques*: A range of core behavioural and cognitive interventions which have been demonstrated to have clinical utility. These include the use of thought records, the use of behavioural experiments, behavioural activation of pleasant event scheduling and the use of exposure therapies
4. *Problem-specific competences and techniques*: CBT practitioners have an advantage when it comes to treating specific disorders such as panic disorder or acute depression. There is a lot of guidance in the literature and specific treatment plans for these and other disorders. See Clark et al. for panic disorder and/or Lewinsohn et al. or Jacobson et al. for depression for examples (Lewinsohn 1974; Lewinsohn et al. 1984, 1985; Clark 1986; Martell et al. 2001).
5. *Metacompetences*: Defined as '…focus on the ability to implement models in a manner that is flexible and tailored to the need of the individual…' (Roth and Pilling 2007, p. 9). There are generic and CBT-specific metacompetences.

Generic competences will be familiar to all. Practitioners should aim to build the capacity to use clinical judgement when implementing treatment interventions and develop the capacity to adapt or amend the treatment in response to patient feedback. CBT-specific competences include a capacity to implement CBT treatment in a manner consistent with the theoretical and philosophical tenets of CBT, the capacity to develop and apply case formulations and to select and skilfully apply the most appropriate interventions to match the needs of the patient and, finally, the ability to pace and structure sessions while overcoming obstacles to the application of CBT in individual cases. See Fig. 6.2 for an overview.

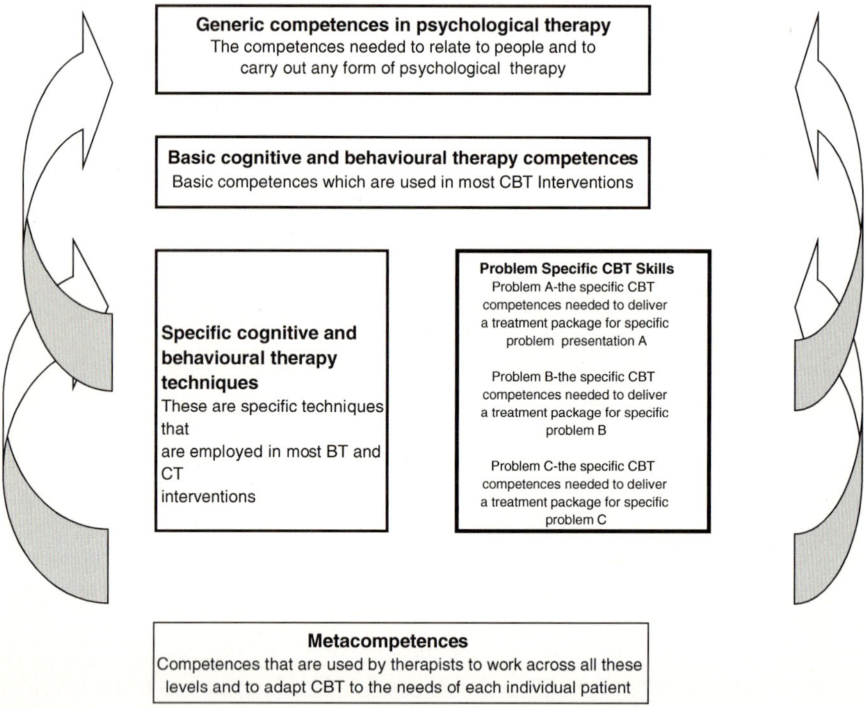

Fig. 6.2 Outline model for CBT competences

6.13 Developing Competence in CBT

To develop these five sets of competences is not an easy task. It takes specific training and guidance. In our training programme, we invite mental health practitioners to come study with us for 2 years. The University of Dundee postgraduate training programme in CBT is consciously structured around the Roth and Pilling framework and coterminous with the British Association of Behavioural and Cognitive Psychotherapies (BABCP) minimum training standards. Throughout the 2 years of training, we aim to provide academic and clinical experiences which foster the development and deepening of these overarching competences and metacompetences. In Year 1 of our programme, we specifically target the development of the generic and core CBT skills. In Year 2 we develop those disorder-specific competences outlined above and in the overview model. This is done in the context of a 1-day training a week integrated with clinical work undertaken back at the trainees' everyday clinical setting. These 'training cases' must be undertaken in the context of clinical supervision with a BABCP-accredited therapist. Supplementary clinical supervision, designed to enhance learning in the five domains of competences, is undertaken with the teaching team here in Dundee as part of the training programme. In our programme we specifically break competences down into their component parts and use actors to provide trainees with an opportunity to develop the capacities outlined above in a more controlled manner than real clinical encounters would allow. Our trainees are encouraged to listen to recordings of their own sessions and to use recognised therapy rating scales to measure the degree to which they are developing these important competences. If after reading this chapter you feel you want to specifically train as a CBT practitioner, use the link *babcp.com* and look for an accredited formal training programme such as ours on the BABCP website. There you will find training programmes which adhere to the development of the capacities discussed in the above section.

6.14 The Central Importance of Clinical Supervision

Clinical supervision is an essential foundation to the provision of optimum psychological therapies (NHS Education for Scotland 2014). Throughout this chapter, the significant role of clinical supervision, in the delivery of effective CBT, has been emphasised. The following definition, from Roth and Pilling's (2008, p. 3) supervision competency framework, helps to clarify its fundamental intention:

> 'This framework conceives supervision as a formal but collaborative relationship which takes place in an organizational context, which is part of the overall training of practitioners and which is guided by some form of contract between a supervisor and a supervisee. The expectation is that the supervisee offers an honest and open account of their work and that the supervisor offers feedback and guidance which has the primary aim of facilitating the development of the supervisee's therapeutic competencies but also ensures that they practice in a manner which conforms to current ethical and professional standards.'

Clinical supervision of CBT is guided by an educational and developmental framework which parallels the therapeutic model. It aims to support and enable the supervisee to increase their therapeutic competence using foci and specific modes of delivery (Sloan et al. 2000).

6.15 P/MH Nurses Using CBT Skills and Techniques in the Mental Health Setting

Numerous authors with a mental health specialism have highlighted continuums of helping (see Davidson et al. 2006). Invariably these differentiate between the different forms of 'helping' (e.g. from professional, sessional psychotherapy sessions) to friendships (i.e. where non-professional help can be offered). The continuum of helping can also be applied to CBT in that CBT can and does occur in formal, sessional, psychotherapy sessions, and yet it can also be used in 'everyday' clinical encounters with mental health clients. Thus, P/MH nurses can:

(a) Use CBT skills and techniques
(b) Work in a counselling way with a CBT theoretical underpinning
(c) Work with a client on specific issues which the evidence shows appear to respond well to CBT—such as addressing phobias, spirals of anxiety and panic

And other P/MH nurses use CBT as they operate as nurse therapists and/or counsellors, nurse practitioners and/or independent practitioners. Furthermore, there is a body of evidence which speaks to the utilisation of CBT skills and techniques by P/MH nurses in various mental health inpatient and community settings (e.g. Brooker et al. 1994; Chan and Leung 2002; Collins and Cutcliffe 2003; Chadwick et al. 2005; Turkington et al. 2006; Clarke and Wilson 2009). P/MH nursing curricula in the Occidental world invariably include material and experience of CBT skills, theory and techniques. And mental health service users overwhelmingly state their desire for more 'talk therapy' (Cutcliffe et al. 2015 raiders…) (not only CBT should be noted). Accordingly, while P/MH nurses might not necessarily use all the skills, techniques and interventions captured in this chapter, there is a broad consensus in the relevant theoretical, clinical, empirical and policy literature that P/MH nurses in various settings can and should consider the more widespread use of CBT skills—even though the authors acknowledge that this is not without challenges and the need for some adaptation.

References

Beck AT, Rush AJ, Shaw BF, Emery G (1979) Cognitive therapy of depression. The Guilford, London

Bennett-Levy J, Butler G, Fennell M, Hackman A, Mueller M, Westbrook D (2004) Oxford guide to behavioural experiments in cognitive therapy. Oxford University Press, Oxford

Bowlby J (1969) Attachment and loss, vol 1 Attachment. Hogarth, London

Brooker C, Falloon I, Butterworth A, Goldberg D, Graham-Hole V, Hillier V (1994) The outcome of training community psychiatric nurses to deliver psychosocial intervention. Br J Psychiatry 165:222–230

Chadwick PDJ, Newman-Taylor K, Abba N (2005) Mindfulness groups for people with distressing psychosis. Behav Cogn Psychother 33(3):351–359

Chan S, Leung J (2002) Cognitive behavioural therapy for clients with schizophrenia: implications for mental health nursing practice. J Clin Nurs 11:214–224

Clark DM (1986) A cognitive approach to panic. Behav Res Ther 24:461–470

Clarke I, Wilson H (2009) Cognitive behaviour therapy for acute inpatient mental health units: working with clients, staff and the milieu. Routledge, London

Collins S, Cutcliffe JR (2003) Addressing hopelessness in people with depression and suicidal ideation: building upon the therapeutic relationship utilising a cognitive behavioural approach. J Psychiatr Ment Health Nurs 10(2):175–186

Cutcliffe JR, Santos JC, Kozel B, Taylor P, Lees D (2015) Raiders of the lost art: have psychiatric/mental health nurses lost, forgotten or abandoned the therapeutic use of self? The case of acute psychiatric settings in the United Kingdom, Portugal, Canada, Switzerland, Germany and Australia. Int J Ment Health Nurs 24:375–385

Davidson L et al (2006) A continuum of helping relationships. Schizophr Bull 32:443–450

Department of Health (2001) Psychological therapies and counselling evidence-based clinical practice guideline. DoH, London

Lewinsohn PM (1974) A behavioural approach to depression. In: Friedman RJ, Katz MM (eds) The psychology of depression: contemporary theory and research. Wiley, New York, NY, pp 157–185

Lewinsohn PM, Antonuccio DO, Breckenridge JS, Teri L (1984) The coping with depression course. Castalia Publishing Company, Eugene, OR

Lewinsohn PM, Hoberman H, Teri L, Hautzinger M (1985) An integrative theory of depression. In: Reiss S, Bootzin RR (eds) Theoretical issues in behavior therapy. Academic, New York, NY, pp 331–359
Martell CR, Addis ME, Jacobson NS (2001) Depression in context: strategies for guided action. Norton, New York, NY
Martell CR, Dimidjian S, Herman-Dunn R (2010) Behavioural activation for depression: a clinician's guide. The Guilford, London
Kazantis N, Deane FP, Ronan KR, L'Abate L (2005) Using homework assignments in cognitive behaviour therapy. Routledge, London
National Health Service Education for Scotland (2014) The matrix 2014: a guide to delivering evidence-based psychological therapies in Scotland. NHS Education for Scotland, Edinburgh
National Institute for Clinical Excellence (2009) Schizophrenia update. Clinical guideline 82. NICE, London
Price J, MacDonald H, Adair KC, Koerner N, Monson CM (2016) Changing beliefs about trauma: a qualitative study of cognitive processing therapy. Behav Cogn Psychother 44(2):156–167
Roth A, Fonaghy P (1996) What works for whom? A critical review of psychotherapy research. The Guilford, New York, NY
Roth AD, Pilling S (2007) The competences required to deliver effective cognitive behavioural therapy for people with depression and anxiety disorders. Improving Access to Psychological Therapies (IAPT) Programme
Roth AD, Pilling S (2008) Using an evidence-based methodology to identify the competences required to deliver effective cognitive and behavioural therapy for depression and anxiety disorders. Behav Cogn Psychother 36:129–147
Schreiber F, Heimlich C, Schweitzer C, Stangier U (2015) Cognitive therapy for social anxiety disorder: the impact of the self-focused attention and safety behaviours experiment on the course of treatment. Behav Cogn Psychother 43(2):158–166
Scottish Intercollegiate Guideline Network (1998) Psychosocial interventions in the management of schizophrenia. No. 30. SIGN, Edinburgh
Scottish Intercollegiate Guideline Network (2010) Management of diabetes. No. 116. SIGN, Edinburgh
Simmons J, Griffiths R (2009) CBT for beginners. Sage, London
Sloan G (1999) The therapeutic relationship in cognitive-behaviour therapy. Br J Commun Nurs 4(2):58–64
Sloan G, White C, Coit F (2000) Cognitive therapy supervision as a framework for clinical supervision in nursing: using structure to guide discovery. J Adv Nurs 32(3):515–524
Turkington D, Kingdon D, Rathod S, Hammond K, Pelton J, Mehta R (2006) Outcomes of an effectiveness trial of cognitive-behavioural intervention by mental health nurses in schizophrenia. Br J Psychiatry 189(1):36–40
Waller G (2009) Evidence-based treatment and therapist drift. Behav Res Ther 47(2):119–127
Waller G, Stringer H, Meyer C (2012) What cognitive behavioral techniques do therapists report using when delivering cognitive behavioral therapy for the eating disorders? J Consult Clin Psychol 80(1):171–175
Westbrook D, Kennerley H, Kirk J (2007) An introduction to cognitive behaviour therapy: skills and applications. Sage, London
White C (2001) Cognitive behaviour therapy for chronic medical problems: a guide to assessment and treatment in practice. Wiley, London
Willson R, Branch R (2006) Cognitive behavioural therapy for dummies. Wiley, London

7 Psychodynamic and Psychoanalytical Theory, Approaches and Clinical Relevance: Applying the Psychoanalytic Principles and Practices to Mental Health Nursing

J. Lopes and John R. Cutcliffe

7.1 Introduction

Spurred by the original contribution of Peplau, who in turn was inspired by Harry 'Stack' Sullivan's work, the notion of interpersonal, psychoanalytical[1]-based psychiatric/mental health (P/MH) nursing has both a relatively long history[2] and contemporary currency. This history notwithstanding examination of the current relevant literature and patterns of P/MH nursing practice in Europe and the rest of the world indicates that psychoanalytical P/MH nursing has 'fallen out of favour', in much the same way that psychoanalytical psychotherapy has passed its zenith. However, psychoanalysis in the twenty-first century now, due mainly to the advances in our understanding of neuroscience over the last 20 years, has an increasing body of work that validates and/or lends credi-

[1] According to the British Psychoanalytic Council (2017), the terms 'psychoanalytic' and 'psychodynamic' are both used to describe psychotherapy based on psychoanalytic principles; as a result, the authors of this chapter use the terms interchangeably. However, we acknowledge that there are other authors who write about differences between psychoanalytical and psychodynamic.

[2] Seminal work in this area started to appear in the 1940s and 1950s.

J. Lopes, Ph.d. (✉)
RN Mental Health Specialist, Psychoanalitic Psychotherapist, School of Health Care, Polithecnical Institute of Setúbal, Setúbal, Portugal
e-mail: joaquimlopes.pessoal@gmail.com

J.R.Cutcliffe
Cutcliffe Consulting, Kingston, Canada

School of Nursing, Coimbra, Portugal
e-mail: jcutcliffe@outlook.com

© Springer International Publishing Switzerland 2018

J.C. Santos, J.R. Cutcliffe (eds.), *European Psychiatric/Mental Health Nursing in the 21st Century*, Principles of Specialty Nursing,
https://doi.org/10.1007/978-3-319-31772-4_7

bility to several traditional psychoanalytic concepts (Solms and Turnbull 2002). With its origins firmly located in mental health/psychological thinking, aspects of psychoanalytical principles can now be detected in some higher education programmes, in analysis of institutional function, in understanding and helping family and group processes/dynamics and in other related domains such as anthropology. Within the domain of mental health care, it is difficult to ignore the significant historical influence that psychoanalytic thinking, principles and practices have had. And concomitantly, in P/MH nursing, this influence is clearly evident in the work of Hildegard Peplau. Peplau established in her book *Interpersonal Relations in Nursing* (1952) the first theoretical and practical bridge between psychoanalysis and nursing under what later came to be known as the school of interpersonal psychoanalysis.

7.2 Core Principles of Psychoanalysis as a Theory and Helping Method

It is well documented that psychoanalytical thinking and counselling can be traced to Sigmund Freud. Freud's thinking and beliefs, after finding no physical cause of 'illness' in some of his patients (at least in part), were that the origin of these 'illnesses' lays in person's own unconscious mind. For Freud (Freud and Breuer 1895; Freud 1915), psychodynamic therapy is based on the idea that true knowledge of people and their problems is possible through an understanding of particular areas of the human mind; these areas are the conscious, the subconscious and the unconscious. These aspects/functions of the mind refer to and include:

- *The conscious*: things that people are aware (or conscious) of—e.g. feelings/emotions, issues or experiences that the person finds anxiety provoking.
- *The subconscious*: elements or phenomena that are currently not at the forefront of our consciousness—or not 'in' a person's current conscious awareness; however, they exist 'just outside of' the person's consciousness, and they are therefore fairly easily accessible.
- *The unconscious*: elements and phenomena that the person is not aware of. The unconscious contains both significant and uncomfortable (or even disturbing) thoughts, memories, etc. It also includes material/memories, wishes and impulses that are too frightening, painful and/or traumatic to the person, that they are 'stored' and, in so doing, mediated or 'kept at bay' by the person's subconscious (hence the process of repression, Bargh 2006). There are at least two other central and critical elements of Freud's view of the unconscious part of a person's mind that must be acknowledged: first is the (for some) uncomfortable truth that the unconscious mind (and the material 'stored' there) actually influences (if not governs or controls) a person's behaviour to a much greater extent than people would expect or know and, second, people 'develop' a range of 'defence mechanisms' (Bargh 2006; Bargh and Morsella 2008; McLeod 2017), for example, repression, projection, rationalization and denial, as a means to avoid having to face or acknowledge these uncomfortable and/or painful feelings, memories, etc. (Bargh 2006; Bargh and Morsella 2008).

For Freud then, psychoanalysis involves a theory of mental functioning and, in particular, of the relationship between people. Psychoanalytic therapy has therefore an objective of transforming this interpersonal relationship, when 'pathological', into a healthier one. The reviewing and revival of emotions related to early-life experiences, being afforded the possibility to think and name the unthinkable (i.e. these repressed feelings, uncomfortable truths held in one's unconscious) and developing the awareness of one's limiting (some might say pathological) patterns developed over time give clients the opportunity to change towards a more satisfactory life. This change is fundamentally based on two main procedures:

(a) The examination, analysis and reconstruction of the past
(b) The development of a new relationship that allows clients to resume the suspended personal development (Coímbra de Matos 2002)

Core principles or rudiments of psychoanalytic perspectives, which appear in the associated literature though not in a consistent or uniformed manner, include (see, e.g. Freud and Breuer 1895; Freud 1915; Bargh 2006; Bargh and Morsella 2008; Safran and Kriss 2014; British Psychoanalytic Council 2017; McLeod 2017; Cramer 2000, 2006, 2015):

- A person's behaviour and feelings are affected, considerably and powerfully, by unconscious motives.
- A person's behaviour and feelings as adults, including especially his/her psychological problems, are rooted in his/her childhood experiences.
- All behaviour has a cause (usually unconscious), even slips of the tongue. Hence, there are no such things as accidents as all behaviour is determined—even though the individual will (often) be unaware of these unconscious determinants.
- A person's individual personality is shaped and modified by different conflicts at different times in childhood, particularly during what Freud referred to as 'psychosexual development'. According to Freud, this process of development has a number of stages—see Table 7.2.
- A person's personality is constituted of three parts: *Id, Ego and Superego.*
- For Freud, this *Id* is the part of our personality that is concerned with urging the organism to satisfy instinctual, basic needs of food, comfort and pleasure.
- For Freud, the *Ego* refers to the logical and common-sense side to our personality.
- For Freud, the *Superego* acts as a 'social conscience'; it moderates, inhibits and controls the basic instincts or drives associated with the *Id*, particularly if/when these drives result in behaviour or actions that are deemed to be socially unacceptable.
- For Freud, everybody will experience tension, conflict and anxiety that result from the competing 'drives' or forces associated with *Id, Ego and Superego*. The drive for sexual pleasure is moderated and restrained by the sense of what is considered to be socially acceptable.[3]
- All human actions are partially driven by material that exists outside of the individual's awareness and/or consciousness.

[3] Other authors use the terms 'right or wrong', given that these are social constructs, culturally.

- Facilitating awareness of unconscious motivations increases the person's awareness of and subsequent capacity to choose and change.
- Change is often hard and raises ambivalent feelings—that's why people tend to avoid painful or threatening feelings, fantasies, experiences, situations and thoughts.
- The therapeutic relationship is an important vehicle for change.
- The therapeutic relationship offers an understanding of the (possible) psychopathological origins and/or causes and development of one's mental health challenges in the 'here and now' (Sundberg et al. 2002).
- Mental health challenges and issues (or for some psychopathology) develop especially as a result of early childhood relational experiences.
- Intrapsychic and unconscious conflicts have a central role in the person's development and in their experiences of mental health problems.
- Unconscious 'life' issues will re-emerge in the context of the client-therapist relationship (transference and countertransference).
- Psychic defences can be used in order to avoid unpleasant consequences of conflict[4] (see Tables 7.1 and 7.2).

[4]Defences are viewed as intrapsychic processes that tend to avoid emotional pain related to

Table 7.1 Common psychoanalytical defence mechanisms

1. Denial	The refusal to accept reality or fact. The person behaves as though their painful experiences, thoughts or feelings did not happen and do not exist
	Commonly used to avoid dealing with painful feelings or areas of their life they don't wish to admit
2. Regression	The return to an earlier stage of development and exhibition of the behaviours associated with that earlier stage, when faced with unacceptable/uncomfortable thoughts or experiences
3. Dissociation	Often (though not unanimously) characterized as the person's defence against trauma. Ranging from 'mild' to more severe detachment, dissociative defence mechanisms are defined by a detachment from 'reality'
	Contemporaneously associated with the Trauma-Informed Care approach (see chapter 9 in this book), people may engage in disassociation from the trauma experienced during childhood
	This can and does then result in 'disassociated' people use often having a disconnected view of themselves in their world
4. Projection	Refers to the inaccurate attribution or 'recognition' of unacceptable, uncomfortable or disagreeable thoughts, feelings or values onto another person—when the person does not have any of these phenomena
	For Freud, when a person has discomforting, embarrassing or disagreeable thoughts, feelings, values, etc., these are unconsciously 'projected' or attributed onto other people. The defence mechanism then serves to make the other person the problem. In so doing, the other person becomes the host or carrier of our own perceived limitations and flaws
	Projection is used especially when the thoughts are considered unacceptable for the person to express or they feel completely ill at ease with having them
	In so doing, a form of temporary relief can be experienced as this displacement makes it easier to live with ourselves because everyone is the problem—not ourselves

Table 7.1 (continued)

5. Repression	The unconscious blocking of unacceptable, disquieting or disagreeable thoughts, feelings and impulses
6. Displacement	Refers to the unconscious redirecting of one's thoughts, feelings, etc. that ought to be directed or targeted at one person but are then displaced and directed at another person
7. Intellectualization	Refers to how, when challenged or confronted with an awareness of our own actions, thoughts or feelings that we find uncomfortable, unacceptable and/or disagreeable and then we may engage in overzealous and overemphasized thinking. In so doing, the person can avoid acknowledging or dealing with emotions that the new awareness produces

Note: Several texts were accessed to populate this table. Thus, the information presented is an amalgam of material drawn from Freud (1938), McWilliams (2008) and Gabbard et al. (2012).

Table 7.2 Freud's stages of psychosexual development

Stage	Features and description	Age range
Oral stage	Freud argues that since an infant's major source of 'exploring' or interacting with the world is via his/her mouth, then rooting/sucking reflex is important	Birth/infancy to about 1 year/18 months
	The infant should develop a sense of trust, comfort and hope, through this oral stimulation if the infant's 'parents' satisfy his/her needs	
	The primary conflict is associated with the weaning process, and for 'healthy' development, the child needs to become less dependent upon caregivers	
Anal stage	The major conflict at this stage is toilet training, as Freud argues that the child has to learn to control his or her bodily needs	About 1 year/18 months old to 3 years old
	According to Freud, how toilet training occurs can have a profound influence on the child	
	Freud links experiences of positive praise/rewards for the 'parents' helps the child (and ultimately the adult) to feel capable and productive	
	On the other hand, Freud links experiences that are lacking in or devoid of support and encouragement that children need during this stage from his/her parents, with negative outcomes, i.e. too lenient an approach for Freud, can lead to messy, wasteful, or destructive personality	
	Too strict an approach, for Freud, can lead to strict, intransigent, stringent, rigid and obsessive personality	
Phallic stage	During this stage, children begin to discover the differences between males and females	About 3 years old to 6 years old
	Freud argues that boys can begin to view their fathers as a rival for the mother's affections (the Oedipus complex)	
	Eventually, the child begins to identify with the same-sex parent	

(continued)

Table 7.2 (continued)

Stage	Features and description	Age range
The latent phase (or period)	A person's *Id*-driven sex drive (or libido for some) is subjugated as the person's *Ego and Superego* develop. This results in a period of calm	From about 6 years old to puberty
	The latent period is a time of exploration in which the sexual energy is still present, but it is directed into other areas such as intellectual pursuits and social interactions	
	This stage is important in the development of social and communication skills and self-confidence	
The genital stage	The individual develops a strong sexual interest in potential sexual partners	From about puberty to death
	(While Freud focuses his theory on sexual attraction to the opposite gender, the authors have broadened this to include twenty-first century understanding around human sexuality)	
	This stage sees a shift in the person from being self-/individually focused to having a greater interest in and concern for others	
	If the other stages have been completed successfully, the individual should now be well balanced, warm and caring	
	The goal of this stage is to establish a balance between the various life areas	

Note: Several texts were accessed to populate this table. Thus, the information presented is an amalgam of material drawn from Freud (1938), McWilliams (2008) and Gabbard et al. (2012)

7.3 Psychiatric/Mental Health Nursing By the Light of Psychoanalysis

Phenomena in P/MH nursing are phenomena of the mind, considering their conscious and unconscious dimensions, and consequently they are non-visible. These phenomena are manifested and expressed in communication and behaviour and require therefore to be interpreted, both in terms of their individual meaning and professional significance. In the linkage between the clinical and theoretical development of psychoanalysis and P/MH nursing, many psychoanalytical concepts have been transplanted and 'applied' to nursing. For instance, such concepts have been applied:

- To the understanding of the intentionality of the therapeutic relationship and its rational for nursing care
- To the possibility of carrying out appropriate referrals of patients

---

thoughts, wishes, feelings or fantasies out of awareness (not conscious) (Safran and Kriss 2014). Research shows that as part of normal development, different defences relate to different developmental periods and that even gender differences can be found in defence use (Cramer 2015).

- To the guidance and supervision of other professionals who deal with particular patients
- To examining 'helpful' communication with the families of individual patients
- To understanding the interpsychic and relational needs of families as collective patients and provide proper collective care
- To the therapeutic adjustment of health unit's organization

7.4 Psychoanalytical Practice and the Psychiatric/Mental Health Nurse

Given the documented goals of psychonalytical counselling, it is necessary to explore if and how these can be operationalized in P/MH nursing practice. Certainly, for Peplau (1991), this was both possible and necessary. A key goal is to bring material and issues from the person's unconscious into his/her conscious (Peplau 1991). A further key goal in psychodynamic counselling is to help people understand and subsequently seek to manage or balance the elements of their personality so that neither the 'id' nor the 'superego' is dominant (Waude 2017). Invariably, attempts to achieve these goals are likely to involve some encouragement of the client to examine his/her childhood or early memory trauma to gain a deeper insight and understanding (Blatt and Levy 2003; McWilliams 2009). This in turn may help the client to release negativities that they still hold, associated with earlier events. Psychoanalysis is based upon the assumption that only by becoming aware of earlier dilemmas, which have been repressed into our unconscious because of painful associations, can we progress psychologically (Blatt and Levy 2003; McWilliams 2009). Accordingly, within the counselling encounter, a psychodynamic orientated P/MH nurse is likely to try and encourage clients to review their emotions, explore their thoughts and recount their early-life experiences. In so doing, the psychodynamic orientated P/MH nurse seeks to help the client gain insight into these formative experiences and explore how such material/experiences held in his/her unconscious might be manifesting and impacting upon his/her life and their present-day problems. It is argued that identifying, recognizing and evaluating any patterns in behaviour can assist people in becoming aware of the ways in which they avoid distress and develop defence mechanisms as a method of coping (Blatt and Levy 2003; McWilliams 2009). Once such patterns are identified and accepted, the psychodynamic orientated P/MH nurse and client can begin to discuss how these limiting or restricting patterns of behaviours might be altered.

As stated previously, psychodynamic orientated P/MH nurse works from a premise that people develop defence mechanisms as a means to keep their painful feelings, memories and experiences in their unconscious. Accordingly, psychodynamic orientated P/MH nurses will seek to encourage clients to speak freely: about themselves, about their childhood and about their emotions, desires and fears (Cramer 2000, 2006, 2015). In so doing, clients reveal vulnerable feelings that have been pushed out of conscious awareness. Thus, for the psychodynamic orientated P/MH nurse, given that behaviour is influenced by unconscious thought, if the counsellor-client dyad can identify, explore and process (and resolve) uncomfortable or painful feelings, then the expectation is that the client's defence mechanisms should diminish or resolve (Cramer 2000, 2006, 2015).

7.5 On Transference in Psychiatric/Mental Health Nursing Therapeutic Relationships

Freud (1938) appears to have first begun to write about the phenomenon of transference when he questioned for the first time the source of the interpersonal relationship pattern that the young Dora (a client of Freud) sought to establish with him. Freud came to theorize that such a relationship pattern was a copy of a previous pattern that Dora had organized in the relationship with her father. The authors pointed out at the beginning of the chapter that evidence emerging from the field of neurosciences serves to corroborate and helps to understand the physiological mechanisms of various traditional psychoanalytic concepts; transference is one of them (Kernberg 2004; Luyten and Blatt 2013). Indeed, findings from neurosciences show today that even before an event happens, our brains have already initiated a series of predictions about what is most likely that might happen, arousing perceptions, behaviours, physiological responses and interpersonal ways of relating to what may best be suitable to those predictions (Pally 2007). These continuous, automatic and unconscious predictions seem to be one of the most important and complex of all brain functions, since they have a purpose geared to survival. To generate these predictions, anticipate future events and prepare the individual for them before they occur, the brain uses the present situation and weaves in past experiences and previous learning. That is, given the anxiogenic character of new forthcoming situations, whereby they are unknown and potentially dangerous, the predictive mechanisms offer the opportunity for the unknown to become more familiar and to prepare and activate a complex prior behaviour intended for stress relieving. Repetition has thus a reducing anxiety function (Freud 1938). In this sense, given that these forecasts incorporate past experiences and previous learning, we can see how past influences present lived experiences. So it can be seen that unconscious 'forecasts' provide a biological mechanism through which ongoing dynamic processes can lead to the unconscious phenomenon of 'repetition', in other words, in terms of interpersonal relationship and psychoanalytic concepts to Transference. In a perhaps more simplified definition, this interpsychic phenomenon is understood today as the unconscious transference of feelings and attitudes experienced with a past person or in a past situation for a present person or situation (Evans, 2007).

7.6 On Countertransference in Psychiatric/Mental Health Nursing Therapeutic Relationships

Despite being a phenomenon that is recognized as inevitable, countertransference in nursing has however been poorly studied, though limited literature exists only in P/MH nursing scientific journals (Jones 2005; Evans 2007). P/MH nursing has been the specialized area of nursing that almost exclusively has turned its attention to the phenomenon of countertransference in clinical nursing. In P/MH nursing encounters, countertransference is expressed in one of two common ways. Given that the P/MH will have his/her own unconscious material, his/her own formative experiences and his/her own sense of 'wounded self', then the client may provoke a transferential reaction in the P/MH nurse. This would be characterized as countertransference. Or, also originating in the P/MH nurse's own unconscious, the P/MH nurse reacts or responds to the client's own transferential actions.

Difficult to identify, since it occurs in himself/herself and given its unconscious character, countertransference in P/MH nursing is characterized by having a quality and intensity that distinguishes it from other feelings that arise in the context of the therapeutic nursing care relationship. Countertransference expresses, in that sense, a set of often inappropriate responses to both the content and the relationship context. It should therefore be presumed and questioned, when the P/MH nurse develops strong emotional and different reactions from those which are usual, recognized by him/her and/or others. As in transference, experiences of countertransference can also create an opportunity for intervention/care. Recognizing and subsequently analysing and interpreting countertransference offer the P/MH nurse 'access' to what the client is unconsciously asking (the unconscious request), thus the importance for P/MH nurses to recognize their own countertransference and, importantly, explore these reactions and their meaning in their ongoing clinical supervision.

7.7 On Projective Identification in Psychiatric/Mental Health Nursing Therapeutic Relationships

Proposed by Klein in 1946, the psychoanalytic concept of projective identification has evolved, thanks to the contribution of several authors. Essentially the concept, enrolled in the object relation school of thought, refers to an intrapsychic movement in which *parts of the self and internal objects are split off and projected into the external object, which then becomes possessed by, controlled and identified with the projected parts* (Segal 1974, quoted by Waska 1999). Projective identification can have multiple purposes, however, since it may be directed towards the *ideal object* in order to try to avoid a fantasized separation or it may be directed towards the *bad object* to, in a paranoid movement, try to gain control of the source of danger, to master it. That is to say that in this complex intrapsychic dynamic, bad parts of the self may be projected in order to get rid of them; bad parts of the self may be projected in order to attack and destroy the object; good parts of the self may be projected to avoid separation; good parts of the self may be projected to keep them safe from bad things inside; or good parts of the self may be projected in order to improve the external object, through a kind of basic projective reparation (ibidem).

Being such a primitive psychic survival mechanism, a form of defence, communication and adaptation, projective identification appears as an unconscious fantasy of feelings of love and hate, intolerable to the patients, which are evacuated in the external object (the other). The possibility of the re-internalization of an injured object, causing depression and fear, or, on the other hand, the re-internalization of an object that has now become hostile and dangerous, causing persecutory anxieties, then takes place. In this context, it's easy to notice that and how projective identification has a significant impact on the intersubjectivity of the relationship, giving place to intense countertransference and pathological interactions: nontherapeutic. This psychic and relational functioning has a prominent place in the schizo-paranoid position proposed by the Kleinian theory and is a frequent finding in patients with psychoses, in particular with paranoid psychoses.

For that matter, the interest of projective identification for mental health nurses arises not only from the possibility to assign a meaning to the conscious and unconscious communication of these patients but also from the possibility to take into account the intense countertransference phenomena it causes. Especially in mental health/psychiatric crisis units and the daily care of various psychotic patients, aspects of intrapsychic and interpersonal communication between mental health nurses and patients can transcend the care settings! These countertransferencial phenomena in response to patient projective identifications can happen to mental health nurses both in an individual and collective form. At the individual level, patients can begin to be felt by the mental health nurse with fear and anxiety, they may be often introduced in domestic conversations, they (or their psychic material) may appear in the mental health nurse dreams, etc. On the other hand, at the collective level, nursing teams of mental health/psychiatric crisis units must take into account and be very aware for the installation of persecutory perceptions/feelings in relation to the hierarchy (the head nurse, etc.) or coworkers, manifestations of a low collective self-esteem, somatization and more frequent sick leaves and signs and symptoms of professional burnout. Being unavoidable in the therapeutic work with psychotic patients, the projective identification and its consequent countertransference need to be unconcealed, in a path that can create a gradual mutual understanding between the patient's needs and the forms it has to communicate them and the interpsychic and interrelational responses given (chosen!) by the mental health nurses, individually and in the context of the health team.

7.8 Towards a "Good-Enough Psychiatric/Mental Health Nurse"

Nightingale (1860) recommended that women, to learn how to be good nurses, should observe how an 'old-fashioned nanny' behaves with the child(ren) in her care; she believed that she alone understands everything the child communicates and that the child can understand everything she tells him/her back and doesn't understand anyone else. Indeed, Winnicott's thinking of a maturational psychoanalysis that takes into account the valuation of both the environment and the care relationship for the child's development offers nursing in general a very attractive spring, both conceptual and practical, in how it almost intuitively allows to connect the child development needs to the health needs of many of our patients, as well as the relational characteristics of maternal care to the relational ones of nursing care. Inspired by Winnicott's works, the possibility of understanding the concept of 'relational sufficiency' applied to nursing care has so been a target of interests of various thinkers and researchers, not all nurses, we must say. Among others, Mello and Lima (2010) highlighted the concepts of holding, enabling environment, transitional space and good-enough relationships to establish the interface with nursing care in maternal and child health. And Allan (2001) went as far as to make an approach to the concept of a "good-enough nurse" in a fertility unit. In mental health nursing, this linkage makes even more sense (Fabricius 1991, 1995; Conran 1991; Correia and Lopes 2014).

In such line of thinking should be noticed that the vast Winnicott's work is organized around two main axes in permanent relation: the emotional development of the baby/child and the environment qualities, desirably good enough. The development and constitution of the individual occur then through various processes of interaction with the environment, referring to the crucial role that the relational caregiver plays in baby's integration, its differentiation and the establishment of a psychism that allows to come to distinguish the boundary between the internal and the external, between the non-self and the self and between confusion and differentiation (Winnicott 1994). Giving great importance to the environment and how it responds to the needs of the child, an environment that blends in earlier stages of maturity with the caregiver himself, the author proposes (1971) the adoption of an acceptance relationship, an attention to the experience of what is proper to each child, sharing even his/her absurdness. It's this initial avoidance of the (adult) need to organize or categorize what may be seen as incoherent that opens the possibility to the unconditional acceptance of the child's psychism and behaviour and to an honest communication with him/her.

In this sense, in the transposition of these principles for the therapeutic relationship with patients with psychiatric disorders and associated changes in thought, perception, behaviour, eccentricities and apparent absurdities, the author argues that some patients need also the therapist to be able to observe the absurdity proper to their at-rest mental state, without being prompted for the need to organize it and to make it intelligible. This reinforces the creation of a relational and acceptance space that allows a freer expression of the psychism and patient's behavior, without the risk of a sense of rejection and consequent withdrawal from the relationship. Interpretation in this sense, not to produce itself such loss of contact, needs to be founded on maturity, on the ability to be vividly understood, otherwise, dramatically premature and invasive, will lead to the loss of contact with the patient and the maintenance of the difficulty for him/her to contact with himself/herself. In his development theory, Winnicott (1971) focuses on the earliest stages of the emotional development of the human being, on the emergence of the self and on the vital importance of the dual relationship. On the baby, he describes an initial state of absolute dependence from the environment that tends, due to the environment/caregiver care, for a relative dependence. Becomes central in this nutrient response of the environment the *Holding* function, mobilized and defined by Winnicott (1971, 1994) as one of the ways the *good-enough mother* protects and integrates the baby. This holding refers to a physical and emotional support, which covers the entire relationship, from the way the mother takes in her arms, feeds, recognizes and understands the baby's needs, offering the possibility to create and grow a sensory integration and a psychosocial skin.

The characteristics of this early relationship find a parallel with the way Winnicott (1994) draws up its psychoanalytical intervention model. Based on the primary model of the mother-baby relationship, the author designed and developed the nature and character of transference and the role of the analytical setting, referring to the psychotherapeutic intervention as a complex derivative of the face that reflects what is there to be seen, an analogy to what the baby finds in his/her good-enough mother's face. The psychotherapeutic intervention thought in these terms converts in returning to the patient, in the long run, what the patient brings to the relationship. For Winnicott (1971, 1994), the essence of psychotherapeutic intervention becomes then the fostering of the integration sustained by the good-enough therapist/environment. The holding function binds strongly to a notion of care mobilized and lived in mental health nursing interventions, a holding that supports, sustains and values the day-to-day care as a basic function of the psychotherapeutic intervention of the mental health nurse. It is vital, in this sense, the creation and maintenance of a therapeutic setting that offers support, a good-enough environment, reliable, which supports and helps patients to metabolize their mental pain, their anguishes, to begin to "name" their needs and turning them into communication.

As part of the psychosocial and internal environment of patients, mental health nurses are the privileged managers of this therapeutic environment, since they know it very well and are able to predict its contingencies in order to promote and maintain its sufficiency. We refer not only the relational holistic provision of mental health nursing care to (with) an individual patient but also to the management of patient groups and even to the inter-professional and interdisciplinary dynamics of mental health teams. In these teams, mental health nurses have a clear leading role in the communication transmission/management and in the linkage it establishes between the various agents of care, maintaining the cohesion and environmental sufficiency (of all the physical and psychosocial environment that responds to patient needs). Promoting a good-enough environment, empathic, which meets patient needs, relates in depth with the very essence of nursing care and, in particular, of mental health nursing care (Correia and Lopes 2014). It takes into account the recognition of the patient's needs, supplying them (meeting the omnipotence illusion); offers an external contention for more disorganized patients such as psychotic patients or with borderline personality disorders; creates a possibility to deal with biographical failures which may become possible to support (facilitating the experience of disappointment); introduces data from reality; and promotes emotional maturation (idem).

References

Aguayo J (2009) On understanding projective identification in the treatment of psychotic states of mind: the publishing cohort of H. Rosenfeld, H. Segal and W. Bion (1946–1957). Int J Psychoanal 90(1):69–92

Allan H (2001) A "good enough" nurse; supporting patients in a fertility unit. Nurs Inq 8:51–60

Alexander F, French TM (1946) Psychoanalytic therapy: principles and application. Ronald, New York
Bargh JA (2006) Social psychology and the unconscious: the automaticity of higher mental processes. Psychology Press, Philadelphia
Bargh JA, Morsella E (2008) The unconscious mind. Perspect Psychol Sci 3(1):73–79
Blatt SJ, Levy KN (2003) Attachment theory, psychoanalysis, personality development, and psychopathology. Psychoanal Inq 23:104–152
British Psychoanalytic Council (2017) Psychoanalytic or psychodynamic? https://www.bpc.org.uk/about-psychotherapy/what-pp. Accessed 22 March 2017
Coímbra de Matos A (2002) Psicanálise e Psicoterapia Psicanalítica. Climepsi, Lisboa
Conran M (1991) Running on the spot or can nursing really change?: Response to Julia Fabricius. Psychoanal Psychother 5(2):109–114
Correia S, Lopes J (2014). Nursing intervention with children with conduct disorder in a psychiatry inpatient unit for children and adolescents (Portuguese edition). Master Thesis in Mental Health Nursing and Psychiatry, School of Health Care, Polytechnic Institute of Setúbal, Portugal. http://comum.rcaap.pt/bitstream/10400.26/6601/1/Trabalho%20de%20Projeto_SusanaCorreia.pdf
Cramer P (2006) Protecting the self: defense mechanisms in action. Guilford, New York
Cramer P (2000) Defense mechanisms in psychology today: further processes for adaptation. Am Psychol 55:637–646
Cramer P (2015) Understanding defense mechanisms. Psychodyn Psychiatry 43(4):523–552. The American Academy of Psychoanalysis and Dynamic Psychiatry
Erikson E, Erikson J (1997) The life cycle completed: extended version. W. W. Norton, New York
Evans A (2007) Transference in the nurse-patient relationship. J Psychiatr Ment Health Nurs 14:189–195
Fabricius J (1991) Running on the spot or can nursing really change? Psychoanal Psychother 5:97–108
Fabricius J (1995) Psychoanalytic understanding and nursing: a supervisory workshop with nurse tutors. Psychoanal Psychother 9:17–29
Freud S, Breuer J (1895) Studies on hysteria. Franz Deuticke, Leipzig
Freud S (1915) The unconscious. SE 14:159–204
Freud S (1938) Basic writings of Sigmund Freud, 38th edn. Modern Library, New York
Gabbard GO, Litowitz BL, Williams P (2012) Textbook of psychoanalysis, 2nd edn. American Psychiatric Publishing, Arlington
Jones AC (2005) Transference, counter-transference and repetition: some implications for nursing practice. J Clin Nurs 14:1177–1184
Kaplan-Solms K, Solms M (2000) Clinical studies in neuro-psychoanalysis: introduction to a depth neuropsychology. Karnac Books, London
Kernberg OF (2004) Contemporary controversies in psychoanalytic theory, techniques, and their applications. Yale University Press, New Haven
Klein M (1946) Notes on some schizoid mechanisms. Int J Psychoanal 27:99–110
Klein M (1952) The origins of transference. Int J Psychoanal 33:433–438
Lopes J (2014) Being cared by a case manager nurse. The lived experience of the person with addition problems (Portuguese Edition). Novas Edições Acadêmicas, Saarbrücken
Luyten P, Blatt SJ (2013) Interpersonal relatedness and self-definition in normal and disrupted personality development. Am Psychol 68:172–183
McLeod S (2017) The unconscious mind. https://www.simplypsychology.org/unconscious-mind.html. Accessed 22 March 2017
McWilliams N (1999) Psychoanalytic case formulation. Guilford, New York
McWilliams N (2008) Psychoanalytic psychotherapy: a practitioner's guide. Guilford, New York
McWilliams N (2009) Psychoanalytic diagnosis, 2nd edn. Guilford, New York
Mello D, Lima R (2010) Nursing care and the Winnicott approach (Portuguese edition). Text Context Nurs Florianópolis Jul-Set 19(3):563–569
Nightingale F (1860) Notes on nursing: what it is, what is not. D. Appleton and Company, New York

Pally R (2007) The predicting brain: unconscious repetition, conscious reflection and therapeutic change. Int J Psychoanal 88:861–881

Peplau H (1991) Interpersonal relations in nursing: a conceptual framework of reference for psychodynamic nursing. Springer Publishing Co, Inc., New York

Safran J, Kriss A (2014) Psychoanalytic psychotherapies. In: Wedding D, Corsini R (eds) Current psychotherapies, 10th edn. Brooks/Cole, Belmont, pp 19–52

Saint-Exupéry A (2000) The little prince (original 1943). Harcourt, Inc., London

Segal H (1974) Introduction to the work of Melanie Klein. Basic Books, New York

Solms M, Turnbull O (2002) The brain and the inner world: an introduction to the neuroscience of subjective experience. Karnac Books, London

Strachey J (ed) (1999) The complete psychological works of Sigmund Freud. The Standard edition, vol 1–24. W. W. Norton & Company, New York. Reprint

Sundberg N, Winebarger A, Taplin J (2002) Clinical psychology: evolving theory, practice, and research. Prentice Hall, Englewood Cliffs

Waska R (1999) Projective identification, countertransference, and the struggle for understanding over acting out. J Psychother Pract Res 8(2):155–161

Waude A (2017) Psychodynamic approach in psychology. https://www.psychologistworld.com/freud/psychodynamic-approach.php. Accessed 22 March 2017

Welfel R, Patterson L (2004) The counseling process: a multitheoretical integrative approach. Brooks/Cole, Cengage Learning, Belmont

Winnicott D (1971) Playing and reality. Tavistock Publication Ltd., London

Winnicott D (1994) Holding and interpretation: fragment of an analysis. Grove, New York

Winship G (1995a) Nursing and psychoanalysis - uneasy alliances? Psychoanal Psychother 9(3):289–299

Winship G (1995b) The unconscious impact of caring for acutely disturbed patients. A perspective for supervision. J Psychiatr Ment Health Nurs 2:227–233

Winship G (1998) Intensive care psychiatric nursing-psychoanalytic perspectives. J Psychiatr Ment Health Nurs 5:361–365

Zimerman D (2008) Manual de Técnica Psicanalítica (Portuguese edition). Artmed, Porto Alegre

The Biopsychosocial Approach: Towards Holistic, Person-Centred Psychiatric/Mental Health Nursing Practice

8

José Carlos Santos, Marie Bashaw, Will Mattcham, John R. Cutcliffe, and Kelly Graziani Giacchero Vedana

8.1 Background and Overview

Somewhat uncomfortable with the then prevailing biomedical orthodox view of people, health and how to respond to health challenges, Engel (1977, 1980) advanced a counter narrative. He made the case if health-care practitioners wanted to offer substantive, adequate and effective responses to a person's suffering, then they needed to consider and respond to needs arising out of the biological, psychological and social dimensions of their experience. As a result, Engel (1977) authored the Biopsychosocial (BPS) model and, in so doing, tried to reverse the dehumanization of health sciences and disempowerment of patients (Borrell-Carrió et al. 2004; Smith et al. 2013). In this context, the BPS model, patient-centred and humanistic approaches can be and have been used in P/MH nursing to bring about improvements in clinical practice

J.C. Santos (✉)
Escola Superior de Enfermagem de Coimbra, Nursing School of Coimbra, Coimbra, Portugal
e-mail: jcsantos@esenfc.pt

M. Bashaw
Assistant Professor of Nursing, Wright State University, Ohio, USA

W. Mattcham
Assistant Professor of Nursing, Cleveland State University, Ohio, USA

J.R. Cutcliffe
Cutcliffe Consulting, Kingston, Canada

School of Nursing, Coimbra, Portugal
e-mail: jcutcliffe@outlook.com

K.G. Giacchero Vedana
Ribeirão Preto College of Nursing - PAHO/WHO Collaborating Centre for Nursing Research Development, University of São Paulo, Butantã, Brazil

© Springer International Publishing Switzerland 2018

J.C. Santos, J.R. Cutcliffe (eds.), *European Psychiatric/Mental Health Nursing in the 21st Century*, Principles of Specialty Nursing,
https://doi.org/10.1007/978-3-319-31772-4_8

(Borrell-Carrió et al. 2004; Henningsen 2015; Smith et al. 2013). This model considers the need to include consideration of individuals' experience, perceptions, function in daily life, intellectual capacity, emotional stability, productivity, performance of social roles and social determinants (Fava and Sonino 2008).

According to Borrell-Carrió et al. (2004), the BPS model is both a philosophy of clinical care and a practical clinical guide. Key philosophical ideas include the notion that suffering, illness and the well-being of the person can be affected and impacted by multiple levels of influence, from the social aspects to the biological. At the practical level, it is a way of attempting to understand the patient's subjective experience and 'weaving' this understanding, as it is an essential consideration, into the care episode (Borrell-Carrió et al. 2004).

The BPS approach can be traced back to Engel's (1977) theoretical and clinical evolution away from the 'one-dimensional' (and linear) Biomedical model. For Engel (1977) restricting or limiting one's conceptualisation of suffering and experiences of 'ill-health' to those available within the Biomedical model did not provide an adequate 'frame' to understand and respond to the person's suffering and experiences. An adequate response from the practitioner, according to Engel (1977), required him/her to understand the person's suffering and to communicate this sense of understanding. And to do so, the practitioner required him/her to be mindful of and respond to the whole multidimensionality of the suffering/experience and thus consider the biological, psychological and social dimensions of suffering/experience/illness (Henningsen 2015).

Engel (1977) can thus be seen to be eschewing reductionist views of the person- and health-related responses. For Engel (1977) there was a further element of this approach; he argued that his ideology might help combat or serve as a counterpoint to the dehumanization of medicine and disempowerment of patients that he perceived. Interestingly, perhaps especially to those Psychiatric/Mental Health (P/MH) nurses that have a 'bent' or preference for qualitative research methods (see Cutcliffe and Goward 2000), his model 'made room' for possibility that the subjective experience of the person was amenable to scientific study (Engel 1977, 1980). Engel's (1977) model subsequently became known as 'the Biopsychosocial model'. As a further interesting element in the origins and early development of the model, Engel (1977) did not focus on mental health; indeed he never tried to demonstrate the models' application or relevance to mental health; rather, he assumed it (Ghaemi 2009). Rather Engel (1977) focused on medical conditions and physiological (rather than psychological) suffering.[1]

As pointed out, Engel posited that to appreciate health in general, one must first consider the psychological, behavioural and social dimensions that contribute to illness-related events (Henningsen 2015). For Engel, the interactions between biological, psychological and social factors determine the cause, manifestation and outcome of wellness and disease. The BPS model posits that any one factor is not sufficient; it is the interaction between people's physical verdure (biology), mental health and behaviour (psychology) and social and cultural context that determine the course of their health-related outcomes (www.boundless.com, n.d.) (Alderfer et al. 2009; Borrell-Carrió et al. 2004; Fava and Sonino 2008; Smith et al. 2013). The BPS approach has been described as an integrative perspective that added patients' psychological and social health

[1] Though this may not be entirely surprising given Engel's background as an internist, with a specialism and interest in gastrointestinal disorders.

concerns to the Biomedical model (Smith et al. 2013), because it considers the relationship between mental and physical aspects of health is complex and health cannot be reducible to laws of physiology (Borrell-Carrió et al. 2004). Thus, this model is directly opposed to a tendency to reductionism and compartmentalization of the variables that influence health conditions (Friedman et al. 2012). This model includes consideration of individuals' experience, perceptions, function in daily life, intellectual capacity, emotional stability, productivity, performance of social roles and social determinants has emerged as a crucial part of clinical investigation and patient care (Fava and Sonino 2008). The Biopsychosocial factors may operate to facilitate, sustain or modify the course of illness because they are important determinants of susceptibility, severity and course of illness (Borrell-Carrió et al. 2004; Fava and Sonino 2008).

8.2 Essential Theoretical Elements of the Biopsychosocial Model

The Biopsychosocial model has a number of theoretical underpinnings. In no order of priority necessarily, the authors can identify:

- The model incorporates holistic views of the person.
- The model draws upon systems theory.
- The model draws upon ecological theory.
- The model draws upon experiential thinking and experiential learning.
- The model emphasizes 'person-centred' health-care approaches.

8.2.1 Holism and Multidimensionality

A clear emphasis in Engel's (1977, 1980) original works is that of rejecting certain pervasive views in medicine at the time, as he wished to 'rehumanize' medical care. Accordingly, he eschewed the dominant, Descartian reductionist views of people and their health. In contrast, a holistic approach, which should be familiar to twenty-first-century P/MH nurses (see, e.g. Long and Baxter 2001; American Holistic Nurses Association and American Nurses Association 2013; Zahourek 2008), refers to a comprehensive view of the person, and his/her health, wherein the person has physical, emotional, social, economic and spiritual domains. Moreover, these domains or dimensions of the person are in intimate contact with one another, to the extent that they have a reciprocal influence on each other and cannot be understood in isolation of the other dimensions. Thus as a further contrast to reductionist philosophy, a holistic view of the person sees him/her as more than the sum of his/her individual parts (Long and Baxter 2001; American Holistic Nurses Association and American Nurses Association 2013; Zahourek 2008).[2] For the authors of this

[2]While some authors appear to have co-opted or adopted the term holism and use this to refer to a collection of 'new age', complimentary and/or 'alternative' health-care 'treatments', the authors deliberately limit their use of the term holism to refer to a holistic approach and a holistic view of the person (ala—Engel's original works).

chapter, holistic P/MH nursing then refers to contemporary nursing practice that expresses and operationalizes this philosophy and view of the person. For Engel, health problems or challenges, including mental health problems, have an origin or antecedent in at least three dimensions. The person's health problem will have a biological component (which considers a person's genes, nutritional status, neuroendocrine and neurological issues), a psychological component (which considers a person's emotions, thoughts, behaviours) and a social component (which considers the person's background and experience of trauma, stress and the environment).

8.2.2 General Systems Theory

The theoretical underpinnings of the biopsychosocial model include 'General Systems theory' (Von Bertalanffy 1976). According to von Bertalanffy, systems theory refers to and is concerned with the structure and properties of systems in terms of 'relationships' the system contains. Understanding these relationships between variables in the system leads to a deeper and more comprehensive understanding of the whole. Interestingly, systems theory is multi- or transdisciplinary in nature as it draws together theory and concepts from various domains of science including physics, philosophy, biology and engineering. In advancing his ideas about systems theory, von Bertalanffy highlighted the interrelatedness and interdependence of phenomena—be they physical, biological, psychological, social and cultural in nature. Systems then, for von Bertalanffy, are integrated wholes, and understanding the properties of the system will not be advanced by adopting a reductionist view.

8.2.3 Ecological Perspectives

Ecological views of health are predicated on the premise that health, behaviour and their determinants are interrelated (Crosby et al. 2013). In recognizing that health is influenced by a range of interrelated factors, ecological views of health consider a combination of individual, social, environmental, interpersonal, organizational, community and public policy issues/factors (Bronfenbrenner 1979; McElroy et al. 1988; Nurse and Edmondson-Jones 2007; Bentley 2013). Ecologically based views of health regard it as axiomatic that no one, single factor can provide an adequate or comprehensive explanation as to why some people or groups are at higher risk of experiencing health challenges and problem. Accordingly, the ecological proposition of the existence of multiple layers of influence, both 'inside' and 'outside' the person, which can have a profound affect and effect on the health and well-being of the person, is highly congruent with the ideas underpinning the BPS approach.

8.2.4 Experiential Knowledge and Experiential Learning

Experiential learning is the process of learning through experience and is often referred to as learning through reflection on doing. As opposed to traditional 'classroom' learning, experiential knowledge is knowledge gained through experience. Dewey (1938), often credited as the originator of experiential learning, argued that it can also be contrasted both with propositional (textbook) knowledge and with practical knowledge. Moreover, experiential learning incorporates the notion that any learning that supports 'students' in applying their knowledge and conceptual understanding to real-world problems, even when this knowledge is acquired in 'classroom' settings (Wurdinger and Carlson 2010). Accordingly, when the BPS refers to the need to consider the person's experience and perceptions as a crucial part of clinical assessment patient care, then the value of client's learning from their own experience of suffering and health challenges can be seen to be woven into the theoretical underpinning of the BPS approach.

8.2.5 Person-Centred Health Care

According to McCance et al. (2011), person-centred (PC) care is a way of thinking about and delivering health care in a manner that sees the people using health and social services as equal partners in planning, developing and monitoring care to make sure it meets their needs. This means an inversion of the traditional models of health care whereby 'patients' (not clients, users or persons) were largely passive recipients of care, not active and 'equal' participants. Person-centred care then means putting people and their families at the centre of decisions and seeing them as experts, working alongside professionals to get the best outcome (Cloninger 2011). The relevant literature shows that there is no consensus on a definition of person-centred care; however, there appear to be some common elements shared across these various definitions and conceptualisations. These include—in no order of priority necessarily:

1. Putting clients at the centre of care.
2. Respecting client values and choices.
3. Power sharing, involving family and/or significant others (if the client wishes).
4. Individualizing responses and care.
5. Communicating empathy, compassion, understanding and being non-judgmental. In order to offer person-centred care, it is argued (see Cutcliffe et al. 2015) that services need to change to be more flexible to meet people's needs in a manner that is best for them. In forming partnerships with clients, the underlying philosophy is enacted—it is about working with people, rather than 'doing to' them (Cutcliffe et al. 2015).

8.3 The Biopsychosocial Approach and Mental Health Care

As stated, the BPS approach presupposes the existence of different hierarchical levels of systems structurally and functionally interconnected. An understanding of the phenomena that can be characterized as 'biological level' (e.g. atoms, molecules, cells, tissues, organs and body systems) is necessary, but not sufficient to explain, let alone respond to health conditions. The higher complex levels such as the psychological (human being perspective, experience and behaviour) and social or environmental (relationships, family context, community, society and environment) also need to be considered. For some authors, these factors are all relevant, in all cases, at all times (Ghaemi 2009).

While the approach does require the P/MH nurse to view the person through a holistic, multidimensional lens, the relevance and contribution of each domain can vary from illness experience to illness experience, from one person to another and even between two different episodes of the same illness in the same person (Fava and Sonino 2008). This is because the relative importance of biological, psychological and social factors in explaining health conditions constantly changes over time (Henningsen 2015). Thus, the model provides a background to the holistic evaluation and practice, but there is no assumption of proportional representation of the domains (Jull 2017). The linear view of causality is substituted by a circular causality considering a complex interaction among psychological, sociological and physiological variables and feedback mechanisms. The literature regarding a biopsychosocial-oriented clinical practice recommends that assistance includes self-awareness, active cultivation of trust, empathy, self-calibration, educating the emotions, using informed intuition and communicating clinical evidence to foster dialogue, not just the mechanical application of protocols (Borrell-Carrió et al. 2004).

There are criticisms of BPS model that consider it not testable (vaguely defined, with unclear boundaries), overly general (non-selective eclecticism, inefficient and time-consuming), without specific method (to be operationalized) (Ghaemi 2009; Smith et al. 2013). In response of these criticisms, the literature regarding BPS model constructed well-defined, consistent and repeatable patient-centred interviewing methods to identify the psychological and social components of the BPS model.

8.4 Evidence of Efficacy: Evaluation and Criticism of the Biopsychosocial Model

Revolta et al. (2016) used the BPS model to help health-care staff to understand, formulate and develop interventions for people with dementia. Through using the BPS model, complex factors that influence a person's well-being can be identified. Through understanding a person's difficulties, the health-care practitioner is able to select appropriate interventions to combat the illness and enhance the patient's wellness. The Biopsychosocial model additionally allows for the consideration of such issues as the belief factors associated with healing and the societal conception of disease. Advantages of the BPS model are found in its holistic awareness of levels in nature and inclusiveness of diverse perspectives. Proponents for BPS advocate that when contemplating illness, one must consider the social and behavioural factors that play a significant role in health overall (e.g. poor eating habits, obesity, smoking, excessive alcohol consumption, recreational drugs, risk taking behaviour, stress, anxiety, depression, etc.). Focusing only on the physical symptoms of illness does not give us the complete picture and understanding of these phenomena. In Habtewold et al. (2016) study on co-morbidity of depression and diabetes, the biopsychosocial variables included marital status, experience of a negative life event in the last 6 months, occupation, diabetic complication and poor social support which significantly increased average depressive symptoms score. Evidence-based interventions focusing on these identified biopsychosocial factors are useful in alleviating depressive symptoms.

The BPS model developed a general framework with the two dominant conceptions of so-called mental illness: (1) the biological psychiatry view that 'mental disorders' arise from faulty biology and (2) the psychodynamic view that emphasizes the psychological dimensions of maladaptive patterns of thinking, feeling and acting and relating could be reconciled. Thus, BPS became the most frequently adopted perspective in psychiatry. As stated by Jensen et al. (2015) in their study on hypnosis, BPS models have proven to be useful in understanding other complex issues, including chronic pain, depression and substance abuse. Importantly, biopsychosocial models allow for the possibility that many factors can play a role and contribute to hypnotic responding. It has been accepted for a long time, in both research and practice, that it is necessary to consider the biological, psychological and social elements of an individual in order to enhance understanding and treatment (Carey et al. 2014). The BPS model is a useful intervention for medical practitioners (Pilgrim 2015).

While there are proponents for the BPS model, it is not without criticism. The most generally cited problem is the inclusiveness of the BPS model that results in an unscientific, pluralistic approach. This model potentially justifies an 'anything goes' approach to psychiatry, medicine and health. This pluralistic approach is quite the opposite of the analytic scientific approach that breaks the world into its component parts. Ghaemi (2009) postulates that the unclear boundaries of BPS can confuse treatment and is a poor model for addressing costs of managed care in the area of psychiatry. Further, Ghaemi (2009) explains that while the biopsychosocial model was valuable in its day as a reaction to biomedical reductionism, its historical role has played out. So-called mental illness is complex; biology is not enough; but the biopsychosocial model is not enough either. In the view of Ghaemi (2009), psychiatry should look to less eclectic, less generic, less vague alternatives.

8.5 Assessment

A number of authors and agencies have advanced guidelines for and/or produced BPS assessment instruments (see, e.g. De Jonge et al. 2001; Pai et al. 2008; Alderfer et al. 2009; Andrasik et al. 2015; MIND 2008). And to a greater or lesser extent, each of these features contain certain rudimentary elements and underpinnings. Not least, given the nature of the BPS approach, the assessment must be holistic and must have assessments of a variety of 'domains' or 'dimensions'. Engel's (1977) original approach focused on the biological, psychological and social dimensions. More contemporary BPS instruments tend to expand the areas of assessment and include additional domains and dimensions. Andrasik et al. (2015), for instance, declare that, within the biological domain, assessment should also focus on physical, physiological, biochemical, nutritional or genetic domains. Similarly, the same authors argue that assessment within the psychological domain should also include focus on emotional, affective, cognitive, behavioural, spiritual and personality domains. And with regard to the social domain, Andrasik et al. state that assessment should include attention to environmental, cultural, family, work and interpersonal domains. While individual BPS assessment instruments share different emphases (Andrasik et al. 2015) and will dedicate more attention to different domains, many of the instruments, in the opinion of the authors, still tend to favour and overemphasize biological/pharmacological—in line with this biomedical emphasis in P/MH care in most parts of the world (see Barkley 2009). Given the focus of this book, however, the authors have advanced an assessment guideline that reflects a more person-centred, less biomedical-orientated approach.

Biopsychosocial assessments, as with other assessments in mental health care, need to occur within the context of a therapeutic relationship; the P/MH assessor will need to establish a healthy degree of rapport (MIND 2008). In so doing, the accuracy of the assessment is enhanced. Indeed, some authors have advanced the argument that to operationalize a genuine BPS assessment, the style of communication needs to move away from 'traditional' assessment methods. For instance, in his paper on interviewing and provider-patient relationships in the BPS approach, Smith et al. (2013) underscore the central role of communication and make the argument that there is a need to educate and train mental health-care providers (Smith focuses on physicians) in patient-centred interviewing methods.

Given that the rationale for an assessment is to gain a comprehensive, holistic 'picture' of the person, his/her specific challenge(s) or mental health problem(s), the P/MH nurse should encourage the person to speak, perhaps initially focusing on recent experiences, stressors, changes and traumatic events, and then the conversation can be widened to include the more historical events and experiences. It would be wise to explore and seek to understand the person's sense of connectedness, his/her relationships and strengths/current limitations. The person should be encouraged to talk about his history—psychiatric (if any) and medical—and, importantly for a BPS assessment, the person's lifestyle (e.g. hobbies, diet, exercise, drug/alcohol use, social support and relationships). And a 'formal' mental health assessment may also be undertaken (see below).

Comprehensive assessments ought to include an exploration of the person's strengths and challenges (MIND 2008), and it is perhaps tautological to point out that accurate and thorough documentation of the assessment must be maintained. And the facility exists for additional, more specific areas, and issues can/could be considered and assessed—such as the potential for or risk of aggression/violence, potential for or risk of self-harm and/or suicidal thoughts/feelings/risk. The authors would advance the view that such specialized areas are perhaps best assessed by a combination of the clinical interview and validated risk assessment instruments (Cutcliffe and Santos 2012). Any assessment interview, for the authors at least, will have increased validity and accuracy, if the P/MH nurse attempts to foster and communicate an atmosphere of understanding and empathy (see also Stein et al. 1998). Indeed, for a genuine application of the BPS approach, then an atmosphere of empathy is necessary (but not sufficient). Creating a permissive atmosphere, one where eliciting the client's perspective is also vital. The assessment should seek the client's ideas and views about his/her situation/experience/health challenge. Ensuring that these qualities, behaviours and attitudes are present and influential during the assessment interview can help establish rapport/build trust, it can further encourage and facilitate the exchange of information, and it both demonstrates and communicates a sense of care, concerns and hope. All of which will, according to Zucarrello (2015), increase the likelihood the client 'buys in' to the agreed treatment plan.

8.6 Example of a Biopsychosocial Assessment

Basic Information:

Name
Date of birth/age
Race/ethnicity
Address/contact details

8.6.1 Presenting Concern(s)

What brought you here today?

What/how would you describe your major (presenting) issues/problems?

What background/history to your problem(s)—if you are aware of any—exists here?

What are you hoping to get from this 'treatment episode'?

What support systems and/or people do you have in your life? Where (to whom) do you go when you need support?

8.6.2 Previous Attempts and/or Experiences with Trying to Resolve Your Issue/Problem

What previous experiences of formal mental health care—if any—do you have?

Please list any 'talk therapy', counselling and psychotherapy you have experienced previously.

Please comment on these previous experiences—how useful/not useful was it? What was particular helpful/unhelpful? What brought this to an end?

What previous experiences of psychotropic medication—if any—do you have?

Please list any 'drugs', dosages and frequency you have taken previously or are currently taking.

Please comment on these previous experiences—how useful/not useful did you find the medication? What was particular helpful/unhelpful? What brought this to an end?

What previous formal psychiatric mental health diagnosis—if any—do you have?

Please list any 'hospitalisations' for psychiatric issues you have had.

Please comment on these previous experiences—how useful/not useful was it? What was particular helpful/unhelpful? What brought this to an end?

What previous or existing medical problems do you have? What previous experiences of formal health care—if any—do you have?

Please list any treatment you have received previously for any/all medical problems.

Please list any (surgical) procedures you have received previously for any/all medical problems.

Please comment on these previous experiences—how useful/not useful was it? What was particular helpful/unhelpful? What brought this to an end?

8.6.3 Previous Use and/or Experiences with Substances and/or Alcohol

Have you ever used drugs or alcohol for recreational purposes? If yes, which substance(s)?

How frequently and what quantity of the substance did you use?

Were there particular experiences or situations that seemed to precipitate your use of the substance/alcohol?

8.6.4 Traumatic and Childhood History

Have you ever been abused or witnessed abuse (physical/emotional/sexual)?

Experience of learning difficulties/impairments or had testing?

How would you describe your childhood?

Educational experience—school experience and highest academic level achieved.

8.6.5 Family History

What, if any, previous experiences of formal mental health care do any of your family members have?

Please list any 'talk therapy', counselling and psychotherapy they have experienced previously.

Please list any 'drugs', dosages and frequency of any psychotropic drugs that your family member has taken previously.

Please list any 'hospitalisations' for psychiatric issues that your family member had.

8.6.6 Employment Status and History

Employed/self-employed/unemployed/student/disabled?

How would you describe your work situation? Work relationships?

Stress related to work situation?

8.6.7 Social/Relationship Status

Single, married, committed relationship?

Do you have children? Relationship with them?

Previous relationships—how did they end?

Living/accommodation situation? Who lives in your home? How adequate/inadequate do you feel your accommodation is?

Exercise? Type, frequency, duration.

Are there any family relationships that are of particular concern for you? Please describe.

Criminal record, history of incarceration?

Do you hold any particular religious/spiritual beliefs—if so—what are these?

How, if at all, do these beliefs help you/add to your current problem(s), issues and challenges?

What do you do to cope with stress?

What do you enjoy doing with your free time?

What do you consider your strengths?

Box 8.1 Mini Mental Health Exam Assessment Areas/Questions

(Adapted from MIND 2008)

Appearance: Age, gender, ethnicity, build, evidence of grooming/personal hygiene

Physical disability, clothing choices

Behaviour: Friendly, hostile, guarded/defensive,

recalcitrant, lascivious, level of eye contact, level of alertness

Motor: Stillness/restlessness/agitation, psychomotor retardation, 'overexuberance', catatonia, dystonia, abnormal movements, gait

Mood/affect: Manic, hypomanic (euphoric), flat affect, depressed, lability, range, appropriate emotional responses, incongruence

Thinking/thoughts: Obsessive thinking, delusional thoughts, ruminations, ideas of reference, intrusive thoughts, persistent thoughts of self-harm and/or suicide, attention/concentration span, coherence, logical, neologisms, thought blocking, thought transmission

Perception: Hallucinations, illusions, depersonalisation

Cognition: Orientated to time, person, place, memory, concentration

References

Alderfer MA, Mougianis I, Barakat LP, Beele D, DiTaranto S, Hwang W-T, Rielly AT, Kazak AE (2009) Family psychosocial risk, distress, and service utilization in pediatric cancer: predictive validity of the Psychosocial Assessment Tool (PAT). Cancer 115(8):S4339–S4349

American Holistic Nurses Association & American Nurses Association (2013) Nursing: scope and standards of practice. In: Nursing books, 2nd edn. Silverspring, San Jose

Andrasik F, Goodie JL, Peterson AL (2015) Biopsychosocial assessment in clinical health psychology. Guilford Press, New York

Barkley J (2009) Biopsychosocial assessment: why the biopsycho and rarely the social? J Can Acad Child Adolesc Psychiatry 18(4):344–347

Bentley M (2013) An ecological public health approach to understanding the relationships between sustainable urban environments, public health and social equity. Health Promotion International. doi: 10.1093/heapro/dat028. First published online: May 9, 2013 http://heapro.oxfordjournals.org/content/early/2013/05/08/heapro.dat028.full

Borrell-Carrió F, Suchman AL, Epstein RM (2004) The biopsychosocial model 25 years later: principles, practice, and scientific inquiry. Ann Fam Med 2(6):576–582. doi:10.1370/afm.245

Bronfenbrenner U (1979) The ecology of human development. Harvard University Press, Cambridge, MA

Carey TA, Mansell W, Tai SJ (2014) A biopsychosocial model based on negative feedback and control. Front Hum Neurosci 8:94. http://doi.org.ezproxy.libraries.wright.edu/10.3389/fnhum.2014.00094

Cloninger CR (2011) Person-centred integrative care. J Eval Clin Pract 17(2):371–372

Crosby RA, Salazar LF, Diclemente RJ (2013) Ecological approaches in the new public health. In. DiClemente RJ, Salazar LF, Crosby RA (eds) Health behavior theory for public health: principles, foundations and applications. Jones and Bartlett, New York, pp 231–252

Cutcliffe JR, Goward P (2000) Mental health nurses and qualitative research methods: a mutual attraction? J Adv Nurs 31(3):590–598

Cutcliffe JR, Santos JC (2012) Suicide and self-harm: an evidence-based approach. Quay Books, London

Cutcliffe JR, Santos JC, Kozel B, Taylor P, Lees D (2015) Raiders of the lost art: have psychiatric/mental health nurses lost, forgotten or abandoned the therapeutic use of self? The case of acute psychiatric settings in the United Kingdom, Portugal, Canada, Switzerland, Germany and Australia. Int J Ment Health Nurs 24:375–385

De Jonge P, Huyse FJ, Stiefel FC et al (2001) Intermed – a clinical instrument for biopsychosocial assessment. Psychosomatics 42(2):106–109

Dewey J (1938) Experience and education. Kappa Delta Pi, USA

Engel G (1977) The need for a new medical model: a challenge for biomedicine. Science 196:129–136

Engel G (1980) The clinical application of the biopsychosocial model. Am J Psychiatr 137:535–544

Fava GA, Sonino N (2008) The biopsychosocial model thirty years later. Psychother Psychosom 77(1):1–2. doi:10.1159/000110052

Friedman RC, Downey JI, Editor D (2012) Editorial: the biopsychosocial model. Psychodyn Psychiatry 40(3):371–376

Ghaemi SN (2009) The rise and fall of the biopsychosocial model. Br J Psychiatry 195(1):3–4. doi:10.1192/bjp.bp.109.063859

Habtewold TD, Islam MA, Radie YT, Tegegne BS (2016) Comorbidity of depression and diabetes: an application of biopsychosocial model. Int J Ment Heal Syst 10:74

Henningsen P (2015) Still modern? developing the biopsychosocial model for the 21st century. J Psychosom Res 79(5):362–363. doi:10.1016/j.jpsychores.2015.09.003

(The) Hunter Institute of Mental Health (HIMH) (2008) *MIND: essentials – a new online resource for nurses and midwives working in hospital and community settings.* file:///C:/Users/jcutc/OneDrive/Documents/bio%20psy%20soc%20paper%20res.pdf

Jensen MP, Adachi T, Tomé-Pires C, Lee J, Osman ZJ, Miró J (2015) Mechanisms of hypnosis: toward the development of a biopsychosocial model. Int J Clin Exp Hypn 63(1):34–75. doi:10.1080/00207144.2014.961875

Jull G (2017) Biopsychosocial model of disease: 40 years on. Which way is the pendulum swinging? Br J Sports Med, bjsports-2016-097362. http://doi.org/10.1136/bjsports-2016-097362

Long A, Baxter R (2001) Functionalism and holism: community nurses' perceptions of health. J Clin Nurs 10(3):320–329

McCance T, McCormack B, Dewing J (2011) An exploration of person-centredness in practice. Online J Issues Nurs 16(2):1

McElroy K, Bibeau D, Steckler A, Glanz K (1988) An ecological perspective on health promotion programs. Health Educ Behav 15(4):351–377

Nurse J, Edmondson-Jones P (2007) A framework for the delivery of public health: the ecological approach. J Public Health Epidemiol 61(6):555–558

Pai AL, Patino-Fernandez AM, McSherry M, Beele D, Alderfer MA, Reilly AT, Hwang W-T, Kazak AE (2008) The psychosocial assessment tool (PAT2.0): psychometric properties of a screener for psychosocial distress in families of children newly-diagnosed with cancer. J Pediatr Psychol 33:50–62

Pilgrim D (2015) The biopsychosocial model in health research: its strengths and limitations for critical realists. J Critical Realism 14(2):164–180. doi:10.1179/1572513814Y.0000000007

Revolta C, Orrell M, Spector A (2016) The biopsychosocial (BPS) model of dementia as a tool for clinical practice. A pilot study. Int Psychogeriatr 28(7):1079–1089. doi:10.1017/S1041610215002379

Smith RC, Fortin AH, Dwamena F, Frankel RM (2013) An evidence-based patient-centered method makes the biopsychosocial model scientific. Patient Educ Couns 91(3):265–270. doi:10.1016/j.pec.2012.12.010

Stein TS, Nagy VT, Jacobs L (1998) Caring for patients on conversation at a time: musings from the interregional clinician patient communication leadership group. Permanente J 2(4):62–68

Von Bertalanffy L (1976) Perspectives on general system theory: scientific-philosophical studies

Wurdinger DD, Carlson JA (2010) Teaching for experiential learning: five approaches that work. Rowman & Littlefield Education, Lanham

Zahourek RP (2008) Integrative holism in psychiatric-mental health nursing. J Psychosoc Nurs Ment Health Serv 46(10):31–37

Zucarrello V (2015) The biopsychosocial interview – the foundation of patient care. https://www.linkedin.com/pulse/biopsychosocial-interview-foundation-patient-care-vic-zuccarello

URLS

http://bjp.rcpsych.org/content/195/1/3

https://www.boundless.com/psychology/textbooks/boundless-psychology-textbook/stress-and-health-psychology-17/introduction-to-health-psychology-85/the-biopsychosocial-model-of-health-and-illness-326-12861/

https://www.psychologytoday.com/blog/theory-knowledge/201510/the-biopsychosocial-model-and-its-limitations

http://www.annfammed.org/content/2/6/576.full

9 Trauma-Informed Care: Progressive Mental Health Care for the Twenty-First Century

John R. Cutcliffe, Rodger Travale, and Tyler Green

9.1 Introduction

At the risk of sounding hyperbolic, perhaps the most significant development in European mental health care in recent decades is the acknowledgement and acceptance of Trauma-Informed Care in mental health-care policy, practice, research and, to a lesser extent, education (Kezelman and Stavropoulos 2012). Such models accentuate the need for mental health-care practitioners, including P/MH nurses, and the organizations that they work within, to recognize and accept the prevalence and pervasive impact that trauma can (and does) have on the lives of the clients they work alongside (SAMHSA 2015; 2016). Further, such models posit the need for mental health services to adapt and become even more trauma-sensitive and trauma-responsive. The significance of this development cannot be understated; for decades mainstream, orthodox psychiatry has denied and ignored how sexual, physical, emotional abuse and/or neglect in children was:

> A genuine and common phenomenon with potentially devastating long-term consequences for the mental health of the survivors. (Hammersley et al. 2007, p. 7/8)

J.R. Cutcliffe (✉)
Cutcliffe Consulting, Kingston, Canada

School of Nursing, Coimbra, Portugal
e-mail: jcutcliffe@outlook.com

R. Travale
Healthcare Manager, Chiron Health Services, Prince George Regional Correctional Centre, British Columbia, Canada

T. Green
Clinical Instructor and Psychiatric Nurse Practitioner, Wright State University Ohio, New York, NY, USA

© Springer International Publishing Switzerland 2018

J.C. Santos, J.R. Cutcliffe (eds.), *European Psychiatric/Mental Health Nursing in the 21st Century*, Principles of Specialty Nursing,
https://doi.org/10.1007/978-3-319-31772-4_9

Yet now, even bastions of mainstream psychiatry are acknowledging this phenomenon and the increasing body of evidence which underscores such models; former president of the American Psychological Association (APA), Steven Sharfstein, for instance, has argued that trauma is to mental health as smoking is to cancer (Franks 2016). Indeed, the evidence which illustrates how the anatomical structure and resultant function of developing brains is altered subsequent to experiences of significant childhood trauma is both substantial and compelling (see Anda et al. 2006; Bremner 2003; Bremner and Vermetten 2001; Cook et al. 2003; 2005; Curtis and Nelson 2003; De Bellis and Thomas 2003; De Bellis et al. 2002; Fan et al. 2011; Heim and Nemeroff 2001, 2002; Larius et al. 2010; Nelson 2011; Shonkoff et al. 2009; Teicher 2000; Teicher et al. 1994, 1997, 2002; Weich et al. 2009).

This body of convergent evidence, drawn from multiple fields of study, shows how childhood experiences, including those occurring during infancy, appear to determine how effectively different areas of the human brain integrate with one another and how well they function together (see Muskett's 2014 review). Perhaps not surprisingly, exposure to 'positive' experiences has been found to be linked with increased and extensive intra-brain connectivity; whereas exposure to negative experiences has been found to suppress neural pathway development (Muskett 2014). Curtis and Nelson's (2003) work for instance showed suppressed pathway development between the cerebral cortex and the limbic system. And while the gradual acknowledgement and acceptance of Trauma-Informed Care within the broader mental health community is encouraging, alas many services/practitioners, including many within the substance misuse and treatment field, have as yet only partially introduced the principles and practices of TIC or not at all. For instance, according to the SAMHSA (2014a) document, most people go through abuse, neglect, loss disaster and/or war without receiving or even having access to TIC services and supports. Further the national survey of substance misuse treatment facilities in the USA (SAMHSA 2010) found that 66% reported incorporating trauma counselling at least some time and none reported fully integrated TIC services. In light of these findings, it may be prudent to remind ourselves of the core components of TIC.

9.2 What Is Trauma

Several definitions, many of which appear to share common elements, have been advanced as to the nature of trauma. According to SAMSHA (2014b, p. 7):

> Trauma results from an event, series of events, or set of circumstances that is experienced by an individual as physically or emotionally harmful or threatening and that has lasting adverse effects on the individual's functioning and physical, social, emotional, or spiritual well-being.

The American Psychological Association (APA) (2016) declares that:

> Trauma is an emotional response to a terrible event like an accident, rape or natural disaster. Immediately after the event, shock and denial are typical. Longer term reactions include unpredictable emotions, flashbacks, strained relationships and even physical symptoms like headaches or nausea. While these feelings are normal, some people have difficulty moving on with their lives.

However, the World Health Organisation's International Classification of Diseases system (ICD-10) (WHO 2016) refers to trauma in their definition of post-traumatic stress disorder (PTSD) as a response to a stressful event of an exceptionally threatening or catastrophic nature, which is likely to cause pervasive distress in almost anyone (e.g. natural or man-made disaster, combat, serious accident, witnessing the violent death of others or being the victim of torture, terrorism, rape or other crime).

While the conceptualisation and definition of trauma has changed over time,[1] current conceptualisations of trauma describe how it can be a single event (e.g. experiencing the 7/7 bombing in London, England), a series of events (childhood neglect or abuse) and/or a chronic condition (PTSD diagnosis) (APA 2016). Contemporary conceptualizations now also recognize the various ways in which a person can encounter or experience the traumatic event, from individually experiencing the event to directly witnessing an event and to vicarious exposure or indeed hearing about an event that affects someone they know (SAMHSA 2014a). Furthermore, conceptualisations of trauma have evolved over the years to now include human-caused events (e.g. trauma associated with war, acts of terror, sexual/physical abuse), or they can be natural events (e.g. weather-based events (flooding, tornados); natural disasters—tsunamis, earthquakes, volcanic eruptions) (SAMHSA 2014a). According to the National Institute for Health and Clinical Excellence (NICE 2015) guidelines for the management of PTSD in adults and children, PTSD is characterized by certain experiences (for some—these are symptoms), and these are listed in Box 1.

Box 9.1 NICE (2005) Guidelines for the Management of PTSD in Adults and Children—Characteristics of PTSD

Sufferers involuntarily re-experience of aspects of the traumatic event in a vivid and distressing way. This can include flashbacks (in which the person acts or feels as if the event is recurring); nightmares and frightening dreams; and repetitive, intrusive and distressing images (or other sensory impressions from the event).

Sufferers avoid of reminders of the trauma—be these be people, situations or circumstances resembling or associated with the event. As a result, the NICE (2005) guidelines add further that people experiencing PTSD often try to push memories of the event out of their mind and avoid thinking or talking about it in detail, particularly about its worst moments. On the other hand, many ruminate excessively about questions that prevent them from coming to terms with the event, for example, about why the event happened to them, about how it could have been prevented or about how they could take revenge.

Sufferers experience hyperarousal, hypervigilance for threat, exaggerated startle responses, irritability, difficulty in concentrating and sleep problems.

Sufferers also describe symptoms of emotional numbing or blunting. These include inability to have any feelings, feeling detached from other people, giving up previously significant activities and amnesia for significant parts of the event.

Sufferers experience other symptoms, including depression, generalized anxiety, shame, guilt and reduced libido (adapted from NICE 2005).

[1] Readers are encouraged to review Wittgenstein (1953), Rodgers (1989) or Cutcliffe and McKenna (2005) on the evolutionary or developmental nature of concepts—they change over time through use. See evidence of this phenomenon also in the changing definitions of diagnoses in progressive iterations of the DSM.

9.3 Understanding the Epidemiology of Trauma: Key Points to Note

Examination of the relevant epidemiological evidence on trauma highlights a number of important particulars:

(a) *Establishing the precise epidemiology of trauma is problematic, especially in children.* According to Saunders and Adams (2014), establishing the precise epidemiology of trauma is bedevilled by a number of issues such as the inherent nature of some of the types of traumatic events that children experience, the assets available to the field for detecting and counting events and the confounding methodological issues between studies. Saunders and Adams (2014) estimate that 8–12% of American youth have experienced at least one sexual assault; 9–19% have experienced physical abuse by a caregiver or physical assault; 38–70% have witnessed serious community violence; one in ten has witnessed serious violence between caregivers; one in five has lost a family member or friend to homicide; 9% have experienced Internet-assisted victimization; and 20–25% have been exposed to a natural or man-made disaster. The WHO's (2013) 'European Region: Preventing Child Maltreatment' report indicates major rises in rates during the 1990s, a slight downward trend in rates since then, but, as yet, no reliable data on how the major economic downtown and associated enforced austerity measures have influenced rates of childhood trauma and maltreatment in Europe.

(b) *Trauma does not discriminate.* People of any gender, race, ethnicity, nationality, sexual orientation, geographical location, socio-economic backgrounds, socio-cultural backgrounds and theological beliefs can and do encounter trauma and experience its potentially[2] deleterious effects on one's holistic well-being (SAMHSA 2014b, 2015).

(c) Perhaps not surprisingly, given the heterogeneous nature of human existence and human experiences, *trauma has been found to produce a range of responses—though many appear to share the commonalities of fear and feelings vulnerability.* Similarly, the same traumatic event or experience does not necessarily produce the same traumatization in different people.

(d) *The degree of trauma appears to be linked to the individual's particular lived experience of the traumatic event* (SAMSHA 2014b, 2015). Similarly, it appears that a range of factors in the individual experiences (e.g. biopsychosocial factors, cultural factors, previous experiences of trauma) influence his/her response to the particular traumatizing event/experience.

(e) *The preponderance of the evidence in this area seems to indicate that the length of the period of recovery following a traumatic event varies considerably* (Yehuda and LeDoux 2007), though it is important to point out that PTSD

---

[2]The author/editors have deliberately used the term 'potentially' here as there is also a body of evidence which shows how in some cases trauma can actually lead to personal development and growth (see Chap. 11).

shows substantial natural recovery in the initial months and years after a traumatic event. The NICE (2005) clinical management guideline indicates that a while a significant number of trauma survivors will likely initially develop some symptoms of PTSD, a substantial proportion of these individuals recover without treatment in the following years, with a steep decline in PTSD rates occurring in the first year. On the other hand, according to the NICE (2005) clinical management guideline, at least a third of the individuals who initially develop PTSD remain symptomatic for 3 years or longer and are at risk of secondary problems such as substance misuse.

9.4 Traumatic Events in Childhood and Substance Misuse Issues in Adult Life: An Overview of the Relevant Literature

Dube et al. (2002, 2003) examined the relationship between illicit drug use in adult life and adverse childhood experiences (ACEs)/traumatic childhood experiences. Their findings indicated that, in comparison to people who had no reported history of childhood traumatic events, people with five or more childhood traumatic events were seven to ten times more likely to report illicit drug use problems, addiction to illicit drugs and parenteral drug use. The authors concluded that higher scores on traumatic childhood event scales had a strong positive correlation with the risk of drug initiation in early adolescence/adulthood and to problems with drug use and drug addiction in later life. In their 2002 paper, Dube et al. report that all the individual childhood traumatic experiences are associated with a higher risk of alcohol abuse as an adult. These authors asserted that, compared to persons with no traumatic history, the risk of heavy drinking, self-reported alcoholism and marrying an alcoholic were increased between two and four times in individuals with a history of traumatic childhood experiences, regardless of parental alcoholism.

Similarly, Grella et al. (2005) explored relationships among exposure to childhood abuse and traumatic events, substance abuse and adult psychological distress in a sample of substance-abusing women offenders ($N = 440$). These authors report that they found direct relationships between several childhood traumatic events and greater adolescent conduct problems and substance abuse. According to Grella et al. (2005), the findings underscore the need to provide trauma-related services for substance-abusing women offenders. Likewise, Simpson and Miller (2002) sought to investigate whether or not there is a connection between childhood sexual or physical abuse (CSA, CPA) and later substance use problems (SUPs) among adolescents and adults. The rates of CSA among females with SUPs were found to be, on average, nearly two times higher than those found in the general population, and the rates of SUPs among women with CSA histories were found to be similarly elevated. Similarly, men with histories of CSA were found to be at greater risk for SUPs than men in the general population.

In a related study, Anda et al. (2002) adopted a retrospective cohort design to examine the relationship between traumatic childhood experiences with risk of alcoholism in adulthood. Their findings suggest that the number of adverse childhood experiences had a graded relationship to alcoholism and depression in adulthood, independent of parental alcohol abuse. And furthermore, these authors concluded that the risk of alcoholism and depression in adulthood increases as the number of reported adverse experiences increases regardless of parental alcohol abuse. In their review of the relevant literature, Guitierres and Van Puymbroeck (2006) found that women substance misusers, more often than men, have been found to have higher rates of violent victimization as children. These victims of childhood sexual and physical abuse exhibit negative psychological outcomes of low self-esteem, depression and anxiety, and they may turn to substance use as a way to cope with these painful psychological consequences. Once women begin to use substances, their experience in the drug world, coupled with their vulnerable psychological state from childhood trauma, puts them at risk for continued victimization from domestic violence and from sexual assault.

Reporting on a major American epidemiological study with 17,000 participants, the ‘Adverse Childhood Experiences study’, Felitti and Anda (2010) declare that the findings in this study provide a remarkable insight into how we become what we are. These authors concluded that it was clear that traumatic childhood experiences have a profound, proportionate and long-lasting effect on emotional well-being and that these experiences very commonly lead to major health risks in adult life—most commonly smoking, alcoholism and substance misuse. In the findings from another nationwide comorbidity survey, Molnar et al. (2001) found significant associations between childhood traumatic experiences and subsequent onset of mood, anxiety and substance use disorders among women and men. They concluded that childhood traumatic events, whether alone or in a larger adversity cluster, are associated with substantial increased risk of subsequent psychopathology.

This brief review of the relevant empirical literature underscores how sexual, physical, emotional abuse and/or neglect in children is a common phenomenon with potentially devastating long-term consequences for the mental health of the survivors (Hammersley et al. 2007). More specifically, the literature also speaks to how traumatic childhood experiences are positively correlated with increased engagement in unhealthy substance misuse and related behaviours in later life. Indeed, the overwhelming consensus in this body of literature supports the existence of this relationship, and so, it is both necessary and prudent to examine how the principles and practices of TIC might be operationalized in a mental health and/or substance misuse treatment facility.

9.5 Assessment

A number of instruments/assessment scales and clinical interview assessment guides have been produced to gauge the severity of the person’s trauma (and even more so for assessing PTSD). The US Department of Veterans Affairs (2016) asserts that assessment is best undertaken using validated measures. However, given the imperfections inherent in all such instrumentation, the authors would urge

Table 9.1 Trauma assessment instruments

Author	Instrument	Available
Paula et al. (recovered 2016)	Brief Trauma Questionnaire (BTQ)	http://www.ptsd.va.gov/professional/pages/assessments/assessment-pdf/brief_trauma_questionnaire.pdf
Kubanyet al. (2000)	Traumatic Life Events Questionnaire (TLEQ).	Development and preliminary validation of a brief broad-spectrum measure of trauma exposure: The Traumatic Life Events Questionnaire. *Psychological Assessment, 12,* 210–224
Foa et al. (2001)	Child Post-traumatic Symptom Scale (CPSS)	The Child PTSD Symptom Scale: A preliminary examination of its psychometric properties. *Journal of Clinical Child Psychology*, 30 (3), 376–384
Steinberg and Beyerlein (recovered 2016).	UCLA Reaction Index	UCLA PTSD reaction index: DSM-5 version http://www.nctsn.org/nctsn_assets/pdfs/mediasite/ptsd-training.pdf

practitioners to use a combination of a through clinical assessment interview (and one's clinical judgement comes to bear here in addition to validated instruments). A number of trauma assessment instruments are listed in Table 9.1.

9.5.1 The Clinical Assessment Interview: Fundamentals and Rudiments

As with any mental health assessment, the accuracy and validity of a trauma assessment is enhanced when the P/MH nurse has established a trusting, therapeutic interpersonal relationship with the client/survivor. However, an argument can be made that asserts how the establishment of such a relationship is both primary and paramount when working with clients with history of traumatic experiences (Ferenick and Rameriz-Hammond 2016). Moreover, even in the presence (or context) of a trusting, therapeutic interpersonal relationship, both the documented evidence and the best practice guidelines for Trauma-Informed Care draw attention to how reluctant traumatized clients can be to talk about their experiences (NICE 2005). Not only is it quite common for clients to find talking about their traumatic experiences to be upsetting (and thus in turn can lead to a reluctance to discuss), but disclosing and discussing the precise nature of the traumatic event(s) can give rise to some re-experiencing symptoms and feelings (Yehuda and LeDoux 2007). As a result, clients can be understandably reluctant, in the beginning, to talk about the most distressing aspects of their experience (Steinberg and Beyerlein 2016).

Similarly, the assessment needs to be comprehensive and holistic and should consider physical, psychological and social issues/needs. Specific attention in the assessment needs to include questions pertaining to re-experiencing the trauma (e.g. flashbacks and nightmares) and experiences of hyperarousal (e.g. exaggerated startle response or sleep disturbance). For assessment of minors, particularly younger children, Ferenick and Rameriz-Hammond (recovered 2016) declare that consideration should be given to asking the child and/or the parents about sleep disturbance or significant changes in sleeping patterns. An assessment should also seek information on whether or not the client is experiencing intrusive symptoms associated with the traumatic event(s) (SAMHSA 2014b). Therefore the P/MH nurse needs to ask about:

- Any recurrent, involuntary and intrusive distressing memories of the event
- Repetitive play with trauma themes
- Recurrent distressing dreams related to the event
- Dissociative reactions (e.g. flashbacks) in which the individual feels/acts as if the event were recurring
- Whether or not there is any evidence of trauma-specific reenactments in the survivor's play
- Psychological distress at cues resembling event
- Persistent avoidance of stimuli associated with the traumatic event(s)
- Attempts to avoid distressing memories/thoughts/feelings about or closely associated with the traumatic event
- Attempts to avoid external reminders (people, places, conversations, activities, objects, situations) that arouse distressing memories/thoughts/feelings about or closely associated with the traumatic event
- Negative alterations in cognitions and mood associated with the traumatic event(s)
- Inability to remember an important aspect of the event (not attributable to altered consciousness, i.e. head trauma, drug/alcohol misuse)
- Persistent and exaggerated negative beliefs or expectations about oneself, others or the world (e.g. 'I deserved it' and 'No one can be trusted')
- Persistent, distorted cognitions about the cause or consequences of the event that lead the individual to blame himself/herself or others
- Persistent negative emotional state (e.g. fear, anger, guilt or shame)
- Significant and detectable diminished interest or participation in significant activities
- Feelings of detachment or estrangement from others
- Persistent inability to experience positive emotions (adapted from SAMHSA 2014a; Ferenick and Rameriz-Hammond recovered 2016; Steinberg and Beyerlein 2016)

Thus, perhaps ironically, an element of an effective assessment process that P/MH nurses need to be mindful of when assessing trauma (and it's impacts) is the client's willingness to and comfort with answering questions about the trauma.

Given that discomfort in talking about the trauma, at least in part because of the client's distrust of others, this behaviour can be a useful proxy indicator of progress/continuing difficulty. Hence, the closeness or degree of openness and trust within the therapeutic relationship also serves as an important piece of the assessment 'picture'. Assessment in Trauma-Informed Care is made more complicated or nuanced by the necessity of respecting the client's rights (and understandable reluctance) to answer questions about trauma. And while this may make assessment more nuanced and protracted, the therapeutic potential and value of treating the relationship as primary (e.g. putting relationship building needs first) outweighs any delay in completing one's assessment.

9.6 Ten Principles of Trauma-Informed Care Services

Elliot et al. (2005) advanced a framework of ten principles of TIC, and they claimed, over a decade ago, that these principles are well understood by those who focus on working with trauma survivors. Significant support for this position can be found in the relevant body of literature; further support for the position is also clearly evident in the large body of work concerned with service user views, experiences and evaluations of mental health-care services. For example, in an examination of mental health service evaluations for the UK, Portugal, Canada, Germany, Switzerland and Australia, the findings indicated that, in many cases, service users encounter a mental health-care inpatient experience that is often devoid of warm therapeutic relationships, respectful interactions, information or choice about treatment and any kind of formal/informal 'talk therapy'. Instead such care experiences are personified by coercion, disinterest, inhumane practices, custodial and controlling practitioners and a gross over-use of pharmacological 'treatments' (Cutcliffe et al. 2015). As a result, one could argue that it is of even greater import to (re)familiarize ourselves with the principles, especially if we wish to nudge our services closer to being truly trauma-informed.

9.6.1 Trauma-Informed Services Recognize the Impact of Violence and Victimization on Development and Coping Strategies

Despite the evidence which highlights the relationship(s) between experiences of childhood trauma and abuse/neglect and mental health problems in later life, there is evidence of limited, not widespread or comprehensive uptake of TIC within mental health-care communities (Reeves 2015). Drawing on the example of Trauma-Informed Care services for women, key national and international articles and reports have continued to identify opportunities and barriers to an integrated and coordinated service response (Barron 2005; Johnson and Zlotnick 2007; Roxburgh et al. 2006; Smith 2004; The Stella Project, (The) Stella Project 2007; United Nations Office on Drugs and Crime. Substance Abuse Treatment and Care for Women 2004). The situation *vis-a-vis* the limited progress on incorporating the principles and practices of TIC into substance misuse facilities leads the British Columbia Centre of Excellence for Women's Health (2009, p. 3) to state that:

> …we have a long way to go towards building a seamless, compassionate, integrated response.

Similarly, the second edition of the so-called Trauma-Informed Toolkit (Klinic Community Health Centre 2013), for instance, states that although trauma may be central to many people's difficulties and awareness of it pivotal to their recovery, in public mental health and social service settings, their trauma is seldom identified or addressed. As several authors have noted (see Grenard et al. 2007; Mitchell and O'Connor 2013; Sypniewski 2016), mental health practitioners report little to no education on and lack of effective guidance on TIC per se. Yet, according to Elliot et al. (2005), when mental health-care staff recognize and acknowledge these formative experiences and the significant effects they can and do have on clients, then client experiences and difficulties are validated. Such is the alleged value of so doing that Elliot et al. (2005) go on to assert that doing so promotes the client's sense of safety and hope.

If one accepts the findings cited above, then there appears to be a need to update and amend relevant curricula, training/education materials and incorporate theoretical models, relevant empirical findings, policy and discursive material pertinent to TIC. Reeves (2015 p. 706) advances a similar argument, stressing the need for additional training and education in TIC stating:

> The empirical and theoretical publications included in this synthesis provide support for the creation of provider training programs on trauma-informed practice.

Such material ought in the view of the authors to be included in all nursing curricula but perhaps has an even more urgent need to be woven into P/MH nursing curricula and substance misuse worker curricula.

9.6.2 Trauma-Informed Services Identify Recovery from Trauma as a Primary Goal

Elliot et al. (2005) make the case that trauma-informed services either offer programs and services to deal with and recover from past trauma or integrate their care delivery with an agency that already provides such services. The authors extend Elliot et al.'s exhortations and advocate that mental health and substance misuse facilities should, similarly, offer programs/interventions to deal with past trauma. Fortunately, there are some examples where this need has been recognized and where this has already occurred (see, e.g. Cutcliffe and Travale 2016; Cutcliffe et al. 2016; United States Department of Veteran Affairs: National Center for PTSD 2016). In such facilities, it is recognized that a reduction (or abstinence) in substance use is a parallel goal to facilitating recovery from one's traumatic background. If one accepts the self-medication hypothesis of substance use and applies this to the context of TIC, then people have developed substance abuse problems in an attempt to manage their distress associated with the effects of trauma exposure and traumatic stress symptoms (National Child Traumatic Stress Network 2016). Accordingly, to address and help the person recover from his/her traumatic past and ipso facto, there could/should be a reduction in substance consumption. Thus, as Jennings (2008) argues, substance misuse facilities must introduce and incorporate services, programs and interventions deigned to facilitate and assist with the client's recovery from specific trauma experiences, for instance, trauma-focused groupwork, personal trauma-focused counselling, somatic experiencing (Levine 1997) or art therapy.

9.6.3 Trauma-Informed Services Employ an Empowerment Model

Empowerment, though bedevilled with various and at times conflicting definitions and conceptualisations (Grant 2003), is (at least partly) concerned with individuals and/or groups gaining more power and control over their lives and choices. It is concerned with a fundamental shift in the (invisible) power imbalance that service users highlight (Cutcliffe and Happell 2009). The authors will not belabour the theoretical and clinical parallels between promoting individual control in TIC services and mental health/substance misuse services. Each domain of practice share increased personal control as a key clinical goal (see also Hipolito et al. 2014). Indeed, Elliot et al. (2008, p. 465) go as far as to state that:

> the empowerment model is essential to recovery from the overwhelming fear and helplessness that is the legacy of victimisation.

9.6.4 Trauma-Informed Services Strive to Maximize a Client's Choices and Control Over His/Her Recovery

Hummer et al. (2010) provide examples of trauma-informed mental health-care services that promote and realize service user choice. Hummer et al. (2010) show how child and youth clients choose their own clothing and food, they have some input into which staff members they work with and children can express their preferences regarding how they wish to be responded to during any de-escalation situations. Similarly, substance use facilities have the capacity to incorporate and promote client choice; indeed a theoretical model of substance misuse treatment (and associated care/responses) predicated on notion of choice was advanced as long ago as 1999 (Glasser 1999). In keeping with the practice example described above, within substance misuse facilities, choices can be offered in terms of the specific program of groups and activities that clients engage in, which 'work program' clients decide on and some choice in which members of staff they work with primarily, and perhaps—most obviously—clients do have choice as to whether or not they engage in recovery per se. And preparation for discharge and aftercare invariably needs to be a consultative, collaborative process involving soliciting the views and preferences of the client. Somewhat ironically, the authors recognize that successful substance misuse programs do require clients to choose to engage and participate, and thus it should be emphasized that clients do indeed have a choice to engage or not.

9.6.5 Trauma-Informed Services are Based in a Relational Collaboration

For many P/MH nurses, situating their clinical work within a therapeutic relationship is *de rigueur* (Cutcliffe 2008); thus, it may seem redundant to emphasize the relational context to mental health and substance misuse facilities that embrace TIC. However, the literature is clear in indicating that there are P/MH nurses who apparently do not share this view (see Cutcliffe 2008; Cutcliffe et al. 2013). The nature and constituency of therapeutic relationships, and more importantly, relationships that promote the growth of trust and help recovery from traumatic experiences have been well described (see Cutcliffe 2008; Cutcliffe et al. 2013, 2015; Hipolito et al. 2014; Hummer et al. 2010; Perry et al. 1995). Similarly, the need for and value of working on and within relationships has been well documented in substance misuse care; the work of Fals-Stewart et al. (1996, 2001) perhaps underscoring how lasting recovery from substance use depends, in part, on making relationships better. Arguably, accepting the primacy of relationships in TIC takes on an even greater significance given that the client's past experiences of abuse and trauma very often occur within the context of a relationship, with well over 40% of cases of child abuse involving a family member and even higher numbers involving someone known to the victim (SAMHSA 2015). The importance of such relationships to Trauma-Informed Care is captured in best practice guidelines, such as those authored by Ferenick and Rameriz-Hammond (2016, p. 81) who state:

> Healing and recovery cannot occur in isolation but within the context of relationships. Relationships fostered with persuasion rather than coercion, ideas rather than force, and empathy rather than rigidity will encourage trust and hope with survivors.

9.6.6 Trauma-Informed Services Create an Atmosphere that is Respectful of Survivors Need for Safety, Respect and Acceptance

Numerous studies and reports have been published during recent years, and in many different nations, regarding the type of services that mental health SUs wish to encounter. The major themes evident in these findings are as follows: (a) SUs prefer a mental health-care experience personified by personal (human-to-human) contacts. (b) SUs want to have a service where they feel they are being listened to, understood and responded to empathically. (c) Similarly, SUs stress the importance of feeling safe and the presence of the 'quality of caring' within interpersonal relationships established with the P/MH professionals as important elements of a successful experience (Cutcliffe et al. 2015). Trauma-informed services have to ensure that staff interactions, program content, the philosophy of care and any procedures/interventions help create a 'space' that is perceived and experienced as welcoming, safe and 'caring' (Elliott et al. 2005). This 'space' refers to both the physical space or environment and the interpersonal 'environment' (see Bloom et al. 2003; Borge and Fagermoen 2008; Green et al. 2005; Hummer et al. 2010; Lowe and Balfour 2015; Mende 2010). Practice guidelines emanating from the Society for the Study of Addiction (2014) stress the same attitudes and skills: stating the need for establishing a positive relationship, one that is empathic and warm; the need to communicate effectively through appropriate use of empathic statements, reflection, clarification and verbal and non-verbal behaviours; and, importantly, the need to be non-judgemental and non-confrontational.

9.6.7 Trauma-Informed Services Emphasize Client's Strengths, Highlighting Adaptations Over Symptoms and Resilience Over Pathology

According to Elliot et al. (2005), some mental health and substance misuse programs too often focus intently on problems that in so doing, practitioners miss the strengths that clients possess. It is unclear if this is an unavoidable outcome of using the medical model, with its emphasis on pathology, trauma-informed services and, as a result, some substance misuse facilities adopt and operationalize a comprehensively different conceptualization. Rather than focusing on the person's pathology and his/her clinical presenting problems, such facilities and approaches (see, e.g. Clark 2002; Manthey et al. 2011; SAMHSA 2009) emphasize a strengths-based approach. Such approaches are underpinned by the belief that clients are most successful at achieving their goals when they identify and utilize their strengths, abilities and assets (Rapp 2006), even when they may not recognize such strengths within themselves (Greene et al. 2005). Supporting this view, Ferenick and Rameriz-Hammond (2016, p. 5) declare that:

> A trauma-informed approach is based on the recognition that many behaviors and responses expressed by survivors are directly related to traumatic experiences.

As a result, so-called symptoms are seen as originating from adaptations to their previous traumatic experience(s) (Elliott et al. 2005; Harris and Fallot 2001; Saakvitne et al. 2000).

9.6.8 The Goal of Trauma-Informed Services is to Minimize the Possibilities of Re-traumatization

It might sound somewhat tautological to state that mental health and substance misuse services ought not to re-traumatize, or traumatize for that matter, the very clients to whom they claim to be providing help and services. However there is, regrettably, a large body of evidence which indicates this is precisely what happens at times (see, for instance, Gallop et al. 1999; Holmes et al. 2004; Larue et al. 2013; McAllister et al. 2002). For mental health/substance misuse services that wish to adopt a trauma-informed approach, the power dynamics present between mental health-care providers and clients have to be acknowledged and minimized if not removed (see Cutcliffe 2008). Given the power differential present in abusive relationships, the contrary experience to this must be provided; P/MH nurses therefore eschew power over clients and seek to empower clients as one way of avoiding repeats of or re-traumatizing experiences.

9.6.9 Trauma-Informed Services Strive to be Culturally Competent and to Understand Each Client in the Context of His/Her Life Experiences and Cultural Background

Culture, according to the relevant literature, can play a significant role both in contributing to/exacerbating a substance misuse problem and in framing the treatment/response (Abbott and Chase 2008). It is well documented that substance misuse consumption is a cultural phenomenon with different patterns in substance of choice and frequency of use, in addition to the presence of risk and protective patterns that can be idiosyncratic to specific cultures, to significant variation in responses to drug users (see for instance, Heath 2001; Horigian et al. 2006; Lombardi and van Servellen 2000; Murphy-Parker and Martinez 2001). Culture in this instance refers to both ethnic- or national-based culture in addition to gender-based cultural nuances and differences. According to Elliot et al. (2005, p. 468):

> understanding the influence of someone's culture is essential to making an effective therapeutic connection…healing takes place within the woman's cultural context.

Accordingly, trauma-informed substance misuse services will then need to be cognizant of both the individual, particularized life story of the client but similarly locate that life story within the client's culture (or cultures).

9.6.10 Trauma-Informed Agencies Solicit Consumer Input and Involve Consumers in Designing and Evaluating Services

In keeping with other exhortations regarding improving formal mental health services, trauma-informed substance misuse services should be informed by the input of the survivors/clients (Rutter et al. 2004; Simpson and House 2002; Tait and Lester 2005). Ideally, this consultation should occur before the services are established, but even where and when this is not possible, formal service evaluation and development must include survivor input. As with the increasing (and most welcome) inclusion of clients on educational program advisory boards and in various educational roles as such as 'expert by experience' (Forest et al. 2000; Simpson et al. 2008), survivors of trauma have invaluable information that needs to be listened to and considered by boards/managers of substance misuse facilities.

9.7 Psychiatric/Mental Health Nursing Responses Within Trauma-Informed Care Models

> As advocates, our role is both to affirm and validate the coping mechanisms that trauma survivors use and also to support survivors in developing new ways to cope with the impact of trauma. (Ferenick and Rameriz-Hammond 2016, p. 5)

At the outset, it needs to be noted that there is currently a paucity of literature, particularly empirical studies, pertaining to Trauma-Informed Care in substance misuse/recovery treatment facilities (and mental health-care facilities per se) (Muskett 2014). What does exist and are the most useful are the various best practice guidelines (e.g. Ferenick and Rameriz-Hammond 2016) and grey literature/documents produced by key stakeholder organizations (e.g. SAMHSA 2014a; b). As a result the final section of this chapter draws together some of these key practice guidelines, and these are listed in Table 9.2.

Table 9.2 How can P/MH nurses enact and operationalize trauma care

• Provide information to the client on what, in all likelihood, to expect after experiencing a trauma
• Explain that mood swings and emotional lability are common in reactions to trauma
• Offer reassurance that this healing or recovery process is certainly possible—but it may take time and may demand a degree of patience on the part of the client
• Discuss how it is not uncommon for clients to have a new 'normal' after recovering from trauma. It is not the same as the 'normal' experienced before the trauma but can be rich and fulfilling in its own right
• It is essential that the P/MH nurse communicate and show respect for the survivor's needs, focus on connecting with the client and remain hopeful regarding their recovery
• Be prepared to listen
• P/MH nurses must be willing and able to work in a collaborative way with survivors, family and friends of the survivor and other human services agencies in a manner that will empower survivors and consumers
• Consider expounding the interrelation between trauma and symptoms of trauma such as substance abuse, eating disorders, depression and anxiety
• Help the survivor explore and identify a range of 'new' coping skills. These activities need to be geared towards helping the survivor create and maintain new, safe connections with others
• Telling the story of the traumatic experiences is essential to healing. The story may well be told more than once. P/MH nurses have to offer an emancipatory opportunity for clients (especially women and children) to shatter the disabling silence that often surrounds experiences of trauma
• Provide reassurance as to the typical 'normal' reaction to trauma; it is very common to be affected by such experiences. Remind the client that experiencing traumatic reactions is not an indication of individual pathology or weakness. Such phenomena are merely indications or manifestations of the client's body and brain attempting to process and heal

(continued)

Table 9.2 (continued)

• Be mindful of, consider and address the client's safety needs
• Work at being trustworthy, genuine, honest open and transparent
• Explore and encourage the option of peer support—formal and informal options
• Always work towards power sharing, seeking collaboration and mutuality.
• Provide choices and options to the client and be respectful of her/his choices
• Be cognizant and respectful of (and work within) the client's cultural, historical and experiential experiences
• Explore and refine alternate, stress-reducing behaviourally based coping skills. These will inevitably be individualized to the client but commonly involve activities such as aerobic exercise, yoga, relaxation exercises and techniques, journaling/blogging/writing, painting/sculpting or other artistic expressions, deep breathing exercises, peer support discussions groups, listening to relaxing music, meditation (or for the more theologically inclined—prayer), cathartic release of emotional pain in a safe environment, warm shower/bath or sports

References

Abbott P, Chase DM (2008) Culture and substance abuse: impact of culture affects approach to treatment. Psychiatric Times 25(1):43–46. Retrieved from http://www.psychiatrictimes.com/articles/culture-and-substance-abuse-impact-culture-affects-approach-treatment

American Psychological Association (2016) Trauma. Retrieved from http://www.apa.org/topics/trauma/

Anda RF, Whitfield CL, Felitti VJ, Chapman D, Edwards VJ, Dube SR, Williamson DF (2002) Adverse childhood experiences, alcoholic parents, and later risk of alcoholism and depression. Psychiatr Serv 53(8):1001–1009

Anda RF, Felitti VJ, Bremner JD, Walker JD, Whitfield C, Perry BD, Dube SR, Giles WH (2006) The enduring effects of abuse and related adverse experiences in childhood: a convergence of evidence from neurobiology and epidemiology. Eur Arch Psychiatry Clin Neurosci 256(3):174–186

Barron J (2005) Multiple challenges in services for women experiencing domestic violence. Housing Care Support 8(1):11

Bloom SL, Bennington-Davis M, Farragher B, McCorkle D, Nice-Martin K, Wellbank K (2003) Multiple opportunities for creating sanctuary. Psychiatry Q 74(2):173–190

Bremner JD (2003) Long-term effects of childhood abuse on brain and neurobiology. Child Adolesc Psychiatr Clin N Am 12:271–292

Bremner JD, Vermetten E (2001) Stress and development: behavioral and biological consequences. Dev Psychopathol 13:473–489

British Columbia Centre of Excellence for Women's Health (2009) Trauma-informed approaches in addictions treatment: gendering the National Framework. Retrieved Nov. 14th 2016 http://bccewh.bc.ca/wp-content/uploads/2014/02/2010_GenderingNatFrameworkTraumaInformed.pdf

Borge L, Fagermoen MS (2008) Patients' core experiences of hospital treatment: wholeness and self-worth in time and space. J Ment Health 17(2):193–205

Clark MD (2002) Strength-based strategies for prevention. In: The blue book. National Catholic Council on Alcoholism and Related Drug Problems, Inc., Lafayette

Cook A, Blaustein M, Spinazzola J, van der Kolk B (eds) (2003) Complex trauma in children and adolescents. National Child Traumatic Stress Network, Los Angeles

Cook A, Spinazzola J, Ford JD, Lanktree C, Blaustein M, Cloitre M (2005) Complex trauma in children and adolescents. Psychiatr Ann 35(5):390–398

Curtis W, Nelson C (2003) Toward building a better brain: neurobehavioral outcomes, mechanisms, and processes of environmental enrichment. In: Luthar S (ed) Resilience and vulnerability: adaptation in the context of childhood adversities. Cambridge University Press, New York, pp 463–488

Cutcliffe JR (2008) The die has been cast? Rediscovering the essence of psychiatric/mental health nursing. Br J Nurs 17(2):88–92
Cutcliffe J, Happell B (2009) Psychiatry, mental health nurses, and invisible power: Exploring a perturbed relationship within contemporary mental health care. Int J Ment Health Nurs 18(2):116–125
Cutcliffe JR, Stevenson C, Lakeman R (2013) Oxymoronic or synergistic: deconstructing the psychiatric and/or mental health nurse. Int J Ment Health Nurs 22:125–134
Cutcliffe JR, Santos JC, Kozel B, Taylor P, Lees D (2015) Raiders of the lost art: a review of published evaluations of inpatient mental health care experiences emanating from the United Kingdom, Portugal, Canada, Switzerland, Germany and Australia. Int J Ment Health Nurs 24:375–385
Cutcliffe JR, Travale R (2016) Unearthing the theoretical underpinnings of 'Green Care' in mental health and substance misuse care: history, theoretical origins and contemporary clinical examples. Issues Ment Health Nurs 3(2):137–147
Cutcliffe JR, Travale RT, Richmond M, Green T (2016) Considering the contemporary issues and unresolved challenges of therapeutic communities for clients with alcohol and substance use problems. Issues Ment Health Nurs 37(9):642–650. doi:10.3109/01612840.2016.1169465
De Bellis M, Keshavan MS, Shifflett H, Iyengar S, Beers SR, Hall J, Moritz G (2002) Brain structures in pediatric maltreatment-related posttraumatic stress disorder: a socio-demographically matched study. Biol Psychiatry 52:1066–1078
De Bellis M, Thomas L (2003) Biologic findings of post-traumatic stress disorder and child maltreatment. Current Psychiatry Rep 5:108–117
Dube SR, Anda RF, Feletti VJ, Edwards VJ, Croft JB (2002) Adverse childhood experiences and personal alcohol abuse as an adult. Addict Behav 27(5):713–725
Dube SR, Felitti VJ, Dong M, Chapman DP, Giles WH, Anda RF (2003) Childhood abuse, neglect, and household dysfunction and the risk of illicit drug use: the adverse childhood experiences study. Pediatrics 111(3):564–572
Elliott DE, Bjelajac P, Fallot RD, Markoff LS, Reed BG (2005) Trauma-informed or trauma-denied: principles and implementation of trauma-informed services for women. J Community Psychol 33(4):461–477
Fals-Stewart W, Birchler GR, O'Farrell TJ (1996) Behavioral couples therapy for male substance-abusing patients: effects on relationship adjustment and drug-using behavior. J Consult Clin Psychol 64:959–972
Fals-Stewart W, O'Farrell TJ, Birchler GR (2001) Behavioral couples therapy for male methadone maintenance patients: effects on drug-using behavior and relationship adjustment. Behav Ther 32:391–411
Fan Y, Shi F, Smith J, Lin W, Gilmore J, Shen D (2011) Brain anatomical networks in early human brain development. NeuroImage 54(3):1862–1871
Felitti VJ, Anda RF (2010) The relationship of adverse childhood experiences to adult medical disease, psychiatric disorders, and sexual behavior: implications for healthcare. In: Ferencik SD, Ramirez-Hammond R (eds) (recovered May 2016) trauma-informed care best practices and protocols for Ohio's domestic violence programs. Ohio Domestic Violence Network, Columbus
Forest S, Risk I, Masters H, Brown N (2000) Mental health service user involvement in nurse education: exploring the issues. J Psychiatr Ment Health Nurs 7:51–57
Franks R (2016) Building a trauma-informed system of care for children in connecticut Retrieved November 14th 2016) http://www.governor.ct.gov/malloy/lib/malloy/SHAC_Doc_2013.04.26_Franks_presentation.pdf
Gallop R, McCay E, Guha M, Khan P (1999) The experience of hospitalization and restraint of women who have a history of childhood sexual abuse. Health Care Women Int 20(4):401–416
Glasser W (1999) Choice theory: a new psychology of personal freedom. Harper, New York
Grella CE, Stein JA, Greenwell L (2005) Associations among childhood trauma, adolescent problem behaviors, and adverse adult outcomes in substance-abusing women offenders. Psychol Addict Behav 19(1):43–53
Green BL, Miranda J, Daroowalla A, Juned S (2005) Exposure, mental health functioning, and program needs of Women in jail. Crime Delinq 51(1):133–151

Greene GJ, Lee MY, Hoffpauir S (2005) The languages of empowerment and strengths in clinical social work: a constructivist perspective. Fam Soc 86(2):267–277
Grenard JL, Ames SL, Wiers R, Thush C, Stacy A, Sussman S (2007) Brief intervention for substance abuse among at-risk adolescents: a pilot study. J Adolesc Health 40:188–191
Guitierres SE, Van Puymbroeck C (2006) Childhood and adult violence in the lives of women who misuse substances. Aggress Violent Behav 11(5:497–513
Hammersley P, Read J, Woodall S, Dillon J (2007) Childhood trauma and psychosis: the genie is out of the bottle. J Psychol Trauma 6(2/3):7–20
Harris M, Fallot R (2001) Using trauma theory to design service systems: new directions for mental health services. Jossey Bass, New York
Heath DB (2001) Culture and substance abuse. Psychiatr Clin N Am 24(3:1479–1496
Heim C, Nemeroff CB (2001) The role of childhood trauma in the neurobiology of mood and anxiety disorders: preclinical and clinical studies. Biol Psychiatry 49(12):1023–1039
Heim C, Nemeroff C (2002) Neurobiology of early life stress: clinical studies. Semin Clin Neuropsychiatry 7(2):147–159
Hipolito E, Samuels-Dennis JA, Shanmuganandapala B, Maddoux J, Paulson R, Saugh D, Carahan B (2014) Trauma-informed care: accounting for the interconnected role of spirituality and empowerment in mental health promotion. J Spiritual Ment Health 16:193–217
Holmes D, Kennedy SL, Perron A (2004) The mentally ill and social exclusion: a critical examination of the use of seclusion from the patient's perspective. Issues Ment Health Nurs 25(6):559–578
Horigian VE, Lage OG, Szapocznik J (2006) Cultural differences in adolescent drug abuse. Adolesc Med Clin 17(2):469–498
Hummer VL, Dollard N, Robst J, Armstrong MI (2010) Innovations in implementation of trauma-informed care practices in youth residential treatment: a curriculum for organizational change. Child Welfare 89(2):79–95
Jennings A (2008) Models for developing trauma-informed behavioral health systems and trauma specific services: an update of the 2004 Report. Retrieved from http://transformation-center.org/wp-content/uploads/2012/06/Trauma-Model-update-2007.pdf
Johnson DM, Zlotnick C (2007) Utilization of mental health treatment and other services by battered women in shelters. Psychiatr Serv 58(12):1595–1597
Kezelman C, Stavropoulos P (2012) Practice guidelines for treatment of complex trauma and trauma informed care and service delivery. Adults Surviving Child Abuse, Kirribilli
Klinic Community Health Clinic (2013) Trauma-informed the trauma toolkit: a resource for service organizations and providers to deliver services that are trauma-informed. Retrieved 14th Nov. 2016 http://trauma-informed.ca/wp-content/uploads/2013/10/Trauma-informed_Toolkit.pdf
Larius RA, Vermetten E, Pain C (2010) The impact of early life on health and disease: the hidden epidemic. Cambridge University Press, Cambridge
Larue C, Dumais A, Boyer R, Goulet M, Bonin J, Baba N (2013) The experience of seclusion and restraint in psychiatric settings: perspectives of patients. Issues Ment Health Nurs 34(5):317–324
Levine PA (1997) Waking the tiger: healing trauma. North Atlantic Books, Berkley
Lombardi EL, van Servellen G (2000) Building culturally sensitive substance use prevention and treatment programs for transgendered populations. J Subst Abus Treat 19(3):291–296
Lowe M, Balfour B (2015) The unheard victims. Psychologist 28(2):118–121
McAllister M, Creedy D, Moyle W, Farrugia C (2002) Nurses' attitudes towards clients who self-harm. J Adv Nurs 40:578–586
Manthey TJ, Knowles B, Asher D, Wahab S (2011) Strengths-based practice and motivational interviewing. Adv Soc Work 12(2):126–151
Mende M (2010) Basic emotional needs: a key concept in the assessment and treatment of trauma. Contemp Hypn 27(2):95–102
Mitchell AM, O'Connor TG (2013) Adverse childhood experiences; translating knowledge into identification of children at risk for poor outcomes. Acad Pediatr 13(1):14–19

Molnar BE, Buka SL, Kessler RC (2001) Child sexual abuse and subsequent psychopathology: results from the National Comorbidity Survey. Am J Public Health 91(5):753–760
Murphy-Parker D, Martinez R (2001) Nursing perspectives of global substance abuse and misuse: US and UK differences. Drug Alcohol Prof 1(1):35–44
Muskett C (2014) Trauma-informed care in inpatient mental health settings: a review of the literature. Int J Ment Health Nurs 23(1):51–59
National Institute for Health and Care Excellence (2005). Post-traumatic stress disorder: management. Retrieved from https://www.nice.org.uk/guidance/cg26
National Child Traumatic Stress Network (2016) Making the connection: trauma and substance abuse. Retrieved from http://nctsnet.org/nctsn_assets/pdfs/SAToolkit_1.pdf
Nelson C (2011) Neural development and lifelong plasticity. In: Keating D (ed) Nature and nurture in early child development. Cambridge University Press, New York, pp 45–69
Perry BD, Pollard RA, Blakley TL, Baker WL, Vigilante D (1995) Childhood trauma, the neurobiology of adaptation, and "use-dependent" development of the brain: how "states" become "traits.". Infant Men Health J 6(4):271–291
Rapp RC (2006) Strengths-based case management: enhancing treatment for persons with substance abuse problems. In: Saleebey D (ed) The strengths perspective in social work practice, 4th edn. Pearson Education, Inc., Boston, pp 128–147
Reeves E (2015) A synthesis of the literature on trauma-informed care. Issues Ment Health Nurs 36:698–709
Roxburgh A, Degenhardt L, Copeland J (2006) Posttraumatic stress disorder among female street-based sex workers in the greater Sydney area, Australia. BMC Psychiatry 6:24–24
Rutter D, Manley C, Weaver T, Crawford MJ, Fulup N (2004) Patients or partners? Case studies of user involvement in the planning and delivery of adult mental health services in London. Soc Sci Med 58(10):1973–1984
Saakvitne KW, Gamble S, Pearlman L, Lev B (2000) Risking connection: a training curriculum for working with survivors of childhood abuse. Sidran Press, Lutherville
Saunders BE, Adams ZW (2014) Epidemiology of traumatic experiences in childhood. Child Adolesc Psychiatr Clin N Am 23(2):167–184
Shonkoff JP, Boyce WT, McEwan BS (2009) Neuroscience, molecular biology, and the childhood roots of health disparities: building a new framework for health promotion and disease prevention. JAMA 301(21):2252–2259
Simpson EL, House AO (2002) Involving users in the delivery and evaluation of mental health services: systematic review. BMJ 325:1265
Simpson TJ, Miller WR (2002) Concomitance between childhood sexual and physical abuse and substance use problems: a review. Clin Psychol Rev 22(1):27–77
Simpson A, Reynolds L, Light I, Attenborough J (2008) Talking with the experts: evaluation of an online discussion forum involving mental health service users in the education of mental health nursing students. Nurse Educ Today 28(5):633–640
Smith E (2004) Nowhere to turn? Responding to partner violence against immigrant and visible minority women. Canadian Council on Social Development, Ottawa
Society for the Study of Addiction: St, Georges London (2014) Communication and substance misuse. Retrieved from https://www.addiction-ssa.org/images/uploads/Clin_111_Communication_treat.pdf
(The) Stella Project (2007) Domestic violence, drugs and alcohol: good practice guidelines (2nd edition)
Substance Abuse and Mental Health Services Administration (2009) Strengths-based case management for substance abuse. Center for Substance Abuse Treatment (CSAT); Substance Abuse and Mental Health Services Administration (SAMHSA), Rockville
Substance Abuse and Mental Health Services Administration (2014a) Concept of trauma and guidance for a trauma-informed approach: SAMHSA trauma and justice strategic initiative (July 2014). Retrieved Nov. 14th 2016 http://store.samhsa.gov/shin/content/SMA14-4884/SMA14-4884.pdf
Substance Abuse and Mental Health Services Administration (2014b). SAMHSA's concept of trauma and guidance for a trauma-informed approach. Retrieved from http://store.samhsa.gov/shin/content/SMA14-4884/SMA14-4884.pdf

Substance Abuse and Mental Health Services Administration (2015). Trauma-informed approach and trauma-specific interventions. Retrieved from http://www.samhsa.gov/nctic/trauma-interventions

Sypniewski RL (2016) Increasing the awareness of trauma informed care in the school setting: giving practitioners the tools to actively participate in trauma related care. Doctor of Nursing Practice Thesis, University of San Francisco. Retrieved from http://repository.usfca.edu/cgi/viewcontent.cgi?article=1083&context=dnp

Tait L, Lester H (2005) Encouraging user involvement in mental health services. Adv Psychiatr 11(3):168–175

Teicher MH (2000) Wounds that time wouldn't heal: the neurobiology of childhood abuse. Cerebrum 2:50–67

Teicher MH, Ito Y, Glod CA, Schiffer F, Ackerman E (1994) Possible effects of early abuse on human brain development, as assessed by EEG coherence. Am J Neuropsychopharmacol 33:52

Teicher MH, Ito Y, Glod CA, Andersen SL, Dumont N, Ackerman E (1997) Preliminary evidence for abnormal cortical development in physically and sexually abused children using EEG coherence and MRI. Ann N Y Acad Sci J 821:160–175

Teicher MH, Andersen SL, Polcari A, Anderson CM, Navalta CP (2002) Developmental neurobiology of childhood stress and trauma. Psychiatr Clin N Am 25:397–426

United Nations Office on Drugs and Crime. Substance Abuse Treatment and Care for Women (2004) Case studies and lessons learned. Drug abuse treatment toolkit. Retrieved Nov. 14th 2016 www.unodc.org/pdf/report_2004-08-30_1.pdf

United States Department of Veterans Affairs: PTSD National Center for PTSD (recovered October 2016) PTSD and problems with alcohol use. Retrieved from http://www.ptsd.va.gov/public/problems/ptsd-alcohol-use.asp

Weich S, Patterson J, Shaw R, Stewart-Brown S (2009) Family relationships in childhood and common psychiatric disorders in later life: systematic review of prospective studies. Br J Psychiatry 194(5):392–398

World Health Organization (2013) European report on preventing child maltreatment. Retrieved from http://www.euro.who.int/__data/assets/pdf_file/0019/217018/European-Report-on-Preventing-Child-Maltreatment.pdf

World Health Organisation (recovered 2016, 3rd October) The global burden WHO management of substance abuse. http://www.who.int/substance_abuse/facts/global_burden/en/

Yehuda R, LeDoux J (2007) Response variation following trauma: a translational neuroscience approach to understanding PTSD. Neuron 56(1):19–32

Competences for Clinical Supervision in Psychiatric/Mental Health Nursing

10

John R. Cutcliffe and Graham Sloan

10.1 Introduction

The term clinical supervision (CS) and its use in nursing contexts date as far back as the 1920s (Burns 1958). It is documented that Florence Nightingale encouraged the supervision of junior nurses by more senior nurses to improve their practical skills (Abel-Smith 1960). Nurse scholars from North America have written about CS since the 1920s with the areas of psychiatric nursing and nurse therapists having the most developed bodies of work (see, e.g. Benfer 1979; Critchley 1987; Day 1925; Farkas-Cameron 1995; Freeman 1952; Muecke 1970; Schmidt 1926; Termini and Hauser 1973; Wolf 1941). Nevertheless, it is only in the comparatively recent past that an interest in formalising CS in nursing has grown. There is now an extensive literature on CS in nursing.

Many of the popular publications, particularly throughout the 1990s, regularly featured articles on CS. The scholarly journals provide a platform for useful debate amongst clinicians, educators, researchers and administrators/managers. A sizeable portion of this literature offers some insight into the ways in which CS has been implemented into a range of clinical settings. But while its implementation appears

J.R. Cutcliffe
Cutcliffe Consulting, Kingston, Canada

School of Nursing, Coimbra, Portugal
e-mail: jcutcliffe@outlook.com

G. Sloan (✉)
Consultant Nurse in Psychological Therapies, Psychological Services,
NHS Ayrshire and Arran, Ayr, Scotland, UK

Psychological Therapies Training Coordinator, NHS Education for Scotland,
NHS Ayrshire and Arran, Ayr, Scotland, UK
e-mail: graham.sloan@aapct.scot.nhs.uk

© Springer International Publishing Switzerland 2018

J.C. Santos, J.R. Cutcliffe (eds.), *European Psychiatric/Mental Health Nursing in the 21st Century*, Principles of Specialty Nursing,
https://doi.org/10.1007/978-3-319-31772-4_10

to be widespread in certain clinical specialty areas (e.g. mental health) and certain countries (Clough 2001; Spence et al. 2002), significant proportions of nurses claim never to have received CS (Davey et al. 2006). Despite its history and breadth of implementation, perhaps it is of surprise that formalised training, competences appropriate to CS and accreditation processes for clinical supervisors in nursing are lacking. In the majority of health-care organisations throughout the UK, for example, no formal qualifications or training are necessarily expected of clinical supervisors (Sloan and Fleming 2011). Presently there are no formalised competences for CS in nursing, nor is there an accreditation process for clinical supervisors in nursing (Lynch et al. 2008; Sloan 2008).

As an attempt to help remedy this situation, this chapter endeavours to stimulate discussion on the value of a minimum competency framework for CS in nursing which would have international relevance and acceptability. Following a systematic literature review, recommendations for specific competences and an associated competency framework are proposed. A number of discussion points and implications arising out of this review and the proposed competency framework are then presented. It is hoped that in the near future, consensus will be established on a formalised competency framework for clinical supervision in nursing.

10.2 Data Sources

A comprehensive search of the literature on CS published from 1996 to 2012 was conducted. Keywords to locate literature on computerised databases—CINAHL, Medline, Psychlit and the British Nursing Index—included CS (610), competences (488), competence (777), nursing (45846) and skills (3531), combining CS with competences and nursing (2); CS competence and nursing (0); CS, nursing and skills (11); and good characteristics (1). Reference lists in the limited literature sourced were also scrutinised for any potentially unlisted or inaccessible sources. A manual scrutiny of textbooks was also conducted to ensure that sources not listed in the computerised databases of journal articles were not overlooked. In an effort to be as comprehensive as possible with our review, the authors also reviewed clinical supervision literature that while originating in related disciplinary areas that are 'outside' of nursing, nurses and nursing had nevertheless endorsed or embraced this literature.

10.3 A Framework for Organising the Findings: Knowledge, Attitudes and Skills

Even a cursory review of the relevant literature will indicate that one of the most common educational frameworks of learning objectives is that of the so-called knowledge, attitudes and skills approach (Bloom et al. 1956). While recognising it's vintage, and some would argue seminal contribution, this framework (and/or others based upon this work) can be found with conspicuous regularity underpinning the curricula of various interpersonally focused disciplines such as psychiatric/mental health nursing, counselling/psychotherapy and general nursing (NMC 2012a; New Zealand 2012b). Perhaps surprisingly, it can also be located in the educational literature of other disciplines such as design and architecture (Bakarman 2004). Given the interpersonal nature of CS and its commonality and congruence with other educational endeavours designed to prepare people for interpersonal focused work (such as nursing, psychology, psychotherapy, social work, etc.), it is logical to organise the findings from our review of the literature according to the knowledge, attitudes and skills framework. Indeed, the authors of this paper contend that it is axiomatic to regard CS training/preparation/education as more than merely the acquisition of knowledge or the refinement of certain skills. However, before so doing, it is necessary to examine Bloom's framework in more detail.

Bloom et al.'s (1956) Taxonomy of Learning Domains identifies three types of learning: cognitive or 'mental' skills, otherwise referred to as k*nowledge*; affective skills whereby there is consideration of growth in feelings or emotional areas, otherwise referred to as a*ttitude*; and psychomotor, manual and physical skills, otherwise referred to as s*kills.* Bloom argued that these learning behaviours can be thought of as the goals of a learning process, and accordingly any effective learning experience can/should result in changes in the 'learner's' knowledge, attitudes and/or skills. Bloom et al. (1956) went further to identify subcategories for each of these three domains. For the cognitive domain, he lists knowledge, comprehension, application, analysis, synthesis and evaluation. Further, Bloom et al. (1956) posited these phenomena in a linear hierarchy, suggesting that knowledge (e.g. the ability to recall facts) is the easiest to acquire in the cognitive domain and evaluation the most difficult. For the affective domain, he lists receiving phenomena, responding to phenomena, valuing, organisation, internalising values (characterisation) and instructional objectives. For the psychomotor domain, he lists perception, set, guided response, mechanism, complex overt response, adaptation and origination.

10.4 Findings

Our review identified a number of specific knowledge, attitudes and skills, and we have collated these into Tables 10.1, 10.2, and 10.3.

Perhaps not surprisingly, there was substantial evidence of 'overlap' or repletion of competencies between literatures; in some cases, the same (or equivalent) competencies were located in many different papers. The other literature reviewed underscored the need for supervisor competencies without distinguishing individual or specific knowledge, attitude or skills.

Arvidsson and Fridlund (2005), for example, reported findings on a study which used the critical incident technique with 25 nurse supervisors, to identify factors that are thought to influence the competency of nurse supervisors. Two main areas were identified: a professional stance and a personal stance. In the professional stance, there were four subcategories: the supervisor creates a secure learning environment, the supervisor facilitates reflection, the supervisor underlines the importance of structure, and the supervisor creates awareness of fundamental nursing values. The personal category included two subcategories: the supervisor expresses doubts regarding her/his own performance as supervisor and the supervisor expresses security regarding her/his own performance as supervisor. Arvidsson and Fridlund (2005) argued that in order for the CS to be effective, supervisors need

Table 10.1 Clinical supervision competencies—knowledge

Knowledge of educational principles which can be applied in supervision
Knowledge of the context within which supervision is provided (including relevant professional, ethical and legal frameworks)
Understanding of the ways in which professional and ethical issues are represented in supervision (e.g. managing boundaries, confidentiality, managing power differentials)
Understanding of issues of difference and diversity in supervision and how these relate both to supervision itself and to the discussion of casework
Knowledge to help supervisees identify the relevance of difference to their practice and to integrate this thinking into their work
Understanding of the importance of a safe environment for facilitating learning and of the factors that affect the development and maintenance of a good supervisory relationship
Knowledge in establishing a professional framework for supervision and in contracting and negotiating boundaries
Knowledge and skills in helping supervisees identify relevant content and to present clinical material
Knowledge of techniques and processes to evaluate supervision, including eliciting feedback
Knowledge of potential sources of bias in evaluation
Knowledge and skills in specifying and applying criteria for gauging competency
Knowledge of relevant criteria/standards set by professional bodies, including assessment procedures relevant to different levels of qualification
Knowledge and skills relevant to supporting the administration and interpretation of objective measures
Knowledge and skills to integrate feedback from objective measures into supervision
Awareness of any limitations in their own training and experience, in the development of supervisory skills and the implications of these for further training
Knowledge and skills to help the supervisee practice specific clinical skills within supervision
Knowledge and skills to make effective use of audio/video recordings and to use in-session direct observation
Knowledge and skills to structure group supervision and to manage group process appropriately
Knowledge of procedures relevant to the assessment of poor performance and failure
Knowledge to help supervisees manage caseload and deliver interventions efficiently
Knowledge to structure supervision sessions
Knowledge to support routine outcome monitoring
Knowledge of the importance of structure in CS, theoretical models, formats, the underpinning philosophy and purpose of CS (and what it is not!), stages of relationship formation and how to form therapeutic working alliances
Knowledge of and about the purpose(s) of CS
Knowledge about clear boundaries of supervision
Knowledge about the management, educative and supportive functions/practices of CS
Knowledge about the various types of contracts in CS
Knowledge of group dynamics
Knowledge of individual and group formats of delivery of CS
Knowledge and skills relevant to certain models/frameworks for CS
Knowledge of ethical challenges, ethical dilemmas and ultimately ethical practice in CS
Knowledge of the necessity, value and centrality of the supervisory relationship
Knowledge pertaining to the importance and practice(s) of evaluating CS
Knowledge of problem-solving frameworks and their associated skills
Knowledge of force field analysis, experiential learning cycles and skills assessment cycles

Table 10.2 Clinical supervision competencies—attitudes (qualities)

Compassion
Supportive
Confirming
Humility
Warmth
Willingness and preparedness to show understanding
Genuineness
Willingness to be open about one's own feelings
A spirit of generosity
A willingness to look for, recognise and acknowledge/reward the successes and ability of the supervisee
A willingness to be open
A willingness to remain open to learning and a corresponding recognition that even though the CS should be focused on the supervisee, there is still a reciprocal learning opportunity for the supervisor
A willingness to be caring (to allow one's humanity to come through)
Respectful—including respecting the opinions of others
Commitment to ongoing (lifelong) development
Commitment to receiving one's own supervision
Committed to updating own practitioner and supervisory skills/knowledge
Committed to the role of supervisor
Comfortable with the authority inherent in the role of supervisor
Appropriate optimism
Sensitivity to supervisee's needs
Sensitivity to individual differences and nuances

(additional) knowledge of relevant theory and an awareness of their own shortcomings coupled with a willingness to acknowledge this.

A small body of work can be located that speaks to the characteristics of a 'good' supervisor. Research conducted in North America (Pesut and Williams 1990), adopting a survey method, focused on the supervisor's perspective. Clinical nurse specialists working in mental health settings require specific knowledge and skills in order to give specific ideas about interventions, provide feedback on performance, create a warm and supportive relationship and promote autonomy. In so doing, for the participants in Pesut and Williams's (1990) study, the supervisor is subsequently regarded as competent and is engaging in 'good' supervision.

Similarly, Severinsson and Hallberg (1996) investigated 18 clinical nurse supervisor's views of their supervisory styles, their personal qualities and their leadership role and the development of these styles. Personal qualities, regarded by these participants, included a willingness and preparedness to show understanding, bringing out genuine feelings and confirming. Confirming was reported as the most important aspect.

Researchers in the UK have also investigated the desirable characteristics of the clinical supervisor by focusing on the supervisee's perspective. Using a combination of quantitative and qualitative methods, Fowler (1995) explored the supervisee's viewpoint of the characteristics of a good clinical supervisor. During the first stage of his study, Fowler employed a questionnaire to 'tease out' issues relating to the supervisor/supervisee relationship. Stage 2 focused on clarifying and

Table 10.3 Clinical supervision competencies—skills

Skills to help supervisees identify the relevance of difference to their practice and to integrate this thinking into their work
Ability to adapt the supervision to the organisational setting in which the supervisee works
Skills and experience in developing and maintaining a supervisory alliance
Skills in establishing a professional framework for supervision and in contracting and negotiating boundaries
Skills in helping supervisees identify relevant content and to present clinical material
Techniques and processes to evaluate supervision, including eliciting feedback
Skills in giving constructive but accurate feedback
Skills in using a range of methods to gain information and give feedback (e.g. self-report, audio and video tapes, colleague and client reports)
Skills relevant to supporting the administration and interpretation of objective measures
Skills to integrate feedback from objective measures into supervision
Skills to help the supervisee practice specific clinical skills within supervision
Skills to make effective use of audio/video recordings and to use in-session direct observation.
Skills to structure group supervision and to manage group process appropriately
Skills to help supervisees manage caseload and deliver interventions efficiently
Skills to support routine outcome monitoring
Skills to structure supervision sessions
Skills to support routine outcome monitoring
Ability to create a secure learning environment
Ability to facilitate and promote reflection in the supervisee
Ability to facilitate and promote self-awareness
Ability to form and maintain an effective supervisory relationship
Ability to give constructive feedback on performance
Ability to promote practitioner autonomy
Ability to hold off being too prescriptive and supervisor—as an expert—let the supervisee find his/her own solutions
Good interpersonal communication skills
Good listening skills
Ability to function as an appropriate role model
Clinically competent in the clinical interventions being supervised
Ability to be thoughtful and thought provoking
Ability to create a trusting environment
Ability to explain the purpose of CS to supervisees
Ability to negotiate a clear and mutually agreed contract
Ability to maintain appropriate boundaries
Ability to set (create) an atmosphere, that is, empathic, genuine, congruent, trustworthy and immediate
Ability to maintain a balance between the managerial, supportive and educative functions of CS
Ability to end a CS session on time and appropriately
Ability to use the following types of intervention: prescriptive, informative, confrontative, cathartic, catalytic and supportive
Ability to give feedback, that is, clear, owned, balanced and specific
Ability to focus on reported content, supervisee's interventions, supervisee/client relationships, supervisee's countertransference, supervision relationship, supervisor's own countertransference
Ability to describe their own way of working
Ability to develop self-supervision skills in supervisees
Ability to collaboratively negotiate a supervision agreement with supervisee
Ability to maintain confidentiality of those issues disclosed during CS

Table 10.3 (continued)

Ability to enable the supervisee to contribute significantly to their supervision
Apply a relevant and useful framework to guide and structure the provision of CS; understand and have the necessary skills to apply the framework
Ability to facilitate the supervisee's reflection on their clinical practice
Ability to evaluate the supervisee's satisfaction with, and usefulness of, the provision of CS
Emotional competencies, emotional skills and emotional literacy

prioritising the characteristics of a good supervisor. A questionnaire based on data from stage 2 was developed (stage 3). In summary, Fowler (1995) informed that good supervisors are knowledgeable and can communicate this knowledge in an understandable way, they discuss their previous knowledge and experience with the student and, in addition to giving criticism, they comment on good practice. Participants in this study identified creating supportive relationships, having the relevant clinical skills and theoretical knowledge and teaching competency as essential characteristics of a good supervisor.

Guided by Fowler's earlier (Fowler 1995) study, Sloan (1999) conducted a descriptive investigation of the characteristics of a good clinical supervisor with staff nurses working in a mental health setting. Sloan (1999) discovered that possessing the ability to form supportive relationships, having relevant knowledge and clinical skills, expressing a commitment to providing CS and having good listening skills were perceived as important characteristics of a 'good' supervisor. These perceptions are consistent with Fowler's (1995) findings.

Prominent in much of the literature identified from the review is the fundamental importance of the supervisory relationship, so much so that it is often cited as being a significant contributor to the experiences of effective supervision. This work accentuates how supervisors require a well-developed skill base in interpersonal relationship formation and maintenance and an understanding of the theory that underpins such actions (see, e.g. Bond and Holland 1998; Chambers and Cutcliffe 2001; Farkas-Cameron 1995; Faugier 1994; Jones 2001; Platt-Koch 1986; Trainor 1978; Sloan 2000). This axiomatic position can be located in many of the existing and significant conceptual frameworks that have been advanced for CS. Faugier (1998), for example, described a growth and support model in an attempt to highlight the purported characteristics of the supervisory relationship. Faugier argued that the role of the supervisor is:

> to facilitate growth and provide essential support to the practice of clinical excellence. (Faugier 1998, p. 25)

According to this model the supervisor needs to possess and communicate certain qualities (in addition to possessing knowledge and skills) in order to facilitate growth in the supervisee (see Tables 10.1, 10.2 and 10.3). Similarly, Proctor's model (Proctor 1987), one of the most frequently cited CS models, at least in UK nursing press (see, e.g. Bartle 2000; Buus and Gonge 2009; Cottrell 2001; Cutcliffe and Proctor 1998; Davey et al. 2006; Faugier and Butterworth 1994; Jones 1995), highlights a variety of supervisor competencies. Supervisors can focus on all or any one of three functions. In nursing's adoption of this model, the *formative* function is concerned with skills development and increasing the supervisee's knowledge; the *normative* function concentrates on managerial issues including the maintenance of professional standards and the *restorative* function is focused on providing support in an attempt to alleviate the stress evoked by doing nursing work. While the original description of the three-function interactive model (Proctor 1987) did not provide any guidance on how a supervisor might operate when working within any of its three functions (Sloan et al. 2000), the supervision alliance model (Proctor 2001) clarifies how supervisors might provide helpful responses when guided by this framework and what knowledge, attitudes and skills are required.

Proctor (2001) highlighted that the supervisor is required to hold (possess) certain values (attitudes). Supervisors need to be enthusiastic (or keen) to work well and are willing to engage in meaningful self-monitoring. Supervisors also need to possess the knowledge and skills to enable them to reflect on experience and practice; similarly they also need to understand (knowledge) that CS is a cooperative enterprise and is distinguished and detached from formal managerial assessment procedures. Proctor also places emphasis on the skills and qualities important to the establishment of an agreement between supervisor and supervisee, given the requirement to create a foundation of a working agreement which is personal and particular. Furthermore, for Proctor, the 'doing' aspect of CS is aided by supervisors having an understanding (knowledge) of the process model of supervision (Hawkins and Shohet 1989), having a familiarity of and fluency with supervisory skills informed by Heron's (2001) six-category intervention analysis framework and the educational practice facilitated by Kolb's learning cycle (Kolb 1984).

In their seminal work, Hawkins and Shohet (1989) described a self-assessment model for supervisors, and this contains reference to (and/or questions regarding) specific knowledge, skills and qualities. While skills and knowledge identified by these authors have subsections, it appears that qualities do not. Another framework taken from psychotherapy and adapted for nursing is the cognitive therapy supervision model (Sloan 2006, 2007; Sloan et al. 2000; Todd and Freshwater 1999). Todd and Freshwater (1999) illustrated the similarities between reflective practice and guided discovery, an important facet of this framework. While it is acknowledged that this approach was devised to help develop the therapeutic competency of cognitive therapists, Sloan et al. (2000) have argued its use in nursing contexts merits consideration. This model differentiates between modes and foci (Padesky 1996). A supervision mode is the means by which supervisee learning and discovery occurs, for example, case discussion, reviewing audio recordings of therapy sessions or the provision of relevant educational material. Consequently, supervisors require an understanding of how to intervene using each of these methods. Additionally, the clinical supervisor requires *knowledge and skills* competency concerning the clinical practice of the supervisee since Padesky's foci include the mastering of new therapeutic skills, conceptualising a client's problems, progressing the therapist's understanding of the client–therapist relationship and working through the therapist's emotional reactions to their clinical work. These modes and foci appear relevant for the practice of CS in nursing where clinical practice has a therapeutic intention and it is recognised that knowledge and skills may develop as a result of practitioners reflecting on their interpersonal relations with clients (Sloan 2007).

As stated previously, our review also included some evidently significant CS textbooks. These were included given the relatively high frequency that they were cited in the other literature reviewed. It is interesting to note that while none of these texts present or expand on particular competencies for CS or offer a formal competency framework for CS in nursing, they each alluded (to a greater or lesser extent) to essential knowledge, attitudes and skills for the effective engagement in CS.

Power (1999, p. 22), for example, lists a range of objectives for CS in nursing. Implied with these objectives are potential competencies which have already been uncovered, for example, supervisors should be able to provide space and enable the supervisee to reflect on their clinical practice, clinical supervisors should understand the principles of adult learning and relevant educational theory to promote supervisee learning, clinical supervisors should be clinically competent in the supervisee's area of practice, and clinical supervisors should be able to initiate and maintain an effective, supportive supervisory relationship.

In Driscoll's (2007) second edition of *Practising Clinical Supervision*, specific standards rather than competencies are highlighted and described by Rafferty, Llewellyn-Davies and Hewitt (Rafferty et al. 2007, p. 219). The provisional standards they suggest include: giving commitment and honouring the time for the task, securing a venue fit for purpose in terms of comfort, privacy, and absence of interruptions, establish a professional working relationship based on mutual trust, attention is given to the expression of professional practice and reflection on its meaning, search for meaning and gathering perspectives driven by empirical knowledge and experience from practice, affirm appropriate practice, support professional esteem and offer achievable challenges to practice based on a secure relationship, provides the necessary will and resources to enable CS, an agreement is reached about the minimum content, ownership and access to any record kept, and use of appropriate authority and recognition of personal and professional boundaries.

The specific contents of Lynch et al.'s (2008) text imply the necessity for a number of potential competencies. They make reference to and give considerable coverage of individual and group formats of delivery of CS (and thus the need for the supervisor to have knowledge of these formats and the requisite skills to operate effectively in both formats), knowledge and skills relevant to certain models/frameworks for CS, ethical practice (which requires a wide range of knowledge, skills and, not least, attitudes) and the supervisory relationship and the importance of evaluating CS.

A further important work which is cited with conspicuous regularity is that of Bond and Holland (1998). Drawing on the work of Heron (1990) and his six-category intervention analysis, Bond and Holland, either directly or implicitly, highlight the need for supervisor competencies. These include knowledge of problem-solving frameworks and their associated skills and more specifically force field analysis, experiential learning cycles and skills assessment cycles. These authors also highlight the need for emotional competencies, emotional skills and emotional literacy and draw particular attention to the need to have self-awareness and thus the skills, knowledge and attitudes associated with perpetual growth in awareness. Significant sections of Bond and Holland's (1998) book are dedicated to specific interpersonal skills and cite the seminal work of Heron (1990).

Heron's framework has been adopted as a supervision framework in nursing (see, e.g. Chambers and Long 1995; Cutcliffe and Epling 1997; Driscoll 2000; Fowler 1996; Johns and Butcher 1993). The six-category system describes six basic kinds of intention a supervisor can have when working with a supervisee. Prescriptive interventions seek to influence and direct the behaviour of the supervisee and include offering advice and making suggestions. To be informative is to offer information or instruction. Confronting interventions directly challenge the rigid and maladaptive ways that limit the supervisee. A confronting intervention tells an uncomfortable truth 'but does so with love, in order that the client concerned may see it and fully acknowledge it' (Heron 1989, p. 45). Cathartic interventions assist the client to abreact painful emotion, for example, grief, fear and anger. Catalytic interventions include encouraging further self-exploration, self-directed living, learning and problem solving in the client. Lastly, to be supportive is to validate or confirm the worth of the client's person, qualities, attitudes or actions.

10.5 Discussion and Implications

As a result of this systematic review of the extant literature, several points for discussion arise and these are listed, in no order of priority (necessarily), in Table 10.4.

Discussion Point 1 The current absence of evidence of a broad consensus regarding the competencies required for clinical supervision.

While there are some commonalities with other interpersonal focused activities and disciplines/professions, there appears to be a growing consensus that there is a specific skill set for CS, though it is important to note that there is currently no consensus on what these are. Indeed in the literature reviewed, the authors could not locate a single text which made the argument that CS does NOT have a unique competency base. It is also noteworthy that some attempts have been made to form or reach some degree of consensus regarding CS competencies within certain

Table 10.4 Points for discussion arising from our systematic review

1. While there appears to be some degree of similarity between the required CS competences advanced by various authors, there is no evidence of broad consensus. Accordingly, the need for some wide-scale research is indicated, perhaps a Delphi study to determine the current extent of the consensus
2. The lack of current consensus appears to be, at least in part, as a result of competencies being advanced for radically different degrees in (or of) clinical supervisor (and supervisee) training/preparation; we appear to be attempting to compare, metaphorically speaking, 'apples with oranges'
3. CS education/training must include attention to the acquisition and/or development or required qualities in addition to skills and knowledge

disciplines or specific domains of practice. See, for example, Roth and Pilling's (2008) competency framework developed for the supervision of psychological therapies which was commissioned by the Care Services Improvement Partnership (CSIP), Skills for Health and NHS Education for Scotland (NES) and the Scottish Government (NES and Scottish Government 2008). The generic supervision competences were developed following a comprehensive review of the psychological therapies' supervision literature in addition to those books and papers viewed as authoritative by professional groups (Roth and Pilling 2008).

Our review also found noticeable overlap and/or repetition of (and/or very closely conceptually related) certain knowledge, attitudes and skills across different authors. By way of an example, several authors made specific reference to knowledge, attitudes and skills related to or concerning the purpose of CS and how this varies according to specific theories/models/approaches. In one such case, broad generic competencies (e.g. 'knowledge of and about the purpose(s) of CS') seems to have a high degree of congruence with introductory-level courses as there is only time/space to offer overviews rather than in-depth, detailed material. Perhaps a more detailed version of the same competencies is the example, 'Knowledge about the management, educative and supportive functions/practices of CS', and this lends itself to a longer, more intensive course/training/preparation. More detailed still and ergo, more fitting with even more intensive, detailed and comprehensive training/courses/preparation is the competency 'Knowledge of: the importance of structure in CS, theoretical models, formats, the underpinning philosophy and purpose of CS (and what it is not!), stages of relationship formation, and how to form therapeutic working alliances'. Accordingly, the authors wish to advance that there are core or basic (entry level?) competencies in CS and at least (probably more) one other 'advanced, specialist' level of competencies. This is hardly surprising given the different levels of degree of training/education in CS and given this corollary with other interpersonally focused health-orientated disciplinary competencies.

Discussion Point 2 The competencies being advanced for radically different degrees in (or of) clinical supervisor (and supervisee) training/preparation.

The findings from our review and related writings found in a recent CS publication illustrate how there is no apparent consensus in the literature as to what is required to prepare practitioners (adequately) to become supervisors (or supervisees). Currently the preparation of supervisors/supervisees for their role(s) within CS varies from no preparation at all (Milne 2009) to in-depth postgraduate-level studies (Sloan and Fleming 2011). While not wishing necessarily to homogenise preparation in/for CS, evidently, this wide variation also tolerates, if not actually encourages, similar variation in curricula (course) content and corresponding differences in emphasis vis-à-vis competency acquisition. Intuitively, it seems logical that there is a relationship between the quality of the CS preparation experience, the focus within the said curricula on competencies and the resultant efficacy of CS subsequently offered by the practitioner. On a related note, in addition to the well-versed argument regarding improvements in CS resulting from experiential learning (e.g. experiential learning as one means to acquire and refine competencies), it seems likely that very short CS preparation courses (with little or no attention to competency acquisition) are very unlikely to produce well-prepared, highly effective supervisors. While the authors acknowledge that this is a somewhat simplistic proposition and the efficacy of the preparation will clearly be influenced by a range of variables, there exists some evidence that supports this proposition (Butterworth et al. 1997).

Now this is not to suggest that there is no utility or value in 1 day workshops on CS. The authors are aware that such educational experience can 'whet the appetite' for more, can provide a brief though interesting glimpse into the world of CS, and can help dispel some of the more common miscomprehensions and misunderstandings. Yet we would argue, and the limited evidence would appear to support our view, that such 1-day workshops are not sufficient to expose would-be supervisors to the wide range of (possibly) required competencies, let alone provide sufficient time and 'space' for competency practice and refinement.

Perhaps what is necessary is a range of CS preparatory 'courses' of different sizes, lengths and intensities, aimed at different groups and with different emphasis on competencies. Drawing on Bloom et al.'s[1] work once more, he described so-called 'higher-level' thinking skills and, importantly, such higher-level thinking skills require prior learning (acquisition) of basic skills, which, according to Bloom, are then integrated into higher-order skills. Further, Bloom declared that skills at different levels must be taught (and evaluated) in different ways. Such central tenets then indicate that CS course designers and instructors need to take these differences into account when considering how competencies are to be covered, acquired and refined in preparatory courses. As a result, if one accepts the cogency of Bloom's position and applies these tenets to CS courses/preparation and training, then there is a strong pedagogical case for having a range of different CS 'courses', some focused on 'basic competencies and others on 'higher level CS competencies'.

There are additional pedagogical lessons and rationales to support the argument for having a range of 'courses' when one considers related (specialist) clinical practices and the different courses available to practitioners. To draw on the example of courses for (in) cognitive behavioural therapy, introductory 'in-house' overviews and study days, short courses and full-time masters' level courses at university are available. While no doubt each deserving of merit, and each serving a particular purpose, the authors sincerely doubt that the recipient of an in-house study day or short course would claim to be proficient[2] as a cognitive behavioural therapist.

The authors are also mindful, particularly in the post-2009 international economic 'meltdown', that any consideration of providing education/training in/for CS will inevitably have to be cognizant of the costs. Interestingly, the costs associated with providing adequate and appropriate training/education in CS were mentioned with conspicuous regularity during the 1990s (see, e.g. Smith 1995). However, the authors would caution against possible shortcuts in CS preparation, expecting disproportionate outcomes and competency acquisition/refinement to financial support and course length. Furthermore, the authors wish to advance the argument that it is a false

[1] And the many fine scholarly works that this original work spawned.

[2] And the authors would argue—safe.

economy to 'shortcut' on CS preparation when there is evidence, albeit limited in scope, size and validity, that shows how receiving high-quality CS can have a positive contribution to well-being (e.g. recipients of CS have lower burnout scores, depersonalisation scores, lower sickness (absence) rates, etc.).[3] Organisations therefore need to be thoughtful about allocating their limited training budgets to CS preparation, perhaps designing strategic plans to provide different courses to different practitioners. That is, while in an ideal world it may be advantageous to provide intensive CS preparation that fully equips supervisors with all the competencies, this is likely to be cost prohibitive, and thus offering a combination of courses to 'train the trainers' and introductory workshops might be a more realistic proposition.

Discussion Point 3 CS education/training must include attention to the acquisition and/or development or required qualities in addition to skills and knowledge.

Competency-based education (and training) is now fairly commonplace in nursing, clinical psychology and counselling/psychotherapy programmes (Arema and McCoy 2010; Catano et al. 2007; Manring et al. 2003; Mulholland 1994). Given the not insubstantial conceptual and practice overlap between CS and the above-listed disciplines, it is perhaps not surprising that a competency-based approach to education and training in CS is starting to emerge (see, e.g. Bagnall et al. 2011; Roth and Pilling 2008). While competency-based education cannot claim to be a unified or homogenised educational approach given the variety of extant conceptualisations in the literature (see, e.g. Arema and McCoy 2010), there is some agreement that the characteristics of competency-based learning include acquisition of essential cognitive, psychomotor and affective skills (Arema and McCoy 2010). The authors of this paper advance the view that some affective skills are clearly related to qualities in the individual. The etymological origins of the word *competent* shed further light on the conceptual similarity of affective skills and qualities as the original Latin word 'competent' means *having essential qualities and abilities to function in specific ways.*

In addition, our review of the extant literature revealed a range of qualities that have been posited as competencies necessary for effective, comprehensive, compassionate and robust CS practice (see Tables 10.1 and 10.3) Accordingly, CS competency training/education must include attention to fostering and developing appropriate qualities in the supervisor. In the absence of this attention, aspirant supervisors acquire only relevant knowledge and particular skills. This has the potential to create CS encounters and interactions that, while maybe technically competent, are devoid of the required, underpinning qualities/attitudes.

By way of an example, demonstrating and communicating an empathic 'felt sense' of the supervisees' difficulty(ies) is often posited as an important element of supervision (see, e.g. Sloan 2006). The literature, both that of a recognised vintage and more contemporary, is clear in pointing out how individuals have different innate levels of empathy or 'empathic maturity' (Carkhuff and Traux 1965; Connor 1994; Cutcliffe and Cassedy 1998; Olsen 2001; Rogers 1975). Further, while equipping supervisors with the technical skills to communicate empathy is an appropriate

[3] Please see Cutcliffe et al. (2011) for a comprehensive review of this evidence.

competency to include, focusing only on skills and knowledge can create a situation where supervisors are able to communicate a feeling (empathy) that they are not necessarily feeling; the skills have no grounding in attitude/quality (Cutcliffe and Cassedy 1998). Bearing in mind the documented need for genuineness or realness in CS (interestingly, another quality) and how such a quality is compromised when practitioners do not possess the affective component or sensitivities that need to underpin the technical skill, the case for ensuring CS education/training incorporates the development of certain required qualities becomes clear.

Conclusion

It is noteworthy that nursing has been remised in establishing a suitable and professionally relevant competency framework for CS in nursing. Arguably the absence of a competency framework with explicit knowledge, attitudes and skills fundamental to the engagement in effective CS has had some contribution to the less than satisfactory outcomes relating to CS in previous research. The authors hope that this paper stimulates debate on the fundamental intention of CS for nursing, and in particular, the guidance a competency framework would offer those engaged in CS (clinical supervisors and supervisees), those providing educational preparation for its participants and to some extent, what process variables evaluators/researchers could measure when investigating outcomes derived from CS. Following on from this, nursing may be able to establish accreditation criteria for clinical supervisors.

Box 10.1 Recommended Reading on Clinical Supervision

Cutcliffe, J.R., Butterworth, T. and Proctor, B. (Eds.) (2001) *Fundamental Themes in Clinical Supervision,* Routledge, London.

(Foreword by Sarah Mullally, Chief Nursing Officer for the UK).

Cutcliffe, J. R., Hyrkas, K., Fowler, J. (2011) *Routledge Handbook of Clinical Supervision: Fundamental International Themes.* Routledge, London.

Hanlon, P., Sloan, G. (2011) Make room for clinical supervision: using an educational DVD resource. *British Journal of Well Being*. 2(3), pp. 27–31.

Lavalette, H., Alexander, J., Gilmour, C., Allan, J., Sloan, G. (2011) Separating clinical and line management supervision in occupational therapy. *British Journal of Well Being*. 2(6), pp. 18–21.

Sloan (1999) Good characteristics of a clinical supervisor: a community mental health nurse perspective *Journal of Advanced Nursing* 30(3), 713–722.

Sloan and Fleming (2011) A literature review of clinical supervision in nursing in the UK. IN: *Routledge Handbook of Clinical Supervision: Global Perspectives on Fundamental Themes—2nd Edition of Fundamental Themes of Clinical Supervision*. Routledge, London.

Sloan and Fleming (2011) Training requirement for clinical supervision in the UK. IN: *Routledge Handbook of Clinical Supervision: Global Perspectives on Fundamental Themes—2nd Edition of Fundamental Themes of Clinical Supervision*. Routledge, London.

Sloan (2006) *Clinical Supervision in Mental Health Nursing*. Wiley & Sons, London.

Acknowledgments This chapter has been reproduced, with kind permission from the publisher. Taylor Francis, from the journal article referenced: Cutcliffe, J.R., & Sloan, G (2014) Towards a consensus of a competency framework for Clinical Supervision in nursing: knowledge, attitudes and skills. *The Clinical Supervisor,* 33(2), 182–203.

References

Abel-Smith B (1960) A history of the nursing profession. Heinemann, London

Anema M, McCoy J (2010) Competency based nursing education: guide to achieving outstanding learner outcomes. Springer, New York

Arvidsson B, Fridlund B (2005) Factors influencing nurse supervisor competence: a critical incident analysis study. J Nurs Manag 13:231–237

Bagnall G, Sloan G, Platz S, Murphy S (2011) NHS education for Scotland training in generic supervision competencies for psychological therapies: pilot course development and evaluation. Ment Health Pract 14(6):18–23

Bakarman AA (2004) Attitude, skill, and knowledge: (ASK) a new model for design education (recovered 2012) http://faculty.ksu.edu.sa/10177/Documents/ASK%20Final%20paper.pdf

Bartle J (2000) Clinical supervision: its place within the quality agenda. Nurs Manag 7(5):30–33

Benfer BA (1979) Clinical supervision as a support system for the care-giver. Perspect Psychiatr Care 17(1):13–17

Bloom B, Englehart M, Furst E, Hill W, Krathwohl D (1956) Taxonomy of educational objectives: the classification of educational goals. Handbook I: cognitive domain. Longmans, Green, New York

Bond M, Holland S (1998) Skills of clinical supervision: a practical guide for supervisees, clinical supervisors and managers. Open University Press, Buckingham

Burns ME (1958) The historical development of the process of casework supervision as seen in the professional literature of social work. Department of Social Work University of Chicago, Chicago

Butterworth T, Carson J, White E, Jeacock J, Clements A, Bishop V (1997) It is good to talk: an evaluation study in England and Scotland. University of Manchester, Manchester

Buus N, Gonge H (2009) Empirical studies of clinical supervision in psychiatric nursing: a systematic literature review and methodological critique. Int J Ment Health Nurs 18(4):250–264

Carkhuff R, Traux C (1965) Training in counselling and psychotherapy: an evaluation of an integrated didactic and experiential approach. J Couns Psychol 29:333–336

Catano V, Darr M, Campbell C (2007) Performance appraisal of behaviour-based competencies: a reliable and valid procedure. Pers Psychol 60:201–230

Chambers M, Cutcliffe J (2001) The dynamics and processes of 'ending' in clinical supervision. Br J Nurs 10(21):1403–1411

Chambers M, Long A (1995) Supportive clinical supervision: a crucible for personal and professional change. J Psychiatr Ment Health Nurs 2(5):311–316

Clough A (2001) Clinical leadership: turning thought into action. Prim Health Care 11(4):39–41

Connor M (1994) Training the counsellor: an integrative model. Routledge, London

Cottrell S (2001) Occupational stress and job satisfaction in mental health nursing: focused interventions through evidence-based assessment. J Psychiatr Ment Health Nurs 8(2):157–164

Critchley DL (1987) Clinical supervision as a learning tool for the therapist in milieu settings. J Psychosoc Nurs 25(8):18–22

Cutcliffe JR, Cassedy P (1998) Empathy, students and the problems of genuineness: can we develop empathy on a short skills-based counselling course? Ment Health Pract 1(9):28–33

Cutcliffe JR, Epling M (1997) An exploration of the use of John Heron's confronting interventions in clinical supervision: case studies from practice. Psychiatr Care 4(4):174–180

Cutcliffe JR, Hyrkas K, Fowler J (2011) Routledge handbook of clinical supervision: fundamental international themes. Routledge, London

Cutcliffe JR, Proctor B (1998) An alternative training approach to clinical supervision: 1. Br J Nurs 7(5):280–285

Davey B, Desousa C, Robinson S, Murrells T (2006) The policy-practice divide: who has CSCS in nursing? J Res Nurs 11(3):237–248

Day GA (1925) Changing competencies of supervision. Mod Hosp 24(5):469–470
Driscoll J (2000) Practising clinical supervision: a reflective approach. Bailliere Tindall, London
Driscoll J (2007) Practising clinical supervision: a reflective approach for health care professionals. Bailliere Tindall, London
Farkas-Cameron MM (1995) Clinical supervision in psychiatric nursing: a self-actualising process. J Psychosoc Nurs Ment Health Serv 33(2):31–37
Faugier J (1994) Thin on the ground. Nurs Times 90(20):64–65
Faugier J (1998) The supervisory relationship. In: Butterworth T, Faugier J, Burnard P (eds) Clinical supervision and mentorship in nursing, 2nd edn. Stanley Thornes, London
Faugier J, Butterworth T (1994) Clinical supervision: a position paper. University of Manchester, Manchester
Fowler J (1995) Nurses perception of the elements of good supervision. Nurs Times 91(22):33–37
Fowler J (1996) Clinical supervision: what do you do after you say hello? Br J Nurs 5(6):382–385
Freeman R (1952) Supervision in the improvement of nursing services. Public Health Nurs 44(7):370–373
Hawkins P, Shohet R (1989) Supervision in the helping professions. Open University Press, Milton Keynes
Heron J (1989) Six category intervention analysis. University of Surrey. Human Potential Resource Group, Guildford
Heron J (1990) Helping the client: a creative practical guide. Sage, London
Heron J (2001) Helping the client: a creative practical guide, 5th edn. Sage, London
Johns C, Butcher K (1993) Learning through supervision: a case study of respite care. J Clin Nurs 2(2):89–93
Jones A (2001) Possible influences on clinical supervision. Nurs Stand 16(1):38–42
Jones A (1995) Clinical supervision in sustaining and developing nursing practice. Int J Palliat Nurs 1(4):211–216
Kolb DA (1984) Experiential learning: experience as the source of learning and development. Prentice-Hall, Englewood Cliffs, NJ
Lynch L, Hancox K, Happell B, Parker J (2008) Clinical supervision for nurses. Wiley, Chichester
Manring J, Beitman BD, Dewan MJ (2003) Evaluating competence in psychotherapy. Acad Psychiatry 27(3):136–144
Milne D (2009) Evidence-based clinical supervision: principles and practice. BPS Blackwell, Oxford
Muecke MA (1970) Video-tape recordings: a tool for psychiatric clinical supervisors. Perspect Psychiatr Care 8(5):200–208
Mulholland J (1994) Competency-based learning applied to nursing management. J Nurs Manag 2(4):161–166
NHS Education for Scotland and The Scottish Government (2008) *The matrix: a guide to delivering evidence-based psychological therapies in Scotland*. Edinburgh
Nursing Midwifery Council (recovered 2012a) *The code: standards of conduct, performance and ethics for nurses and midwives* http://standards.nmc-uk.org/PreRegNursing/statutory/background/Pages/more-background-and-context.aspx
Nursing Midwifery Council (recovered 2012b) *Guidance on professional conduct for nursing and midwifery students* http://www.nmc-uk.org/Documents/Guidance/NMC-Guidance-on-professional-conduct-for-nursing-and-midwifery-students.pdf
Olsen DP (2001) Empathetic maturity: theory of moral point of view in clinical relations. Adv Nurs Sci 24(1):36–46
Padesky C (1996) Developing cognitive therapist competency: teaching and supervision models. In: Salkovskis PM (ed) Frontiers of cognitive therapy. The Guilford Press, London
Pesut DJ, Williams CA (1990) The nature of clinical supervision in psychiatric nursing: a survey of clinical specialists. Arch Psychiatr Nurs 4(3):188–194
Platt-Koch LM (1986) Clinical supervision for psychiatric nurses. J Psychosoc Nurs 24(1):7–15
Power S (1999) Nursing supervision: a guide for clinical practice. Sage Publications, London

Proctor B (1987) Supervision: a co-operative exercise in accountability. In: Marken M, Payne M (eds) Enabling and ensuring: supervision in practice. National Youth Bureau and the Council for Education and Training in Youth and Community Work, Leister, pp 21–34

Proctor B (2001) The supervision alliance model. In: Cutcliffe JR, Butterworth T, Proctor B (eds) Fundamental themes of clinical supervision. Routledge, London

Rafferty M, Llewellyn-Davies B, Hewitt J (2007) Setting standards for the practice of clinical supervision – a Welsh perspective. In: Driscoll J (ed) Practising clinical supervision: a reflective approach for health care professionals. London, Bailliere Tindall

Rogers C (1975) Empathic: an unappreciated way of being. Couns Psychol 2:2–10

Roth T, Pilling S (2008) www.ucl.ac.uk/clinical-psychology/CORE/Supervision framework.htm

Schmidt E (1926) Principles and practices of supervision. Am J Nurs 27(2):119–120

Severinsson EI, Hallberg IR (1996) Clinical supervisors' views of their leadership role in the clinical supervision process within nursing care. J Adv Nurs 24(1):151–161

Sloan G (1999) Good characteristics of a clinical supervisor: a community mental health nurse perspective. J Adv Nurs 30(3):713–722

Sloan G (2000) The supervisory relationship: are we forgetting something? Netlink Psychiatr Nurs Res Netw 14:7–8

Sloan G (2006) Clinical supervision in mental health nursing. Wiley, London

Sloan G (2007) Psychological approaches to the supervision encounter. In: Driscoll J (ed) Practising clinical supervision: a reflective approach for healthcare professionals. Bailliarie Tindall, London

Sloan G (2008) Clinical supervision in mental health nursing: accreditation anyone? Ment Health Nurs 28(3):18–20

Sloan G, Fleming M (2011) Training requirements for clinical supervision in the United Kingdom. In: Cutcliffe JR, Hyrkas K, Fowler J (eds) Routledge handbook of clinical supervision: fundamental international themes. Routledge, London

Sloan G, White C, Coit F (2000) Cognitive therapy supervision as a framework for clinical supervision in nursing: using structure to guide discovery. J Adv Nurs 32(3):515–524

Smith JP (1995) Clinical supervision: conference by the NHSE. J Adv Nurs 21(5):1029–1031

Spence C, Cantrell J, Christie J, Samet W (2002) A collaborative approach to the implementation of clinical supervision. J Nurs Manag 10(2):65–74

Termini M, Hauser MJ (1973) The process of the supervisory relationship. Perspect Psychiatr Care 11(3):121–125

Todd G, Freshwater D (1999) Reflective practice and guided discovery: clinical supervision. Br J Nurs 8(20):1383–1389

Trainor MA (1978) A helping model for clinical supervision. Superv Nurse 9(1):30–36

Wolf L (1941) Development of floor nursing and supervision *Hospital* March pp. 53–56

European and Worldwide Mental Health Epidemiology and Trends

11

Evanthia Sakellari

11.1 Introduction: Mental Health Problems Across the Lifespan

Promoting and maintaining mental health remain a major public health challenge for nations all around the globe. Methodological and epistemological limitations notwithstanding our best evidence indicate that hundreds of millions of people worldwide are affected by mental health problems. Mental health problems are prevalent in all societies, among women and men, at all stages of life.

Wittchen et al. (2011) claim that their prevalence findings underline that mental health problems must be considered to be Europe's foremost health-care challenge of the twenty-first century. This challenge is complex, with dozens of group of so-called disorders and hundreds of imprecise diagnoses that might require preventive, therapeutic, and rehabilitative interventions of different types and intensities in different age groups (Wittchen et al. 2011). In the European Union, over one-third of the population suffers from some form of mental health problem at some point in their life. Almost 50 million European Union (EU) citizens (about 11% of the population), on average at a single point in time, are estimated to be living with a mental health problem (European Union 2008). The most frequent so-called disorders are anxiety "disorders" (14.0%), insomnia (7.0%), major depression (6.9%), somatoform (6.3%), alcohol and drug dependence (4%), ADHD (5%) in the young, and dementia (1–30%, depending on age) (Wittchen et al. 2011).

E. Sakellari
Department of Public Health and Community Health, Athens University of Applied Sciences, Athens, Greece

Department of Nursing Science, University of Turku, Turku, Finland
e-mail: evasak@utu.fi

© Springer International Publishing Switzerland 2018
J.C. Santos, J.R. Cutcliffe (eds.), *European Psychiatric/Mental Health Nursing in the 21st Century*, Principles of Specialty Nursing,
https://doi.org/10.1007/978-3-319-31772-4_11

In 2014, there were an estimated 43.6 million adults in the USA with a formal mental health problem in the past year, and this number represented 18.1% of all US adults (Center for Behavioral Health Statistics and Quality 2015). Of the 16 million Australians aged 16–85 years, almost half (45% or 7.3 million) had a mental health problem at some point in their life, and one in five (20% or 3.2 million) Australians had a mental health problem that endured longer than 12 months. More than a quarter (26%) of people aged 16–24 years and a similar proportion (25%) of people aged 25–34 years had a 12-month (or longer) mental health problem compared with 5.9% of those aged 75–85 years old. Among all age groups, 12-month so-called anxiety disorders had the highest prevalence, with the highest rate in the 35–44 years age group (18%) (Australian Bureau of Statistics 2007).

The overall 1-year prevalence of mental health problems, within 14 countries worldwide, ranges from 4 to 26% (WHO World Mental Health Survey Consortium 2004). Later, the estimated lifetime prevalence of having one or more of the so-called disorders considered here varies widely across the World Mental Health surveys, from 47.4% in the USA to 12.0% in Nigeria (Kessler et al. 2007). A meta-analysis for the years 1980–2013 (Steel et al. 2014) concluded that on average one in five adults (17.6%) experienced a common mental health problem within the past 12 months and 29.2% across their lifetime. Countries within North and Southeast Asia in particular displayed consistently lower 1-year and lifetime prevalence estimates than other regions, and 1-year prevalence rates were also low among sub-Saharan Africa. The so-called disorders of the brain and mental health problems, in particular, contribute 26.6% of the total all-cause burden. The three most important contributors to burden of disease are depression (7.2% of the overall burden of disease in Europe), Alzheimer's disease/dementia (3.7%), and alcohol/misuse (3.4%). There are clear gender differences: women were disproportionally affected by depression (1 in 10 healthy years of life lost is due to this disorder or 10.3% of all the DALYs), while for men alcohol/misuse is the biggest relative contributor to the mental health disease burden in Europe (Wittchen et al. 2011).

According to the WHO (2016), approximately 15% of adults aged 60 and older suffer from a mental health problem, and so-called neuropsychiatric disorders among the older adults account for 6.6% of the total disability (DALYs) for this age group. However, more than half of all adults with existing mental health problems were diagnosed in their childhood (WHO Regional Office for Europe 2014). Analysis of age-of-onset reports shows that many mental health problems begin in childhood-adolescence and have significant adverse effects on subsequent role transitions. Adult mental health problems are found in the World Mental Health data to be associated with high levels of role impairment. Despite this burden, the majority of mental health problems go untreated (Kessler et al. 2009a). Worldwide, the leading causes of years lost because of disability (YLDs) for 10–24-year-olds were so-called neuropsychiatric disorders (45%) (Gore et al. 2011). More than 10% of children and adolescents in Europe have some form of mental health problem (European Public Health Alliance 2014).

Wittchen et al. (2011) have concluded that the most frequent mental health problems in EU, in terms of the estimated number of persons affected across all age groups, are so-called anxiety disorders (69.1 million) with the unipolar depression (30.3 million) being next. The so-called anxiety disorders, which include panic "disorder," generalized anxiety "disorder," post-traumatic stress "disorder," phobias, and separation anxiety "disorder," are the most common class of mental health problems presenting in the general population; the estimated lifetime prevalence of any so-called anxiety disorder is over 15%, while the 12-month prevalence is more than 10% which is generally higher in developed countries than in developing countries (Kessler et al. 2009b). Moreover, most so-called anxiety disorders are more prevalent in women than in men (McLean et al. 2011).

A meta-analysis for the years 1980–2013 showed that women had higher rates of mood (7.3%:4.0%) and anxiety (8.7%:4.3%) problems during the previous 12 months (Steel et al. 2014). An earlier study showed that phobias and separation anxiety "disorder" all have very early ages of onset (medians in the range 7–14 years), while generalized anxiety "disorder," panic "disorder," and post-traumatic stress "disorder," in comparison, have much later age-of-onset distributions (median 24–50 years), and the median age of so-called onset of mood disorders ranges between the late 20s and the early 40s (29–43 years) (Kessler et al. 2007). In New Zealand and the USA, prospective measurement yielded lifetime estimates that suggest the experience of certain so-called DSM-defined disorders by age 32 may be very common: anxiety disorder (49.5%) and depression (41.4%) (Moffitt et al. 2010). A nationwide cross-sectional study which was conducted among Nepalese adults showed that prevalence of anxiety, depression (HADS-D), and comorbid of anxiety and depression were 16.1%, 4.2%, and 5.9%, respectively (Risal et al. 2016).

Mathers and Loncar (2006) support that by 2030, depression is likely to be the second highest cause of disease burden. Almost all studies show a higher prevalence of depression among women than men, with a ratio of between 1.5:1 and 2:1 (Hyman et al., Hyman et al. 2006). The World Mental Health survey showed a 2.4% lifetime prevalence of bipolar spectrum and 1.5% 12-month prevalence (Merikangas et al. 2011). A recent systematic review found that the prevalence of bipolar disorder ranges from 0.1 to 7.5% (Caetano Dell'Aglio et al. 2013). Moreover, unipolar depression occurs in 7% of the general elderly population, and it accounts for 5.7% of YLDs among over 60-year-olds (WHO 2016).

Moreover, depression is the predominant cause of illness and disability for both boys and girls aged 10–19 years (WHO 2014a), while so-called major depressive disorders are the most frequent conditions in children and adolescents, followed by so-called anxiety disorders, so-called behavioral or emotional disorders, and substance misuse problems (European Public Health Alliance 2014). In Australia (Australian Bureau of Statistics 2007) approximately 15% of young people (aged 16–24) have so-called anxiety disorders, and 6% have so-called affective disorders (such as depression). The World Mental Health surveys estimate that the prevalence of 12-month serious mental illness is 4–6.8% in half of the countries, 2.3–3.6% in one-fourth, and 0.8–1.9% in one-fourth (Kessler et al. 2009b). Assuming conservatively that the main age range of risk is between ages 15 and 55, researchers estimate lifetime risk is in the range of 0.08 to 0.44 percent for schizophrenia. Although schizophrenia is a relatively uncommon mental health problem, estimates of disease burden are high – around 2,000 DALYs lost per one million total population (because the condition is associated with early onset, long duration, and severe disability) (Hyman et al. 2006).

11.2 Perinatal Mental Health

A review on the studies on the prevalence of common perinatal mental health problems in women in low- and lower-middle-income countries revealed that the weighted mean prevalence was 15.6% antenatally and 19.8% postnatally (Fisher et al. 2012). The prevalence of mental health problems in the perinatal period in low- and middle-income countries is higher than in high-income countries (WHO 2008). The WHO confirmed the high percentage of suicides among women in Vietnam during the perinatal period to be 8–16.5%, depending on the province (WHO 2005a). Studies in the United Kingdom on the causes of death in women up to 1 year after giving birth concluded that suicide was the leading cause of death which is responsible for 10% of all deaths (Oates 2003) and similar findings in Australia too (Austin et al. 2007).

Postpartum depression affects 10–15% of new mothers, while many of these cases remain undiagnosed (Thurgood et al. 2009). A review of the literature on prevalence of postpartum depression identified studies reporting prevalence in 40 countries demonstrating a wide range of reported prevalence from almost 0% to almost 60% (Halbreich and Karkun 2006). An analysis among Canadian women found that the national prevalence of minor and major postpartum depression symptomatology was 8.46% and 8.69%, respectively (Lanes et al. 2011). In the USA data from 25 states participating in the 2011 Pregnancy Risk Assessment Monitoring System showed that about one out of ten women experienced frequent postpartum depressive symptoms (CDC 2016).

11.3 Trends in Rate of Mortality Due to Mental Health Problems

According to the WHO (2014b), over 800,000 people die due to suicide every year, and there are many more who attempt suicide. Suicide is a global phenomenon in all regions of the world; in 2012, 75% of global suicide occurred in low- and middle-income countries. In 2012, worldwide, suicide accounted for 1.4% of all deaths, making it the 15th leading cause of death. Suicide occurs throughout the lifespan and is the second leading cause of death among 15–29-year-olds globally which accounts for 8.5% of all deaths (WHO 2014b). Among younger people aged 10–24 years worldwide, suicide is included in one of the prominent causes of all deaths (6%) (Patton et al. 2009) and one of the top three causes of adolescent deaths globally (WHO 2014a) with at least 100,000 youths who kill themselves each year worldwide (European Child Safety Alliance 2014). In European countries of low and middle income, suicide was one of the major causes of deaths (14%) in males aged 10–24 years. In high-income countries, suicide accounted for 15% of male mortality, and in females suicide (12%) is also one of the main causes of death (Patton et al. 2009). Among adults aged 30–49 years, it accounts for 4.1% of all deaths and is ranked the fifth leading cause of death (WHO 2014c).

In 2012, there were 164 thousand deaths in the EU-28 resulting from mental and so-called behavioral disorders, equivalent to 3.3% of all deaths. The highest prevalence is met in the United Kingdom (7.2%) which is more than double of the EU average and Sweden, the Netherlands, Denmark, and Switzerland, while in Greece, Bulgaria, and Romania was the lowest (0.1%) (Eurostat 2015). A review (Bremberg 2015) examining the time trends for mental health problems in the Nordic countries and the Netherlands between 1990 and 2010 revealed that the average suicide rate among 15–24-year-olds in the period 1990–2010 varied between 6 per 100,000 in the Netherlands and 20.7 per 100,000 in Finland. The average annual decrease per 100,000 was −0.27 in Denmark, −0.42 in Finland, 0.09 in the Netherlands, and −0.20 in Norway, but in Sweden there was an annual increase of +0.04.

Among low- and middle-income countries in the six WHO regions, there is an almost threefold range in the age-standardized suicide rate, from a low of 6.1 per 100,000 in the Region of the Americas to a high of 17.7 per 100,000 in the Southeast Asian Region (WHO 2014c). In a cross-sectional study across 17 countries (Kokkevi et al. 2012), the median prevalence of self-reported suicide attempts was 10.5% (range 4.1–23.5%), and among of those who reported having attempted suicide, the majority also reported self-harm thoughts (range 80.9–93.9%) with the median of frequent self-harm thoughts (at least five times) was 7.4% (range 2.1–15.3%). Self-harm was one (13th) of the top 20 leading causes of years of life lost (YLL) – globally in 2012, while the YLL for self-harm decreased by 12% from 2000 to 2012 (WHO 2014d).

Finally, suicide is estimated to contribute more than 2% to the global burden of disease by the year 2020 (WHO 2012). The global, age-standardized rate of suicide in 2012 was estimated to be 11.4 per 100,000 population (WHO 2015a). Suicide remains a significant cause of premature death, with over 50,000 deaths per year in the European Union (European Public Health Alliance 2014).

11.4 The Impact of the Global, Financial Crisis

The financial crisis has had a clear impact on mental health. In addition to an introduction of overall cuts to social and (mental) health services (childcare, child, and family benefits), some EU countries have seen significant decline in budgets designated specifically to mental health priorities (including of the child population) (European Child Safety Alliance 2014). For example, in Greece, an increase in psychosocial problems in child and adolescent patients was reported in hospitals between 2007 and 2011 (Anagnostopoulos and Soumaki 2013).

A workshop entitled “Mental Health in Times of Economic Crisis” organized by the European Parliament’s Committee on Environment, Public Health and Food Safety concluded that Europe is facing a mental health crisis and recognized that every 1% increase in unemployment correlates to a 0.8% rise in suicides (European Union 2012). It is clear that the health and well-being of people are not considered when decisions on measures are taken (Sakellari and Pikouli 2013). One of the most reported outcomes of the austerity measures due to the financial crisis has been an increase in the suicide rate; between 2009–2011 there was a substantial increase in the rates of people stating they had suicidal ideation and in actual attempts (Economou et al. 2013) and a significant impact on the mental health provision (Pikouli et al. 2013).

11.5 Mental Health-Care Trends

Globally, there was a slight decrease of 5% in the number of mental hospitals between 2011 and 2014. A more significant decrease is observed for the number of mental hospital beds, which has dropped by nearly 30% compared to 2011 (WHO 2015a). Most mental health problems remain undetected and untreated, resulting in a substantial – and largely avoidable – burden to patients, families, and communities (WHO and WONCA 2008). Most of the people with mental health problems – 75% in many low-income countries – do not have access to the treatment they need (WHO 2015b). Not only are resources for mental health scarce, but they are also distributed inequitably: between countries, between regions, and within local communities. Need and access tend to vary inversely – those with highest need have least access to care (Saxena et al. 2007). It is estimated that up to one-half of those with depression (Bland et al. 1997) and one-third to one-half of those affected by anxiety (Andrews et al. 2001) seek professional help, while people often seek help from informal sources, such as friends or family, rather than from formal sources (Rickwood et al. 2007).

Despite often higher disability, mental health problems are undertreated compared to physical disorders both in developed and developing countries (Ormel et al. 2008), due to the fact that almost one-third of countries worldwide do not have a budget for mental health services, while one-fifth of countries spend less than 1% of their total health budget on mental health services (WHO 2005b). Later reports (WHO 2015a) show that the expenditure levels in low-, lower-middle-, and upper-middle-income country groups are very low (less than US$ 2) and fall far below levels estimated for high-income countries (over US$ 50 per head of population).

Regarding help-seeking intentions, a recent study (Suka et al. 2016) found that psychological problems (such as depressed mood) were less likely to induce help-seeking intentions than a physical problem (such as dizziness), when 85.9% of the participants reported a positive help-seeking intention and 42.7% gave first priority to seeking help from formal sources, while these percentages were smaller in the cases of depressed mood (74.9 and 18.7%).

Across all WHO regions, the large majority of mental health workers counted in the Atlas 2014 survey are working in inpatient and day care services (82% globally) (WHO 2015a). The WHO Mental Health Atlas 2014 reports that globally, the median number of mental health workers is 9 per 100,000 population, but there is extreme variation (from below 1 per 100,000 population in low-income countries to over 50 in high-income countries). More specifically, there are 6.6 psychiatrists per 100,000 population in the sampled high-income countries, compared to less than 0.5 per 100,000 population in low- and lower-middle-income countries. Similarly, there are over 30 nurses working in mental health per 100,000 population in high-income country settings compared to 0.4 in low-income countries, 2.5 in lower-middle-income countries, and 7.1 in upper-middle-income countries (WHO 2015a).

Conclusion

To conclude, robust arguments have been advanced which point out that being mentally healthy is central to achieving full potential, both within the individual and where everyone can contribute to society; however, despite this awareness mental health problems have a high prevalence in Europe and the rest of the world. The recent financial crisis, which had significant and major impacts in Europe, and which for many continues, appears to have increased the demand for mental health services. Psychiatric/mental health nurses, as members of the interdisciplinary team, have an important role to play in mental health by providing high-quality health care focused on primary health care and prevention, as well as taking action in developing proper strategies and policies in order to decrease inequalities. One of the challenges for psychiatric/mental health nurses is community mental health care since nowadays most mental health issues have to be addressed in primary health care. The psychiatric/mental health nurses may have multiple roles within the interdisciplinary team, such as care provider, counselor, case manager, crisis worker, and advocate, all of which are a valuable contribution in community mental health care. Thus, the development of new competencies and evidence-based practices is always needed in order to provide skilled professional services with the best outcomes in the context of community mental health.

References

Anagnostopoulos DC, Soumaki E (2013) The state of child and adolescent psychiatry in Greece during the international financial crisis: a brief report. Eur Child Adolesc Psychiatry 22:131–134

Andrews G, Issakidis C, Carter G (2001) Shortfall in mental health service utilisation. Br J Psychiatry 179:417–425

Austin MP, Kildea S, Sullivan E (2007) Maternal mortality and psychiatric morbidity in the perinatal period: challenges and opportunities for prevention in the Australian setting. Med J Aust 186(7):364–367

Australian Bureau of Statistics (2007) National survey of mental health and wellbeing: summary of results. [Online]. Retrieved 15 May, 2016, from www.abs.gov.au

Bland RC, Newman SC, Orn H (1997) Help-seeking for psychiatric co-called disorders. Can J Psychiatr 42(9):935–942
Bremberg S (2015) Mental health problems are rising more in Swedish adolescents than in other Nordic countries and the Netherlands. Acta Paediatr 104:997–1004
Caetano Dell'Aglio J, Basso LA, Iracema de Lima Argimon I, Arteche A (2013) Systematic review of the prevalence of bipolar disorder and bipolar spectrum co-called disorders in population-based studies. Trends Psychiatry Psychother 35(2):99–105
CDC (2016) Depression among women. Retrieved 15 May, 2016, from http://www.cdc.gov/reproductivehealth/depression/
Center for Behavioral Health Statistics and Quality (2015) Behavioral health trends in the United States: results from the 2014 National survey on drug use and health. Retrieved 15 May, 2016, from http://www.samhsa.gov/data/
Economou M, Madianos M, Peppou LA, Theleritis C, Patelakis A, Stefanis C (2013) Suicidal ideation and reported suicide attempts in Greece during the economic crisis. World Psychiatry 12(1):53–59
European Child Safety Alliance (2014) Preventing youth suicide and self-directed violence. Retrieved 15 May, 2016, from http://www.childsafetyeurope.org/publications/info/factsheets/youth-suicide.pdf
European Public Health Alliance (2014) Growing up in the unhappy shadow of the economic crisis: mental health and well-being of the European child and adolescent population. [Online]. Retrieved 15 May, 2016, from www.epha.org
European Union (2008) European pact for mental health and well-being 2008. [Online]. Retrieved 15 May, 2016, from http://ec.europa.eu/health/ph_determinants/life_style/mental/docs/pact_en.pdf
European Union (2012) European Parliament's Committee on environment, public health and food safety workshop mental health in times of economic crisis, proceedings. [Online]. Retrieved 15 May, 2016, from http://www.europarl.europa.eu/RegData/etudes/workshop/join/2012/492440/IPOL-ENVI_AT(2012)492440_EN.pdf
Eurostat (2015) Mental health and related issues statistics. Retrieved 15 May, 2016, from http://ec.europa.eu/eurostat/statistics-explained/index.php/Mental_health_and_related_issues_statistics#Mental_healthcare
Fisher J, Cabral de Mello M, Patel V, Rahman A, Tran T, Sara Holtona S, Holmes W (2012) Prevalence and determinants of common perinatal mental health problems in women in low- and lower-middle-income countries: a systematic review. Bull World Health Organ 90:139–149
Gore FM, Bloem PJN, Patton GC, Ferguson J, Joseph V, Coffey C, Sawyer SM, Mathers CD (2011) Global burden of disease in young people aged 10–24 years: a systematic analysis. Lancet 377:2093–2102
Halbreich U, Karkun S (2006) Cross-cultural and social diversity of prevalence of postpartum depression and depressive symptoms. J Affect Disord 91:97–111
Hyman S, Chisholm D, Kessler R, Patel V, Whiteford H (2006) Mental health problems. In: W.H.O., disease control priorities related to mental, neurological, developmental and substance abuse co-called disorders. World Health Organization, Geneva, pp 1–20. [Online]. Retrieved 15 May, 2016, from http://www.who.int/mental_health/publications/financing/disease_control_priorities_mental_neurological_co-called disorders/en/
Kessler RC, Aguilar-Gaxiola S, Alonso J, Chatterji S, Lee S, Ormel J, Ustün TB (2009a) The WHO world mental health (WMH) surveys. Psychiatrie (Stuttg) 6(1):5–9
Kessler RC, Aguilar-Gaxiola S, Alonso J, Chatterji S, Lee S, Ormel J et al (2009b) The global burden of mental health problems: an update from the WHO World Mental Health (WMH) Surveys. Epidemiol Psichiatr Soc 18(1):23–33
Kessler RC, Angermeyer M, Anthony JC, De Graaf R, Demyttenaere K, Gasquet I et al (2007) Lifetime prevalence and age-of-onset distributions of mental health problems in the World Health Organization's World Mental Health Survey Initiative. World Psychiatry 6:168–176
Kokkevi A, Rotsika V, Arapaki A, Richardson C (2012) Adolescents' self-reported suicide attempts, self-harm thoughts and their correlates across 17 European countries. J Child Psychol Psychiatry 53(4):381–389

Lanes A, Kuk JL, Tamim H (2011) Prevalence and characteristics of postpartum depression symptomatology among Canadian women: a cross-sectional study. BMC Public Health 11:302
Mathers CD, Loncar D (2006) Projections of global mortality and burden of disease from 2002 to 2030. PLoS Med 3(11):2011–2030
McLean CP, Asnaani A, Litz BT, Hofmann SG (2011) Gender differences in anxiety co-called disorders: prevalence, course of illness, comorbidity and burden of illness. J Psychiatr Res 45(8):1027–1035
Merikangas KR, Jin R, He JP, Kessler RC, Lee S, Sampson NA et al (2011) Prevalence and correlates of bipolar spectrum disorder in the World Mental Health survey initiative. Arch Gen Psychiatry 68(3):241–251
Moffitt TE, Caspi A, Taylor A, Kokaua J, Milne BJ, Polanczyk G, Poulton R (2010) How common are common mental health problems? Evidence that lifetime prevalence rates are doubled by prospective versus retrospective ascertainment. Psychol Med 40(6):899–909
Oates M (2003) Suicide: the leading cause of maternal death. Br J Psychiatry 183:279–281
Ormel J, Petukhova M, Chatterji S, Aguilar-Gaxiola S, Alonso J, Angermeyer MC et al (2008) Disability and treatment of specific mental and physical co-called disorders across the world. Br J Psychiatry 192:368–375
Patton GC, Coffey C, Sawyer SM, Viner RM, Haller DH, Bose K et al (2009) Global patterns of mortality in young people: a systematic analysis of population health data. Lancet 374:881–892
Pikouli K, Konstakapoulus G, Ioannidi N, Sakellari E, Ploumpidis D (2013) The impact of financial crisis on the services of a community mental health center in Athens, Greece: 2008–2011. Poster presentation Horatio Congress, Istanbul
Rickwood D, Deane F, Wilson C (2007) When and how do young people seek professional help for mental health problems? Med J Aust 187(7 Suppl):S35–S39
Risal A, Manandhar K, Linde M, Steiner TJ, Holen A (2016) Anxiety and depression in Nepal: prevalence, comorbidity and associations. BMC Psychiatry 16:102
Sakellari E, Pikouli K (2013) Assessing the impact of the financial crisis in mental health in Greece. Ment Health Nurs 33(6):19–21
Saxena S, Thornicroft G, Knapp M, Whiteford H (2007) Resources for mental health: scarcity, inequity, and inefficiency. Lancet 370:878–889
Steel Z, Marnane C, Iranpour C, Chey T, Jackson JW, Patel V, Silove D (2014) The global prevalence of common mental health problems: a systematic review and meta-analysis 1980-2013. Int J Epidemiol 43(2):476–493
Suka M, Takashi Yamauchi T, Sugimori H (2016) Help-seeking intentions for early signs of mental illness and their associated factors: comparison across four kinds of health problems. BMC Public Health 16:301
Thurgood S, Avery DM, Williamson L (2009) Postpartum depression (PPD). Am J Clin Med 6(2):17–22
WHO (2005a) Maternal mortality in Vietnam 2000–2001. An in-depth analysis of causes and determinants. [Online]. Retrieved 15 May, 2016, from http://www.who.int/reproductivehealth/publications/monitoring/9789290611912/en/
WHO (2005b) Mental health atlas. [Online]. Retrieved 15 May, 2016, from http://www.who.int/mental_health/evidence/atlas/global_results.pdf
WHO (2008) Maternal mental health and child health and development in low and middle income countries: report of the meeting held in Geneva, Switzerland, 30 January to 1 February, 2008. [Online]. Retrieved 15 May, 2016, from http://www.who.int/mental_health/prevention/suicide/mmh_jan08_meeting_report.pdf
WHO (2012) Public health action for the prevention of suicide. [Online]. Retrieved 15 May, 2016, from http://apps.who.int/iris/bitstream/10665/75166/1/9789241503570_eng.pdf
WHO (2014a) New global report: depression predominant cause of illness and disability among adolescents. Retrieved 15 May, 2016, from http://www.euro.who.int/en/health-topics/noncommunicable-diseases/mental-health/news/news/2014/05/new-global-report-depression-predominant-cause-of-illness-and-disability-among-adolescents
WHO (2014b) Suicide data. Retrieved 15 May, 2016, from http://www.who.int/mental_health/prevention/suicide/suicideprevent/en/

WHO (2014c) Preventing suicide: a global imperative. Retrieved 6 May, 2016, from http://www.who.int/mental_health/suicide-prevention/world_report_2014/en/
WHO (2014d) World Health Statistics 2014. [Online]. Retrieved 15 May, 2016, from apps.who.int/iris/bitstream/10665/112738/1/9789240692671_eng.pdf
WHO (2015a) Mental health atlas 2014. Retrieved 15 May, 2016, from http://www.who.int/mental_health/evidence/atlas/mental_health_atlas_2014/en/
WHO (2015b) WHO Mental Health Gap Action Programme (mhGAP). Retrieved 15 May, 2016, from http://www.who.int/mental_health/mhgap/en/
WHO (2016) Mental health and older adults. Retrieved 15 May, 2016, from http://www.who.int/mediacentre/factsheets/fs381/en/
WHO, WONCA (2008) Integrating mental health into primary care. A global perspective. [Online]. Retrieved 15 May, 2016, from http://www.who.int/mental_health/resources/mentalhealth_PHC_2008.pdf
WHO World Mental Health Survey Consortium (2004) Prevalence, severity, and unmet need for treatment of mental health problems in the World Health Organization World Mental Health Surveys. J Am Med Assoc 291:2581–2590
WHO Regional Office for Europe (2014) Investing in children: the European child and adolescent health strategy 2015–2020. [Online]. Retrieved 15 May, 2016, from http://www.euro.who.int/__data/assets/pdf_file/0010/253729/64wd12e_InvestCAHstrategy_140440.pdf?ua=1
Wittchen HU, Jacobi F, Rehm J, Gustavsson A, Svensson M, Jönsson B et al (2011) The size and burden of mental health problems and other co-called disorders of the brain in Europe 2010. Eur Neuropsychopharmacol 21:655–679

Mental Health Nurses and Responding to Suffering in the Twenty-first Century Occidental World: Accompanying People on Their Search for Meaning

12

John R. Cutcliffe, Jan Kare Hummelvol, Arild Granerud, and Bengt Erikson

12.1 Introduction

Much of contemporary health and mental health practice pays little attention to suffering (Cassell 1991). While a close examination of some of the (earlier) literature associated with the recovery movement appears to link recovery and suffering, the majority of this work pays scant or no attention to this relationship (see, for example, World Health Organisation 2001; Borg and Kristiansen 2004; Bonney and Stickley 2008). Indeed, contemporary, occidental life is often depicted as suffering-free or rather, in societies that espouse hedonistic tendencies such as the United States of America (consider, for example, the "Declaration of Independence" reference to "life, liberty and the pursuit of happiness"), suffering is frequently depicted as antagonistic to the pursuit of happiness. Within the somewhat limited discourse on suffering, the focus is invariably concerned with healthcare practitioners stopping, and/or curing suffering (Cassell 1991). From a superficial perspective, these views have an intuitive logic, after all, why would any healthcare practitioner want clients to suffer? However an alternative perspective would perhaps take issue with this position; such a view sees suffering as an inevitable aspect of the human condition and experience; as something to be expected and unavoidable and often something that cannot always be 'cured' or

J.R. Cutcliffe (✉)
Cutcliffe Consulting, Kingston, Canada

School of Nursing, Coimbra, Portugal
e-mail: jcutcliffe@outlook.com

B. Eriksson • A. Granerud • J.K. Hummelvol
Inland Norway University of Applied Science, Faculty of Public Health,
Hedmark University College, Elverum, Norway
e-mail: bengt.eriksson@hihm.no; arild.granerud@hihm.no

© Springer International Publishing Switzerland 2018

J.C. Santos, J.R. Cutcliffe (eds.), *European Psychiatric/Mental Health Nursing in the 21st Century*, Principles of Specialty Nursing,
https://doi.org/10.1007/978-3-319-31772-4_12

'removed.' It sees suffering as something that might need to be endured, minimized, relieved, explored for meaning, and maybe even learned from (Deegan 2003).

Literature from a range of pertinent disciplines indicates that while these ideas may seem 'out of step' with those embedded in contemporary healthcare practice, they are actually deep-rooted and have long been recognized (see for instance Gabriel 1984; Hall 1986; Kleinman 1988; Tedeschi and Calhoun 1995; Miller 2004). Tedeschi and Calhoun (1995, p. ix), for instance, write that

> This volume is an attempt to weave together material from various writings in philosophy, religion and especially psychology to account for a phenomenon *that has been recognized since ancient times but given little attention by psychologists: the experience of growth or strengthening that often occurs in persons who have faced traumatic events* (emphasis added).

The mental health care community's response(s) to suffering has profound implications for clients and professionals. Accordingly, this chapter begins with an examination of definitions and conceptualizations of suffering, and pays particular attention to the under-reported view *vis a vis* the potential therapeutic and developmental value of suffering. We then examine how suffering is conceptualized and responded to in the twenty-first century occidental world. And we outline a range of interventions that Psychiatric/Mental Health (P/MH) nurses can use when attempting to help persons experiencing mental health-related suffering. We conclude by highlighting how the problem is most pronounced when this arguably inevitable and potentially developmentally beneficial aspect of the human condition morphs into or is replaced by the view that there is something wrong with the individual if he/she experience suffering.

12.2 Definition and Conceptualizations

A number of definitions and conceptualizations of suffering have been advanced and as the authors wish to draw on original source materials, we recognize that some of the references could be regarded as being of a 'recognized vintage.' The Merriam-Webster Dictionary (2014) defines suffering as

The state or experience of one that suffers or pain.

Similarly, the Online Dictionary (2014) defines suffering as

> the condition of one who suffers; the bearing of pain or distress or an instance of pain or distress.

Kahn and Steeves (1986) define suffering as an individual's experience of threat to self via events such as pain or loss. Similarly, a number of authors with a medical background consider suffering to be inextricably linked to pain (see, for instance, Scarry 1985; Chapman and Garvin 1985). In these definitions, suffering is conflated with pain and it is perhaps no surprise then that the primary effort in medical research on suffering has been to alleviate pain (Roy 1998). According to Cassell (1991), this is an unhelpful conflation as pain and suffering are not the same phenomena. Similarly, Eriksson (1993, p. 186) states that suffering

> differs from pain in that it does not speak the same language. Suffering and pain are often present in the same life situation, and it may be difficult to define the point where suffering ends and pain begins.

In his classic work Cassell (1991, p. 32/33) states that suffering is

> 1. a holistic, multi-dimensional phenomenon, that is not limited or restricted to physical suffering. 2. …unfortunately suffering can (and is) also an iatrogenic phenomenon—it can be caused by healthcare intervention(s), even those designed to begin relief. 3. While there appear to be some commonalities across phenomenological antecedents of suffering, ultimately, suffering remains an individualized experience.

Classic works with a noted vintage such as Frankl (1963) and Zborowski (1969) highlight how suffering also occurs in response to the meaning of the symptoms to the sufferer. A number of authors have demonstrated how suffering can be a response to a variety of different types of loss (Charmaz 1983; DeBellis et al. 1986; Morse and Johnson 1991; Chapman and Garvin 1985). And a limited literature on suffering has emanated from nursing scholars (Morse and Johnson 1991; Eriksson 1993; Eriksson 1993; Morse and Carter 1996, Morse et al. 1996; Hummelvoll 2010), and this body of work advances a number of positions: (a) relieving suffering is a nursing imperative; (b) relieving suffering is bound up with the nurse sharing the suffering experience; (c) nurses have a moral obligation to speak of suffering; (d) suffering appears to have two distinct process or phases: enduring and emotional suffering. And that there appear to be at least four, related modes of suffering: (a) *Disease suffering*—related to the experience and consequences of disease or illness. (b) *Existential suffering*—suffering as a result of the loss of meaning in life. (c) *Care and treatment suffering*—arising from relationships between the person seeking help and the helper. And (d) *Social suffering*—related to reduced opportunities for social participation and societal reactions to the individual's expression of illness in public spaces. Lastly Eriksson's (1993) work draws together a number of important theoretical elements to capture the essence of suffering—this is displayed in Box 12.1.

Box 12.1 The Essence of Suffering According to the Finish Nurse Scholar Eriksson's (1993)

1. Suffering is an inseparable part of life and therefore also consistent with health, i.e. human being can bear endurable suffering and still experience health.
2. The opposite of suffering is pleasure, which explains why there can be joy and pleasure in suffering.
3. Suffering has no given basis for determination, or cause, and suffering has many faces.
4. Suffering cannot be defined. We can only give it characteristics. Suffering often lacks an explicit language.
5. Suffering is in its ontological essence a unique, isolated, total experience and it does not have an immediate referent in concrete reality. This means that the suffering person is lonely and in one respect unapproachable. It is

difficult to understand another's suffering in its deepest dimension. Although we do not understand suffering, we can see and understand that the other is suffering.

6. Suffering as such has no meaning, but the human being can ascribe meaning to it by reconciling it with his/her suffering.
7. Suffering in its deepest essence is a form of dying. To suffer is to die from something, but it can also lead to something new.
8. In his/her isolation and suffering the human being is searching for communion. But often through symbols and metaphors.
9. Every suffering human being has his/her own dramas of suffering. He/she must find a co-actor to confirm it as it really is (pp. 186–87)

12.3 The Psychological and Existential Literature on Suffering: An Unavoidable Yet Developmentally Invaluable Experience

Even a cursory review of the relevant psychological and existential literature on suffering posits a significantly different conceptualization to the view that suffering and pain are isomorphic. This conceptualization has two key points: (1) that suffering is an unavoidable feature of the human condition or human experience (Frankl 1961; Nietzsche 1992; 1963; Oreopoulos 2005), indeed, for Eriksson (1993) it is the deepest, most tacit, and most "naked" mode of human existence, and (2) that suffering can lead to personal growth and development, and for some, may even be necessary for full growth and development (Fromm 1947; Frankl 1961, 1963; Kierkegaard 1983; Kahn and Steeves 1986; Tedeschi and Calhoun 1995; Mandella accessed 2014; and to a lesser extent Cassell 1991). A summary of these authors' statements which underscore the experiential nature of suffering is provided in Table 12.1.

With regard to the first key point, Nietzsche (1992) argued that to live (as a human) is to suffer and to survive is to find some meaning in the suffering. Roberts (2008) draws on the Nietzschean concept "eternal return" or "eternal recurrence" and discusses the relationship between suffering and recovery. In essence, the argument posits that if one is given the choice to live one's life again, over and over, with no alterations, many people would choose to do so, although being aware that it would include recurrent parts of suffering and pain. Fromm (1947) similarly advances the position that psychological growth only occurs because the individual faces up to the inescapable realities and tragedies of life (see also Tedeschi and Calhoun 1995). Frankl (1961, 1963) declared that people need to confront the primordial facts of existence: suffering, guilt, and transitoriness. For Frankl, suffering is inextricably linked to personal meaning and despair regarded, not as the direct product of suffering but rather the outcome when the suffering is viewed as devoid of meaning. With regard to the second point, a number of authors, both academic and secular, refer to and explore the transformative processes that occur when the meaning of suffering is realized. According to Råholm (2008), the drama or experience of suffering can be described by the following concepts: to

Table 12.1 Quotes and contributions pertaining to the potential for personal growth and development that can be found in suffering

Author	Quote
Frankl (1963)	"We must never forget that we may also find meaning in life even when confronted with a hopeless situation, when facing a fate that cannot be changed. For what then matters is to bear witness to the uniquely human potential at its best, which is to transform a personal tragedy into triumph, to turn one's predicament into a human achievement. When we are no longer able to change a situation--just think of an incurable disease such as inoperable cancer, we are challenged to change ourselves"
Helen Keller (accessed February 2014)	"Character cannot be developed in ease and quiet. Only through experience of trial and suffering can the soul be strengthened, ambition inspired, and success achieved."
Kierkergard (1983)	"Experiences of crisis are necessary for full personal development"
Paul Tournier (accessed Feb 2014)	"Acceptance of one's life has nothing to do with resignation; it does not mean running away from the struggle. On the contrary, it means accepting it as it comes, with all the handicaps of heredity, of suffering, of psychological complexes and injustices"
Oreopoulos, D.G. (2005)	"It seems that every illness and misfortune in life holds within its shadow a life-affirming lesson, if we are willing to be taught by it. Suffering is life's most effective and profound teacher of development and growth and it furthers our efforts to find meaning in our lives"
Tedeschi and Calhoun (1995, p. 3)	"If we ourselves suffer, we must find our own words for this experience and the way this experience illuminates life mystery; thus enabling us to benefit from it as the audience may benefit from the performance of tragedy"
Nelson Mandela (accessed Feb 2014)	"Our human compassion binds us the one to the other—not in pity or patronizingly, but as human beings who have learnt how to turn our common suffering into hope for the future"

endure, to struggle, to sacrifice life and health, and to become. Becoming implies that a degree of reconciliation is achieved, i.e., being on the road towards a new unity. Gustafsson et al. (2011) found that the meaning of reconciliation for women suffering from grief is like a process that leads to *new sight* and to an *opening* in life, that is, reconciliation as opening up new sights. In addition reconciliation has a progressive form and is a *transition* from the experience of grief and suffering to the experience of health and wholeness. Interestingly, Calhoun and Tedeschi (2006) operationalizing these philosophical and theoretical positions into clinically meaningful applications pioneered the concept of posttraumatic growth; a construct underscored by the view that change occurs as the result of one's struggle with a highly challenging, stressful, and traumatic events (Moore 2014). These authors designed the Post Traumatic Growth Inventory (Tedeschi and Calhoun 1995), a 21-item instrument for assessing positive outcomes in people who have experienced traumatic events (Tedeschi and Calhoun 2004; Moore 2014).

Captivatingly the limited empirical and anecdotal literature in this area, such as it is, seems to underscore the potential therapeutic (or developmental) value of suffering. Focusing on the suffering associated with mental health problems, the testimonies of creative, successful, and inspirational individuals refer to how they missed aspects/all of their mental health problem(s) when they were 'well' and how without this suffering, they would not be as successful, as creative, or as inspirational as they are. A summary of these authors' testimonies is provided in Table 12.2.

Table 12.2 Quotes and contributions from "famous" people pertaining to the potential for personal growth and development that can be found in mental health experiences/suffering

Author	Quote
Steven Fry (2006)	"I love my condition too. It's infuriating I know, but I do get a huge buzz out of the manic side. I rely on it to give my life a sense of adventure, and I think most of the good about me has developed as a result of my mood swings"
John Nash (accessed Feb 2014)	"I wouldn't have had good scientific ideas if I had thought more normally"
Spike Milligan (accessed 2014)	"It's a gift and a curse (so-called mental illness). You get the pain much worse than anybody else, but you see a sunrise much more beautiful than anybody else"
Sir Winston Churchill	Storr (2005) on Churchill and so-called mental illness *"Had he been a stable and equable man, he could never have inspired the nation. In 1940, when all the odds were against Britain, a leader of sober judgment might well have concluded that we were finished"*
Kay Radfield Jamison (1996)—Psychologist, author and sufferer of so-called bi-polar disorder	"These are very difficult ethical issues, because manic-depressive illness can confer advantages on both the individual and society. The disease, in both its severe and less severe forms, appears to convey its advantages not only through its relationship to the artistic temperament and imagination, but through its influence on many eminent scientists, as well as business, military, religious and political leaders" p. 195
John Cleese (2008)	"I feel that it must be acknowledged that misery is a necessary condition for great humour in the vast majority of cases"

12.4 Suffering in the Contemporary, Occidental World: Missed Opportunities and the Allure of the Pharmacological Quick Fix

Some years ago, the psychiatrist and psychotherapist Weiskopf-Joelson (1980, p. 3), in reference to Logotherapy and the search for meaning in suffering, stated that such a search,

> may help counteract certain unhealthy trends in the present day culture of the United States, where the incurable sufferer is given very little opportunity to be proud of his suffering and to consider it ennobling rather than degrading.

Frankl (1961, p. 136) offered very similar remarks, referring to how the United States had a "mental hygene philosophy" that communicated the central message that

> people ought to be happy.

Were these seminal contributors alive today, we doubt that the emphasis in contemporary mental health policy would give them any cause for celebration or optimism; quite the contrary. If one examines trends or patterns in contemporary life within the occidental world, one can detect a pervasive message regarding happiness. 'Hollywood' and/or the movie industry produces countless movies where happy endings are the norm. Self-help and self-improvement books proliferate, daytime television bombards the viewer with stories of how to be happier, so-called motivational speakers abound, many of whom offer guarantees for increased happiness. And in our view, perhaps the most pervasive and pernicious marketing/pushing of perpetual happiness emanates from the pharmaco-psychiatric nexus (Whittaker 2002; Healy 2005; Szasz 2007).

Concerns regarding the increased pathologizing of 'everyday life' in the contemporary occidental world appear to increasing (Szasz 2007; Frances 2013) and may have reached a new zenith following the publication of the DSM V (Greenberg 2014; Sykes Wylie 2014). Moreover, such medicalization of normal and with that an eschewing of suffering as a potential valuable, developmental experience, is perhaps evidenced by data pertaining to rates of prescription of antidepressant (ADs) medications over recent years, most notably Selective Serotonin Reuptake Inhibitors (SSRIs). According to (Currie 2005),

> Prior to the advent of SSRIs, depression was considered *to be a self-limiting phenomenon which was likely to resolve itself, without treatment, in the vast majority of cases* (emphasis added). Now, according to researcher and author, Charles Medawar, it is almost heresy to say that most episodes of depression are self-limited and will end without treatment. Drug intervention is seen to be so imperative that the failure to prescribe would be thought of as negligent, even perhaps legally indefensible.

Evidence of rates of prescription from several countries seems to support Currie's point. In a study of antidepressant prescription in the USA for instance, Olfson and Marcus (2009) report that the years 1995–2006 saw a marked and broad expansion in antidepressant prescription (over 200%), and that individuals treated with ADs became more likely to also receive treatment with antipsychotic medications and less likely to undergo psychotherapy. Drawing on Centers for Disease Control and Prevention (CDCP) data, Mojtabail and Olfson (2011) report that 73 percent of AD prescriptions, for 230,000 visits by adults to offices of primary care doctors, were written for patients with no formal diagnosis of depression in 2007 and that this number is increasing. Interestingly, Mojtabail and Olfson (2011) argue that people (prescribing physicians) should recognize the difference between the sadness and grief that becomes more common with age and 'real' major depression.

In their analysis of antidepressant (AD) drug sales in Italy over the years 1988–1996, Barbui et al. (1999) found an increase of 53%. They concluded that while SSRIs gave a new impetus to AD sales, any possible public health benefits have yet to be demonstrated. Middleton et al. (2001) report a 200–300% increase in prescription of ADs in the United Kingdom. Also in the UK, Munoz-Arroyo et al. (2005) analyzed Scottish Health Surveys and General Practitioner (GP) consultation data for 1995–1998, a total of 175,955 patients. They concluded

> There is no evidence of an increase in incidence, prevalence, care-seeking behaviour or identification of depression during the period of a sharp increase in anti-depressant prescribing. Further work is required to explain the increase.

Then in Canada, prescriptions for all ADs increased by 353% from 3.2 to 14.5 million during the years 1981–2000 (Currie 2005). And lastly, in a major report for the Irish Ministry of Health, (recovered O'Mahony 2014) which highlights an 84% increase in recent rates of prescription of SSRIs, the author states that

> The 'medicalisation' of society is not in its best interests and it is unsustainable. The belief that every problem requires medical treatment is false. This overuse can cause distress, ill-health and even death.

If the population of the occidental world is becoming more 'depressed' and therefore warrant these substantial increases in use of SSRIS, there ought logically to be a corresponding measurable change in outcomes for depressed people. A proxy measure commonly used to measure the efficacy (or otherwise) of ADs is that of national suicide rates; and yet despite the surge in rates of prescription in SSRIs there is no corresponding inverse reduction in national rates of suicide. Data collected by the USA CDCP (accessed 2014; AFSP, accessed 2014) indicates that between 1990 and 2000, the suicide rate decreased from 12.5/100,000 to 10.4/100,000 suicide deaths per 100,000. Over the next 10 years, however, the rate generally increased and by 2010 stood at 12.1 deaths per 100,000. Similarly, Hall et al. (2003) found a steep increase in AD prescribing in Australia from 1991 to 2000, though this was not accompanied by a decline in overall rates of suicide. Data from many parts of the world are unequivocal in showing a distinct and pronounced global trend in the rate of prescription of psychotropic medications, including SSRIs. And yet, epistemological limitations notwithstanding, the data pertaining to suicide rates do not indicate any proportionate, corresponding reductions and in some cases, the rates have actually increased. This disconnect and contradiction has been highlighted by the former chief psychiatrist of New York state (van Praag 2005, p. 254) who states

> Over the past decades the rate of completed suicide has remained quite stable, and that of suicide attempts seems to have increased. These are puzzling observations, since (it is often purported) that depression the major precursor of suicide and antidepressants have been used increasingly in the treatment of depression. These observations have not attracted sufficient attention, possibly because they do not accord with consensus opinions about depression treatment in psychiatry today.

While we remain open-minded to alternative explanations, we believe that the data included above can be regarded as evidence of the increasing pathologizing and medicalization of the human experience—one that includes or is even personified by the pathologizing of periods of unhappiness and suffering.

12.5 Accompanying the Person on His/Her Journey Through Suffering and Recovery: Possible Therapeutic Strategies and Interventions of Psychiatric/Mental Health Nurses

It should be acknowledged that the pursuit of continuous happiness is an unrealistic goal, given all the challenges, vagaries, and problems that life can contain. The human condition is not and never has been an existential experience defined or captured by only one singular 'state of being' or one affective state. Consider the poignant remarks of Maltsberger (Maltsberger et al. 1992, p. 86) who writes that

> successful adulthood demands that one must passively endure disappointment over and over again. Maturity demands that one must accept suffering without flying into rages against life or against one's body.

Similarly, Maris (1981, p. xviii) contends that

> from the existential perspective under the best conditions, life is short, painful, fickle, often lonely and anxiety-generating.

As a result, in place of an automatic, almost inconsiderate pharmacological response to the person who reports suffering we argue that a more considered response is required; one which is at least mindful of the potential value of the experience of suffering. In the interests of clarity, in no way are we suggesting that nurses should cause, encourage or 'turn a blind eye' to suffering. Nor are we advancing some pseudo-theological viewpoint on the experience of suffering. What we are suggesting is that where suffering is occurring as a result of a mental health problem(s), then we (P/MH nurses) can act as a balm and work with the person in helping him/her discover meaning in the experience. P/MH nurses can accomplish this utilizing a number of actions.

Firstly, P/MH nurses need to change their perception of suffering and how they respond to it. How nurses conceptualize experiences and phenomena relevant to their care provides the foundation and direction for their practice (McKenna 1997). Such conceptualizations, whether formalized into nursing theory or remaining more implicit, nevertheless indicate what should form the basis for nursing care and interventions (Cutcliffe et al. 2010). They help nurses decide what they need to know; how to frame or contextualize the care offered and legitimize/delegitimize what is appropriate and what is not. The view that suffering is something to be avoided at all costs and the view that sees pain and suffering and isomorphic, may paradoxically, limit the person's growth and development. When suffering is conceptually conflated with pain, which Cassell (1991) reminds us is not uncommon, then understandably the focus of the care becomes alleviating and controlling the pain at the potential expense of the other domains or dimensions of suffering. When nurses seek to cure or stop the suffering, this leaves no room for exploring how the experience of suffering might actually benefit the person. P/MH nurses need to be able to understand that while they cannot cure the suffering, there are still valuable and potentially therapeutic, developmentally valuable things they can do. Accordingly, there appears to be a distinct need for nurses to radically re-think their view(s) of suffering and open their minds to the possibilities that while long recognized have been overlooked and paid little attention of late (Tedeschi and Calhoun 1995).

Secondly, P/MH nurses need to support and help the person explore and find meaning in the experience of suffering. According to Frankl (1961, 1963) there are three ways to discover meaning in one's life: (1) by creating a work or doing a deed; (2) by experiencing something or encountering someone; and (3) by the attitude we take toward unavoidable suffering. For Frankl, it is the experience of suffering itself that sets up the opportunity to discover meaning. He argues that if people can accept the challenge to suffer bravely, then life has a meaning up to the last moments of one's life. Finding meaning and value in one's experience of suffering can be beneficial, though difficult and painful developmental experience(s). Yet enduring and finding meaning in suffering gives the person access to life lessons and personal development that are otherwise 'out of reach' (see Table 12.2). The P/MH nursing role in such situations then must include helping the person search for and explore this meaning, and 'travel' (metaphorically) with the person on their journey of discovery. This necessitates the need for nurses to be able to bear (vicariously) the suffering without feeling the need to abandon the person. Further, the P/MH nurse can use specific techniques associated with 'Meaning-centred counselling' (see Wong 1998; recovered 2014): contextualise the problem, attributional probing, life review and playing back, fast forwarding, magical thinking, constructing a personal meaning profile, targeting and contracting, effective coping, overcoming the 'Achilles heel.'

Thirdly, P/MH nurses should help the person find an alternative central cognitive schema. Exploring and finding meaning can be brought about via so-called "caring conversations" in which a narrative approach can be utilized (Fredriksson and Lindström 2002). Time is spent listening and hearing the client; encouraging cathartic release and the client can experience the presence of another who encourages him/her to move through a situation of pain to moments of healing. This requires finding a voice for suffering (Råholm 2008). The person who is suffering needs to articulate and reformulate his/her story as a way through their suffering (Råholm 2008). And so clients should be encouraged to create a narrative that also makes room for and includes notions of hope, growth, and reconciliation. Narratives of suffering, as Lorem (2008) reminds us, have the potential of making the suffering person more visible as a human being—and in this way opening him/her up to relationships with others. Alteration of the central, cognitive schema can also involve helping the person understand that despite the contemporary, occidental world view on suffering and corresponding pre-occupation with happiness, life is and can be often about suffering. Ergo—to suffer does not mean you need fixing; these experiences mean that you are human.

Fourthly, P/MH should encourage the person to reflect, explore, and discuss more about what is <u>really</u> important to them. Within the body of work on subjective well-being, we are reminded that people have not and do not often spend large amounts of time and energy reflecting and exploring what is really important to them (see Dolan et al. 2008), which results in under-developed or/and incomplete personal constructs. The experience of suffering then provides the opportunity for a deeper consideration of what really matters; it is a time for reflection and increasing self-awareness. According to accounts located in the relevant literature (such as Emblen and Pesut 2001; Hall 2001; Egnew 2005; DeMichelle 2009) the epiphanies and gestalts that result can be something of a surprise to the person, with reference to new perspectives and hitherto unexplored areas. Or the reflection leads to re-examination and reiteration of previously held (and diminished) constructs and values. In these explorations, rather than halt at the surface or superficial description of what is thought to be important, P/MH nurses seek to focus on the deeper meanings, help access the clients (often hidden or obscured) core values, existential anxieties, and unique thinking processes (Wong 1998). And they can facilitate this by means of reflection, critical examination, and life review (Wong 1998). Frankl (1961, p. 36) offers the following example of discovering what was really important to him.

> Then I grasped the meaning of the greatest secret that human poetry and human thought and belief have to impart: The salvation of man is through love and in love. I understood how a

> man who has nothing left in this world still may know bliss, be it only for a brief moment, in the contemplation of his beloved.

Fifthly, P/MH nurses need to have a holistic presence with the person who is suffering and accompany him/her on his/her journey. In keeping with Cassell's (1991) position, the limited literature in this area (see Kogstad et al. 2009; Gustafsson et al. 2011; Berglund et al. 2012) warns that the experience of suffering can be exacerbated as a result of healthcare experiences; more specifically: from feeling mistreated; from struggling to have one's healthcare needs and autonomy respected; to feeling powerless and to feel fragmented and objectified (Berglund et al. p. 5/12). Similarly, Rusner et al. (2010) argue that the suffering person desires: to be needed; to be able to be oneself; and to be valued and confirmed. Thus the need for P/MH nurses to have a presence, emotionally and physically to the sufferer. In so doing the P/MH nurse becomes aware of the client's particular needs, wishes, and desires. He/she can involve the client in all care-related discussions and decisions, communicates a sense that the client is not powerless, is valued and confirmed. And the presence of this compassionate other can combat the sense of isolation and alienation that often accompanies suffering. Priya (2012, p. 213) perhaps captures the essence of this intervention when he refers how

> suffering and healing are not two disjointed experiences. Despite experiencing distress or suffering, a humanizing space created by empathetic witnessing of a listener may initiate a new enabling meaning and value for the afflicted person.

Sixthly, P/MH nurses can facilitate access to fellow 'sufferers' (e.g., support groups) where additional support can be found; where the sense of isolation or alienation associated with suffering can be countered. It has long been recognized that peer support is synonymous with groups as these can harness the power of shared experiences to provide support to group members (see Yallom 2005; Diefenbeck et al. 2014). Erdner et al. (2005) assert that the experience of suffering a mental health problem often leads to a sense of isolation and alienation; a feeling of alienation described by Erdner et al. (2005, p. 378) as "existential loneliness." As a result, P/MH nurses need to provide or facilitate access to material, accounts, testimonies, of the many others who have experienced suffering—perhaps in the form of peer support or therapeutic groups. Such access can expose the person who is suffering to others who have found meaning in their own suffering and are better for this.

Seventhly, P/MH can facilitate the person's movement further towards self-transcendence. According to Oreopoulus (Oreopoulos 2005), the healing power of suffering is an awe-inspiring mystery. Life's insurmountable obstacles, he argues, can give rise to hitherto unknown potentials and usher the person towards a new purpose. An awareness arising from the experience of suffering, namely that control over one's life is a myth, enables the person to learn humility and accept life's limitations. Oreopoulus (Oreopoulos 2005) argues that

> by enduring suffering, rather than fighting it, we discover the solitary path of an inward journey…We feel grounded in something deeper, wiser and more powerful than the previous sense of self; no longer do we take life for granted. By clarifying our priorities and

values, we live more wisely. While respecting the separateness of others, we feel closer to them and experience a new mutuality in relationships with loved ones.

For seminal contributors such as Maslow (1972), self-transcendence is concerned with full 'spiritual' awakening; with extreme wellness or optimal well-being. Maslow (1972) purports that self-transcendence captures the person's expansion of sense of self and personal, individual identity. In essence, moving the individual away from less developed, more ego-centric views of self to being more consciously and purposefully 'meta-motivated.' The self-transcendent individual for Maslow (1972) then becomes concerned with what he describes as the values of being, e.g., perfection, truth, beauty, goodness, unity, etc. And Maslow (1972) declares that there is a strengthening of the person's engagement with synergy, with intra-psychic, with interpersonal relations, with acting and thinking intra-culturally and internationally. P/MH nurses can then help the person understand that, perhaps paradoxically for some, the experience can actually propel the person into new heights of personal growth; into an expanded sense of identity and consciousness expansion.

Conclusion

In this paper we have identified two conceptualizations of suffering: one sees it as something that needs to be cured or fixed and that it is isomorphic to pain; the other sees it as an unavoidable feature of the human condition or experience and that it can lead to personal growth (and may even be necessary for full growth and development). We have shown how the former conceptualization is highly congruent with the increased pathologizing of 'everyday life,' with an eschewing of suffering as a potential valuable, developmental experience, and with the inexorable proliferation of pharmacological 'treatment.'

The current orthodoxy of mental health care leaves little, if any, room for the sufferer to be proud of his suffering and to consider it ennobling rather than degrading (Weiskopf-Joelson 1980). Yet there is a sizeable body of literature both of a recognized vintage and more contemporary that draws attention to the major problems associated with the over-zealous medicalization of society and human experiences. Not least these orthodox views restrict the opportunity for the transformative processes that can occur in the individual when the meaning of suffering is realized. Accordingly, we assert that there is a clear need for P/MH nurses to re-think their views of suffering, to explore with the person, the meaning in his/her suffering experience and how they might accompany the individual on his/her suffering journey. And we have included a range of approaches and interventions that P/MH nurses can use when attempting to help those experiencing mental health-related suffering. While the wish to remove a person's suffering can be understood as laudable and maybe even the act of a moral agent, the preponderance of the evidence seems to indicate that in so doing, we may actually deny the person's chance for growth and development, propel him/her towards further ignobility, and reinforce unhelpful conceptualizations of what it is to be human in the twenty-first century.

References

American Foundation for Suicide Prevention (2014) Facts and figures: suicide deaths. Available at Http://www.afsp.org/understanding-suicide/facts-and-figures. Accessed 12 Feb 2014
Barbui C, Campomori A, D'Avanzo B, Negri E, Garattini S (1999) Antidepressant drug use in Italy since the introduction of SSRIs: National trends, regional differences and impact on suicide rates. Soc Psychiatry Psychiatr Epidemiol 34(3):152–156
Berglund M, Westin L, Svanström R, Sundler AJ (2012) Suffering caused by care – Patients' experiences from hospital settings. Int J Qual Stud 7. doi:10.3402/qhw.v7io.18688
Bonney S, Stickley T (2008) Recovery and mental health: a review of the British literature. J Psychiatr Ment Health Nurs 15(2):140–153
Borg M, Kristiansen K (2004) Recovery-orientated professionals: helping relationships in mental health services. J Ment Health 13(5):493–505
Cassell EJ (1991) The nature of suffering and the goals of medicine. Oxford University Press, Oxford
Calhoun LG, Tedeschi RG (2006) Handbook of post-traumatic growth: research and practice. Lawrence Erlbaum Associates, New York
Chapman RC, Garvin J (1985) Suffering: the contributions of persistent pain. Lancet 353:2233–2237
Charmaz K (1983) Loss of self: a fundamental form of suffering in the chronically ill. Sociol Health Illn 5(2):168–195
Cleese J (2008) Why being funny is no joke. The independent. Available at http://www.independent.co.uk/life-style/health-and-families/health-news/why-being-funny-is-no-joke-769859.html. Accessed 18 Feb 2014
Currie J (2005) The marketization of depression: the prescribing of SSRI antidepressants to women. Available at www.whp-apsf.ca/pdf/SSRIs.pdf. Accessed 30 Mar 2014
Cutcliffe JR, Hyrkas K, McKenna HP (2010) Nursing models: application to practice. Quay Books, London
DeBellis R, Marcus E, Kutscher AH et al (1986) Suffering: psychological and social aspects in loss grief, grief and care. Haworth Press, New York
DeMichelle KA (2009) Memories of suffering: exploring the life story narratives of twice-widowed elderly women. J Aging Stud 23(2):103–113
Deegan P (2003). Recovery: the experience and the evidence. Available at http://www.recoverydevon.co.uk/download/2justflower.ppt. Accessed 6 Jan 2014
Diefenbeck CA, Klemm PR, Hayes ER (2014) Emergence of Yalom's therapeutic factors in a peer-led, asynchronous, online support group for family caregivers. Issues Ment Health Nurs 35(1):21–32
Dolan P, Peasgood T, White M (2008) Do we really know what makes us happy? A review of the economic literature on the factors associated with subjective well-being. J Econ Psychol 29(1):94–122
Egnew TR (2005) The meaning of healing: transcending suffering. Ann Fam Med 3(3):255–262
Emblen J, Pesut B (2001) Strengthening transcendent meaning: a model for the spiritual nursing care of patients experiencing suffering. J Holist Nurs 19(1):42–56
Erdner A, Magnusson A, Nyström M, Lützén K (2005) Social and existential alienation experienced by people with long-term mental illness. Scand J Caring Sci 19:373–380
Eriksson K (ed.) (1993). Möten med lidanden. Åbo: Åbo Akademi, Institutionen för vårdvetenskap. Report no. 4
Frances A (2013) Saving normal: an insider's revolt against out-of-control psychiatric diagnosis, DSM-5, Big pharma, and the medicalization of ordinary life. Harper Collins, New York
Frankl V (1961) Logotherapy and the challenge of suffering. Rev Existent Psychiatry 1:3–7
Frankl V (1963) Man's search for meaning: an introduction to logotherapy. Pocket Books, New York
Fredriksson L, Lindström U (2002) Caring conversations – psychioatric patients' narratives about suffering. J Adv Nurs 40(4):396–404
Fromm E (1947) Man for himself. Holt, Rinehart & Winston, New York

Fry S (2006) Steven fry: my battle with mental illness. The independent. Available at http://www.independent.co.uk/life-style/health-and-families/health-news/stephen-fry-my-battle-with-mental-illness-416386.html. Accessed 19 Feb 2014
Gabriel Y (1984) A psychoanalytical contribution to the sociology of suffering. Int Rev Psychoanal 11(4):467–480
Greenberg G (2014) The cult of DSM: ending our allegiance to the Great Gazoo. Psychotherapy Networker, March/April, 21–27
Gustafsson L-K, Wiklund-Gustin L, Lindström UÅ (2011) The meaning of reconciliation: women1s stories about their experience of reconciliation with suffering from grief. Scand J Caring Sci 25:525–532
Hall DJ (1986) God and human suffering: an exercise in theology of the cross. Augsburg Publishing House, Minneapolis
Hall VP (2001) Bearing witness to suffering in AIDS: constructing meaning from loss. J Assoc Nurses AIDS Care 12(2):44–55
Hall WD, Mant A, Mitchell PB, Rendle VA, Hickie IB, McManus P (2003) Association between antidepressant prescribing and suicide in Australia, 1991–2000: trend analysis. Br Med J 10(326):1008
Healy D (2005) Psychiatric drugs explained, 5th edn. Elsevier, Edinburgh
Hummelvoll JK (2010) Møte med mennesket i psykiatrien; implikasjoner for psykiatrisk sykepleie. Tidsskrift for Sygeplejeforskning 1:13–20
Kahn DL, Steeves RH (1986) The experience of suffering: conceptual clarification and theoretical definition. J Adv Nurs 11(6):623–631
Keller H (2014) The quotations page. Available at http://www.quotationspage.com/quote/30186.html. Accessed 21 Feb 2014
Kierkegaard S (1983) Fear and trembling. (HV Long & EH Long Trans.) Princeton University Press, New Jersey
Kleinman A (1988) The illness narratives: suffering, healing and the human condition. Basic Books, New York
Kogstad R, Hummelvoll JK, Eriksson B (2009) User experiences of different treatment cultures in mental health care. Ethical Hum Psychol Psychiatry 11(2):97–111
Lorem GF (2008) Making sense of stories: the use of patient narratives within mental health care research. Nurs Philos 9:62–71
McKenna HP (1997) Nursing theories and models. Routledge, London
Maltsberger J (1992). cited in Maris RW, Berman AL, Silverman MM. Comprehensive textbook of suicidology. New York: Guildford Press
Mandela N (2014) Brainy quote. Available at http://www.brainyquote.com/quotes/quotes/n/nelsonmand447262.html. Accessed 22 Feb 2014
Maris RW (1981) Pathways to suicide: a survey of self-destructive behaviors. John Hopkins University Press, Baltimore
Maslow A (1972) The farther reaches of human nature. Viking, New York
Merriam-Webster Dictionary (2014). Available at http://www.merriam-webster.com/dictionary/suffering. Accessed 13th Jan 2014
Middleton N, Gunnell D, Whitley E, Dorling D, Frankel S (2001) Secular trends in antidepressant prescribing in the UK, 1975–1998. J Public Health 23(4):262–267
Miller RB (2004) Facing human suffering: psychology and psychotherapy as moral engagement. APA, Washington DC
Milligan S. (2014) Mental health forum. Available at http://www.mentalhealthforum.net/forum/thread75495.html. Accessed 20 Feb 2014
Mojtabail R, Olfson M (2011) Proportion of antidepressants prescribed without a psychiatric diagnosis is growing. Health Aff 30(8):1434–1442
Moore M (2014) Can good come from bad? Do suicide survivors experience growth after their loss? In: Cutcliffe JR, Santos JC, Links P, Zaheer J, Harder HG, Campbell F, McCormick R, Harder K, Bergmans Y, Eynan R (eds) Routledge international handbook of clinical suicide research. Routledge, London, pp 298–307

Morse JM, Johnson JL (eds) (1991) The illness experience: dimensions of suffering. Sage, Newbury Park Ca

Morse JM, Carter BJ (1996) The essence of enduring and expressions of suffering: the reformulation of self. Sch Inq Nurs Pract 10:43–60

Morse JM, Whittaker H, Tason M (1996) The caretakers of suffering. In: Chesworth J (ed) Transpersonal healing: essays on the ecology of health. Sage, Newbury Park, pp 91–104

Munoz-Arroyo R, Sutton M, Morrison J (2005) Exploring potential explanations for the increase in antidepressant prescribing in Scotland using secondary analysis of routine data. Br J Gen Pract 56(527):423–428

Nash J. (2014) Schizophrenia daily blog. Available at http://www.schizophrenia.com/sznews/archives/001617.html. Accessed 20 Feb 2014

Nietzsche, F. (1992). Beyond good and evil. In: Basic writings of Nietzsche. (Trans. and Ed. Walter Kaufman.) New York, The Modern Library

Olfson M, Marcus SC (2009) National patterns in antidepressant medication treatment. Arch Gen Psychiatry 66(8):848–856

Online Dictionary (2014). Available at http://www.thefreedictionary.com/suffering. Accessed 20 Jan 2014

O'Mahony N (2014) Executive report for the Oireachtas subcomittee for health: main concerns to investigate regarding the influence of the pharmaceutical industry in the island of Ireland. Holistic action group/MINDFREEDOM Ireland. Available at http://psychrights.org/Countries/UK/ExecReport4HealthComm.pdf. Accessed 25 Mar 2014

Oreopoulos DG (2005) Is there meaning in suffering? Hum Med, 5, 2. Available at http://www.humanehealthcare.com/Article.asp?art_id=830. Accessed 18 Feb 2014

Priya KR (2012) Social constructionist approach to suffering and healing: Juxtaposing Cassell, Gergen and Kleinman. Psychol Stud 57(2):211–223

Redfield-Jamison K (1996) An unquiet mind: a memoir of moods and madness. Vintage Books, New York

Roy DJ (1998) The relief of pain and suffering: ethical principles and imperatives. J Pallaitive Care 14(2):3–5

Roberts M (2008) Facilitating recovery by making sense of suffering: a Nietzschean perspective. J Psychiatr Ment Health Nurs 15:743–748

Rusner M, Carlsson G, Brunt D, Nyström M (2010) A dependence that empowers – the meaning of the conditions that enable a good life with bipolar disorder. Int J Qual Stud Health Well-Being 5:4653

Råholm M-B (2008) Uncovering the ethics of suffering using a narrative approach. Nurs Ethics 15(1):62–72

Scarry E (1985) The body in pain. Oxford University Press, Oxford

Storr A (2005) Black dog, Kafka's mice, and other phenomena of the human mind. Ballantine Books, New York

Sykes Wylie M (2014) The book we love to hate: Why DSM-5 makes nobody happy Psychotherapy Networker, March/April, 28–35

Szasz T (2007) The medicalization of everyday life: selected essays. Syracuse University Press, Syracuse

Tedeschi RG, Calhoun LG (1995) Trauma and transformation: growing in the aftermath of suffering. Sage, Thousand Oaks

Tedeschi RG, Calhoun LG (2004) Posttraumatic growth: conceptual foundations and empirical evidence. Psychol Inq 15(1):1–18

Tournier P (2014) Brainy quotes. Available at http://www.brainyquote.com/quotes/quotes/p/paultourni112268.html. Accessed 20 Feb 2014

Van Praag H (2005) Why haven't antidepressants reduced suicide rates? In: Hawton K (ed) Prevention and treatment of suicidal behavior: from science to practice. Oxford University Press, Oxford, pp 239–260

Weiskopf-Joelson E (1980) The place of logotherapy in the world today. Int Forum Logother 1(3):3–7

Whittaker R (2002) Mad in America: bad science, bad medicine, and the enduring mistreatment of the mentally ill. Perseus Publishing, Philadelphia
Wong PT (1998) Meaning-centred counselling. In: Wong PT (ed.) The quest for human meaning: a handbook of theory, research and application. pp. 72–110
World Health Organisation (2001) The World health report: 2001: mental health: new understanding, new hope. World Health Organization, Geneva
Yallom I (2005) The theory and practice of group psychotherapy, 5th edn. Basic books, New York
Zborowski M (1969) People in pain. Jossey-Bass, San Francisco

Part II

Settings and Contexts

13 Acute Inpatient Psychiatric/Mental Health Nursing: Lessons Learned and Current Developments

Roland van de Sande

13.1 Introduction

At the macro level, psychiatric/mental health (P/MH) nurses are facing several challenges in providing safe and therapeutic inpatient nursing care. Across Europe the number of available beds per 100,000 population varies considerably (van de Sande et al. 2011); however, in most European regions, the number of inpatient beds has reduced during recent years (in some cases, quite dramatically—see Nolan and Brimblecombe 2012). Such 'developments' have had significant impacts on what care can be provided by P/MH nurses, most notably, how these challenges have eroded the potential and/or opportunities for psychotherapeutic P/MH nursing with many clients. Most remaining beds are now situated in acute psychiatric wards, and the pressure on available beds is accompanied by the principle 'the worst in and the best out'. In some parts of Europe, including the author's nation, this means that nowadays 'inpatient' care is more focused on stabilization rather than allowing patients to take time to recover from the consequences of a crisis in a clinical environment.

13.2 Engaging Therapeutically in Inpatient Settings

Unfortunately a considerable number of clients that disengaged from community psychiatric services are facing relapses and lack informal social support to manage their own distress. This results in some countries experiencing an increase of

R. van de Sande
Institute of Nursing Studies, Utrecht University of Applied Sciences, Utrecht, The Netherlands

Parnassia Psychiatric Institute, The Hague, The Netherlands
e-mail: roland.vandesande@hu.nl

© Springer International Publishing Switzerland 2018

J.C. Santos, J.R. Cutcliffe (eds.), *European Psychiatric/Mental Health Nursing in the 21st Century*, Principles of Specialty Nursing,
https://doi.org/10.1007/978-3-319-31772-4_13

involuntary admissions, for instance, the USA (Figueroa et al. 2004; Tulloch et al. 2011), the UK (Barker et al. 2011; Hayes et al. 2013), New Zealand (Chai et al. 2013), Australia (Bastiampillia et al. 2010), Norway (Hustoft et al. 2013) and the Netherlands (Schoevaerts et al. 2013). In addition to their mental health challenges, such clients will also have to cope with the stress of admission and adjusting to involuntary care. In such situations, P/MH nurses can make a difference in terms of engaging therapeutically. Melartin et al. (2005), for instance, emphasize the need for persistent psychotherapeutic approaches given the fact that many, newly admitted acute clients have destabilized and/or stopped taking medication. Therefore, forming, nurturing and building up a new therapeutic relationship are one of the first priorities. This position is supported by at least two studies concluding that symptom reduction outcomes after inpatient psychotherapy seem to be more associated with the quality of the therapeutic alliance rather than individual patient characteristics (Dinger et al. 2008; Marcus et al. 2011). These findings indicate that self-reflection and therapeutic skills of P/MH nurses can indeed make a difference in the acute phase even when the client is destabilized and difficult to engage with. They can, for example, bridge the gap to a community-based recovery process and start working on combatting hopelessness and regaining self-control.

13.3 Promising Intervention? Engagement as a Counteraction to Containment

In the last decade some evidence emerged that the ongoing investment in practice development and especially enhancing the therapeutic engagement in acute psychiatric wards can reduce containment measures (Mistral et al. 2002; Bowers et al. 2006; Bowers et al. 2014). Another interesting study conducted by O'Malley et al. (2007) showed that containment measures went down by 23% following therapeutic skills improvements in the nursing workforce in acute psychiatric wards. These competences can, for example, be used in engaging the client in establishing joint de-escalation prevention plans to avoid last resort interventions. There is promising evidence that joint early recognition plans designed with patients can be helpful (Fluttert et al. 2010; Smith et al. 2005). In fact a meta-analysis (de Jong et al. 2016) on RCTs of interventions to reduce compulsory admission revealed that joint crisis plans are one of the few options that could be effective in bringing about this reduction. The process of co-creating a joint crisis plan can start during the admission phase and be refined with the community mental health nurse after discharge to prevent a future compulsory hospitalization. In this process clients are asked which circumstances could trigger escalations and what would be the preferred approaches of mental health staff and relatives or friends in these situations.

For clients that are temporarily unable to collaborate in establishing a joint crisis plan, structured short-term risk assessment by nurses can be beneficial to prevent unnecessary escalations. In this way P/MH nurses can consistently objectify the early signs of the risks of escalations and discuss these in a nonjudgemental way with the patient and colleagues. This approach can promote safety for clients, visitors and staff. Given the significant results of two-cluster randomized clinical trial (RCT) in the nursing domain conducted by Abderhalden et al. (2008) and van de Sande et al. (2011), this evidence-based approach could inform 'best practice' guidelines and/or standards. There is robust evidence that such structured approaches can result in fewer escalations and containment measures in acute psychiatric wards. Once the client is more stable, the step of co-creating a joint crisis plan can be tried again. In this context P/MH nurses could also discuss the risk patterns that they have observed to support a sound joint crisis plan.

For acute psychiatric wards that host mainly involuntary clients, establishing and maintaining therapeutic engagement may face additional difficulties. One of the impeding factors is that clients in the peak of a psychotic crisis can temporarily lose psychological insight (Pini et al. 2001). On the other hand McEvoy et al. (2006) found that ongoing attempts to invest during this crisis phase in therapeutic engagement can work once the symptoms are in remission. An example of co-creation of inpatient therapeutic care is perhaps how service users, carer umbrella organizations, P/MH nurses and doctors form a new consensus framework for high and intensive care by means of mapping methodology (Trochim 1989; van Mierlo et al. 2014). In the Netherlands this consensus process was followed by several pilots and factor analysis rounds that eventually resulted in the national validation of a high and intensive care accreditation evaluation scale. Below, an overview how these criteria may be transferred to 21 essential competences that P/MH nurses based should demonstrate in such settings:

1. Demonstrate low-threshold initiatives to engage with patients (early recognition of alarming signs and be truly available).
2. Using transparent clinical reasoning when protocols are not applicable in a certain situation.
3. Tailor-made clinical use of evidence-based intervention and research-based theories.
4. Support the patient's individual recovery process.
5. Empower the patient's strengths and capacities as much as possible.
6. Utilizing the admission as an important part of the recovery process.
7. Systemic approaches in care co-ordination created together with relatives and community health services.
8. Tailor-made use of relevant evidence-based multidisciplinary guidelines.
9. A proficient contribution in the diagnostic process and the evaluation of the stabilization process.
10. Adequate use of risk evaluation instruments.
11. Using best practice approaches in negotiating, conflict mitigation and de-escalation interventions.
12. Safeguarding the person's safety of patients and colleagues.

13. Safe practice of break away and manual restraint techniques.
14. Using adequate protocols for medication, using patient information and monitoring side effects.
15. Monitoring and guidance in addiction issues.
16. Using proficient knowledge on health-care law including patient's rights.
17. Ability to provide adequate psychoeducation about stress, coping and mental illness.
18. Supporting the patient to co-create joint crisis plans.
19. Reflection on action and the provision of adequacy to colleagues.
20. Adequate use of suicide prevention strategies according to evidence-based guidelines.
21. Adequate registration of containment measures and debrief and evaluation of these with the patients.

In any western country, mental health practitioners have the moral obligation to follow relevant guidelines to manage crisis behaviour in the least restrictive way (Glick et al. 2008; NICE 2015). In this context the four principles of biomedical ethics (Beauchamp and Childress 2013) are also important to keep in mind:

1. Non-maleficence
2. Autonomy
3. Beneficence
4. Confidentiality

For example, self-inflicted injuries can result in containment measures when clinicians assess that the client has temporary control and that his/her behaviour will harm himself/herself. In these types of escalations, psychosocial stressors are not isolated from dysfunctional neurobiological processes; in fact both often play a key role in aggressive and self-destructive outbursts (Doihara et al. 2008; Groholt and Ekeberg 2009). Therefore P/MH nursing staff need to minimize/prevent unnecessary self-harm if the client becomes overwhelmed by acute psychosocial stressors, severe mood or anxiety symptoms (Soloff and Chiapetta 2012). For example, impulse control problems are well-known manifestations in clients suffering from (so-called) post-traumatic stress (Elbogen et al. 2008), borderline personality problems (Benvenuti et al. 2005) and severe mood symptoms (Hendin et al. 2010). Neglecting these aspects may result in a decline of psychosocial functioning, stigma and a vicious cycle of the use (increase) of containment measures. This may well become problematic for the client and P/MH nurses and can seriously impede the therapeutic relationship or even provoke patients to disengage from mental health services in the future.

13.4 Further Challenging Situations Encountered in Inpatient Acute Mental Health Settings

Some authors have reported that almost 5% of clients suffering from so-called psychotic disorders will eventually die from fatal self-destructive acts (Palmer et al. 2005). Other authors dispute these findings arguing that 5% is an overestimate. Self-destructive behaviour is sometimes acutely provoked by aggressive command hallucinations or guilt-induced delusions (Glick et al. 2008). In this context P/MH nurses sometimes need to use intrusive interventions to prevent further life threatening damage. The risk of fatal outcomes is higher for schizophrenia patients that also suffer from severe mood problems (Large et al. 2011) and co-morbid drug and alcohol addiction (Suokas et al. 2010). However, the overall inpatient prevalence of fatal outcomes of self-destructive behaviour appears to be relatively low (Combs and Romm 2007). In half of the fatal cases hospitals will face, litigation (Robbert 2006) which often implicates inquiries focused on the nursing process in the ward. Some relevant evidence indicates that a high proportion of fatal self-destructive incidents occur directly after absconding: often jumping from heights or being hit by large vehicles (Spiessl et al. 2002). Inside the wards most fatal destructive incidents occur by self-asphyxiation: plastic bags or hangings (Knoll 2012; Meehan et al. 2006; Mann et al. 2005).

The clinical and policy picture regarding acts of self-harm and mental health-care agency responses to the same is confusing. There are some data that show how a sizeable percentage of all acute psychiatric admissions were related to self-destructive acts. There are also data available that do indicate how some suicide attempts, including successful attempts, do occur on inpatient settings (REFs). And there exist a multitude of studies that have shown an elevated risk of suicide being associated with certain mental health problems and experiences (for some—diagnoses). Yet, despite the relatively low number of those fatal incidents, the attention paid to risk management/prevention, the human resources poured in to attempts to keep people physically safe and the print space (number of articles, papers, guidelines published, etc.) dedicated to writing about preventing acts of self-harm are all considerably disproportionate to the scope/size of the problem. Further, according to Owen et al. (2002), the provision of continuity of care in this client group can be very complicated. Research findings suggest that clients demonstrating repetitive self-destructive behaviour are seriously in need of long-lasting therapeutic relationships (Kapur et al. 2000; Simon and Petch 2002; Stringer et al. 2013). As nurses are spending more time in direct contact/direct patient care than any other discipline, they can make a difference in promoting continuity of care and use the admission episode as a start for building up therapeutic engagement and promote other help-seeking behaviour.

During a crisis clients disengage or even abscond driven by the perception that the ward is unsafe (Muir-Cochrane et al. 2011). One of the fears that many P/MH nursing staff report is the absconsion of self-destructive clients; the prevalence of this problem in acute psychiatric wards varies from 13 to 38% of all admitted patients; most of them return without any severe incidents (Meehan et al. 1999; Bowers et al. 1998; Stewart and Bowers 2011). Nevertheless, the risk of absconding is often reported to be an important reason for the use of a variety of containment measures (Van der Merwe et al. 2009). Conversely, Lang et al. (2010) found that absconding decreased after the introduction of less restrictive and open-door policy in a former locked ward in Germany. According to the findings from Bailey et al. (2016) study, the promotion of therapeutic engagement and calculated risk taking by P/MH is crucial to minimize absconding from the wards. One of the successful factors of overcoming a self-destructive crisis is the way clients experience the therapeutic engagement of P/MH nurses (REFS). Therefore, P/MH nurses need to take into account that therapeutic engagement needs to build up carefully. The psychopathological experiences of admitted clients, such as paranoid delusions, elevated mood and blunted affect, may complicate and hinder any nurse-client communication (Lobbestael et al. 2013; Miczek et al. 2007; Siever 2008; Soyka 2011; Krakowski 2003).

13.5 Further Challenges

A number of studies report that many inpatients encounter traumatic experiences (e.g. physical/verbal aggression violence or sexual harassment) during previous admissions (Kumar et al. 2001; Walsh et al. 2003; Dean et al. 2007; Choe et al. 2008; Sturup et al. 2011; Hodgins et al. 2007; Katsikidou et al. 2013; van der Post et al. 2014). Sometimes this is one of the main reasons why clients disengage from mental health services (REF). Therefore, Walsh et al. (2003) highly recommend including routine victimization questions in admission interviews and during P/MH nurse-client encounters and interactions. The proportion of victimized clients appears to be higher than the number of violent patients in acute psychiatric wards. For example, Fortugno et al. (2013) found a 38% victimization rate in a sample of 537 psychotic inpatients across Europe. They also found that patients in a state of mania appear the most likely victims due to their own temporary impulsive behaviour and misjudging the boundaries of interpersonal actions.

Although the phenomenon of victimization is still under researched, some studies give more detailed insights in the proportion of both verbal threats and physical violence among fellow patients. A British study conducted by Hodgins et al. (2007) found that almost 50% of the clients experienced serious verbally or physically threatening behaviour by fellow inpatients: this happened both to males (57%) and females (48%). In Greece, Katsikidou et al. (2013) found even higher victimization rates (59%). Urban inpatients appear to be much more at risk for victimization before and during the admission (Hodgins et al. 2007; Sturup et al. 2011). A study in a number of North American acute psychiatric wards reveals that approximately 22% of client population has been assaulted by fellow patients, at least once (Choe et al. 2008).

Maintaining a safe and therapeutic environment is an ongoing challenge for P/MH nurses in acute psychiatric wards. Not surprisingly most involuntary admitted clients have mixed emotions about their stay in these settings (van der Post et al. 2014). Some clients can understand the clinical and legal decisions and believe that such actions prevented them from further harm, whereas others perceive the level of coercion as disproportionate and as a consequence of stay in an acute ward that is disengaged from the psychiatric services normally offered (Katsakou et al. 2012). These disclosures indicate the importance of the continuous promotion of therapeutic engagement in acute psychiatric wards. Therefore, the prevention of boredom, hopelessness and lack of therapeutic options needs to be balanced with the prevention of overstimulation by overcrowded wards, violence and aggression or sexual harassment of fellow patients and illegal drug use (Quirk and Lelliot 2001). All these problems have been associated with poor treatment outcomes and unsafe situations in psychiatric wards.

Cutcliffe and Stevenson (2008) state that P/MH nurses have a long frontline tradition with caring for people in the peak of a crisis. The challenge for P/MH nurses in this context is to integrate relevant scientific knowledge with interpersonal and personified therapeutic approaches. This needs to be demonstrated in a nonjudgemental way and focused on the understanding of hidden meaning of crisis behaviour. On the other hand P/MH nursing care can be more effective when good practices are shared in the team and are replicable by most of the colleagues. According to Berg and Hallberg (2000), high-quality therapeutic engagement implicates intensified presence in which preventing from gliding away in an overload of distress is the core element of our work. However, these therapeutic qualities often remain implicit and difficult to share in teamwork in caring for acute patients. Dziopa and Ahern (2009) argue that if these interpersonal attributes remain vague, these will seriously impede high-level practice standards. Bowers et al. (2014) attempred to brigde some of these gaps by synthesizing the available evidence to minimize escalations in acute psychiatric wards. This research process led to the creation of the so-called "Safeward" model. In this process the materials were reviewed by a panel of experts. Eventually they found six conflict domains that can be influenced by P/MH nurses: (1) the group dynamics in the patient community, (2) patient characteristics, (3) regulatory frameworks, (4) staff characteristics, (5) physical environment in the hospital and (6) influences from outside the hospital. In those domains there are several triggers for imminent escalations that need to be addressed by nurses therapeutically. Early and preliminary attempts to evaluate the model using a cluster RCT, imitations notwithstanding, were undertaken by Bowers et al. (2015). Staff and clients, in 31 randomly chosen wards, participated in 15 randomly chosen hospitals. In the experimental condition, a reduced rate of conflict events of 15% was found, and the rate of containment events was reduced by 26.4%. These findings encouraged some psychiatric settings in certain parts of Europe to embrace the model. Currently the Safewards model (Bowers et al. 2014) is translated in at least five other European languages and actively used in clinical practice and nurse education. The Safewards toolkit enables P/MH nurses, for example, to coach daily group sessions in a structured way. The following agenda are used during those sessions:

1. Round of thanks and news, for example.
2. Round of news; staff explain events that have happened that might be confusing or distressing. This is used to assist the patients to psychologically understand each other's behaviour or to understand the reasons why the staff act the way they do and ask everyone to watch over each other and keep each other safe.
3. Round of suggestions.
4. Requests: to offer the chance to offer suggestions as to how to get along with each other over the next period and pay attention to the requests and offers of each other.

13.5.1 Implementation of Sustainable Good Practices to Enhance Therapeutic Inpatient Care

Rix and Sheppard (2003) argue that although relevant evidence-based interventions to reduce coercive practices are available, they are infrequently used in acute psychiatric wards. They state that new approaches in such settings only seem to be used if there is an immediate clinical benefit for frontline workers, and supportive organizational conditions are promoted by all managers at various levels. This includes clinical leadership and management support and the involvement of patient representatives. Similar premises are echoed by Huckshorn (2004) and Colton (2010), both of whom have applied these views within organizational models to minimize coercion in acute psychiatric wards in the USA. These six core strategies led to an impressive reduction of seclusion in Pennsylvania (Smith et al. 2005) and were subsequently adopted internationally in New Zealand (O'Hagan et al. 2008), Australia (Ryan and Happell 2009) and Canada (Larue et al. 2009) and were more recently also tested successfully in Finland (Putkonen et al. 2013). In the USA, lessons learned from seclusion reduction programmes revealed that if the board of the hospital did not embrace interventions to reduce seclusion, all the efforts vanished in the end (Huckshorn 2004; Colton and Xiong 2010). Those authors state that organizational factors and leadership of administrators may have as much if not even more influence on coercion reduction as knowledge about the individual being exposed to containment measures.

Given the previously discussed findings, the following three major goals continuously need to be on the radar of P/MH nurses working on acute inpatient units/wards:

1. Retention of the therapeutic, interpersonal relationship as the primary goal of care, with the knowledge and understanding that such actions serve as an intervention themselves in addition to creating the conditions in which other interventions are contextualized/embedded.
2. Assessment and psychotherapeutic efforts targeted on the client's previous, unhelpful experiences during crisis episodes.
3. Prevention of under stimulation (especially boredom) and avoidance of overstimulation.

13.6 Conclusion and Recommendations

For many years, P/MH nurses have served in the role of 'critical companion' of clients during the peak or apex of their mental health crisis. Performing effectively and therapeutically in this role requires the formation and maintenance of an interpersonal, therapeutic relationship. Though it should be acknowledged that doing so is not without significant challenges, many current mental health systems are at least in part antagonistic to this goal and that such efforts make substantial demands on the P/MH nurse. Acute P/MH nursing care requires a focus on preserving and promoting the client's dignity, which appears to be bound up with a range of attitudes, qualities and behaviours in the nursing staff, namely, being there for the patient without too many formal/informal barriers, balancing calculated therapeutic risk taking with client's safety issues and limiting setting, all occurring within the context and boundaries of a therapeutic relationship. The complexity of psychologically induced crisis behaviour needs a holistic understanding to inform the approaches of the P/MH nurse. Clients often haven't chosen to rely on clinicians; therefore, it is our moral duty to minimize harm during the admission. The bed reduction campaigns in many countries implicate short admissions focusing on stabilizing the client to enable the recovery process at home. Nevertheless the psychosocial skills of inpatient P/MH nurses can make a big difference in the prognosis of the admitted client. Somewhat paradoxically for some, even these 'crises' that precipitate admission can become opportunities for growth and development. Fortunately these psychosocial skills used in psychiatric wards are increasingly scientifically evaluated. The relevant findings are increasingly disseminated and are finding their way into substantive 'therapeutic toolkits' and 'best practice guidelines' for clinical practice and advanced training. This improves the consistency of the therapeutic climate in acute care. This may reduce the risk of re-traumatizing vulnerable patients and disengagement from any mental health care in the future.

References

Abderhalden C, Needham I, Dassen T, Halfens R, Haug HJ, Fischer JE (2008) Structured risk assessment and violence in acute psychiatric wards: randomized controlled trial. Br J Psychiatry 193(1):44–50

Bailey J, Page B, Ndimande N, Connell J, Vincent C (2016) Absconding: reducing failure to return in adult mental health wards. BMJ Qual Improv Rep 5(1):u209837.w5117

Barker V, Taylor M, Kader I, Stewart K, Le Fèvre P (2011) Impact of crisis resolution and home treatment services on user experience and admission to psychiatric hospital. Psychiatrist 35(3):106–110

Bastiampillia T, Bidargaddi N, Dhilon R, Schroder G, Strobel J, Galley P (2010) Implications of bed reduction in an acute psychiatric service. Aust Med J 193(7):383

Beauchamp T, Childress J (2013) Principles of biomedical ethics, 7th edn. Oxford University Press, New York

Benvenuti A, Rucci P, Ravani L (2005) Psychotic features in borderline patients: is there a connection to mood dysregulation? Bipolar Disord 7(4):338–343

Berg A, Hallberg I (2000) Psychiatric nurses' lived experiences of working with inpatient care on a general team psychiatric ward. J Psychiatr Ment Health Nurs 7:323–333

Bowers L, Jarrett M, Clark N (1998) Absconding: a literature review. J Psychiatr Ment Health Nurs 5(5):343–353
Bowers L, Brennan G, Flood C, Lipang M, Oladapo P (2006) Preliminary outcome of a trial to reduce conflict and containment on acute psychiatric wards: city nurses. J Psychiatr Ment Health Nurs 13:165–172
Bowers L, Alexander J, Bilgin H, Botha M, Dack C, James K, Papadopoulos C (2014) Safewards: the empirical basis of the model and a critical appraisal. J Psychiatr Ment Health Nurs 21(4):354–364
Bowers L, James K, Quirk A, Simpson A, Stewart D, Hodsoll J (2015) Reducing conflict and containment rates on acute psychiatric wards: the safewards cluster randomised controlled trial. Int J Nurs Stud 52(9):1412–1422
Chai Y, Wheeler Z, Herbison P, Gale C, Glue P (2013) Factors associated with hospitalization of adult psychiatric patients: cluster analysis. Australas Psychiatry 21(2):141–146
Choe J, Teplin L, Abram K (2008) Perpetration of violence, violent victimization, and severe mental illness: balancing public health concerns. Psychiatr Serv 59:153–164
Colton D (2010) Checklist for assessing your organization's readiness for reducing seclusion and restraint. Available at https://www.livesinthebalance.org/sites/default/files/S&R%20Checklist%20-%202010.pdf
Colton D, Xiong H (2010) Reducing seclusion and restraint: questionnaire for organizational assessment. J Psychiatr Pract 16(5):358–362
Combs H, Romm S (2007) Psychiatric inpatient suicide: a literature review. Primary Psychiatry 14(12):67–74
Cutcliffe JR, Stevenson C (2008) Feeling our way in the dark: the psychiatric nursing care of suicidal people—a literature review. Int J Nurs Stud 45(6):942–953
de Jong MH, Kamperman AM, Oorschot M, Priebe S, Bramer W, van de Sande R, van Gool A, Mulder CL (2016) Interventions to reduce compulsory psychiatric admissions: a systematic review and meta-analysis. JAMA Psychiat 73(7):657–664
Dean K, Moran P, Fahy T, Tyrer P, Leese M, Creed F, Burns T, Murray R, Walsh E (2007) Predictors of violent victimization amongst those with psychosis. Acta Psychiatr Scand 116(5):345–353
Dinger U, Strack M, Lechenring F, Wilmers F, Schaunberg H (2008) Therapist effects on alliance in inpatient psychotherapy. J Clin Psychol 64(344–354):2008
Doihara C, Kawanishi C, Yamada T, Sato R, Hasegawa H, Furuno T (2008) Trait aggression in suicide attempters: a pilot study. Psychiatry Clin Neurosci 2008(62):352–354
Dziopa F, Ahern K (2009) Three different ways mental health nurses develop quality therapeutic relationships. Issues Ment Health Nurs 30(1):14–22
Elbogen E, Beckham J, Butterfield M, Swartz M, Swanson J (2008) Assessing risk of violent behavior among veterans with severe mental illness. J Trauma Stress 21(1):113–117
Figueroa R, Harman J, Engberg J (2004) Use of claims data to examine the impact of length of inpatient psychiatric stay on readmission rate. Psychiatr Serv 55(5):560–565
Fluttert F, Meijel B, Nijman H, Bjorkly S, Grypdonk M (2010) Preventing aggressive incidents and seclusions in forensic care by means of the 'Early Recognition Method'. J Clin Nurs 19(11–12):1529–1537
Fortugno F, Katsakou C, Bremner S, Kiejna A, Kjellin L, Nawka P, Raboch J, Kallert T, Priebe S (2013) Symptoms associated with victimization in patients with schizophrenia and related disorders. PLoS One 8(3):e58142
Glick R, Berlin R, Fishkind A (2008) Emergency psychiatry, principle and practice. Lippincott Williams & Wilkins, Philadelphia
Groholt B, Ekeberg O (2009) Prognosis after adolescent suicide attempt: mental health, psychiatric treatment, and suicide attempts in a nine-year follow-up study. Suicide Life Threat Behav 39(2):125–136
Hayes J, Gibbons R, Outim F, Tang S, Chakraborty A (2013) A new model for quality improvement in acute inpatient psychiatry: observational data from an acute assessment unit. JRSM Short Rep 3(9):65
Hendin H, Al Jardin R, Houck P, Hughes S, Turner B (2010) Role intense affects in predicting short term risk for suicidal behavior, a prospective study. J Nerv Ment Dis 198(3):220–225

Hodgins S, Alderton J, Cree A, Aboud A, Mak T (2007) Aggressive behaviour, victimisation and crime among severely mentally ill patients requiring hospitalization. Br J Psychiatry 191(4):343–350

Huckshorn K (2004) Reducing seclusion and restraint use in mental health settings: core strategies for prevention. J Psychosoc Ment Health Nurs 42(9):22–41

Hustoft K, Larsen T, Auestad B, Joa I, Johannessen J, Ruud T (2013) Predictors of involuntary hospitalizations to acute psychiatry. Int J Law Psychiatry 36(2):136

Kapur K, Young A, Murata D (2000) Risk adjustment for high utilizers of public mental health care. J Ment Health Policy Econ 3:129–137

Katsakou C, Rose D, Amos T, Bowers L, McCabe R, Oliver D, Wykes T, Priebe S (2012) Psychiatric patients' views on why their involuntary hospitalisation was right or wrong: a qualitative study. Soc Psychiatry Psychiatr Epidemiol 47(7):1169–1179

Katsikidou M, Samakouri M, Fotiadu M, Arvatini A, Vorvolakos T, Xenitidis K, Livaditis M (2013) Victimization of the severely mentally ill in Greece: the extent of the problem. Int J Soc Psychiatry 59(7):706–715

Knoll J (2012) Inpatient suicide: identifying vulnerability in the hospital setting. Psychiatric Times May 22, http://www.psychiatrictimes.com

Krakowski M (2003) Violence and serotonin: influence of impulse control, affect regulation, and social functioning. J Neuropsychiatry Clin Neurosci 15(3):294–305

Kumar S, Guite H, Thornicroft G (2001) Service users experience of violence within a mental health system: a study using grounded theory approach. J Ment Health 10(6):597611

Lang U, Hartmann S, Schulz-Hartmann S, Gudlowski Y, Munk R, Haebler von I, Gallinat J, Heinz A (2010) Do locked doors in psychiatric hospitals prevent patients from absconding? Eur J Psychiatry 2(4):199–204

Large M, Smith G, Sharma S, Nielssen O, Singh S (2011) Systematic review and meta-analysis of the clinical factors associated with the suicide of psychiatric in-patients. Acta Psychiatr Scand 124:18–29

Larue C, Dumais A, Ahern E et al (2009) Factors influencing decisions on seclusion and restraint. J Psychiatr Ment Health Nurs 16:440–446

Lobbestael J, Maaike C, Arntz A (2013) The relationship between adult reactive and proactive aggression, hostile interpretation bias, and antisocial personality disorder. J Personal Disord 27:53–66

Mann J, Apter A, Bertolote J et al (2005) Suicide prevention strategies: a systematic review. JAMA 294(16):2064–2074

Marcus DK, Kashy DA, Wintersteen MB, Diamond GS (2011) The therapeutic alliance in adolescent substance abuse treatment: a one-with-many analysis. J Couns Psychol 58(3):449–455

McEvoy J, Johnson J, Perkins D, Lieberman J et al (2006) Insight in first-episode psychosis. Psychol Med 36(10):1385–1393

Meehan T, Morrison P, McDougall S (1999) Absconding behaviour: an exploratory investigation in an acute inpatient unit. Aust N Z J Psychiatry 33(4):467–472

Meehan T, McIntosh W, Bergen H (2006) Aggressive behaviour in the high-secure forensic setting: the perceptions of patients. J Psychiatr Ment Health Nurs 13:19–25

Melartin TK, Rytsälä HJ, Leskelä US, Lestelä-Mielonen PS, Sokero TP, Isometsä ET (2005) Continuity is the main challenge in treating major depressive disorder in psychiatric care. J Clin Psychiatry 66(2):220–227

Miczek KA, de Almeida RM, Kravitz EA, Rissman EF, de Boer SF, Raine A (2007) Neurobiology of escalated aggression and violence. J Neurosci 27(44):11803–11806

Mistral W, Hall A, McKee P (2002) Using therapeutic community principles to improve the functioning of a high care psychiatric ward in the UK. Int J Ment Health Nurs 11(1):10–17

Muir-Cochrane E, Mosel K, Gerace A, Esterman A, Bowers L (2011) The profile of absconding psychiatric inpatients in Australia. J Clin Nurs 20(5–6):706–713

NICE (2015) Violence and aggression: short-termViolence and aggression: short-term management in mental health, health andmanagement in mental health, health and community settingscommunity settings, NICE guideline, Published: 28 May 2015 nice.org.uk/guidance/ng10

Nolan P, Brimblecombe N (2012) Mental health care services in europe: provision and practice. Radcliffe, London
O'Hagan M, Divis M, Long J (2008) Best practice in the reduction and elimination of seclusion and restraint; seclusion: time for change. Te Pou Te Whakaaro Nui: the National Centre of Mental Health Research, Information and Workforce Development, Auckland
O'Malley J, Frampton C, Wijnveld A, Porter R (2007) Factors influencing seclusion rates in an adult psychiatric intensive care unit. Journal of Psychiatric Intensive Care 3(2):93–100
Owens D, Horrocks J, House A (2002) Fatal and non-fatal repetition of self-harm systematic review. Br J Psychiatry 181(3):193–199
Palmer B, Pankratz V, Bostwick J (2005) The lifetime risk of suicide in schizophrenia: a reexamination. Arch Gen Psychiatry 62:247–253
Pini S, Cassano G, Dell'Osso L, Amador X (2001) Insight into illness in schizophrenia, schizoaffective disorder, and mood disorders with psychotic features. Am J Psychiatry 158(1):122–125
Putkonen A, Kuivalainen S, Louheranta O, Repo-Tiihonen E, Ryynänen OP, Kautiainen H, Tiihonen J (2013) Cluster-randomized controlled trial of reducing seclusion and restraint in secured care of men with schizophrenia. Psychiatr Serv 64:850
Quirk A, Lelliott P (2001) What do we know about life on acute psychiatric wards in the UK? A review of the research evidence. Soc Sci Med 53(12):1565–1574
Rix S, Sheppard G (2003) Acute wards: problems and solutions. Implementing real change in acute in-patient care, more than just bringing in the builders. Psychiatrist 27:108–111
Robbert S (2006) Imminent suicide: the illusion of short-term prediction. Suicide Life Threat Behav 36(3):296–301
Ryan R, Happell B (2009) Learning from experience: using action research to discover consumer needs in post-seclusion debriefing. Int J Ment Health Nurs 18(2):100–107
Schoevaerts K, Bruffaerts R, Mulder CL, Vandenberghe J (2013) Stijging van het aantal gedwongen opnames in België en Nederland: een epidemiologische analyse. Tijdschr Psychiatr 55(1):45–55
Siever L (2008) Neurobiology of aggression and violence. Am J Psychiatr 165:429–442
Simons L, Petch A (2002) Needs assessment and discharge: a Scottish perspective. J Psychiatr Ment Health Nurs 9(4):435–445
Smith G, Davis R, Bixler E, Lin H, Altenor A, Altenor R, Hardentstine B, Kopchick G (2005) Pennsylvania state hospital system's seclusion and restraint reduction program. Psychiatr Serv 56(9):1115–1122
Soloff P, Chiapetta L (2012) Prospective predictors of suicidal behaviour in borderline personality disorder at 6-year follow up. Am J Psychiatr 169:484–490
Soyka M (2011) Neurobiology of aggression and violence in schizophrenia. Schizophr Bull 37(5):913–920
Spiessl H, Hubner-Liebermann B, Cording C (2002) Suicidal behaviour of psychiatric inpatients. Acta Psychiatr Scand 106(2):134–138
Stewart D, Bowers L (2011) Absconding and locking ward doors: evidence from the literature. J Psychiatr Ment Health Nurs 18:89–93
Stringer B, van Meijel B, Eikelenboom M, Koekkoek B, Verhaak PF, Kerkhof AJ, Penninx BW, Beekman AT (2013) Perceived need for care and health care utilization among depressed and anxious patients with and without suicidal ideation. Crisis 34(3):192–199
Sturup J, Sorman K, Lindqvist P, Kristiansson M (2011) Violent victimization of psychiatric patients: a Swedish case–control study. Soc Psychiatry Psychiatr Epidemiol 46(1):29–34
Suokas J, Perälä J, Suominen K, Saarni S, Lönnqvist J, Suvisaari J (2010) Epidemiology of suicide attempts among persons with psychotic disorder in the general population. Schizophr Res 124:22–28
Trochim W (1989) An introduction to concept-mapping for planning and evaluation. Eval Program Plann 12:1–16
Tulloch A, Fearon P, David A (2011) Length of stay of general psychiatric inpatients in the United States: systematic review. Admin Pol Ment Health 38(3):155–168

van de Sande R, Nijman H, Noorthoorn EO, Wierdsma AI, Hellendoorn E, van der Staak C, Mulder CL (2011) Aggression and seclusion on acute psychiatric wards: effects of short term risk assessment. Br J Psychiatry 199:473–478

Van der Merwe M, Bower L, Jones J, Simpson A, Haglu K (2009) Locked doors in acute inpatient psychiatry: a literature review. J Psychiatr Ment Health Nurs 16:293–299

van der Post L, Peen J, Visch I, Mulder CL, Beekman A, Dekker J (2014) Patient perspectives and the risk of compulsory admission: the Amsterdam Study of Acute Psychiatry V. Int J Soc Psychiatry 60(2):125–133

van Mierlo T, Bovenberg F, Voskes Y, Mulder N (2014) Werkboek HIC high en intensive care in de psychiatrie. de Tijdstroom, Utrecht

Walsh E, Moran P, Scott C, McKenzie K, Burns T, Creed F, Tyrer P, Murray R, Fahy T (2003) UK 700 group: prevalence of violent victimization in severe mental illness. Br J Psychiatry 183:233–238

Community Psychiatric/Mental Health Nursing: Contexts and Challenges—The Case of Nurse Prescribing and Recovery-Focused Interventions

14

Steve Hemingway and Neil Brimblecombe

14.1 Psychiatric/Mental Health Nursing and Mental Health Services: Historical Developments in England, the UK and Europe

Psychiatric/mental health (P/MH) nursing across Europe shares much in terms of historical origins and, today, shares much in common in terms of culture and practice. Yet behind these similarities, details of historical differences and national contexts have had effects on the current practice and professional position of nursing (Brimblecombe and Nolan 2012). During the nineteenth and first half of the twentieth century institutions for the care and treatment of people with so-called mental illness opened up across Europe (Brimblecombe and Nolan 2012; Shorter 2006). A range of factors influenced this process:

- The centralisation of authority and the development of bureaucracy in nation states
- The wish of such states to, both, better care for and better control their populations
- Evidence produced at the time that seemed to demonstrate the beneficial effects of compassionate care in asylums—the result to which was that the 'admission to a hospital' was 'the benchmark of quality care' (Shorter 2006)
- The strengthening of the medical profession and its (successful) attempt to take authority over the field of so-called mental illness

S. Hemingway (✉)
University of Huddersfield, Huddersfield, UK
e-mail: s.j.hemingway@hud.ac.uk

N. Brimblecombe
South London and Maudsley NHS Foundation Trust, London, UK

© Springer International Publishing Switzerland 2018

J.C. Santos, J.R. Cutcliffe (eds.), *European Psychiatric/Mental Health Nursing in the 21st Century*, Principles of Specialty Nursing,
https://doi.org/10.1007/978-3-319-31772-4_14

The medicalisation of asylums created a powerful lobby expounding the necessity of 'medical care' which excluded non-medics from authority in talking about so-called mental illness (and running asylums). Medicalisation ultimately led to 'therapeutic nihilism' when the physical interventions that were increasingly emphasised over the earlier 'moral' (psychological and social) treatments achieved so little. The occasional spectacular biomedical success, such as that of the treatment of general paralysis of the insane (GPI) (Braslow 1995), encouraged otherwise unsuccessful physical treatments to be pursued.

14.2 The Shift to Deinstitutionalisation

Community psychiatric/mental health nursing in Europe developed as a result of changes in the approach to psychiatric healthcare, with a shift away from institutionally based care and an overall expansion in the number of people seen by mental health services. There were a range of factors driving this change:

- Psychiatric institutions had grown larger, and were no longer perceived as therapeutic in themselves,
- New anti-psychotic drugs introduced in the early 1950s potentially made living outside the hospitals possible for many patients. However, in reality this was not always closely correlated with reducing bed numbers. In England, there were significant reductions in the numbers of inpatients prior to the routine introduction of the new medications (reference), whilst in Norway reduction in hospital beds only started in the early 1970s (Pedersen and Kolstad 2009)
- A combination of scandals regarding ill treatment in institutions and evidence of the ill effects of prolonged hospital stays created a general rejection of large scale institutions (Goffman 1968),
- Increased professional focus on active and acute treatment and less emphasis on long-term care of the chronically ill,
- From the 1960s onwards, consumer and social rights campaigner movements challenged the status quo (Brown 1981),
- Not only was the detention of large numbers of individuals, who could have potentially been cared for at home, increasingly seen as morally undesirable, there were also questions as to the financial costs of such systems (Knapp et al. 2011).

Across Europe the speed and degree of the shift from institutional to community focused care has varied considerably, as has the role of P/MH nurses in such moves. Local factors, such as financial resources and social acceptance of deinstitutionalisation, have led to marked variation in the quality of the community mental care systems (Fakhoury and Priebe 2002) even when ministers of health from all the European World Health Organisation states have publicly committed to developing community based services to replace care in large institutions.

14.3 The Shift to Community-Focused Care and Nursing: The Development of Community Mental Health Nursing in the UK

The variation in approach to deinstitutionalisation and the varying roles of P/MH nurses in different healthcare systems have both influenced the major shift/no shift of nurses to work in community settings across Europe. For example, very early approaches to community care in the Netherlands involved P/MH nurses (Koekkoek et al. 2009), whilst in Germany, the role of P/MH nurses has remained predominantly one of inpatient care, with other professions taking on community roles. In many countries, national plans for major community based developments have simply not been delivered in practice (Brimblecombe and Nolan 2012).

In the United Kingdom (UK) the inpatient population in the hospitals peaked in 1954/55, and was from then on rapidly reduced. To support this change, staff from psychiatric hospitals began to work the community with the first 'community mental health nurse' (CPMHN) posts in England being established at Warlingham Park Hospital during the 1950s (May 1965). The subsequent growth in community P/MH nursing roles was gradual with only 1000 CPMHNs by 1977 and 2000 by 1980. It was, however, a catalyst for change amongst P/MH nurses, as those working in the community were working outside of the direct supervisory influence of psychiatry (Brimblecombe 2005), and this gave an opportunity for P/MH nurses to develop an agenda of professionalisation and independence (Godin 1996) and to become more recognised as a professional group in their own right (Brimblecombe 2005).

Hunter (1974) describes the early development of the role of the CPMHN as having two phases—the first being concerned with what has come to be known as the after-care or continuing care stage, and the second of more diverse functions. These include the incorporation of skills gradually being developed by some P/MH nurses in the more progressive services, particularly psychotherapeutic and behavioral treatment methods. For the first 20 years of the development of community care services, CPMHNs worked almost exclusively with people suffering from schizophrenia or older people with mental health problems. The P/MH nursing role being, largely, to prevent relapse or readmission. From the 1980s onwards, this changed with P/MH nurses increasingly working in primary health-care settings (rather than focusing on work with people in specialist mental health services with severe and enduring mental health problems). By the mid-1990s, there was a strong policy push back against this trend, as there was little evidence that much of this primary care work was clinically effective and that people with so-called severe mental illness were often not receiving adequate services (Gournay 1994; Department of Health 1994). A similar change of emphasis also took place in the Netherlands (Koekkoek et al. 2009).

In 2006 in England, a government-led review of P/MH nursing was undertaken. Its first recommendation was that the 'principles and values of the Recovery

Approach will inform P/MH nursing practice in all areas of care and inform service structures, individual practice and educational preparation'.

Accordingly nurses were to:

- Value the aims of service users.
- Work in partnership and offer meaningful choice.
- Be optimistic about the possibilities of positive change.
- Value social inclusion.

The focus on a recovery model was a confirmation (if one was needed) that nurses were not to pursue a narrow 'medicalised' model of care, focusing on symptom reduction, but should be working in partnership to meet the service users' own goals wherever possible.

14.4 Nurse Prescribing in Mental Health

Historically, the professional demarcations for providing medication were that the doctor prescribed, the pharmacist dispensed and the nurse administered (Hemingway and Ely 2009). The idea of CPMHNs extending their role into prescribing was introduced late in the last century (Hemingway and Flowers 2000). There were a series of arguments as to why this was both logical and was potentially in the best interests of service users. Firstly, P/MHNs were undeniably already heavily involved with medications related issues, with an estimated 22% of the inpatient P/MHNs' time being spent on medicines related interventions (Whittington and McLaughlin 2000), and a significant amount of time also spent on medication related issues in community settings (Hemingway 2016). Nurses also reported that they often 'defacto' prescribed, by explicitly advising doctors on exactly what to actually prescribe (Ramcharan et al. 2001). The potential benefits of P/MHNs prescribing were set out by the National Prescribing Centre (2005):

- To allow service users quicker access to medication
- To provide services more efficiently and effectively
- To increase service user choice
- To make better use of nurses' skills and knowledge

14.5 Becoming a Nurse Prescriber

In the UK, since 2003 P/MH nurses have potentially been able to prescribe, initially from a plan drawn up by a medical practitioner and more recently independently, i.e. the nurse diagnoses and can prescribe any drug within their area of competence and the limits of their knowledge (Hemingway and Ely 2009). Take up of the prescribing role is, therefore, dependent on organisational governance ownership and support (Hemingway and Ely 2009). In order to be able to legally register as prescribers, nurses in the UK are required to attend a generic 26-day university-based training programme and undergo a period of supervised practice with an experienced doctor (Nursing and Midwifery Council 2006).

14.6 Nurse Prescribing Internationally

As well as within the UK, NP has become legally permissible in other countries including Australia (Elsom et al. 2007), New Zealand (Chaston and Seccombe 2009) and the USA, where nurse practitioners have been prescribing for four decades (Kroezen et al. 2011), although different models exist across individual states. In 2011, Kroezen et al. (2011) additionally identified a further four Western European and Anglo-Saxon countries that had implemented nurse prescribing: Canada, Ireland, Sweden and the UK. Since that time, Finland, the Netherlands and Spain have also now introduced models of NP. Reports from New Zealand and Ireland suggest very small numbers of NPs practice in mental health settings as of yet (Chaston and Seccombe 2009; McBrien 2015). In contrast, a survey in 2014 (Dobel-Ober and Brimblecombe 2016) identified 817 nurse prescribers working in nationally funded mental health services in England (with 75% of organisations responding to the survey).

14.7 Research Evidence

Overall, research evidencing that NP is safe and therapeutic specifically in mental health settings has lagged behind service developments. Only one empirical study has been conducted to date comparing outcomes between those patients treated by nurses using supplementary prescribing and those treated by psychiatrists (Norman et al. 2010). All participants in this study had a diagnosis of 'psychosis'. As with medication adherence, the primary outcome measures were equivocal across all participants. Participants treated by NPs were more satisfied with their treatment by health-care services generally. No differences in clinical or cost outcomes were elicited.

Further evidence has subsequently been published regarding service users' experience of nurse prescribing. Jones et al. (2007) reported positive views of service users to the idea of NP in a small-scale qualitative study, whilst Ross et al. (2014) carried out interviews and focus groups with 57 service users who experienced nurse prescribing. The researchers concluded that service users liked to have their nurse prescribe for them as they valued the pre-established relationship. They also valued the consistency of seeing the same person and the relative ease of access to appointments.

A series of national surveys have mapped the characteristics and growth of nurse prescribing in nationally funded mental health services (Dobel-Ober et al. 2010; Dobel-Ober and Brimblecombe 2016). These have shown a steady growth over the 10-year period studied but with marked variation between individual organisations as to the level of adoption of nurse prescribing. The model of nurse prescribing favoured by mental health-care organisations has increasingly been that of 'independent prescribing', which allows greater flexibility and responsiveness rather than a 'supplementary prescribing model'.

14.8 CPMHN Work: A Changing Portfolio of Complexity

The development of CPMHNs work has closely followed the political, social and economic realities of the time and related policy initiatives (Brimblecombe and Nolan 2012). Thus, from the closure of asylums to the development of specialist community teams, CPMHNs have developed their role and skill sets in order to meet the increasing number of people diagnosed with a mental health problem and the complexity of service user needs (Norman and Ryrie 2013).

In recent times, countries around the world have faced challenges following the 2008 financial crash. The 'Austerity agenda' has led to health and social care budgets have been cut in real terms, meaning the reality now for any MHNs across Europe providing care in increasingly complex situations with decreased resources (Hemingway et al. 2013; Sakellari and Pikouli 2013; Santos and Cutcliffe 2013). However, these changes have also created possibilities to provide services in different and more creative ways (McDaid and Park 2010; Santos and Cutcliffe 2013).

14.9 Non-medical Prescribing: A Biological, Reductionist or Recovery-Focused Initiative—A Critical Analysis of the Outcomes of CMHN Prescribing

Critiques of P/MHNs taking on prescribing roles relate to their skills, knowledge and training and to the risk of a refocusing of the nursing role away from one that focuses on engagement and recovery-oriented care to one that is aligned with a medicalised view of care and mental health problems themselves.

14.9.1 The Right Knowledge and Skills?

There have been long-standing criticisms that P/MHNs do not have the requisite skills and knowledge to engage with the prescription of medicines (Duxbury et al. 2010; Hemingway et al. 2015). Education and skill deficits as well as other lapses in practice can also lead to errors been made, impacting negatively upon experiences for service users (Haw et al. 2015). Against this background, the evidence is that P/MHNs have been prescribing for over a decade now without any notable increase in error rate in line with showing P/MHNs can prescribe as safely and effectively as psychiatrists (Earle et al. 2011; Fisher and Vaughan-Cole 2003; Gumber et al. 2012; Norman et al. 2010).

14.9.2 Will the Addition of Prescribing Inhibit, Thwart or Negate CPMHN Therapeutic Engagement with Service Users?

The extension of roles of CPMHNs and increased pressure from reduced hospital beds and more emphasis on community-based treatment have resulted in increased caseloads (Happell et al. 2012). Pressures to extend their role have also come with the austerity agenda (Hemingway et al. 2013). Concern has been raised that such changes may provide a barrier to actually spending time with the service user and focusing on therapeutic engagement (Barker and Buchanan-Barker 2012; Simpson 2005). When, irony notwithstanding, the overwhelming theme in mental health service user evaluation literature is for more interpersonal, 'talk therapy' time with mental health professionals and less emphasis on drugs! Alternatively, a more positive reframe is that advanced practice nursing roles can be shaped to address complex and dynamic health-care system needs and demands for flexibility in service delivery (Bryant-Lukosius et al. 2004), for example, in meeting specific skills' shortages in workforce, particularly in challenging economic circumstances (Buchan et al. 2015). Within the UK, the focus on attempting to provide a 24 h service outside of hospital, as well as within, has been seen as requiring a multi-skilled workforce which brings a 'new way of working' (Brimblecombe 2009).

The evidence is that the extension of prescribing into P/MHN or CPMHNs roles is sustainable and increasing (Dobel-Ober et al. 2010). Gumber et al. (2012) report nurse prescribers as believing that their input had benefited patients, whilst there is reported success in meeting clinical targets in particular services through the development of nurse prescribing (Boyd 2013; Earle et al. 2011). These reports would be meaningless without a service user perspective, but what we know so far suggests a generally favourable experience of nurse prescribing, at least compared with that of doctors (Jones et al. 2007; Ross et al. 2014).

14.9.3 Prescribing and Recovery?

The same national review of mental health nursing that reiterated the importance of nurses adopting a recovery focus, based on working to service users' rather than professionals' goals, and the need for a 'holistic' approach to the individual to take account of psychological, social, physical and spiritual needs also recommended increased implementation of nurse prescribing based on local need (Department of Health 2006, p. 47). Are these recommendations incompatible with each other? The recovery model aims to work with the service user to reconstruct a sense of identity, feel socially included, gain power and control over their lives and feeling optimistic about life (Bonney and Stickley 2008). A recovery focused approach should move beyond symptom alleviation and understand the experiential aspect of mental distress and facilitate an individualised notion of recovery (Gale and Marshall-Lucette 2012).

The arguments for and against prescribing have been taking place since the inception of nurses being able to prescribe (Ross et al. 2014). McCann and Clark

(2008) framed this debate as arising from a care or curing conceptual dichotomy. Thus the biologically deterministic intervention of prescribing may be framed as negating the caring aspect that CPMHNs should focus on with service users (Wells et al. 2009; Ross et al. 2014). An emphasis on person-centred care or recovery focus for CPMHNs has been the guiding philosophy in P/MH nursing for the last decade (Gale and Marshall-Lucette 2012). Nurse prescribing has been characterised by some as undermining a nursing focus on recovery and service user choice (Snowden 2010). Nurse prescribing can be seen as reflecting a dominant 'medical approach' which emphasises tablets and injections to obtain symptom relief or medical recovery, rather than engaging with the service user about their needs and aspirations about the care they receive (Barker and Buchanan-Barker 2012; Edward et al. 2014).

A counter view is that the marginalising of the importance of medication, with the major focus on psychosocial interventions, may negate the ability of P/MH nurses to implement truly holistic interventions as necessary to support the service user towards their own recovery (Bailey and Hemingway 2006; Snowden 2010). The context of this is that 80% of service users in community settings in the UK are already prescribed psychotropic medication (Care Quality Commission 2013). Psychotropic medication is, for some at least, prescribed to alleviate mental distress but is associated with a range of side-effects, including some that can reduce life expectancy (Hemingway 2016). The efficacy of antipsychotic medication is criticised as having short-term efficacy but no real long-term gain (Harris and Shattell 2012; Moncrieff et al. 2013). Similarly, the overuse of antidepressants has been criticised, with their efficacy being questioned, as well as distressing side-effects being identified (Middleton and Moncrieff 2011). This evidence can be used to argue against over reliance on medication as a treatment or, alternatively, to recognise that the prescription of psychotropic medication needs real expertise to balance the risks and benefits of treatment (Snowden 2010). Nurse prescribers can not only prescribe medication, but they can also choose to not prescribe or, indeed, stop existing medication based on individual need. Where a nurse is already in a relationship with an individual service user, they may be best placed to help balance the needs of that person rather than referring all prescribing issues to a doctor who may know the service user less well, or indeed in some cases, not at all (Ross et al. 2014). Whether or not P/MHNs prescribe, they have a moral, legal and ethical duty to ensure that people, who take antipsychotics to aid their recovery or those who choose to discontinue them, do so based on an informed decision (Bressington and White 2015).

14.10 Conclusion: The Future

Nurse prescribing in mental health settings seems to be likely to continue to grow, both in the UK and internationally. Concerns that this may adversely affect the relationship between P/MH nurses and service users do not seem to be reflected in their reported experience of this relationship. It seems likely that, as with most innovations, the outcome will depend as much on the manner of use rather than the innovation itself. Nurse prescribing may lead the P/MH nurse to a narrow focus on a biomedical intervention or become part of a truly holistic approach to the individual to help them towards their own personal recovery.

References

Bailey K, Hemingway S (2006) Psychiatric/mental health nurses as non-medical prescribers: validating their role in the prescribing process. In: Cutcliffe JR, Ward MW (eds) Key debates in psychiatric/mental health nursing. Elsevier, Edinburgh, pp 220–235

Barker P, Buchanan-Barker P (2012) First, do no harm: confronting the myths of psychiatric drugs. Nurs Ethics 19:451

Bonney S, Stickley T (2008) Recovery and mental health: a review of the British literature. J Psychiatr Ment Health Nurs 15(2):140–153

Boyd R (2013) Early diagnosis and access to treatment for dementia patients. Nurs Prescr 11(4):174

Braslow JT (1995) Effect of therapeutic innovation on perception of disease and the doctor-patient relationship: a history of general paralysis of the insane and malaria fever therapy, 1910-1950. Am J Psychiatr 152(5):660–665

Bressington D, White J (2015) Recovery from psychosis: physical health, antipsychotic medication and the daily dilemmas for mental health nurses. J Psychiatr Ment Health Nurs 22(7):549–557

Brimblecombe NR (2005) The changing relationship between mental health nurses and psychiatrists in the United Kingdom. J Adv Nurs 49(4):344–353

Brimblecombe N (2009) New Ways of Working for nurses. J Ment Health Train Educ Pract 4(3):4–9

Brimblecombe N, Nolan P (eds) (2012) European mental health services described. Radcliffe, Oxford

Brown P (1981) The mental patients' rights movement and mental health institutional change. Int J Health Serv 11(4):523–540

Bryant-Lukosius D, DiCenso A, Browne G, Pinelli J (2004) Advanced practice nursing roles: development, implementation and evaluation. J Adv Nurs 48(5):519–529

Buchan J, Twigg D, Dussault G, Duffield C, Stone PW (2015) Policies to sustain the nursing workforce: an international perspective. Int Nurs Rev 62(2):162–170

Care Quality Commission (2013) Community mental health survey 2013. http://www.cqc.org.uk/public/publications/surveys/community-mental-health-survey-2013. Accessed 11 May 2014

Chaston D, Seccombe J (2009) Mental health nurse prescribing in New Zealand and the United kingdom: comparing the pathways. Perspect Psychiatr Care 45:17–23

Department of Health (1994) Working in partnership: a collaborative approach to care. Report of the Mental health review team. HMSO, London

Department of Health (2006) From values to action: the chief nursing officer's review of mental health nursing. Department of Health, London

Dobel-Ober D, Brimblecombe N (2016) National survey of nurse prescribing in mental health services; a follow up six years on. J Psychiatr Ment Health Nurs 23:378

Dobel-Ober D, Brimblecombe N, Bradley E (2010) Nurse prescribing in mental health: national survey. J Psychiatr Ment Health Nurs 17:487–493

Duxbury JA, Wright K, Bradley D, Barnes P (2010) Administration of medication in the acute mental health ward: perspective of nurses and patients. Int J Ment Health Nurs 19(1):53–61

Earle EA, Taylor J, Peet M, Grant G (2011) Nurse prescribing in specialist mental health (part 1): the views and experiences of practising and non-practising nurse prescribers and service users. J Psychiatr Ment Health Nurs 18(3):189–197

Edward K, Welch A, Elsom S, Edward K, Munro I, Welch A (2014) Resilience, recovery, reconnection and therapeutic optimism. In: Mental health nursing. Dimensions of praxis. Oxford University Press, Melbourne

Elsom S, Happell B, Manias E (2007) Exploring the expanded practice roles of community mental health nurses. Issues Ment Health Nurs 28(4):413–429

Fakhoury W, Priebe S (2002) The process of deinstitutionalization: an international overview. Curr Opin Psychiatry 15(2):187–192

Fisher SE, Vaughan-Cole B (2003) Similarities and differences in clients treated and in medications prescribed by APRNs and psychiatrists in a CMHC. Arch Psychiatr Nurs 17(3):101–107

Gale J, Marshall-Lucette S (2012) Community mental health nurses' perspectives of recovery-oriented practice. J Psychiatr Ment Health Nurs 19(4):348–353

Godin P (1996) The development of community psychiatric nursing: a professional project? J Adv Nurs 23(5):925–934

Goffman E (1968) Asylums: essays on the social situation of mental patients and other inmates. AldineTransaction, New Brunswick

Gournay K (1994) Redirecting the emphasis to severe mental illness. Nurs Times 90(25):40–41

Gumber R, Khoosal D, Gajebasia N (2012) Non-medical prescribing: audit, practice and views. J Psychiatr Ment Health Nurs 19(6):475–481

Happell B, Hoey W, Gaskin CJ (2012) Community mental health nurses, caseloads, and practices: a literature review. Int J Ment Health Nurs 21(2):131–137

Harris BA, Shattell MM (2012) A critical nursing perspective of pharmacological interventions for schizophrenia and the marginalization of person-centered alternatives. Issues Ment Health Nurs 33(2):127–129

Haw C, Stubbs J, Dickens G (2015) Medicines management: an interview study of nurses at a secure psychiatric hospital. Journal of Advanced Nursing 71(2):281–294.

Hemingway S (2016) Mental health nurses' medicines management role: a qualitative content analysis. Nurs Prescr 14(2):84–91

Hemingway S, Ely V (2009) Prescribing by mental health nurses: the UK perspective. Perspect Psychiatr Care 45(1):24–35

Hemingway S, Flowers K (2000) Nurse prescribing in the field of community mental health nursing. Nurs Times 96(43):40–41

Hemingway S, Coxon G, Munday D, Ramsay M (2013) Austerity is bad for mental health: implications for mental health nurses. Ment Health Nurs 33(6):7–9

Hemingway S, McCann T, Baxter H, Smith G, Burgess-Dawson R, Dewhirst K (2015) The perceptions of nurses towards barriers to the safe administration of medicines in mental health settings. Int J Nurs Pract 21(6):733–740

Hunter P (1974) Community psychiatric nursing in Britain: an historical review. Int J Nurs Stud 11(4):223–233

Jones M, Bennett J, Lucas B, Miller D, Gray R (2007) Mental health nurse supplementary prescribing: experiences of mental health nurses, psychiatrists and patients. J Adv Nurs 59(5):488–496

Knapp M, Beecham J, McDaid D, Matosevic T, Smith M (2011) The economic consequences of deinstitutionalisation of mental health services: lessons from a systematic review of European experience. Health Soc Care Community 19(2):113–125

Koekkoek B, Van Meijel B, Schene A, Hutschemaekers G (2009) Community psychiatric nursing in the Netherlands: a survey of a thriving but threatened profession. J Psychiatr Ment Health Nurs 16(9):822–828

Kroezen M, van Dijk L, Groenewegen PP, Francke AL (2011) Nurse prescribing of medicines in Western European and Anglo-Saxon countries: a systematic review of the literature. BMC health services research 11(1):127

McBrien B (2015) Personal and professional challenges of nurse prescribing in Ireland. Br J Nurs 24:524–528

McCann TV, Clark E (2008) Attitudes of patients towards mental health nurse prescribing of antipsychotic agents. Int J Nurs Pract 14(2):115–121

McDaid D, Park A (2010) Economics and public mental health. In: Goldie I (ed) Public mental health: a handbook. Pavilion, Brighton

Middleton H, Moncrieff J (2011) 'They won't do any harm and might do some good': time to think again on the use of antidepressants? Br J Gen Pract 61(582):47–49

Moncrieff J, Cohen D, Porter S (2013) The psychoactive effects of psychiatric medication: the elephant in the room. J Psychoactive Drugs 45(5):409–415

National Prescribing Centre, the National Institute for Mental Health in England, and the Department of Health (2005). Improving mental health services by extending the role of nurses in prescribing and supplying medication. National Prescribing Centre, Liverpool

Norman I, Ryrie I (2013) Mental health nursing: an art and a science. In: The art and science of mental health nursing: a textbook of principles and practice. McGraw-Hill Education (UK), London, pp 33–47

Norman IJ, Coster S, McCrone P, Sibley A, Whittlesea C (2010) A comparison of the clinical effectiveness and costs of mental health nurse supplementary prescribing and independent medical prescribing: a post-test control group study. BMC Health Serv Res 10(1):1

Nursing and Midwifery Council (2006) Standards of proficiency for nurse and midwife prescribers. NMC, London

Pedersen PB, Kolstad A (2009) De-institutionalisation and trans-institutionalisation-changing trends of inpatient care in Norwegian mental health institutions 1950-2007. Int J Ment Heal Syst 3(1):1

Ramcharan P, Hemingway S, Flowers K (2001) A client centred case for nurse supplementary prescribing. Ment Health Nurs 21(5):6–11

Ross JD, Clarke A, Kettles A (2014) Mental health nurse prescribing: using a constructivist approach to investigate the nurse–patient relationship. J Psychiatr Ment Health Nurs 21:1–10

Sakellari E, Pikouli K (2013) Assessing the impact of the financial crisis in mental health in Greece. Ment Health Nurs 33(6):19–21

Santos JC, Cutcliffe J (2013) The recent global socioeconomic crisis and its effects on mental health in Portugal. Ment Health Nurs 33(6):33–35

Shorter E (2006) The historical development of mental health services in Europe. In: Knapp M, McDaid D, Mossialos E (eds) Mental Health Policy and Practice across Europe. McGraw-Hill Education (UK), London, p 16

Simpson A (2005) Community psychiatric nurses and the care co-ordinator role: squeezed to provide 'limited nursing'. J Adv Nurs 52(6):689–699

Snowden A (2010) Integrating medicines management into mental health nursing in UK. Arch Psychiatr Nurs 24(3):178–188

Wells J, Bergin M, Gooney M, Jones A (2009) Views on nurse prescribing: a survey of community mental health nurses in the Republic of Ireland. J Psychiatr Ment Health Nurs 16(1):10–17

Whittington D, McLaughlin C (2000) Finding time for patients: an exploration of nurses' time allocation in an acute psychiatric setting. J Psychiatr Ment Health Nurs 7(3):259–268

15 Unearthing the Theoretical Underpinnings of "Green Care" in Mental Health and Substance Misuse Care: History, Theoretical Origins, and Contemporary Clinical Examples

John R. Cutcliffe and Rodger Travale

15.1 Introduction

While the term 'Green Care' (GC) may not be familiar to some associated with contemporary approaches to mental health and addictions care, or for others the term may conjure images of '1970s hippies,' 'tree huggers,' or even so-called potheads or stoners, the principles and practices of GC can be located in mental health-care facilities as long ago as the late eighteenth and early nineteenth centuries (Sempik 2010). Arguably, the origins of GC in formal mental health care can be traced back to two historical facilities: Pinel's Bicêtre facility in Paris, France, and Tuke's 'Retreat' in York, Northern England, both of which emphasized much of the philosophy and practice that can still be located in current conceptualizations of GC (see, e.g., 'Epidaurus' in Greece, Gesler 1992; Haigh 2012; 'Soteria project' Mosher 1999).

Rather than being seen as the latest iteration of complimentary health care, the latest non-mainstream health kick fad,[1] GC needs to be taken seriously, studied systematically, understood, and ultimately tested. Indeed, as with any bona fide science-driven discipline, both clinical practice and research activity in psychiatric/mental health (P/MH) nursing and mental health care are legitimized (at least to

[1] Such as the "cabbage soup diet" of the 1990s, the use of magnets for joint pain, or routine colonic irrigations or enemas—none of which have a robust scientific evidence base.

J.R. Cutcliffe (✉)
Cutcliffe Consulting, Kingston, Canada

School of Nursing, Coimbra, Portugal
e-mail: jcutcliffe@outlook.com

R. Travale
Healthcare Manager, Chiron Health Services, Prince George Regional Correctional Centre, British Columbia, Canada

© Springer International Publishing Switzerland 2018

J.C. Santos, J.R. Cutcliffe (eds.), *European Psychiatric/Mental Health Nursing in the 21st Century*, Principles of Specialty Nursing,
https://doi.org/10.1007/978-3-319-31772-4_15

some extent) by grounding such activities in theory (McKenna and Slevin 2008). Indeed, for many, the theories we hold must guide our practice, and without such theory, there is no evidence-based practice (Cutcliffe et al. 2010; McKenna 1997; McKenna and Slevin 2008; Meleis 2012). The importance of theoretical underpinnings for mental health care has long been acknowledged (see Sullivan 1953). Robust theoretical constructs are required which in turn give rise to testable hypotheses (Cutcliffe and Harder 2012). Indeed, in the absence of robust, preferably parsimonious theory, practitioners lack a conceptual scaffolding upon which to build their practice (see, e.g., Phillips et al. 2012), and some have even postulated that without such theory, questions arise as to whether or not psychiatry is a legitimate branch of medicine or science (see Phillips et al. 2012).

As a result, if the mental health and addictions care "community" are to take "GC" seriously and further elevate it from the level of pseudoscience, then its theoretical underpinnings need to be unearthed, examined, and articulated. Accordingly, what this will paper intends to do is (a) situate current GC definitions in a brief introduction to the history and background of GC in mental health and addictions, (b) identify and articulate the principle theoretical propositions of GC, (c) consider the cogency and validity (or otherwise) of these theoretical propositions by reviewing their use in related contexts and where it exists, draw on empirical findings, and (d) provide real clinical examples of how these theoretical underpinnings are actualized and operationalized in a therapeutic community that provides care for residents with alcohol or/and substance abuse problems.

15.2 The Historical Roots of Contemporary Positions on "Green Care"

Among the earliest examples of a mental health-care institution that operationalized a 'Green Care' philosophy is the so-called York Retreat facility. Pioneered by William Tuke, treatment at the facility was based on personalized attention, benevolence, and restoring the self-esteem/self-control of its residents (Sempik et al. 2010). Additionally, a strong emphasis was placed on 'treatments' such as farm laboring in pleasant, outdoor surroundings, and walks in picturesque and quiet 'countryside' surroundings (Tuke 1882—see also Rush 1912). Residents were 'allowed' if not encouraged to wander around the grounds and gardens, which were maintained by the residents themselves, and the grounds were also stocked with various domestic farm animals which again were tended to by the residents. Interestingly, the social environment and sense of 'brotherhood' or being part of a large family was fostered by the staff and seen as a key part of the treatment (Tuke 1882). Captivatingly, even a cursory examination of the twenty-first-century facilities that operationalize such practices will show two things:

1. GC, either in part or more fully, has been transplanted or introduced in a wide range of care settings such as prisons/correctional facilities, shelters, community residents, and psychiatric treatment facilities/hospitals (De Leon 1994).
2. The term 'Green Care' seems to be used as a broad, capacious, 'catch all' term that encompasses a range of activities, therapies, and interventions—all linked by their use of nature and the natural environment (Sempik et al. 2010).

Contemporary definitions of GC seem to underscore its capacious nature and invariably define it as being composed of several related concepts and practices. According to Hine et al. (2008), while there is much diversity under the broader umbrella of GC, the common linking ethos is essentially to use nature to produce health, social, or educational benefits. Haubenhofer et al. (2010) define GC as:

> A link between traditional healthcare and other sectors of human societies, like agriculture, gardening, landscape and nature conservation, animal keeping and animal husbandry, and different combinations lead to different types of green care. (p107)

Whereas Sempik (2010) purports that a common understanding of the concept GC sees it as the:

> Use of nature and nature environments to provide health and social and educational benefits for various groups of vulnerable or socially excluded persons. (Sempik 2010, p16)

Similarly, Berget et al. (2012, p. 1) declare that:

> GC is an inclusive term for a wide range of complex interventions e.g. care farming, animal-assisted therapy, and therapeutic horticulture. (Berget et al. 2012, p. 1)

While a more precise definition asserts that:

> 'Green care' is the utilisation of agricultural farms - the animals, the plants, the garden, the forest, and the landscape - as a base for promoting human mental and physical health, as well as quality of life, for a variety of client groups. (Austrian Horticultural Society 2015)

'Green care' and the various activities subsumed within the broader term are a specific collection of interventions. The term captures targeted processes that are designed to have a positive effect on the holistic health and well-being of the individual, and as such, it should not be confused with any reported improvements in health/well-being that may arise from a passive experience of nature. In other words, the natural environment is not simply a backdrop for GC, and while the health benefits of experiencing nature are increasingly being recognized, everything that is green is not GC.

15.3 Key Theoretical Approaches/Elements: 1. Connectedness

The first theoretical element that is embedded within the overall GC theoretical framework is that of connectedness, the proposition that humans have an innate need to feel connected. Further, this need to feel connected is found in both interpersonal (i.e., the need to connect with other people) and the more metaphysical, some might say existential, i.e., the need to feel connected to the world and or the universe. Far from being esoteric or fringe, the human need for connectedness is well documented in the literature of a number of linked disciplines such as psychology (Maslow 1962), philosophy (Marcel 1948), sociology (Durkheim 1951), psychiatry (Sullivan 1953), psychiatric/mental health nursing (Cutcliffe and Stevenson 2007; Peplau 1988), and theology (Lisack 2009).

To focus on the notion of feeling connected to the world or universe first, the philosopher Gabriel Marcel (1948) constructed a persuasive argument about the nature of human existence and what he referred to as the "ontological *exigence*." *According to Marcel, exigence refers to the person's* need/demand for some level of coherence in the cosmos and more importantly (in terms of the issue of connectedness) for some understanding of one's place and role within this coherence. For Marcel, ontological *exigence* is not simply a wish or desire; it is not reducible to some psychological state, mood, or attitude. It is more central to existence than that; it is a movement of the human spirit that is inseparable from being human. To paraphrase, there is an in alienable element of the human condition that is concerned with experiencing a sense of knowing one's place in the world, feeling connected to the world and others in it, and feeling that one has a place and purpose (Cutcliffe and Stevenson 2007).

To then consider interpersonal connectivity or to cite an oft-used synonym, social integration, the body of extant work is so robust and has withstood innumerable tests to the extent that Berkman et al. (2000, p. 843) state:

> It is now widely recognized that social relationships and affiliation have powerful effects on physical and mental health for a number of reasons.

An early, if not seminal, contribution to this area was that of Durkheim (1951) who advanced an argument showing how social integration and cohesion can influence mortality (suicide rates). Interestingly, more contemporary research has confirmed or perhaps rediscovered the significant influence of so-called 'upstream determinants' of health on psychological well-being (e.g., Burrow 1992; Platt et al. 2005). On a more interpersonal rather than societal level, Bowlby's (1969, 1973, 1980) highly influential work on attachment, separation, and loss included the proposition that there is a universal human need to form close interpersonal bonds. Moreover, according to Bowlby, this need afforded the same or equivalent degree of significance and meaning in the individual as other primary needs such as feeding and staying warm. According to Berkman et al. (2000), the strength of Bowlby's theory lies in its premise of the individual's need for secure attachments—and thus connectivity—for its own sake. While acknowledging the vintage (if not seminal) nature of Bowlby's work, more contemporary findings are highly supportive of Bowlby's proposition. For instance, neuroscientist Lieberman's (2013) work highlights how a growing body of research shows that the need to connect socially with others is as basic as our need for food, water, and shelter. Lieberman argues that being socially connected is the human brain's lifelong mission and that this has evolved over millions of years resulting in major differences in the brain that distinguish us from our ancestors. Lieberman points out how mammals are more socially connected than reptiles, primates more than other mammals, and humans more than other primates, and from this, he infers that becoming more socially connected is essential to human survival.

Psychiatric/mental health nurses have long asserted the primacy of interpersonal connection as the bedrock of their practice and philosophy (Barker 1999; Cutcliffe 2008; Peplau 1988; Sullivan 1953). Described by some as the 'founding mother of psychiatric nursing,' Peplau (1988) situates P/MH nursing squarely within an interpersonal context and considers the formation and development of therapeutic interpersonal relationships as the core function of P/MH nurses and the medium by which other therapeutic activities and engagements are manifest. And while an emphasis on interpersonal relationships can be found underpinning P/MH nursing curricula throughout the world, there also exists a body of empirical work which has attempted to operationalize and measure the effects of such relationships on service user (SU) outcomes (Cahill et al. 2013; Forchuk et al. 1998; Martin et al. 2000; Sheehan et al. 2011; Thibeault 2012).

A further body of work that supports the notion of the basic human need for connection, and what's more, describes what can result when the interpersonal connection is absent, is that of Orbach's work on human touch and suicidality. Orbach (2003) summarizes his findings and reports results that point to suicidal youngsters having lower tactile sensitivity and responsiveness and lower emotional investment in the body. These suicidal youngsters were found to be disconnecting from the normal, required, basic human need of connection through touch and touching (see also Harlow and Soumi 1970). Related findings have been uncovered in associated areas, such as the empirical correlation reported between the increased use of touch and physical comforting and survival rates in low birth weight infants (Feldman et al. 2002; Sloan et al. 1994). Accordingly, the theoretical element of GC, termed here "connectedness," appears to be grounded on a sound and robust theoretical underpinning. The body of extant work, both historical and more contemporary, has withstood innumerable tests to the extent that the powerful effects of connectedness and social relationships are now considered to be axiomatic.

15.4 Key Theoretical Approaches/Elements: 2. Contact with Nature

The next theoretical element that is embedded within the overall GC theoretical framework is that of contact and interaction with nature, the proposition that such contact can improve psychological health and well-being—not least by reducing stress and enhancing a person's mood (i.e., having an antidepressant effect) (Bird 2007; Burls 2007; Kaplan and Kaplan 1989; Pretty 2004, 2007; Sempik et al. 2010).

A sizeable and increasing body of work now exists which identifies and supports the proposition that exposure to and subsequent contact with 'green space' can have powerful positive effects on a person's mental health (Beyer et al. 2014; Pretty 2004). In his review paper, Pretty (2004) identified and described three levels of exposure to nature:

1. Viewing nature, e.g., looking out through one's window to see nature or reading a book about nature
2. Being in the presence of nature, e.g., walking in the countryside or sitting in your garden
3. Active participation and involvement in nature, e.g., gardening or farming

While Pretty (2004) could not describe the precise mechanism or process of how such exposure leads to improvements in psychological well-being, he summarized the evidence that shows how all three levels appear to lead to significant mental health benefits. In their 2010 study, Van de Berg et al. report findings that highlight how contact with nature or even access to nature can act as a possible protective factor against developing mental health problems. Their study examined responses to stressful life events and found that respondents with more access to green spaces within a three mile radius were significantly less impacted by stressful life events, after controlling for a variety of variables such as age, gender, income, etc.

In their recent population health-based, state-wide survey of the health of Wisconsin (USA) residents, Beyer et al. (2014, p. 3468) convey some persuasive findings regarding access to and contact with nature. They state:

> We found in our sample that higher levels of neighborhood green space correspond to better mental health outcomes, when controlling for a wide range of confounding factors. The associations between green space and mental health are significant and sizeable and persist with different measurement techniques. Furthermore, the estimated effect of environmental green space is similar in magnitude to that of other well-known and studied contributors to symptomology for depression, anxiety and stress.

While much of contemporary mental health practice and policy appears not to have embraced the empirical evidence exemplified above, which draws attention to a possible causal relationship between access to and or contact with nature and improved mental health, this is not a new argument per se (see, e.g., Wilson 1984). Furthermore, US federal-level research funding institutes appear to have accepted the possibility of this relationship(s). For instance, in 1984 Wilson (1984) described his theory of "biophilia" and advanced the argument that this need for people to be in contact with nature is an innate and powerful instinct, a basic drive like other human basic drives. Theories that posit the need to be in contact with nature as a basic human need are most often couched in the form of some legacy of our evolutionary/developmental origins. That is to say that theorists postulate that early human existence was inextricably tied to nature. Kellert and Wilson (1993) describe this as a primal biological need of our species, a part of our species' evolutionary heritage. Whether or not humankind's need to be in contact with nature does indeed turn out to be yet another example (with apologies to Darwin 1871) of the indelible stamp of humankind's lowly origin, there does exist a reasonably well-developed body of empirical findings pertaining to the positive correlation between the amount of accessible green space and improved psychological health (Barton and Pretty 2010; Beyer et al. 2014; De Vries et al. 2003; Takano et al. 2002; Van de Berg et al. 2010).

Lastly in this section, it is noteworthy that within the United States, a separate institute within the National Institute of Health has been established—the National Institute of Environmental Health Sciences (NIEHS), the remit of which is concerned with obtaining a deeper and more sophisticated understanding of the interactions between the environment(s) and health. Similarly, a discrete field of psychology has emerged which is concerned with the direct study of the relationship between an environment and how that environment affects its inhabitants, namely, "environmental psychology" (De Young 2013). Accordingly, while our understanding and knowledge base of such interactions requires further development, there appears to be widespread consensus that such relationships do exist. Accordingly, as with the previous theoretical element of GC, contact with nature or green space appears to be grounded on a sound and robust theoretical underpinning and an emerging though expanding empirical evidence base.

15.5 Key Theoretical Approaches/Elements: 3. Benefits of Exercise

The next embedded theoretical element that is embedded within GC is that of the therapeutic value of exercise. And while it would seem somewhat redundant or superfluous to restate the very well-established physiological benefits associated with engaging in exercise, the psychological benefits may be less well known. Engaging in physical exercise appears to have a therapeutic effect for people experiencing depression (Craft and Perna 2004). Indeed, many studies have been undertaken to investigate the possible relationship between exercise and symptoms of depression, and it is noteworthy that the overwhelming majority of these studies have reported a positive benefit, to the extent that engaging in exercise is now regarded as an excellent antidote for mild to moderate depression (see Paluska and Schwenk 2000 for an excellent review of this evidence). Indeed, Paluska and Schwenk (2000, p. 169) noted:

> Recent meta-analyses of clinically depressed men and women of all age groups found substantial decreases of depressive symptoms following both short and long courses of exercise.

The therapeutic effects have been found in studies where the exercise regimen could hardly be described as exhaustive or harsh. For instance, even engaging in 30 minutes of treadmill walking, for 10 consecutive days, produced clinically and statistically significant reductions in depression rating scores (Dimeo et al. 2001). Furthermore, when exercise was combined with psychological care, even greater improvements in mental health scores were recorded (Craft and Landers 1998; Jacquart et al. 2014; North et al. 1990). To clarify, both exercise and talk therapy have repeatedly and consistently been found to have an antidepressant effect when used individually. However, the most significant effect appears to occur when exercise and talk therapy are combined. Jacquart et al. (2014, p. 8), for instance, concluded that:

> Overall, these results indicate that patients' post-treatment depression scores were significantly lower in those receiving the STEP treatment compared with those receiving individual psychotherapy only or standard care.

According to Craft and Perna (2004), findings from studies in this area also suggest that the therapeutic psychological benefits arising from engaging in exercise are long lasting with subjects reporting the maintenance of beneficial effects through the 12-month follow-up period. While the precise mechanisms of the action of exercise on depression are not currently understood, the current state of the evidence allows Paluska and Schwenk (2000, p. 169) to conclude the following:

> Physical activity appears to be as effective as other therapeutic modalities for the treatment of mild or moderate depressive symptoms.

There exists a large body of evidence that shows how engaging in exercise can also result in therapeutic effects for the person experiencing anxiety. Indeed, many studies have been undertaken to investigate the possible relationship between exercise and symptoms of anxiety, and it is noteworthy that the overwhelming majority of these studies have reported a positive benefit and that these findings appear to be relatively consistent over time (see, e.g., the meta-analyses of Herring et al. 2013; Petruzzello et al. 1991). Petruzzello et al. (1991) undertook three meta-analyses of studies that examined the relationship between exercise and anxiety. These authors report that across all three meta-analyses, the overall effect sizes were significantly greater than zero. This indicates that no matter how anxiety is assessed (i.e., state, trait, or a psychophysiological measure), exercise is associated with a reduction in anxiety. Petruzzello et al. (1991) conclude that their results substantiate the hypothesis that exercise is associated with reductions in anxiety but only for aerobic forms of exercise. These effects were generally independent of both subjects (i.e., age and health status). Similarly, Herring et al. (2013) undertook review of the extant evidence of the effects of exercise training on anxiety among healthy adults, adults with a chronic illness, and individuals diagnosed with an anxiety disorder. As with previous and earlier reviews and meta-analyses, Herring et al. (2013) declared that the bulk of the available empirical evidence indicates that exercise training reduces symptoms of anxiety among healthy adults, chronically ill patients, and patients with panic disorder (see also Wipfli et al. 2008). A number of theoretical explanations for these consistent findings have been advanced, and these have some supporting evidence, to a greater or lesser extent, but the scientific community currently does not possess a precise and verified model of the therapeutic effects of exercise on anxiety.

Interestingly, while it should be noted that this body of work remains in its relative infancy, there is currently a dearth of methodologically robust and generalizable studies that illustrate a therapeutic effect of exercise on alcohol and drug use (Zschucke et al. 2012). Engaging in regular exercise may have a prophylactic effect whereby Smith and Lynch (2012) draw attention to the epidemiological studies which have shown that individuals who engage in regular aerobic exercise are less likely to engage in illicit drug use or abuse. However, Zschucke et al. (2012) summarize the state of the science as thus:

> So far, no methodologically firm studies are present to verify the long-term effects of exercise interventions with regards to craving, abstinence, relapse and psychological variables. Although beneficial effects induced by exercise are theoretically plausible, clinically admitted and highly intuitive, well-designed studies need to be conducted to empirically corroborate these assumptions.

15.6 Key Theoretical Approaches/Elements: 4. Occupational Work

The next theoretical element that is embedded within the overall GC theoretical framework is that of occupation or work as a therapeutic, meaningful, and, some would argue, (see, e.g., Kielhofner 2009) transformative activity. As with the three previous theoretical elements, the use of occupation or work can be traced back to the early therapeutic communities. And yet, such modest beginnings are now eclipsed by the well-developed body of work and associated policy positions that place occupation or work not only as a key theoretical/practice element of therapeutic communities but embed such programs as part of mental health recovery per se (Becker and Drake 2003; NAMI, 2015).

Early pioneers of occupational work as a therapeutic activity, such as William Rush Dunton, advanced the view that occupation is a basic human need (Dunton 1919). In this seminal work, he argued that all mental health patients should have occupations which they enjoy as he believed that so-called sick minds may be healed through occupation. For Dunton, occupation creates structure and organizes time; it brings meaning to life, culturally and personally, and occupational activity needed to be personalized as it is particularized to the individual; different people value different occupations; thus, one size will not fit all. Such views were then operationalized in the occupational therapy treatment model, "Habit Training," initiated at Johns Hopkins Hospital in the early twentieth century. For Dunton and his acolytes, the lack of structure and balance in the lives of clients with mental health problems meant that these individuals would benefit from occupational activities such as work, rest, and play. As a result, the theoretical position was that such goal-directed activities should be used to help individuals learn new skills, become more productive, and experience the therapeutic benefits of a balanced daily schedule.

Far from being esoteric or peripheral views, occupation and employment are now firmly embedded in the mental health recovery discourse and associated policy positions, in many parts of the world (Becker and Drake 2003; Becker et al. 2001; NAMI 2015; SAMSHA, 2015). Empirical findings from studies of supported employment paint an encouraging though as yet equivocal picture regarding occupation and employment as therapeutic activity. Continuous employment has been found to be positively correlated with improved psychological and physical health (Bartley et al. 2004). In drawing together this emerging body of work, Sempik et al. (2010) declare that work and employment are not just a source of financial income, but engaging in work seems to foster a sense of belonging. Moreover, according to NAMI (2015), while supported employment has not been found to lead to increased risk for rehospitalization, employment programs have not been found to increase quality of life or self-esteem. That being said, NAMI (2015) also reports that mental health service consumers who are employed for a meaningful length of time demonstrate significant improvements in self-esteem and symptom management compared with clients who do not work. According to Kielhofner (2009), the theoretical underpinnings of occupation, work, and employment have multiplied and varied over the last 100 years or so, with theoretical approaches apparently failing in and out of favor (see Kielhofner 2009), so much so that the underpinning theoretical model of occupation or work as a therapeutic activity appears to have come full circle whereby contemporary theory once more posits occupation as occupying a central role in human well-being. For Kielhofner (2009, p. 3):

> When someone engages in an occupation, that person's unique characteristics interact with the specific occupation being done, creating a dynamic that leads people to think, feel and behave in ways that they would not otherwise.

Accordingly, the element of GC, termed here "occupation/work," has, over the years, given rise to a wide range of theoretical explanations, some that appear to have withstood the test of time better than others. And the contemporary view of occupation/work—in and of itself—occupying a central role in human well-being appears to have an emerging, though as yet, somewhat equivocal body of empirical evidence.

15.7 Clinical Examples: Nascent Examples of the Operationalization in Mental Health and Substance Misuse Care

In the absence of an abundance of robust empirical findings to draw upon, perhaps especially findings that indicate causal relationships between GC interventions and improvements in holistic well-being (Haigh 2012), one way that helps further validate GC as bona fide care paradigm for substance misusers is providing real clinical examples of how the theoretical elements have been operationalized. Accordingly, we draw on the example of the "BC New Hope Recovery Society: Baldy Hughes (BH) Therapeutic Community," a unique facility in Northern British Columbia, Canada.

At this facility, *connectedness* is promoted through having community activities, functions, and environment(s). The facility is replete with identified common areas for holding group and other shared, communal activities, engineered to help create and foster a joint sense of community. Community meetings for each dormitory are held every week, and each resident is encouraged to attend and participate. Issues, problems, and successes are also addressed, at times, through community meetings for all the residents. Regular peer group meetings are offered where activities and interactions are aimed at heightening residents' awareness of their attitudes and behaviors that are limiting, constraining, or even damaging. Theoretical and policy elements of "recovery" are practiced such as gentle and constructive confrontation (Heron 2001), experiencing and communicating compassion and responsible concern for one another, a shift toward acting honestly with one's self and others, and acknowledging and confronting the reality of their addiction.

Connectedness is further promoted by forming identified dyads consisting of a senior resident and a more junior resident, wherein senior residents are expected to demonstrate the desired behaviors and reflect the values and teachings of the community. Moreover, the senior resident serves as a support, confidant, encourager, and advocate for the more junior resident, and this results in the formation and development of a robust interpersonal connection.

A greater sense of connectedness to the community and to one another is fostered through the emphasis on group work, whereby the majority of all activities occur in groups or meetings where residents can interact and learn from one another. For example, meals are prepared by groups of residents and shared by the entire community; a variety of therapeutic groups occur each day (except weekends), and jobs are organized and undertaken in groups; the whole community comes together to acknowledge, honor, and celebrate personal and community "milestones" via participation in group ceremonies, rituals, birthday celebrations, and stages of graduation, program goal attainment.

Connectedness is further encouraged by eradicating traditional power differentials between staff and residents (see Cutcliffe and Happell 2009; Cutcliffe et al. 2013). Staff members are considered to be part of, rather than separate from, the community; they share many communal activities with the residents. This interestingly often necessitates a significant philosophical shift in the staff's attitudes from those frequently espoused in both mainstream psychiatry and many entry-level educational programs, whereby power differentials between staff and residents are minimized rather than encouraged (Cutcliffe and Happell 2009).

15.7.1 Contact with Nature

Baldy Hughes Therapeutic Community is situated in rural Northern British Columbia. It is surrounded on all four sides by wilderness. As soon as one leaves the grounds, then one encounters rural, unspoiled country side—mostly evergreen forests and some "prairies/pastures." In such geographical and topographical surroundings, one cannot help but be exposed to nature; one cannot help but be struck by the tranquility. This location, as with some other therapeutic communities for clients with substance use issues, has the added advantage of removing residents from their alcohol/drug "networks" and "connections."

The facility runs a number of "animal care" or animal husbandry programs. These range from programs to care for chickens and goats to pigs and, perhaps more specialized, horses and even beekeeping. Residents can take part in vegetable cultivation programs, making use of the commercial-sized greenhouses and/or large outdoor vegetable gardens. The beekeeping program is more technical than some and requires specialized equipment (and some training); nevertheless, it remains a further example of contact with nature. Formal and informal activities make use of the surrounding "green areas" and wilderness; thus, hikes are quite common during the summer. Beautification projects and working with the flower beds and plants are another example and outdoor meditation, and Yoga sessions might also be considered as providing contact with nature.

Occupation and work are woven into the individualized recovery plans of each resident and are tailored according to his stage of recovery, abilities, and interests (where possible). The work opportunities take many forms, ranging from informal "domestic" work in and around the facility to specific employment programs. Residents are responsible for and actively involved in the day-to-day operation and maintenance of the facility. More specific work activities are associated with each dorm where residents learn, through communal living and functioning, to work at maintaining a "homely" residential living experience. As residents move into the second half of their year-long program, a variety of employment programs become available. Baldy Hughes has established agreements and signed memos of understanding with local employers and local postsecondary educational facilities. As a result residents can engage in apprenticeship electrician programs, woodwork and woodshop programs, working with heavier machinery (e.g., tractors), and vehicle maintenance/repairs—garage/mechanic programs. The authors of this paper will also not belabor the work involved in the animal husbandry and horticulture programs which often required some hard physical labor.

And lastly to consider examples of *benefits of physical exercise*, in addition to the physical exercise involved with the occupation/work and animal husbandry/horticultural programs, additional and separate exercise opportunities and programs are also available. The facility has a large and well-equipped gymnasium which residents may use with or without structured exercise programs and designed workouts. Community walks and hikes are commonplace (not during the winter so much). Aerobic exercises are made available sometimes, and formal/informal "pick up" floor hockey games—indoors and outside—are a fairly regular occurrence.

Conclusion

This paper has identified four principle theoretical propositions that appear to underpin the contemporary practice of Green Care, and these are connectedness, contact with nature, benefits of exercise, and occupation/work as therapeutic. Examination of the literature, from a range of relevant disciplines, shows that "connectedness" appears to be grounded on a sound and robust theoretical underpinning. The body of extant work, both historical and more contemporary, has withstood innumerable tests to the extent that the powerful effects of connectedness and social relationships are now considered to be axiomatic. Similarly, "contact with nature" appears to be grounded on a sound and robust theoretical underpinning and an emerging though expanding empirical evidence base. "Occupation/work" has, over the years, given rise to a wide range of theoretical explanations, some that appear to have withstood the test of time better than others. And the contemporary view of occupation/work occupying a central role in human well-being appears to have an emerging, though as yet, somewhat equivocal body of empirical evidence. And with regard to the fourth and final proposition, the psychological therapeutic value of exercise appears to have a solid and robust theoretical underpinning, in addition to empirical findings which highlight the value of exercise in helping to combat mild to moderate depression. However, we currently do not possess a precise and verified model of the therapeutic effects of exercise on anxiety.

References

Austrian Horticultural Society (2015) Green care: Health effects, economics and policies: COST Action 866 - Green Care in Agriculture: http://archive.healtheconomics.org/conferences/2007/06/20/green-care-heal-1.html. Recovered 6 Nov 2015

Barker P (1999) The philosophy and practice of psychiatric nursing. Churchill Livingstone/Elsevier, Edinburgh

Bartley M, Sacker A, Clarke P (2004) Employment status, employment conditions and limiting illness: prospective evidence from the British household panel survey 1991-2001. Journal of Epidemiology and Community Health 58:501–506

Barton J, Pretty JN (2010) What is the best dose of nature and green exercise for improving mental health: a multi-study analysis. Environ Sci Technol 44:3947–3955

Becker DR, Drake RE (2003) A working life for people with severe mental illness. Oxford University Press, New York

Becker DR, Smith J, Tanzman B, Drake RE, Tremblay T (2001) Fidelity of supported employment programs and employment outcomes. Psychiatr Serv 52(6):834–836

Berget B, Lidfors L, Pálsdóttir AM, Soini S, Thodberg K (2012) Green care in the Nordic countries – a research field in progress: report from the Nordic research workshop on green care in Trondheim, June 2012. HealthUMB, Norwegian University of Life Sciences, Ås

Berkman LF, Glass T, Brissette I, Seeman TE (2000) From social integration to health: Durkheim in the new millennium. Social Science Medicine 51(6):843–857

Beyer KMM, Kaltenbach A, Szabo A, Bogor S, Nieto FJ, Malecki KM (2014) Exposure to neighborhood green space and mental health: evidence from the survey of health of Wisconsin. Int J Environ Res Public Health 11(3):3453–3472

Bird W (2007) Natural thinking: investigating the links between the natural environment, biodiversity and mental health. Royal Society for the Protection of Birds. Retrieved from http://www.rspb.org.uk/Images/naturalthinking_tcm9-161856.pdf. Accessed 20 June 2015)

Bowlby J (1969) Attachment. attachment and loss (volume 1), 2nd edn. Basic Books, New York

Bowlby J (1973) Separation: anxiety & anger. Attachment and loss (volume 2). International psycho-analytical library, no.95. Hogarth Press, London

Bowlby J (1980). Loss: sadness & depression. Attachment and loss (volume 3). Hogarth Press, London

Burls A (2007) People and green spaces: promoting public health and mental well-being through ecotherapy. J Public Ment Health 6(3):24–39

Burrow S (1992) The deliberate self-harming behaviour of patients within a British special hospital. J Adv Nurs 17(2):138–148

Cahill J, Paley G, Hardy G (2013) What do patients find helpful in psychotherapy? Implications for the therapeutic relationship in mental health nursing. J Psychiatr Ment Health Nurs 20(9):782–791

Craft LL, Landers DM (1998) The effect of exercise on clinical depression: a meta-analysis. Med Sports Sci Exerc 30(Suppl 5):S117

Craft LL, Perna FM (2004) The benefits of exercise for the clinically depressed. Prim Care Companion J Clin Psychiatry 6(3):104–111

Cutcliffe JR (2008) The die has been cast? Rediscovering the essence of psychiatric/mental health nursing. Br J Nurs 17(2):88–92

Cutcliffe JR, Happell B (2009) Psychiatry, mental health nurses and invisible power: exploring a perturbed relationship within contemporary mental health care. Int J Ment Health Nurs 18(2):116–125

Cutcliffe JR, Harder H (2012) Methodological rigor in qualitative research: slavish adherence or 'following the yellow brick road?'. Qual Rep 17(81):1–19

Cutcliffe JR, Stevenson C (2007) Care of the suicidal person. Churchill Livingstone/Elsevier, Edinburgh

Cutcliffe JR, McKenna HP, Hyrkas K (2010) Nursing models: application to practice. Quay Books, London
Cutcliffe JR, Stevenson C, Lakeman R (2013) Oxymoronic or synergistic: deconstructing the psychiatric and/or mental health nurse. Int J Ment Health Nurs 22:125–134
Darwin C (1871) The descent of man, and selection in relation to sex, 1st edn. John Murray, London
De Leon G (1994) Modern therapeutic communities for addiction: the quest for "right living" in modern TCs. Available from http://www.thefix.com/content/therapeutic-communities-George-De-Leon-professional-voices0514. Accessed 12 May 2015
De Vries S, Verheij RA, Groenewegen PP, Spreeuwenberg P (2003) Natural environments- healthy environments? An exploratory analysis of the relationship between greenspace and health. Environ Plan A 35:1717–1731
De Young R (2013) Environmental psychology overview. In: Klein SR, Huffman AH (eds) Green organizations: driving change with IO psychology. Routledge, New York, pp 17–33
Dimeo F, Baurer M, Varahram I et al (2001) Benefits from aerobic exercise in patients with major depression: a pilot study. Br J Sports Med 35:114–117
Dunton WR (1919) Occupational therapy: a manual for nurses. W. B. Saunders, Philadelphia
Durkheim E (1951) Suicide: a study in sociology. Free Press, Glencoe. (Original work 1897)
Feldman R, Feldman AI, Sirota L, Weller A (2002) Effects of skin-to-skin contact on parenting and infant development in premature infants. Pediatrics 110:16–26
Forchuk C, Jewell J, Schofield R, Sircelj M, Valledor T (1998) From hospital to community: bridging therapeutic relationships. J Psychiatr Ment Health Nurs 5:197–202
Gesler W (1992) Therapeutic landscapes: medical issues in light of new cultural geography. Soc Sci Med 34(7):735–746
Haigh R (2012) The philosophy of Green Care: why it matters for our mental health. Ment Health Soc Incl 16(3):127–134
Harlow HF, Soumi SJ (1970) The nature of love simplified. Am Psychol 25:161–168
Haubenhofer DK, Elings M, Hassink J, Hine RE (2010) The Development of Green Care in Western Countries. Explore 6:106–111
Heron J (2001) Helping the client: a creative and practical guide, 4th edn. Sage, London
Herring MP, Lindheimer JB, O'Connor PJ (2013) The effects of exercise training on anxiety. Am J Lifestyle Med 8(6):388–403
Hine R, Peacock J, Pretty J (2008) Care farming in the UK – evidence and opportunities. Report for the National Care Farming Initiative (UK). Department of Biological Sciences and Centre for Environment and Society, University of Essex
Jacquart SD, Marshak HH, Dos Santos H, Luu SM, Berk LS, McMahon PT, Riggs M (2014) The effects of simultaneous exercise and psychotherapy on depressive symptoms in inpatient, psychiatric older adults. Adv Mind Body Med 28(4):8–17
Kaplan R, Kaplan S (1989) The experience of nature: a psychological perspective. Cambridge University Press, New York
Kellert SR, Wilson EO (1993) The biophilia hypothesis. Island Press, Washington
Kielhofner G (2009) Conceptual foundations of Occupational therapy practice, 4th edn. FA Davis, Philadelphia
Lieberman M (2013) Social: why our brains are wired to connect. Crown, New York
Lisack T (2009) Continuous partial attention and human connectedness: A grounded theory study. Dissertation, University of Phoenix. Available from http://gateway.proquest.com/openurl?url_ver=Z39.88-2004&res_dat=xri:pqdiss&rft_val_fmt=info:ofi/fmt:kev:mtx:dissertation&rft_dat=xri:pqdiss:3428556. Accessed 8 Aug 2015
Marcel GG (1948) Blackham HJ (1986) Six existentialist thinkers. Routledge, London, pp 140–159
Martin DJ, Garske JP, Davis KM (2000) Relation of the therapeutic alliance with outcome and other variables: a meta-analytic review. J Consult Clin Psychol 68(3):438–450
Maslow A (1962) Toward a psychology of being. Princeton, D van Nostrand
McKenna HP (1997) Nursing theories and models. Routledge, London
McKenna HP, Slevin OD (2008) Nursing models, theories and practice. Blackwell, Oxford

Meleis AI (2012) Theoretical nursing: development and progress, 5th edn. Lippincott, Philadelphia
Mosher L (1999) Soteria and other alternatives to acute psychiatric hospitalization: a personal and professional review. J Nerv Ment Dis 187:142–149
National Alliance on Mental Illness (recovered 2015) Supported employment. Available from http://www2.nami.org/template.cfm?template=/contentManagement/contentDisplay.cfm&contentID=8364. Accessed 22 July 2015
North TC, McCullagh P, Tran ZV (1990) Effect of exercise on depression. Exerc Sports Sci Rev 18:379–415
Orbach I (2003) Suicide and the suicidal body. Suicide Life Threat Behav 33(1):1–8
Paluska SA, Schwenk TL (2000) Physical activity and mental health: current concepts. Sports Med 29(3):167–180
Peplau H (1988) Interpersonal relations in nursing, 2nd edn. Macmillan, New York
Petruzzello SJ, Landers DM, Hatfield BD, Kubitz KA, Salazar W (1991) A meta-analysis on the anxiety reducing effects of acute and chronic exercise. Outcomes and mechanisms. Sports Med 11(3):143–182
Phillips J, Frances A, Cerullo MJ et al (2012) The six most essential questions in psychiatric diagnosis: a pluralogue part 2: issues of conservatism and pragmatism in psychiatric diagnosis. Philos Ethics Humanit Med 7:8. http://www.ncbi.nlm.nih.gov/pmc/articles/PMC3390269/
Platt S, Davis S, Sharpe M et al (2005) Contextual effects in suicidal behavior: evidence, explanation and implications. In: Hawton K (ed) Prevention and treatment of suicidal behaviour: from science to practice. Oxford University Press, Oxford, pp 53–70
Pretty J (2004) How nature contributes to mental and physical health. Spiritual Health Int 5:68–78
Pretty J (2007) The Earth only endures: on reconnecting with nature and our place in it. Earthscan, London
Rush B (1912) Medical inquiries and observations upon diseases of the mind. Reproduced as (1962) The History of Medicine Series. No. 15. Hafner, New York
Sempik J (2010) Green care and mental health: gardening and farming as health and social care. Ment Health Soc Incl 14(3):15–22
Sempik J, Hine R, Wilcox D (eds) (2010) Green care: a conceptual framework, a report of the working group on the health benefits of green care, COST action 866, green care in agriculture. Centre for Child and Family Research, Loughborough University, Loughborough
Sheehan KA, Phil D, Burns T (2011) Perceived coercion and the therapeutic relationship: a neglected association? Psychiatr Serv 62(5):471–476
Sloan N, Leon-Camacho WL, Rojas PE et al (1994) Kangaroo mother method: randomized control trial of alternative method of care for stabilizing low birth weight infants. Lancet 344:782–785
Smith MA, Lynch WJ (2012) Exercise as a potential treatment for drug abuse: evidence from preclinical studies. Front Psychiatry 2:82. Available at http://www.ncbi.nlm.nih.gov/pmc/articles/PMC3276339/. Accessed 10 June 2015
Substance Abuse and Mental Health Services Administration – U.S.A. Department of Health and Human Services (2015) Transforming Lives Through Supported Employment. Available from http://www.samhsa.gov/grants/grant-announcements/sm-14-011. Accessed 21 June 2015
Sullivan H (1953) The interpersonal theory of psychiatry. Tavistock, New York
Takano T, Nakammura K, Watanbe M (2002) Urban residential environments and senior citizen's longevity in megacity areas: the importance of walkable green spaces. J Epidemiol Environ Health 56:913–918
Thibeault C (2012) The relationships of hospitalized persons with acute mental illness and their nurses: an interpretive inquiry. ProQuest information & learning. Diss Abstr Int: Sect B: Sci Eng 72(9):5230–5230
Tuke DH (1882) Chapters in the history of the insane in the British Isles. Kegan Paul Trench, London
Van de Berg AE, Maas J, Verheij RA, Groenewegen PP (2010) Green space as a buffer between stressful life events and health. Soc Sci Med 70:1203–1210
Wilson EO (1984) Biophilia: the human bond with other species. Harvard University Press, Cambridge

Wipfli BM, Rethorst CD, Landers DM (2008) The anxiolytic effects of exercise: a meta-analysis of randomized trials and dose–response analysis. J Sport Exerc Psychol 30:392–410
Zschucke E, Heinz A, Strohle A (2012) Exercise and physical activity in the therapy of substance use disorders. Sci World J 2012:1. Available from http://www.ncbi.nlm.nih.gov/pmc/articles/PMC3354725/

Nursing People in Prisons, Forensics and Correctional Facilities

16

Tommy Dickinson, Amrita Mullan, Kirsty Lippiatt, and Julie Ann Owen

16.1 Introduction

Nursing within a secure environment can be traced back to the days of 'Bedlam'[1] (Dale et al. 2001), where so-called care was torturous and patients were victims. In the UK, forensic psychiatric/mental health (P/MH) nursing has emerged as a distinct field of practice since the opening of 'Broadmoor'[2] Hospital in 1863 and developed substantially over the decades (Mason 2002). Forensic mental health care refers to the care of mentally disordered offenders: people who have been in contact with the criminal justice system and who have been transferred to secure hospitals (Rutherford and Duggan 2007). The so-called 'secure beds' are a huge cost to the National Health Service (NHS). One medium secure bed costs around £483 per day (Centre for Mental Health 2013). NHS England (2013) reported that within the UK, there are 795 high secure beds, 3192 medium secure beds and 3732 low secure beds, and the average length of stay in such settings is 2 years (Centre for Mental Health 2013). In the UK, offenders with mental health problems can be detained in secure settings under the Mental Health Act 1983 [as amended]. The standards for medium and low secure services are currently set out by the Quality Network for Forensic Mental

[1] 'Bedlam' refers to the first London hospital to specialise in the so-called 'mentally ill' and origin of the word "bedlam" describing chaos or madness.

[2] Broadmoor Hospital is a high-security psychiatric hospital in England.

T. Dickinson (✉)
The University of Manchester, Manchester, UK
e-mail: tommy.dickinson@kcl.ac.uk

K. Lippiatt • J.A. Owen
King's College London, London, UK

A. Mullan
Sheffield Health & Social Care NHS Foundation Trust, Sheffield, UK

© Springer International Publishing Switzerland 2018

J.C. Santos, J.R. Cutcliffe (eds.), *European Psychiatric/Mental Health Nursing in the 21st Century*, Principles of Specialty Nursing,
https://doi.org/10.1007/978-3-319-31772-4_16

Health Services (Royal College of Psychiatrists 2016). Additionally, the Ministry of Justice has produced guidance relating to mentally disordered offenders that covers offenders who are detained in hospital, those who have been discharged to the community and those transferred from prison to hospital (Ministry of Justice 2016).

Safeguarding the public remains the priority of the criminal justice system. However, there is increasing concern that prison is not always an appropriate environment for prisoners (Her Majesty's Inspectorate of Prison, 2006). The primary principles of punishment, control and security may have a detrimental impact not only on vulnerable individuals who have pre-existing mental health problems but also on those who are considered mentally well. This can result in deterioration in mental health, exacerbation of vulnerability and increased risk of self-harm (Dickinson 2009). Indeed, Lord Bradley (2009) highlights that over 90% of prisoners had one or more of the psychiatric disorders: psychosis, neurosis, personality disorder, hazardous drinking and drug dependence. Therefore, although challenging it is crucial a balance is struck between the health needs of prisoners and the prison's guiding principles (Goomany and Dickinson 2015).

Following impassioned calls from many distinguished modern figures (see, e.g. Dostoyevsky, Pope John Paul II, Churchill), the humane treatment of prisoners has come to define a civilised society, and the improvements in prison conditions have been advanced by the European Convention on Human Rights and subsequent incorporation into UK law and the Human Rights Act 1998. However, the provision of care within secure environments is problematic owing to the complexities of the prison regime and high (particular) needs of patients (Dickinson and Hurley 2012; Offender Health Research Network 2010). This chapter aims to explore some of the key practice issues that P/MH nurses working within secure environments may experience and envisions alternative possibilities for constructive and caring interventions.

16.2 Key Practice Issues

16.2.1 The Therapeutic Alliance

The role of the nurse in any setting is complex. In a secure environment, there is the added pressure of maintaining security (Mason 2002). Perimeter walls and contemporary surveillance and security procedures provide a continuous thread to the historic forensic landscape of containment and control (Foucault 1975; Scull 1993). While the importance of physical and procedural containment in the provision of safe forensic service delivery and public protection is understood and acknowledged, the complex equation and interplay of so-called mental illness, psychopathology and offending behaviour require the contemporary nurse working in prisons, forensics and correctional facilities to integrate an understanding of emotional containment in the context of the nurse-patient relationship (Aiyegbusi and Clarke-Moore 2008). However, inculcating an integrated approach to therapeutic containment has not been without its challenges.

Unfortunately, the concluding decades of twentieth century secure care in England are in part characterised by criticism of high secure services via public inquiry and independent review (Blom-Cooper 1992; Fallon 1999). The Blom-Cooper public inquiry (Blom-Cooper 1992) exposed Ashworth Hospital as operating institutionalised, brutal and dehumanising practices with the behaviour of some nurses called into question or seriously criticised. The Fallon public inquiry highlighted that significant breaches in security had taken place in the Personality Disorder Unit at Ashworth Hospital alongside allegations of serious offending behaviour by hospital patients (Fallon 1999). Meanwhile at Broadmoor Hospital the report into the deaths of three men of African-Caribbean origin, Michael Martin, Joseph Watts and Orville Blackwood who all died in seclusion following restraint and the forced administration of medication (Blackwood Inquiry 1993) raised considerable concern about the care and treatment of patients from black and minority ethnic communities.

Forensic P/MH nurses often work with patients who have a history of complex trauma and profound emotional deprivation and neglect where the origins of trauma are rooted in early life experiences and played out in relationships with others (De Zulueta 2006). Additionally, the patient group they serve are subject to societal 'othering' and marginalisation owing to their offending histories (Cohen 2011). Subsequently, the dynamics inherent in the forensic nurse-patient relationship requires expert navigation through something of an ethical and moral maze (Barker 2011).

Security versus therapy is a constant dilemma within secure settings, and balancing security with nursing care is a challenge. Gildberg et al. (2012) found that a significant role of the nurse in secure settings was to maintain security and that security conduct is linked to all aspects of interaction with patients. Jacob and Holmes (2011) posit that security and nursing care not only coexist within the forensic environment but also rely on each other in order to take place and that a secure mind-set can dictate how nursing care is delivered. Moreover, Martin and Street (2003) identified that nurses' notes maintained a custodial orientation where surveillance was a priority over a therapeutic stance.

The therapeutic alliance plays a pivotal role in the recovery of mental health patients, and within a secure setting, this alliance is just as essential, if not more so. Arguably, forensic P/MH nursing is primarily concerned with interpersonal relationships, and owing to the level of risk within the field, the ability to develop such relationships is one of the most important skills a nurse may possess (Dale et al. 2001; Dickinson et al. 200b), Dickinson 2009. Indeed, Peternejli-Taylor (2003) states that forming therapeutic relations with patients is one of the most important competencies for a forensic nurse as it influences the nursing process and ultimately the quality of care.

The nurse-patient relationship is widely viewed to form the cornerstone of interpersonal therapeutic endeavour and the role of therapeutic boundaries is central (Aiyegbusi and Clarke-Moore 2008). Arguably, the translation of boundaries that are supportive and protective for the patient and the nurse requires a conceptual lens moving beyond the overt signposts of rules, regulations and security protocols, towards an integrated understanding, which encompasses the problems inherent in 'therapeutic' over-involvement and under-involvement (Peternelj-Taylor 2002; Sheets 2001).

Arguably, with few exceptions (see Aiyegbusi and Clarke-Moore 2008; Aiyegbusi and Kelly 2011) forensic nurses have paid limited attention to attachment patterns and psychodynamic interpretations of distress, trauma and offending behaviour. Recognition of the intense emotional experiences of practitioners working with forensic patients has been elegantly described (Cordess and Cox 1995). However, appreciation of the part that exposure to destructive psychopathology may have on the conscious and unconscious responses of nurses in their day-to-day work with forensic patients requires sustained exploration. Working with people who have a diagnosis of personality disorder is now part and parcel of mental health services in prisons and correctional and forensic mental health settings (NIMHE, 2003). Nonetheless, significant challenges for practitioners have been identified in the research literature (Bowers 2002) and in a highly critical public inquiry (Fallon 1999).

A recent study (Aiyegbusi and Kelly 2015) used a mixed method approach incorporating a quantitative Delphi study and qualitative methods to explore the lived experience of nurses and patients via the nurse-patient relationship. This groundbreaking study explores and formulates via a psychoanalytic model of understanding, the highly painful emotional phenomena arising from the traumatic history of the patient which then manifests in the nurse-patient relationship. This approach represents a seismic shift in the exploration of complex dynamic processes anchored by the nurse-patient relationship and will hopefully help form a platform and paradigm for ongoing work into the forensic nurse-patient relationship.

It is important that nurses working within secure settings are non-judgemental and demonstrate unconditional positive regard. Nevertheless, Jacob and Holmes (2011) identify that remaining non-judgemental in a secure environment is challenging owing to the nature of patients' crimes, e.g. murder and sex offences. Martin and Street (2003) elaborate stating that nurses can be judgemental when they impose moral standards on patients and the nurse-patient relationship becomes compromised when they thought of the patient's offence (Martin and Street 2003). However, Jacob and Holmes (2011) offer strategies to overcome this. Strategies include meeting the patient before reading their file and entering 'clinical mode', whereby values are set aside, disconnecting the person from the crime and focusing on the task at hand.

Closely allied with respect are the nurses' availability, presence and willingness to invest time engaging with patients. Where staff are not available, this translates to perceptions of lack of interest, which serves as a barrier to the development of a positive therapeutic relationship (MacInnes et al. 2014). Moreover, offering little or no time to engage with patients and nursing from a distance is viewed to be demonstrative of a lack of respect (Olofsson and Jacobsson 2001). To foster a therapeutic relationship, nurses need to spend time with patients (clients) and to enable them to open up and disclose their story, so appropriate interventions can be formulated. Scanlon (2006), however, found that there were differences in what individual P/MH nurses considered to be enough time. Furthermore, the nature of the forensic environment can be restricting, and so opportunities to interact with patients can be limited which can negitively impact on nurses' ability to form therapeutic relationships with people in their care (Jacob and Holmes 2011, Dickinson and Wright 2008). Indeed, Martin and Street's (2003) study exploring evidence of the therapeutic relationship in forensic psychiatric nursing found that there were few file entries that actually indicated the nurse had spent significant time engaging with patients. Therefore, it is pertinent that nurses make time to engage with patients/clients. Nurses can use informal activities and 'small talk' as a way to get to know patients and enable them to begin to trust staff. Additional methods include participating in activities such as sport and talking with patients about everyday topics such as television and the weather.

Patients may demonstrate violent and aggressive behaviour if they perceive their concerns are not listened to (Goomany and Dickinson 2015). Therefore, the ability to listen is vital. Patients report they want staff to demonstrate true empathy as this illustrates their needs can be anticipated. Additionally and importantly as forensic patients are treated under the Mental Health Act 1983 [as amended], giving correct and relevant information regarding legal rights and treatment is viewed as a key skill associated with respect (MacInnes et al. 2014). The therapeutic relationship is significantly linked to patient satisfaction and engagement, with the main areas of importance to patients being treated with respect and staff being available. However, the constructs of the therapeutic relationship have been shown to have overlapping concepts.

16.3 Prevention and Management of Violence and Aggression

Violence and aggression are a global problem in many areas of health and social care – including mental health care, with the greatest number of incidences occurring in inpatient psychiatric units and these incidents being consistently higher across forensic settings (NICE 2015; The British Psychological Society/The Royal College of Psychiatrists 2014). A survey of an independent secure service recorded 2137 incidents involving 56.4% of patients. The incident rate was found to be greater in medium secure in comparison to low secure, and in high secure environments, 5658 incidents were recorded over a 16-month period (Dickens et al. 2013; Uppal and McMurran 2009). It is unsurprising therefore that a crucial role for nurses working within secure milieus is the therapeutic prevention and management of violent and aggressive behaviour to maintain the safety of patients while ensuring a safe and therapeutic environment.

Assaults against staff affect both their physical and emotional wellbeing and contribute to low job satisfaction, an increase in sickness absence and staff turnover, increase in anxiety and reduced psychological wellbeing (Cacciacarne et al. 1986; Dickinson and Wright 2008). Therefore, it is imperative that our understanding of the causes, prevention and management of violence and aggression is increased.

16.4 Causes

Many theories have been put forward to explain the cause of aggression and ultimately violence; however, for the authors of this chapter, psychological theories appear to be most helpful as they attempt to understand the complexities of human behaviour (Dickens et al. 2013). From this aggression can be categorised into three aetiological models: factors internal to the person, external environmental factors and situational/interactional factors. (*See Chap. 33 which features a systemic, four quadrant model of violence and aggression*). Translated to mental health settings, aggression and violence are seen to lie within the person; some suggest individuals are predisposed to be more aggressive than others, due to their so-called mental illness or personality (Nijman and Rector 1999). Other individual factors said to influence aggressive behaviour include sex, age, socioeconomic status, index offence and non-compliance with medication (Health and Service Executive [HSE] n.d.). Conversely, external explanations look towards both social and physical environmental influences, for example, the layout of the ward and the skill mix of staff. Knowles et al. (2008) found within a medium secure setting that patients were more likely to be aggressive to staff of the same gender. Lastly, situational/interactional factors, which are founded on Bandura's social learning theory, suggest aggression is learnt and maintained by operant conditioning (Dickens et al. 2013). One particular focus of research in this area has been the interaction between staff and patients. The way in which staff speak to patients has been asserted as a strong influential factor of violence and aggression (Camerino et al. 2008). Furthermore, inconsistencies among staff and the imposition of regimes and feelings that staff do not understand or are listening to their concerns may also contribute the violent and aggressive behaviour (Jansen et al. 2005). Situational/interactional factors are considered to lead to better prediction of violence and aggression when compared to internal or external factors. However, the complexity of such behaviour makes it difficult to determine its source, and it is likely that all three factors interplay (Dickens et al. 2013).

16.5 Prevention, Prediction and Risk Management"

Although risk cannot be completely eliminated, risk assessment and management is an essential part of good P/MH nursing clinical practice. P/MH nurses are obliged to put into place reasonably practicable preventive and protective measures and to foster a safe and therapeutic environment for both staff and patients. One way by which professionals are expected to achieve this is through the formulation and frequent review of systematic risk assessment. These assessments are used to inform implementation of measures to minimise associated risk (HSE). The way in which risk is assessed is the source of much debate, with some favouring actuarial methods over clinical assessment while others placing importance on intuition and clinical judgement in assessments for violence (Barry et al. 2007). However, when performing risk assessments and forming management plans, Wood (2006) asserts professional judgement must be underpinned by a strong evidence base.

'Static' factors or characteristics such as gender, past violent and/or aggressive behaviour and forensic history are important considerations when predicting violent risk; however, as they are not changeable, they play a lesser role when seeking to reduce risk (Elbogen et al. 2006). Arguably, it is 'dynamic' factors, which may have greater influence when predicting violence as these maybe vary, for example, with environment, personal relationships and changes in personality (Health Service Executive n.d.). The Historical, Clinical and Risk Management Assessment Scheme (HCR-20) is a commonly used risk assessment tool and assists in the identification of dynamic risk factors, which require intervention and treatment. Edens et al. (2005) argue, even where structured risk assessments are used, it has limited accuracy when predicting whether an individual poses a continuing threat to society as they simply provide a score of the likely risk of reoffending. Therefore, it is crucial to formulate a risk assessment for the purposes of management that is individualised and dynamic and that can be reviewed and developed.

Attitudes and beliefs held by nursing staff about the causes of aggression were influential when deciding upon the most appropriate intervention to resolve an incident (Dickens et al. 2013; Pulsford et al. 2013). Broadly, psychological, physical and pharmacological interventions are drawn upon, and one or more of these may be employed to manage violence and aggression in any one incident. National guidelines together with local policies stress nurses must exhaust their resources and skill set before turning to other more coercive interventions. In practice, this means using psychological interventions such as verbal de-escalation, observing for signs and symptoms of anger, distraction and using low stimulus environments. These techniques help to develop rapport with the patient, strengthening the therapeutic alliance with the result of increasing self-efficacy and job satisfaction and maintaining patient autonomy and dignity (Cowin et al. 2003).

16.6 Self-Harm

The extent of mutilation and the determination exhibited by people in prisons, forensics and correctional facilities to engage in serious acts of self-harm is astonishing. Individuals have 'swallowed pens, inserted pencils into their penises and paperclips into their abdomens, bitten chunks of flesh from their arms, slashed and gashed themselves' (Human Rights Watch 2003, p. 174). Nurses' responses to people who self-harm have traditionally focussed on stopping the self-harm, sometimes involving extreme responses such as force or constant observation (Shaw and Shaw 2008). Forensic nurses have been shown to be more likely to utilise special observations more frequently than their counterparts in non-forensic settings (Whitehead and Mason 2006). However, it has been recognised that this may have a paradoxical effect, with respondents in one study stating that they felt confined, they had limited privacy, and in some cases it exacerbated their symptoms by increasing anxiety and irritability (Cardell and Rogers-Pitula 1999). Hoping for the cessation of self-harm might be an unrealistic aim, given that self-harm is often a strategy for coping, surviving and transcending intolerable distress; it can even be a way to avert suicide. Other studies have shown that patients have positive associations with self-harm (McLaughlin 2007; Pardoe and Trainor, 2017). Further, according to Shaw and Shaw (2008), in some cases, it can be better simply to limit damage while self-harm continues. Indeed NICE (2004, p. 35) offers the following guidance:

> consider giving advice and instructions on harm minimisation issues and techniques.

Nurses are in an ideal position to give this information (Pembroke 2006). It involves nurses accepting the need of patients to self-harm as a method of survival until this is possible by other means. This is not to condone or encourage self-harm but to face the reality of it, so that eventually, the safety of the patient is maximised. Here, patients are educated on basic anatomy and physiology and the correct use of dressings, as well as how to access first aid and wound care services (Pembroke 2006). Harrison (1998) posits the concept of therapeutic risk-taking to encourage people who self-harm to take responsibility for their behaviour. In addition, Pembroke (1998) has gone so far as to advocate that inpatient facilities should offer clean blades to patients to minimise infection. Nevertheless, the evidence base on the use of harm minimisation to prevent self-harm and suicide is limited.

The Nursing and Midwifery Council (2015) states that patient autonomy must be upheld; however, it also states that nurses must manage and assess risk; therefore, in this particular case, the code could indeed contradict itself. This leaves nurses in somewhat of a dilemma. On the one hand, they are aware that increasing individuals' responsibility is beneficial in the management of self-harm, but on the other hand, they are seen as being responsible for their care and cannot really be seen to be advocating that patients continue to harm themselves. Rumbold (2000, p.57) states that:

> acts of interference with other persons' autonomy are often justified by the claim that these acts are for the benefit or welfare of those who are being interfered with.

Therefore, it could be asserted that by failing to facilitate a harm minimisation approach, nurses are not upholding patients' autonomy.

It is clear that this is a controversial issue and it is difficult to understand how a facilitative approach to self-harm (particularly giving clean blades to patients) could be applied within prisons, forensics and correctional facilities. Indeed, there is a risk to others if self-harmers have access to blades, which could be significant given that many of the people within these environments have serious convictions, including assaults on others. In addition, there is the need to consider public perception should a serious incident such as suicide or assault on a fellow patient or prisoner occur with professionals having provided the means for the incident to take place.

Facilitating patients by providing the means to self-harm within these environments is not an option. There could be a definite benefit to educating the patients on harm minimisation strategies such as safer cutting techniques, correct use of dressings and wound care; despite nurses' best efforts, clinical experience has shown that patients are sometimes able to find means to self-harm. Moreover, Pembroke (2006) states that with such information, patients have a choice about the way they self-harm, making it safer. Arguably, paradoxically, with this information, patients are given more autonomy. Nurses must accept that facilitating patient improvement and autonomy will engender a small but significant risk (Pauker and Cooper 1990). However, nurses' scope for autonomous practices such as those discussed above, can only be fostered if the policies of the clinical setting in which they are working advocate such an approach. Consequently, nurses need to take an active role in influencing and structuring the political agenda that governs the clinical setting.

Conclusion

P/MH nurses working within secure milieus are generally striving to provide patient-centred and high-quality care in an often challenging, stressful and frustrating environment. Patients within prisons, forensics and correctional facilities should receive a holistic assessment that endeavours to promote health, among those with a so-called mental illness and ensure a state of mental, social and emotional wellbeing for all. The evidenced link between mental health, substance misuse and crime demonstrates the potential for P/MH nurses to have a positive impact on reoffending and the running of secure milieus (Norman and Parrish 2002). While the guiding principles of the secure system will remain, there is a need for P/MH nurses to be innovative and imaginative in the application of interventions to minimise any negative impact that confinement may exert on individuals.

The secure environment can have a negative impact on the psychological health of patients contained within them, and such patients are an exceptionally socially excluded group. Therefore, P/MH nurses must look to interventions beyond pharmacotherapy and become more recovery focussed to support patients to meet some of their basic needs. Additionally, they must draw on their skills, experience and intuition to identify those patients who are at greater risk of their mental health deteriorating as a result of one or more of these aspects.

Nurses working within secure environments tend to work with patients who hold complex and multifaceted needs. Therefore, these P/MH nurses often need to become case managers and plan and implement composite care packages. A large part of the P/MH nurses' role in secure environments is risk assessment, management and reduction. Indeed risk management is as much about providing inclusive and holistic care as it is concerned with implementing any specialist risk assessment skills. Fundamentally, it also necessitates patients being actively involved in their own care (Duncan 2013). Finally, the nurses' therapeutic alliance with people within prisons, forensics and correctional facilities is paramount. Therefore, P/MH nurses working with patients in secure settings should seek to re-evaluate their core nursing skills of therapeutic communication, listening and being non-judgemental, and demonstrate that they empathise with the challenging situation that their patients are in.

References

Aiyegbusi A, Clarke-Moore J (2008) Therapeutic relationships with offenders: an introduction to the psychodynamics of forensic mental health nursing. (Forensic focus). Jessica Kingsley, London

Aiyegbusi A, Kelly G (2011) Professional and therapeutic boundaries in forensic mental health practice. Jessica Kingsley, London

Aiyegbusi A, Kelly D (2015) 'This is the Pain I feel!' Projection and emotional pain in the nurse-patient relationship with people diagnosed with personality disorder in forensic and specialist personality disorder services: findings from a mixed method study. Psychoanal Psychother 29(3):276

Barker P (2011) Mental health ethics the human context. Routledge, Oxon

Barry M, Loucks N, Kemshall H (2007) Serious violent offenders: developing a risk assessment framework [pdf]. Available from: http://www.rmascotland.gov.uk/files/5512/7263/5813/Serious%20Violent%20Offenders%20-%20Developing%20a%20Risk%20Assessment%20Framework.pdf. Accessed 8 Apr 2016

Blackwood Inquiry. (1993) Report of the committee of inquiry into the death of orville blackwood and a review of the deaths of two other Afro-Caribbean patients 'big, black and dangerous?'. Special hospital services authority

Blom-Cooper L (1992) Report of the committee of inquiry into complaints about Ashworth hospital, Vols 1 and 2, Cmnd 2028–1. HMSO, London

Bowers L (2002) Dangerous and severe personality disorder: response and role of the psychiatric team. Routledge, London

Bradley K (2009) The Bradley report. https://www.rcpsych.ac.uk/pdf/Bradley%20Report11.pdf. Accessed 7 Jan 2014

Cacciacarne M, Resnick PJ, MaArthur C, Althot SE (1986) Burnout in forensic psychiatric staff. Med Law 5(4):303–308

Camerino D, Estryn-Behar M, Conway PM, Heijden BIJM, Hasselhorn HM (2008) Work-related factors and violence among nursing staff in the European NEXT study: a longitudinal cohort study. Int J Nurs Stud 45:35–50

Cardell R, Rogers-Pitula C (1999) Suicidal inpatients' perceptions of therapeutic and nontherapeutic aspects of constant observation. Psychiatr Serv 50(8):1066–1070

Centre for Mental Health (2013). Briefing note: Secure care services. Centre for Mental Health, London. Available at: http://www.centreformentalhealth.org.uk/secure-care-a-briefing-note. Accessed 22 Mar 2016

Cohen S (2011) Folk devils and moral panics, 4th edn. Taylor Francis, New York

Cordess C, Cox M (1995) Forensic psychotherapy: crime, psychodynamics and the offender patient. Jessica Kingsley Publihsers, London

Cowin L, Davies R, Estall G, Berlin T, Fitzgerald M, Hoot S (2003) De-escalating aggression and violence in the mental health setting. Int J Ment Health Nurs 12(1):640–673

Dale C, Thompson T, Woods P (2001) Nursing. In: Dale C, Thompson T, Woods P (eds) Forensic mental health: issues in practice. Harcourt, London, pp 19–30

De Zulueta F (2006) From pain to violence: the traumatic roots of destructiveness. Wiley-Blackwell, West Sussex

Dickens G, Piccirillo M, Alderman N (2013) Causes and management of aggression and violence in a forensic mental health service: perspectives of nurses and patients. Int J Ment Health Nurs 22(6):532–544

Dickinson T (2009) The attitudes of nurses and healthcare workers within secure environments towards young people who self-harm. M.Sc. Thesis, University of Bradford

Dickinson T, Hurley MA (2012) Exploring the antipathy of nursing staff who work within secure healthcare facilities across the United Kingdom to young people who self-harm. J Adv Nurs 68(1):147–158

Dickinson T, Wright KM (2008) Stress and burnout in forensic mental health nursing: a review of the literature. Br J Nurs 17(2):82–87

Dickinson T, Ramsdale S, Speight G (2009a) Managing aggression and violence using rapid tranquillisation. Nurs Stand 24(7):40–49

Dickinson T, Wright KM, Harrison J (2009b) The attitudes of nursing staff in secure environments to young people who self-harm. J Psychiatr Ment Health Nurs 16(10):947–951
Duncan G (2013) Forensic mental health care. In: Norman I, Ryrie I (eds) The art and science of mental health nursing: principles and practice. Oxford University Press, pp 640-656
Edens J, Buffington-Vollum J, Keilen A, Roskamp P, Anthony C (2005) Predictions of future dangerousness in capital murder trials: is it time to disinvent the wheel? Law Hum Behav 29(1):55–86
Elbogen EB, Van Dorn RA, Swanson JW, Swartz MS, Monohan J (2006) Treatment engagement and violence risk in mental disorder. Br J Psychiatry 189:354–360
Fallon P (1999) Report of the Committee of Inquiry into the Personality Disorder Unit, Ashworth Hospital. The Stationary Office, London
Foucault M (1975) (Translated 2nd Edition, 1995) Discipline and punish: the birth of the prison. Random House, New York
Gildberg FA, Bradley SK, Fristed P, Hounsgaard L (2012) Reconstructing normality: characteristics of staff interactions with forensic mental health inpatients. Int J Ment Health Nurs 21(2):103–113
Goomany A, Dickinson T (2015) The influence of prison climate on the mental health of adult prisoners: a literature review. J Psychiatr Ment Health Nurs 22(6):413–422
Harrison A (1998) Self-harm. A harmful procedure. Nurs Times 94(27):37–38
Health Service Executive (n.d.) Risk management in mental health services [pdf]. Available from: https://www.hse.ie/eng/services/publications/Mentalhealth/RiskManagementinMentalHealth.pdf. Accessed 4 Apr 2016
Her Majesty's Inspectorate of Prisons (2006) Inquiry into the quality of healthcare at Yarl's Wood Immigration Removal Centre. HM Prison Service, London
Human Rights Watch (2003) Ill-equipped: US prisons and offenders with mental illness [online]. Human Rights Watch, USA. Available from: www.hrw.org/reports/2003/usa1003/. Accessed 24 Apr 2016
Jacob JD, Holmes D (2011) Working under threat: fear and nurse-patient interactions in a forensic psychiatric setting. J Forensic Nurs 7(2):68–77
Jansen GJ, Dassen TWN, Jebbink GG (2005) Staff attitudes towards aggression in health care: a review of the literature. J Psychiatr Ment Health Nurs 12:3–13
Knowles SF, Coyne SM, Brown SL (2008) Sex differences in aggressive incidents towards staff in secure services. J Forensic Psychiatry Psychol 19(4):620–631
MacInnes D, Courney H, Flanagan T, Bressington D, Beer D (2014) A cross sectional survey examining association between therapeutic relationships and service user satisfaction in forensic mental health settings. BMC Res Notes 7(1):657. doi:10.1186/1756-0500-7-657. Accessed 25 Jan 2016
Martin T, Street AF (2003) Exploring evidence of the therapeutic relationship in forensic psychiatric nursing. J Psychiatr Ment Health Nurs 10(5):543–551
Mason T (2002) Forensic psychiatric nursing: a literature review and thematic analysis of role tensions. J Psychiatr Ment Health Nurs 9(5):511–520
McLaughlin C (2007) Suicide-related behaviour, understanding, caring and therapeutic responses. Wiley, Chichester
Ministry of Justice (2016) Mentally disordered offenders. Available at: http://www.justice.gov.uk/offenders/types-of-offender/mentally-disordered-offenders. Accessed 4 Apr 2016
National Institute for Clinical Excellence (2004) Self-harm: the short-term physical and psychological management and secondary prevention of self-harm in primary and secondary care. NICE, London
National Institute for Health and Care Excellence (2015) Violence and aggression: short-term management in mental health, health and community settings [pdf]. Available from: https://www.nice.org.uk/guidance/ng10/resources/violence-and-aggression-shortterm-management-in-mental-health-health-and-community-settings-1837264712389. Accessed 17 Mar 2016
National Institute for Mental Health England (2003) Personality disorder: no longer a diagnosis of exclusion. NIMHE, Bethesda
NHS England (2013) 2014/15 NHS standard contract for high secure mental health services (adults). NHS England, Redditch
Nijman HLI, Rector G (1999) Crowding and aggression and inpatient psychiatric wards. Psychiatr Serv 50(6):830–698

Norman A, Parrish A (2002) Prison nursing. Blackwell, Oxford
Nursing and Midwifery Council (2015) The code: professional standards of practice and behaviour for nurses and midwives. Available at: https://www.nmc.org.uk/standards/code/. Accessed 11 Feb 2016
Offender Health Research Network (2010) The pathway of prisoners with mental health problems through prison health services and the effect of the prison environment on the mental health of prisoners. http://www.ohrn.nhs.uk/OHRNResearch/EnvPath.pdf. Accessed 22 Mar 2016
Olofsson B, Jacobsson L (2001) A plea for respect: involuntarily hospitalized psychiatric patients' narratives about being subjected to coercion. J Psychiatr Ment Health Nurs 8(4):357–366
Pardoe, J & Trainor, G. (2017) Transgender youths who self-harm: perspectives from those seeking support. Mental Health Today. Available from: https://www.mentalhealthtoday.co.uk/transgender-youths-who-self-harm-perspectives-from-those-seeking-support
Pauker SL, Cooper AM (1990) Paradoxical patient reactions to psychiatric life support: clinical and ethical considerations. Am J Psychiatr 147(4):488–491
Pembroke L (1998) Only scratching the surface. Nurs Times 94:38–39
Pembroke L (2006) Limiting self harm. Emerg Nurse 14(5):8–10
Peternelj-Taylor C (2002) Professional boundaries. A matter of therapeutic integrity. J Psychosoc Nurs Ment Health Serv 40:4,22–4,29
Peternelj-Taylor C (2003) Guest editorial: incarceration of the vulnerable. J Psychosoc Nurs 41(9):6–7
Pulsford D, Crumptom A, Baker A, Wilkins T, Wright K, Duxbury J (2013) Aggression in a high secure hospital: staff and patient attitudes. J Psychiatr Ment Health Nurs 20(4):296–304
Royal College of Psychiatrists (2016) Quality network for forensic mental health services. Available at: http://www.rcpsych.ac.uk/workinpsychiatry/qualityimprovement/ccqiprojects/forensicmentalhealth/publications.aspx. Accessed 4 Apr 2016
Rumbold G (2000) Ethics in nursing practice. Balliere Tindall, London
Rutherford M, Duggan S (2007) Forensic mental health services: facts and figures on current provision. Sainsbury Centre for Mental Health, London. Available at: www.scie-socialcareonline.org.uk. Accessed 22 Mar 2016
Scanlon A (2006) Psychiatric nurses perceptions of the constituents of the therapeutic relationship: a grounded theory study. J Psychiatr Ment Health Nurs 13(3):319–329
Scull A (1993) The most solitary of afflictions: madness and society in Britain, 1700–1900. Yale University Press, New Haven
Shaw C, Shaw T (2008) Harm-minimisation for self-harm [online]. Available from: http://www.harm-ed.com/PDF/Harm-Minimisation-for-Self-Harm.pdf. Accessed 01 Apr 2016
Sheets VR (2001) Professional boundaries: staying in the lines. Dimens Crit Care Nurs 20(5):36–40
The British Psychological Society and The Royal College of Psychiatrists (2014) Violence and aggression. The short-term management of violence and physically threatening behaviour in mental health, health and community settings [pdf]. Available from: https://www.nice.org.uk/guidance/ng10/documents/violence-and-aggression-update-draft-full-guideline2. Accessed 17 Mar 2016
Uppal G, McMurran M (2009) Recorded incidents in a high-secure hospital: a descriptive analysis. Crim Behav Ment Health 19(4):265–276
Whitehead E, Mason T (2006) Assessment of risk and special observations in mental health practice: a comparison of forensic and non-forensic settings. Int J Ment Health Nurs 15:235–241
Wood J (2006) Profiling high-risk offenders: a review of 136 cases. Howard J Crim Just 45(3):307–320

eHealth, Telematics and Telehealth

17

Nina Kilkku

17.1 Introduction

Earlier in 2016, the World Health Organization (WHO) launched their interim report on global strategy for people-centred and integrated health services. This report includes the notion that while a lot has been accomplished, we still have a way to go to provide person-centred services (WHO 2016a). The implementation of different technological solutions is seen as one possibility to support person-centred care and research (Salvador-Carulla et al. 2013). eHealth development is strongly supported internationally and in the EU. In the EU-level eHealth action plan 2012–2020 is guiding this development process (European Commission 2012). Several aspects are highlighted in the latest WHO (2016b) eHealth report with recommendations for the future. eHealth is considered to encompass more than just technology, and therefore recommendations are also made from a variety of viewpoints. Many of these are also affecting psychiatric/mental health nurses, and the need for education programmes was strongly emphasized in the report (WHO 2016b).

The Internet has become one of the main environments in which people search for information, share their experiences and spend time. It is seen as a part of daily life for many people; around 40% of the world's population has an Internet connection (www.internetlivestats.com). While both the benefits of and problems related to the Internet have been recognized, it seems that there is no going back (Deslich et al. 2013); however, we need to remember that not all people have access to digital solutions (Cleary et al. 2008). People are using the Internet to search for information on mental health issues (Horgan and Sweeney 2010). There might be some generational issues, but as technology increasingly becomes integrated into our daily lives with smartphones,

N. Kilkku
School of Health Care, Tampere University of Applied Sciences,
Pirkanmaa, Finland
e-mail: minat@utu.fi

© Springer International Publishing Switzerland 2018

J.C. Santos, J.R. Cutcliffe (eds.), *European Psychiatric/Mental Health Nursing in the 21st Century*, Principles of Specialty Nursing,
https://doi.org/10.1007/978-3-319-31772-4_17

tablets and other easy-access technological solutions, e-solutions in health care, especially in mental health, are also becoming increasingly common (Perle and Nierenberg 2013). From a medicinal point of view, psychiatry is one area where the use of eHealth solutions could be beneficial (Lopez and Lustig 2015). P/MH nurses have been considered latecomers to this field (Repique 2007), while at the same time there are many different forms of technology already used in practice, education, management and research. Blended learning often includes web-based methods (Rigby et al. 2012). In the context of research, there are several possibilities (Cleary et al. 2008), for example, in data gathering (Baker et al. 2010; Engqvist et al. 2011; Oates 2015).

17.2 eHealth: Its Benefits and Problems

In this chapter, the concept of eHealth is adapted to cover a variety of terms, including 'ICT-based nursing', 'telematics', 'telemedicine', 'telepsychology' and 'telepsychiatry'. This follows the ideas of Della Mea (2001) as well as the following description of eHealth provided by Eysenbach (2001, p. e20):

> e-health is an emerging field in the intersection of medical informatics, public health and business, referring to health services and information delivered or enhanced through the Internet and related technologies. In a broader sense, the term characterizes not only a technical development, but also a state-of-mind, a way of thinking, an attitude, and a commitment for networked, global thinking, to improve health care locally, regionally, and worldwide by using information and communication technology.

According to the results of the systematic review of the definitions of eHealth conducted by Oh et al. (2005), while technology is not a substitute for human activities, it can provide something more. In general, in these definitions eHealth was seen in a positive light. However, more research should be integrated in eHealth developments to show the benefits of eHealth (Black et al. 2011). This lack of research is clearly evident in a systematic review on the effectiveness of social media interventions for people with schizophrenia in which only two studies were found on the issue (Välimäki et al. 2016). In Donker et al.'s (2013) systematic review of the use of smartphones to deliver mental health programmes, only a couple of evidence-based apps were found.

For service provision and to ensure access to care, different technological solutions are considered highly beneficial (Salmoiraghi and Hussain 2015), especially in rural areas (Bhandari et al. 2011; Paulson et al. 2015; Wilshire 2012), in developing countries (Blaya et al. 2009) and in situations where low-intensity interventions are either sufficient or can provide a first step in a stepped-care approach (Milgrom and Gemmill 2014). The need to transfer patients between services could be decreased (Buckley and Weisser 2012), and staff shortages might be helped (Ellington 2013) when eHealth solutions are implemented in practice. Internet-based interventions could also increase knowledge and decrease stigma (Finkelstein et al. 2008; Kiropoulos et al. 2011). These benefits are connected with ideas of active participation, social inclusion and recovery; information enables decision-making and active participation. New innovations, such as personal health records and the possibility to follow your own activity, mood etc., are available for those who want and have the technological resources to use them. In fact, many clients/patients and nurses do want to use such innovations. A recent study on an eHealth application to implement an illness and recovery management programme provides one example of this kind of approach (Beentjes et al. 2016).

However, there are also critical voices regarding a variety of ethical issues, including privacy, security and patient safety (Deslich et al. 2013), and different prerequisites, like training and organizational support. Critical voices are important and understandable as not all people have access to technological solutions or are willing to use them. Professionals in mental health care are also responsible for treating some of the negative consequences of technology, such as cyberbullying, which is linked also with some mental health problems (Carpenter and Hubbard 2014; Magaud et al. 2013), pathological Internet use (Morahan-Martin and Schumacher 2000) and Internet addiction (Fitzpatrick 2008; Wieland 2014). Guest editorial associate professor Wieland (2014) is actually shaking us, P/MH nurses, on this issue; there is addiction developed around the Internet and there are several other disciplines studying, writing and treating clients, but P/MH nurses are quite invisible when actually we should take the lead in education, prevention and treatment of Internet disorders and accept that technology is not going away (Wieland 2014).

Although not all of the previous studies clearly demonstrate the positive significance of using eHealth, but sometimes it might be also the only option as García-Lizana and Muñoz-Mayorga (2010, p. 119) concluded in their systematic review on the use of eHealth solutions with depression:

> There is a well-founded hypothesis that videoconference produces the same results as face-to-face treatment and that self-help Internet programs could improve symptoms. More research is needed; nevertheless, when traditional care is not possible, telemedicine could be used.

17.3 Psychiatric/Mental Health Nurses and eHealth

There are already some encouraging studies that show the processes involved in using ICT solutions in different P/MH nursing contexts. Anttila (2012) studied information-based patient education in nearly 500 sessions and concluded that while information technology could be adapted with patients who have severe mental health disorders, time is needed to fit these activities in clinical practice; furthermore, the context, circumstances and training of the staff must be taken into consideration. Nurses' positive viewpoint regarding the use of technology in their practice is a good basis for further development (Kurki 2014). However, support and evaluation from the organizations are required; there will be changes in the nurses' work styles, and therefore organizations should offer more flexible possibilities for nurses to adapt information technology in direct patient care. This might also enhance P/MH nurses' positive attitudes towards information technology, increase job satisfaction and decrease stress (Koivunen et al. 2013).

Nurses' competences, skills and readiness to use technology are often mentioned as the key factors which might have an effect on the use of eHealth possibilities in practice (Koivunen et al. 2007; Perle and Nierenberg 2013). The first step would be to know and understand how the Internet works to enable its use in clinical nursing practice and to be able to prevent negative consequences (Fetter 2009). Concerns from the patients' viewpoint could also prevent nurses from implementing eHealth solutions (Koivunen et al. 2007). It might also be a question of cultural change rather than technological skills (De Weger et al. 2013) as there is a need to adapt different roles and styles of practice in the virtual environment (Bhandari et al. 2011). It is important that professionals find themselves these ways of working comfortable (Callahan and Inckle 2012).

It might also be important for us to recognize that we are actually already using a lot of technology in our daily practices. Callan et al. (2009) used a case example to describe how we can use different technologies with service users. As this example is already 7 years old, some technical solutions have changed, but the ideas are still evident in practice today, such as in the use of emails, reminders about medication by smartphone and programmes for time management and psychoeducation.

17.4 eHealth Solutions for Mental Health Practice

Some very practical instructions and tips are described in the literature, such as in De Weger et al. (2013) review of the use of video conferencing in mental health practice. They conclude with recommendations on implementation, staff and service user consultations, training and technical specifications. For the usage of video conferencing in mental health practice, they provide detailed information on a variety of ethical issues, including confidentiality, data protection and informed consent, and on clinical specifications and the practicalities of meetings (De Weger et al. 2013). This kind of sharing of knowledge is highly beneficial as other people have probably had similar questions when planning video conferences for consultations or other purposes. They also highlight the need to clarify if these kinds of new solutions are found important not only by managers but also by staff and service users (De Weger et al. 2013). Similarly, Kane et al. (2012) have described different considerations and viewpoints when technology is utilized in medical team meetings.

There are already many mobile apps for nurses to use and to guide patients. Elias et al. (2014) gathered information on some apps, such as those developed for optimism and PSTD (Elias et al. 2014). Another example is a mobile app called Oiva which is based on acceptance and commitment therapy (ACT). Oiva was designed to support active learning of skills connected with mental wellness, and it includes brief ACT-based exercises. The results of the feasibility study were positive and thus encourage the use of the app (Ahtinen et al. 2013).

There are also positive results regarding the use of a telephone- and text message-based telemedicine concept for patients with mental health disorders, especially those with symptoms of anxiety and depression (van den Berg et al. 2015). Studies have also shown that telephone-based care management of medication is beneficial for older adults (Maust et al. 2013).

17.5 Some Specific Areas of eHealth

Internet- or mobile-based solutions are enabling a different kind of person-centred health monitoring for persons themselves and different kinds of interventions also in a preventive manner. Lappalainen et al. (2013) described the positive results of a personal health technology-based psychological intervention with men who had stress and mood problems in terms of addressing stress, burnout and job satisfaction.

Adolescents with mental health problems are one group of patients with whom different technological options have been used and studied (Kurki et al. 2011; Horgan and Sweeney 2010). Some specific diagnosis-based studies with adolescents (Paing et al. 2009) and their parents (Binford Hopf et al. 2013) have been conducted. Adolescents are often more accustomed to technology, and the adaptation of these solutions might thus be easier. Adolescents might also have difficulties with accessing mental health services (Horgan and Sweeney 2010), which indicates the importance of using eHealth solutions. One important area for eHealth is patient education. Promising results have been found, for example, with adolescent suicide survivors (Hoffmann 2006). It seems that mental health nurses are motivated to use Internet-based psychoeducation in different contexts, including in acute wards, but support from organization is needed (Anttila et al. 2011), also with policy-making (Anttila et al. 2008).

17.6 Other Mental Health Contexts: Psychotherapy and eHealth

In the field of psychotherapy, there have been several studies about the use of technology, of which only some examples are mentioned here. These studies are often diagnosis-based and conducted in different comparative settings, e.g. the use of Internet-based cognitive behaviour therapy versus cognitive behavioural group therapy in the treatment of social anxiety disorder (Hedman et al. 2011). Most of these studies conclude that more research is needed as the number of studies in general is still quite low. Richards and Richardson (2012) described a review and meta-analyses of computer-based psychological treatments for depression and concluded that the efficacy and effectiveness of these treatments were supported. According to a pilot study, Internet-based CBT could also be beneficial in the treatment of obsessive compulsive disorders (Andersson et al. 2011) as it is efficacious and increases accessibility to treatment (Andersson et al. 2012). For adults' anxiety disorders, it might be important to have therapist-supported Internet-based cognitive behavioural therapy, but there might not be any difference between face-to-face and

Internet-based practice. However, more research is also needed on this subject (Olthuis et al. 2015).

Technological care solutions for psychosis also seem to be acceptable and feasible and have the potential to improve clinical and social outcomes, but again, more research is still needed (Alvarez-Jimenez et al. 2014). Social media can also offer new possibilities to recognize negative symptoms and impairments in social cognition related to schizophrenia; however, the risks, such as unintended disclosure and stigma, should be recognized (Torous and Keshavan 2016). Researchers have recognized that certain patient groups, like men and younger patients with problematic drug use, women or older patients with combined substance use problems, require extra caution when using Internet-based CBT (Gajecki et al. 2014). There are also psychotherapists who are reluctant to adapt technological solutions in practice. The reasons for such reluctance include the need for training and equipment, costs and unfamiliarity with the possible benefits (Schwartzman et al. 2012).

17.7 Postgraduate Education

In the field of education, there are good examples of e-learning possibilities for postgraduates, including a study about the practicing mental health nurses using the e-learning course nursing interventions to manage distressed and disturbed patients. Encouraging results show that changes occurred in nurses' knowledge and attitudes; furthermore, the transfer of knowledge into practice led to changes in nurses' behaviour (Lahti 2014). More of these kinds of evaluations and information are needed for eHealth education purposes (WHO 2016b). One example of the postgraduate e-learning possibilities is the EU-funded eMenthe project. This project aimed to enhance masters-level education in mental health practice by developing e-learning materials through European cooperation. These materials have been produced in international co-operation between higher education institutes from Finland, Sweden, the United Kingdom, Ireland and the Netherlands. The results of this project are materials, not courses or programmes, which are available to everyone online. Reliable content has been produced based on critical reviews and numerous interviews with key stakeholders in participating countries (ementhe. Tamk.fi; ementhe.eu; Stickley et al. 2016; WHO 2016b). As the challenges in the mental health field are quite similar in different countries, these kinds of enterprises may be beneficial for bringing knowledge and knowhow together for the mutual benefit of those in the profession.

Simulation is one rapidly growing method in nursing education. For example, virtual patient simulation could be beneficial, not only for mental health nurse students but also for other professionals coming into contact with service users (Guise et al. 2012). Virtual patients have also been studied in the context of postgraduate nurses' education focusing on clinical reasoning with positive results (Forsberg et al. 2011; Forsberg et al. 2014). As in the field of education in general (and not only in higher education), technology has already been adapted in various ways; it is thus likely that we will see more developments in mental health nursing education with a blended learning approach. Future students might already be used to studying using different methods of learning provided by different technical solutions. Updates might be needed in the nurse education curricula to ensure that they are 'evidence-based computer and Internet curricula' (Koivunen et al. 2008).

17.8 New Arrivals

Serious health gamification is one of the novel and fastest developing eHealth developments. Some studies have been conducted already, but more are needed regarding the use of games in health-care practice (Blakely et al. 2008). New games have also been developed specifically related to mental health, including the video game PlayMancer, which was developed in a European multicentre study (Fernández-Aranda et al. 2012). Biofeedback has been integrated in some of the games and in some mobile apps. One example of these kinds of apps is Ginger.io, which recognizes if a mental health service user is acting in a symptomatic way; when the user does behave in such a way, the app sends text messages to the user and the care provider (http://news.mit.edu/2014/mental-health-monitoring-goes-mobile-0716).

From the standpoint of research, big data is one of the more interesting possibilities for the future. Digital health records and biofeedback data are examples of continuous data gathering possibilities for health-care research. This kind of data provides new possibilities for different research designs but also demands new kinds of thinking from the researchers. The WHO's eHealth report (2016b) noted that only six member states have national policies or recommendations on the use of big data in the health sector, while only four member states have a policy to guide the use of this kind of data by private companies. There is thus clearly a need for future research on eHealth as privacy and safety issues need to be clarified and secured (WHO 2016b).

Conclusion

As this chapter has shown, more research is needed on eHealth to be able to demonstrate the long-term impacts. Reliability issues are important as several programmes, mobile applications and games are now available, but evidence-based information is either lacking or could only be found in a few studies (Donker et al. 2013). We also need more research from various viewpoints; several research reviews mentioned the need for efficacy studies and studies conducted from the viewpoint of staff, organizations and costs, but we also need more studies like Hanley's (2012) that are conducted from the service user-viewpoint. It is also important that users of these kinds of technologies are participating in development processes (Välimäki et al. 2008). Adaptation of eHealth is a challenge for mental health nurses to remain updated and capable of finding the most suitable technological solution with patients and families. With respect to the service system, organizations and educators, this change demands support, training possibilities and a vision for the future. As eHealth is a rapidly growing and developing area in health care, it became clear while writing this article that some references from even a few years ago might already include outdated information, especially when describing the technological solutions. This rapid development also presents challenges for our research designs and publication processes in the future.

Acknowledgements I would like to thank the information specialist Taina Peltonen at the Tampere University of Applied Sciences for her support in the literature searches.

References

Ahtinen A, Mattila E, Välkkynen P, Kaipainen K, Vanhala T, Ermes M, Sairanen E, Myllymäki T, Lappalainen R (2013) Mobile mental wellness training for stress management: feasibility and design implications based on a one-month field study. JMIR Mhealth Uhealth 1(2):e11

Alvarez-Jimenez M, Alcazar-Corcoles MA, González-Blanch C, Bendall S, McGorry PD, Gleeson JF (2014) Online, social media and mobile technologies for psychosis treatment: a systematic review on novel user-led interventions. Schizophr Res 156(1):96–106

Andersson E, Ljótsson B, Hedman E, Kaldo V, Paxling B, Andersson G, Lindefors N, Rück C (2011) Internet-based cognitive behavior therapy for obsessive compulsive disorder: a pilot study. BMC Psychiatry 11:125

Andersson E, Enander J, Andrén P, Hedman E, Ljótsson B, Hursti T, Bergström J, Kaldo V, Lindefors N, Andersson G, Ruck C (2012) Internet-based cognitive behaviour therapy for obsessive-compulsive disorder: a randomized controlled trial. Psychol Med 42:2193–2203

Anttila M, Koivunen M, Välimäki M (2008) Information technology-based standardized patient education in psychiatric inpatient care. J Adv Nurs 64(2):147–156

Anttila M, Välimäki M, Koivunen M, Luukkala T, Kaila M, Pitkänen A, Kontio R (2011) Adoption of an Internet-based patient education programme in psychiatric hospitals. J Psychiatr Ment Health Nurs 18:914–923

Anttila M (2012) Adoption of information technology based patient education in psychiatric nursing. Annales Universitatis Turkuensis, D 1005. Department of Nursing Science. University of Turku, Finland. http://urn.fi/URN:ISBN:978-951-29-4921-2. Accessed 25 Apr 2016

Baker J, Playle J, Nelson P, Lovell K (2010) An evaluation of the impact of the recommendations of the chief nursing officer's (England) review of mental health nursing in mental health trusts and universities in England: findings from stage one, an e-survey. J Clin Nurs 19(17–18):2590–2600

Beentjes TAA, van Gaal BGI, Goossens PJJ, Schoonhoven L (2016) Development of an e-supported illness management and recovery programme for consumers with severe mental illness using intervention mapping, and design of an early cluster randomized controlled trial. BMC Health Serv Res 16:20

Binford Hopf RB, Le Grange D, Moessner M, Bauer S (2013) Internet-based chat support groups for parents in family-based treatment for adolescent eating disorders: a pilot study. Eur Eat Disord Rev 21(3):215–223

Bhandari G, Tiessen B, Snowdon A (2011) Meeting community needs through leadership and innovation: a case of virtual psychiatric emergency department (ED). Behav Inform Technol 30(4):517–523

Black AD, Car J, Pagliari C, Anandan C, Cresswell K, Bokun T, McKinstry B, Procter R, Majeed A, Sheikh A (2011) The impact of eHealth on the quality and safety of health care: a systematic overview. PLoS Med 8(1):e1000387

Blakely G, Skirton H, Cooper S, Allum P, Nelmes P (2008) Educational gaming in the health sciences: systematic review. J Adv Nurs 65(2):259–269

Blaya J, Fraser H, Holt B. (2010) E-health technologies show promise in developing countries. Health Aff (Millwood) 29:244–51. https://doi.org/10.1377/hlthaff.2009.0894

Buckley D, Weisser S (2012) Videoconferencing could reduce the number of mental health patients transferred from outlying facilities to a regional mental health unit. Aust NZ J Public Health 36:478–482. https://doi.org/10.1111/j.1753-6405.2012.00915.x
Callahan A, Inckle C (2012) Cybertherapy or psychobabble? A mixed methods study of online emotional support. Br J Guid Couns 40(3):261–278
Callan JA, Howland RH, Puskar K (2009) Using computers and the Internet for psychiatric nursing intervention. J Psychosoc Nurs 47(1):13–14
Carpenter LM, Hubbard GB (2014) Cyberbullying: implications for the psychiatric nurse practitioner. J Child Adolesc Psychiatr Nurs 27:142–148
Cleary M, Walter G, Matheson S (2008) What is the role of e-technology in mental health services and psychiatric research? J Psychosoc Nurs 46(4):42–28
Della Mea V (2001) What is e-Health (2): The death of telemedicine? J Med Internet Res 3(2):e22
Deslich S, Stec B, Tomblin S, Coustasse A (2013) Telepsychiatry in the 21st century: transforming healthcare with technology. Perspectives in Health Information Management 10 (Summer). http://mds.marshall.edu/cgi/viewcontent.cgi?article=1096andcontext=mgmt_faculty. Accessed 5 Apr 2016
De Weger E, Macinnes D, Enser J, Francis J, Jones FW (2013) Implementing video conferencing in mental health practice. J Psychiatr Ment Health Nurs 20:448–454
Donker T, Petrie K, Proudfoot J, Clarke J, Birch MR, Christensen H (2013) Smartphones for smarter delivery of mental health programs: a systematic review. J Med Internet Res 15(11):e247
Gajecki M, Berman AH, Sinadinovic K, Andersson C, Ljotsson B, Hedman E, Ruck C, Lindefors N (2014) Effects of baseline problematic alcohol and drug use on Internet-based cognitive behavioral therapy outcomes for depression, panic disorder and social anxiety disorder. PLoS One 9(8):e104615
García-Lizana F, Muñoz-Mayorga I (2010) Telemedicine for depression: a systematic review. Perspect Psychiatr Care 46(2):119–126
Guise V, Chambers M, Välimäki M (2012) What can virtual patient simulation offer mental health nursing education? J Psychiatr Ment Health Nurs 19:410–418
Hoffmann WA (2006) Telematic technologies in mental health caring: a web-based psychoeducational program for adolescent suicide survivors. Issues Ment Health Nurs 27:461–474
Horgan A, Sweeney J (2010) Young students' use of the Internet for mental health information and support. J Psychiatr Ment Health Nurs 17:117–123
Elias BL, Fogger SA, McGuiness TM, D'Alessandro KR (2014) Mobile apps for psychiatric nurses. J Psychosoc Nurs 52(4):42–47
Ellington E (2013) Telepsychiatry by APRNs: an answer to the shortage of pediatric providers? Issues Ment Health Nurs 34:719–721
Engqvist I, Ferszt G, Ahlin A, Nilsson K (2011) Women's experience of postpartum psychotic episodes—analyses of narratives from the Internet. Arch Psychiatr Nurs 25(5):376–387
European Commission (2012) eHealth action plan 2012–2020—Innovative healthcare for the 21st century. https://ec.europa.eu/digital-single-market/en/news/ehealth-action-plan-2012-2020-innovative-healthcare-21st-century. Accessed 1 Apr 2016
Eysenbach G (2001) What is e-health? J Med Internet Res 3(2):e20
Fernández-Aranda F, Jiménez-Murcia S, Santamaría JJ, Gunnard K, Soto A, Kalapanidas E, Bults RGA, Davarakis C, Ganchev T, Granero R, Konstantas D, Kostoulas TP, Lam T, Lucas M, Masuet-Aumatell C, Moussa MH, Nielsen J, Penelo E (2012) Video games as a complementary therapy tool in mental disorders: PlayMancer, a European multicenter study. J Ment Health 21(4):364–374
Fetter MS (2009) The internet: backbone of the world wide web. Issues Ment Health Nurs 30:281–282
Finkelstein J, Lapshin O, Wasserman E (2008) Randomized study of different anti-stigma media. Patient Educ Couns 71(2):204–214
Fitzpatrick JJ (2008) Internet addiction: recognition and interventions. Arch Psychiatr Nurs 22(2):59–60
Forsberg E, Georg C, Ziegert K, Fors U (2011) Virtual patients for assessment of clinical reasoning in nursing – a pilot study. Nurse Educ Today 31:757–762
Forsberg E, Ziegert K, Hult H, Fors U (2014) Clinical reasoning in nursing, a think-aloud study using virtual patients – a base for an innovative assessment. Nurse Educ Today 34:538–542

Hanley T (2012) Understanding the online therapeutic alliance through the eyes of adolescent service users. Couns Psychother Res 12(1):35–43

Hedman E, Andersson G, Ljótsson B, Andersson E, Rück C et al (2011) Internet-based cognitive behavior therapy vs. cognitive behavioral group therapy for social anxiety disorder: a randomized controlled non-inferiority trial. PLoS One 6(3):e18001

Kane B, Groth K, Randall D (2012) Medical team meetings: utilising technology to enhance communication, collaboration and decision-making. Behav Inform Technol 30(4):437–442

Kiropoulos LA, Griffiths KM, Blashki G (2011) Effects of a multilingual information website intervention on the levels of depression literacy and depression-related stigma in Greek-born and Italian-born immigrants living in Australia: a randomized controlled trial. J Med Internet Res 13(2):e34

Koivunen M, Välimäki M, Jakobsson T, Pitkänen A (2008) Developing an evidence-based curriculum designed to help psychiatric nurses learn to use computers and Internet. J Prof Nurs 24(5):302–314

Koivunen M, Välimäki M, Pitkänen A, Kuosmanen L (2007) A preliminary usability evaluation of Web-based portal application for patients with schizophrenia. J Psychiatr Ment Health Nurs 14:462–469

Koivunen M, Kontio R, Pitkänen A, Katajisto J, Välimäki M (2013) Occupational stress and implementation of information technology among nurses working on acute psychiatric wards. Perspect Psychiatr Care 49:41–49

Kurki M (2014) Nurses' acceptance of an Internet-based support system in the care of adolescents with depression. Annales Universitatis Turkuensis D 1124. Department of Nursing Science. University of Turku Finland. http://urn.fi/URN:ISBN:978-951-29-5803-0. Accessed 15 Mar 2016

Kurki M, Koivunen M, Anttila M, Hätönen H, Välimäki M (2011) Usefulness of Internet in adolescent mental health outpatient care. J Psychiatr Ment Health Nurs 18:265–273

Lahti M (2014) Evaluation of an e-learning course: coercion practices in psychiatric nursing. Annales Universitatis Turkuensis D 1121. Department of Nursing Science. University of Turku, Finland. http://urn.fi/URN:ISBN:978-951-29-5778-1. Accessed 1 Apr 2016

Lappalainen P, Kaipainen K, Lappalainen R, Hoffrén H, Myllymäki T, Kinnunen ML, Mattila E, Happonen AP, Rusko H, Korhonen I (2013) Feasibility of a personal health technology-based psychological intervention for men with stress and mood problems: randomized controlled pilot trial. JMIR Res Protoc 2(1):e1

Lopez WM, Lustig SL (2015) Telepsychiatry: watching your back while staying in the black. Psychiatr Times 32(8):41–44

Magaud E, Nyman K, Addington J (2013) Cyberbullying in those at clinical high risk for psychosis. Early Interv Psychiatry 7(4):427–430

Maust DT, Mavandadi S, Benson A, Streim JE, DiFilippo S, Snedden T, Weber AL, Oslin DW (2013) Telephone-based care management for older adults initiated on psychotropic medication. Int J Geriatr Psychiatry 28:410–416

Milgrom J, Gemmill A (2014) Feasibility and efficacy of an Internet treatment for postnatal depression utilising a behavioural activation approach. Evid Based Nurs 17(4):102. https://doi.org/10.1136/eb-2013-101636

Morahan-Martin J, Schumacher P (2000) Incidence and correlates of pathological Internet use among college students. Comput Hum Behav 16:13–29

Oates J (2015) Use of Skype in interviews: the impact of the medium in a study of mental health nurses. Nurse Res 22(4):13–17

Oh H, Rizo C, Enkin M, Jadad A (2005) What Is eHealth (3): A Systematic Review of Published Definitions. 7(1):e1. Published online 2005 Feb 24. https://doi.org/10.2196/jmir.7.1.e1

Olthuis JV, Watt MC, Bailey K, Hayden JA, Stewart SH (2015) Therapist-supported Internet cognitive behavioural therapy for anxiety disorders in adults. Cochrane Database Syst Rev 5(3):CD011565. https://doi.org/10.1002/14651858.CD011565

Paing WW, Weller RA, Welsh B, Foster T, Birnkrant JM, Weller EB (2009) Telemedicine in children and adolescents. Curr Psychiatry Rep 11:114–119

Paulson LR, Casile WJ, Jones D (2015) Tech it out: implementing an online peer consultation network for rural mental health professionals. J Rural Ment Health. Advance online publication. https://doi.org/10.1037/rmh0000034. Accessed 25 Apr 2016

Perle JG, Nierenberg B (2013) How psychological telehealth can alleviate society's mental health burden: a literature review. J Technol Hum Serv 31:22–41

Repique R (2007) Computers and information technologies in psychiatric nursing. Perspect Psychiatr Care 43(2):77–83.

Richards D, Richardson T (2012) Computer-based psychological treatments for depression: a systematic review and meta-analysis. Clin Psychol Rev 32(4):329–342

Rigby L, Wilson I, Baker J, Walton T, Price O, Dunne K, Keeley P (2012) The development and evaluation of a 'blended' enquiry-based learning model for mental health nursing students: 'making your experience count'. Nurse Educ Today 32:303–308

Salmoiraghi A, Hussain S (2015) A systematic review of the use of telepsychiatry in acute settings. J Psychiatr Pract 21(5):389–393

Salvador-Carulla L, Cloninger CR, Thornicroft A, Mezzich JE, Geneva Declaration Consultation Group (2013) Background, structure and priorities of the 2013 Geneva declaration on person-centered health research. Int J Pers Cent Med 3(2):109–113

Schwartzman D, Segal R, Drapeau M (2012) Perceptions of virtual reality among therapists who do not apply this technology in clinical practice. Psychol Serv 9(3):310–315

Stickley T, Higgins A, Meade O, Sitvast J, Doyle L, Ellilä H, Jormfeldt H, Keogh B, Lahti M, Skärsäter I, Vuokila-Oikkonen P, Kilkku N (2016) From the rhetoric to the real: a critical review of how the concepts of recovery and social inclusion may inform mental health nurse advanced level curricula—the eMenthe project. Nurse Educ Today 37:155–163

Torous J, Keshavan M (2016) The role of social media in schizophrenia: evaluating risks, benefits, and potential. Curr Opin Psychiatry 29(3):190–195

van den Berg N, Grabe H-J, Baumeister SE, Freyberger HJ, Hoffmann W (2015) A telephone- and text message-based telemedicine concept for patients with mental health disorders: results of a randomized controlled trial. Psychother Psychosom 84:82–89

Välimäki M, Anttila M, Hatonen H, Koivunen M, Jakobsson T, Pitkanen A, Herrala J, Kuosmanen L (2008) Design and development process of patient-centered computer-based support system for patients with schizophrenia spectrum psychosis. Inform Health Soc Care 33(2):113–123

Välimäki M, Athanasopoulou C, Lahti M, Adams CE (2016) Effectiveness of social media interventions for people with schizophrenia: a systematic review and meta-analysis. J Med Internet Res 18(4):e92

Wieland DM (2014) Internet addiction–opportunities for assessment and treatment by psychiatric-mental health nurses. J Psychosoc Nurs 52(7):3–5

Wilshire TW (2012) Telepsychiatry services at a tribally run behavioral health clinic. Psychol Serv 9(3):318–319

Wolrld Health Organisation (2016a) WHO global strategy on people-centred and integrated health services. Interim report. http://apps.who.int/iris/bitstream/10665/155002/1/WHO_HIS_SDS_2015.6_eng.pdf?ua=1&ua=1. Accessed 26 Apr 2016

Wolrld Health Organisation (2016b) From innovation to implementation. eHealth in the European region. www.euro.who.int/en/eHealth. Accessed 26 Apr 2016

18 Public Health and Ecological Approaches: The Example of eHealth for Adolescent Mental Health Support

Anttila Minna, Kurki Marjo, and Välimäki Maritta

18.1 Introduction

There is no health without mental health. The state of mental well-being and health-related behaviour during adolescence has crucial impacts on mental well-being and performance later in adulthood. Still, mental health problems are the most common health disorders among adolescents in Europe (World Health Organization 2012a) and every fifth adolescent has some type of mental health problem (Costello et al. 2011). Research exploring measures that can be taken to prevent so-called mental health disorders among adolescents and on how to promote mental health in this age group, as well as appropriate types of programmes that can be used to do this, can improve adolescent mental health and prevent social exclusion (Wykes et al. 2015).

Recently, information technology (IT) has been developed and used to support mental well-being in everyday life among adolescents (Corrieri et al. 2014). At the same time, there is an increasing debate over whether or not IT is actually usable in the field of mental health. Some have concerns about its usability in vulnerable populations, such as young people (Allison et al. 2012), and others may doubt its possible harms for patients with mental health problems (Kaplan et al. 2011). Despite rapid progress in the development of IT for health promotion and disease treatment, so-called mental disorders remain highly prevalent (Sander et al. 2016). On the other hand, its potential utility has been recognised in the promotion of mental health and

A. Minna, PhD (✉)
Department of Nursing Science, University of Turku, FI-20014 Turku, Finland
e-mail: anna.onnela@ouka.fi

K. Marjo, RN, PhD
Department of Child Psychiatry, University of Turku, Turku, Finland

V. Maritta, RN, PhD
Department of Nursing Science, University of Turku, Turku, Finland

School of Nursing, Hong Kong Polytechnic University, Hung Hom, Hong Kong

© Springer International Publishing Switzerland 2018

J.C. Santos, J.R. Cutcliffe (eds.), *European Psychiatric/Mental Health Nursing in the 21st Century*, Principles of Specialty Nursing,
https://doi.org/10.1007/978-3-319-31772-4_18

prevention of so-called mental disorders (Hayes et al. 2016). In this chapter, our aim is to introduce readers to adolescent mental health and the promotion of such in daily life, using IT. First, we will describe the most common mental health problems reported among adolescents. Second, we will facilitate a deeper understanding of the promotion of mental health in this age group. Third, eHealth as a tool that can be used to support adolescent mental well-being will be introduced.

18.2 Adolescents and So-Called Mental Disorders

It has been estimated that mental health problems affect 10–20% of adolescents worldwide (World Health Organization 2012a). They have a significant impact on adolescents' daily lives, including aspects such as life management, studying, and relationships with friends (Kieling et al. 2011). The most common so-called mental health disorders among adolescence are mood disorders (depression), anxiety, conduct disorders, substance abuse, and eating disorders (Marttunen and Haravuori 2015). Out of all so-called mental health disorders among adolescents, depression most heavily burdens society.

Despite the high prevalence of depression among this age group, health care systems have difficulties in recognising the problem (Thapar et al. 2012). At the same time, early recognition of adolescents' mental health problems proves difficult in many European countries, and the problems often go untreated (Kieling et al. 2011). In Finland, approximately 20–40% of adolescents with mental health problems have received treatment from health care services (Marttunen and Haravuori 2015), and less than 50% of adolescents with depression receive sufficient treatment (Lindberg 2010). Due to functional impairment, lower production levels and early disability pensions, it is reasonable to say that depression is a high-cost mental health problem on many levels (Olesen et al. 2012).

Depression has been found to be associated with adolescents' suicidal ideation and attempts (Nock et al. 2013) and Rahme et al. (2015) found that those students who had attempted suicide were younger, and fewer students had a history of substance abuse but were otherwise not different from nonstudents in their history of other mental problems. There are various reasons why adolescents have difficulties in seeking help for mental health problems. Some reasons include a reluctance to share thoughts about problems face-to-face with adults (Marttunen and Karlsson 2013). Another reason is the fear of stigma. About one-third of adolescents with mental health problems experience stigmatisation by school staff and half of them by friends or family members. Such stigmatisation is related to negative behaviours, such as under-estimation of adolescents' skills, gossiping and avoidance (Haddad and Tylee 2013). Adolescents may perceive a danger of losing friendships if real feelings are shared with friends (Anttila et al. 2015).

18.3 Adolescents and Mental Health Promotion

There are several reasons that investing in the promotion of positive mental health of adolescents can be said to have a great impact on their futures. The Mental Health Action Plan for 2013–2020 highlights actions that improve the mental health of adolescents as well as evidence-based interventions. Adolescents with mental health problems should be provided early intervention support through psychosocial and other non-pharmacological interventions, which are based on evidence-based knowledge and realised in community care (World Health Organization 2013). Promoting adolescents' mental health at an early stage has a significant influence on an individual's future on many levels. It can impact educational achievement, psychosocial well-being, physical health, quality of life and work performance (World Health Organization 2012a). It has been estimated that approximately half of the so-called mental health disorders in adults begin before the age of 14 (World Health Organization 2013). Therefore, mental health promotion and early intervention and prevention programmes are vital in avoiding later adult mental health problems that tend to continue if not treated. These kinds of programmes also improve individual well-being and functionality of people in different life areas (Kieling et al. 2011).

Positive mental health includes the idea that mental health is a resource. It is related to an adolescent's positive sense of well-being, as in their self-esteem, optimism and ability to develop and maintain relationships (Stengård and Appelqvist-Schmidlechner 2010). The concept of resilience is also included in positive mental health. Resilience means that an adolescent is able to cope well with challenges, adversity or stress. Adolescents who are resilient can flexibly deal with problems and find ways to reduce the negative effects of stress. Adolescents can also promote resilience and positive mental health through different strategies, such as practising problem solving, social skills and an optimistic thinking style (Murphey et al. 2013).

Growing evidence shows that the mental health of adolescents could be affected by a variety of environmental factors, including family and school environments, friendships, and social and economic factors. Compared to adults, adolescents are especially at risk of developing mental health disorders. This is due to developmental challenges, such as biological and sexual maturation, the development of individual identity, and the establishment of independence and autonomy when leaving the parental home for the first time (Stengård and Appelqvist-Schmidlechner 2010).

Identifying factors that may be associated with adolescent mental health is important because it is possible for these factors to be supported. Focusing on improving the social skills, problem-solving skills and self-confidence of adolescents can aid in the prevention of mental health problems (World Health Organization 2012a). Low-threshold, easy-access services and early programmes are important for strengthening the life management skills and mental well-being of adolescents (Carral et al. 2009). Schools with multidisciplinary personnel have a key role in identifying both protective and risk factors related to adolescent mental health and in providing low-threshold support and mental health care for their students (Ramos et al. 2013). Schools are natural places where adolescent mental health can be promoted and preventive programmes initiated as early as possible. Strengthening protective factors related to mental health in schools can make important contributions to improving developmental outcomes for adolescents (World Health Organization 2012a). Supportive programmes should therefore be used actively in school environments to help to prevent mental health problems among adolescents and also help them deal with difficulties in their daily lives. Besides health promotion programmes, school health care services have the possibility to be more accessible and less stigmatising for adolescents than mental health specialty care (Pryjmachuk et al. 2011).

18.4 eHealth and Adolescent Mental Well-Being

According to World Health Organization (2012b), eHealth is concerned with improving the flow of information, through electronic means, to support the delivery of health services and the management of health systems. Its potential has been seen as an alternative to conventional programmes in health care at lower costs (Andersen and Svensson 2013). For example in Finland, 89% of 16- to 24-year-olds use the internet several times a day (Official Statistics of Finland 2014), which makes eHealth an appropriate method. Generally, eHealth is seen as the future for various areas of services, especially in mental health support for adolescents (Clarke et al. 2015). It can be used to support a smooth care process and to improve and provide early mental health promotion (Kurki et al. 2011). Recently, eHealth has reshaped the routines of daily life for many people (Hayes et al. 2016). Social media can offer a channel for social networking with bulletin boards, chat rooms, or mailing lists (Griffiths et al. 2009) and offer opportunities for adolescents to be in contact with their friends (Carral et al. 2009).

Within the context of mental health, eHealth can offer support for self-management; one can find problem-solving skills training, help coping with negative thoughts and symptom follow-up (Kaltenhaler et al. 2006). Various eHealth programmes have been developed for adolescents for the prevention of depression, anxiety or stress, and emotional distress (Slone et al. 2012). eHealth programmes (Renton et al. 2014) have also been developed to support adolescent mental well-being at school (Corrieri et al. 2014). Other positive aspects of eHealth have been identified, including its appropriateness for those with no one to discuss their problems with (Mitchell et al. 2014). Adolescents want to be part of a peer group (Anttila et al. 2015), and eHealth provides them with an anonymous way to share experiences (Andersen and Svensson 2013).

eHealth can be effective in preventing or reducing depressive symptoms in adolescents and young adults (Dick and Ferguson 2015; Rice et al. 2014). Participating in eHealth programmes has reduced adolescents' depressed moods (Saulsberry et al. 2013) and symptoms of depression (van der Zanden et al. 2014). Calear and Christensen (2010) found that the programmes that targeted students exhibiting elevated levels of depression were the most effective. In general, adolescents evaluate eHealth as being helpful, and they express appreciation for an opportunity to share their problems with peers (Iloabachie et al. 2011). In addition to networking, adolescents have appreciated the possibility for anonymity and self-tests (Havas et al. 2011). Variety of eHealth programmes such as mobile phones (Slone et al. 2012), website feedback (Välimäki et al. 2012), and video games have found to be potential for health behaviour change (Montanaro et al. 2015).

On the other hand, various risk factors have been raised in relation to the use of eHealth by adolescents. Perhaps one real-life concern is the fear of adolescents becoming problematic internet user. Kilik et al. (2016) found in Turkey that the factors associated with internet addiction were being male, having low academic achievement, and having inadequate social support and communication skills. Other risk factors related to pathological internet use have also been identified, including poor sleeping habits, tobacco use, poor nutrition and physical inactivity (Durkee et al. 2016). Adolescents have also been found to display their alcohol use on social media (Moreno et al. 2016), pro-anorexia websites have been postulated as more harmful than traditional media (Juarez et al. 2012) and variety of problems have been discussed such as a danger that teens may become targets of sexual harassment online, victim of pedophiles and cyber bullying (Meena et al. 2012). Other problems regarding eHealth are a lack of engagement (O'Kearney et al. 2009), which may be due to technical problems, large amounts of reading materials, and the sense that the programme and its appearance are more suitable for an age group other than the user (Stasiak et al. 2014). Further, there is also the danger that adolescents are left to use eHealth with too little supervision (Kaltenhaler et al. 2006).

To ensure that eHealth is user-centred (de Boer et al. 2013) and accessible, adolescent participation in the development of future services should be guaranteed (Nair et al. 2015). This would also improve the quality of health services in adolescent support (National Health Service 2009) which is highly required in order to avoid non-effective programme use (Leigh and Flatt 2015). By developing more user-friendly health services for adolescents (World Health Organization 2012a), it is also possible to offer new communication channels for those who may have difficulties with sharing their views with others (Slone et al. 2012).

18.5 Discussion

In this chapter, our aim was to introduce readers to adolescent mental health and its promotion using IT. Mental health problems in adolescence have a significant impact on adolescents' daily lives (Kieling et al. 2011). These adolescents should be provided early support (World Health Organization 2013) using low-threshold easy-access services and early programmes which strengthen their life management and mental well-being (Carral et al. 2009). eHealth is future method in mental health support for adolescents (Clarke et al. 2015) and it can be used to support smooth care process and to improve and provide early mental health promotion (Kurki et al. 2011). eHealth has the potential to be helpful among adolescents if it is safely carried out and the confidentiality of adolescents has been taken into account (Farnan et al. 2013). This is the case especially at schools (O'Kearney et al. 2009; Calear and Christensen 2010) where a wide range of preventive programmes have already been implemented. It is important that in school settings adolescents can discuss everyday events, personal concerns and problems. This can help them to develop intimate and affectionate relationships that support and protect them (Goldbaum et al. 2003) as well as promote their inclusion into society.

Adolescent support at school using eHealth requires that it is included in curricula as part of health education studies. Support is especially useful when adolescents are finishing their basic education (Marttunen and Haravuori 2015). Therefore, school and student health services could benefit from eHealth, which increases knowledge about adolescent well-being and offers support in the daily lives of these students. This is important because adolescents need to learn mental health skills for later in life. There is an urgent need to find out new ways how adolescents could receive support and share their concerns without fear. Even though adolescents with mental disorders may be withdrawn from social contacts, they still desire for people to take care of them, ensure their well-being, and understand them (Woodgate 2006). It is important to consider how to tackle stigma, try to prevent discrimination and social exclusion, and provide a more humanistic perspective to mental health problems.

References

Allison S, Bauermeister JA, Bull S, Lightfoot M, Mustanski B, Shegog R et al (2012) The intersection of youth, technology, and new media with sexual health: moving the research agenda forward. J Adolesc Health 51(3):207–212

Andersen AJW, Svensson T (2013) Internet-based mental health services in Norway and Sweden: characteristics and consequences. Admin Pol Ment Health 40(2):145–153

Anttila K, Anttila M, Kurki M, Hätönen H, Marttunen M, Välimäki M (2015) Concerns and hopes among adolescents attending adolescent psychiatric outpatient clinics. Child Adolesc Mental Health 20(2):81–88

Calear AL, Christensen H (2010) Review of internet-based prevention and treatment programs for anxiety and depression in children and adolescents. Med J Aust 192(11 Suppl):S12–S14

Carral V, Braddic F, Jane Llopis E, Jenkins R (2009) A snapshot of child and adolescent mental health in Europe: infrastructures, policy and programmes. In: Braddick F et al (eds) Child and adolescent mental health in Europe: Infrastructures, policy and programmes. European Communities, Luxembourg, pp 7–25. http://ec.europa.eu/health/ph_determinants/life_style/mental/docs/camhee_infrastructures.pdf. Accessed 4 May 2016

Clarke AM, Kuosmanen T, Barry MM (2015) A systematic review of online youth mental health promotion and prevention interventions. J Youth Adolesc 44(1):90–113

Corrieri S, Heider D, Conrad I, Blume A, Konig H-H, Riedel-Heller S (2014) School-based prevention programs for depression and anxiety in adolescence: a systematic review. Health Promot Int 29(3):427–441

Costello EJ, Copeland W, Angold A (2011) Trends in psychopathology across the adolescent years: what changes when children become adolescents, and when adolescents become adults? J Child Psychol Psychiatry 52(10):1015–1025

de Boer D, Delnoij D, Rademakers J (2013) The importance of patient-centered care for various patient groups. Patient Educ Couns 90(3):405–410

Dick B, Ferguson BJ (2015) Health for the world's adolescents: a second chance in the second decade. J Adolesc Health 56(1):3–6

Durkee T, Carli V, Floderus B, Wasserman C, Sarchiapone M, Apter A et al (2016) Pathological internet use and risk-behaviors among European adolescents. Int J Environ Res Public Health 13(3):E294

Farnan JM, Snyder SL, Worster BK, Chaudhry HJ, Rhyne JA, Arora VM (2013) Online medical professionalism: patient and public relationships: policy statement from the American College of Physicians and the Federation of State Medical Boards. Ann Intern Med 158(8):620–627

Goldbaum S, Craig W, Pepler D, Connolly J (2003) Developmental trajectories of victimization: identifying risk and protective factors. In: Elias MJ, Zins JE (eds) Bullying, peer harassment, and victimization in the schools: the next generation of prevention. Haworth, New York, pp 139–156

Griffiths KM, Calear AL, Banfield M (2009) Systematic review on Internet Support Groups (ISGs) and depression (1): do ISGs reduce depressive symptoms? J Med Internet Res 11(3):e40

Haddad M, Tylee A (2013) The development and first use of the QUEST measures to evaluate school nurses' knowledge and skills for depression recognition and management. J Sch Health 83(1):36–44

Havas J, de Nooijer J, Crutzen R, Feron F (2011) Adolescents' views about an Internet platform for adolescents with mental health problems. Health Educ 111(3):164–176

Hayes JF, Maughan DL, Grant-Peterkin H (2016) Interconnected or disconnected? Promotion of mental health and prevention of mental disorder in the digital age. Br J Psychiatry 208(3):205–207

Iloabachie C, Wells C, Goodwin B, Baldwin M, Vanderplough-Booth K, Gladstone T et al (2011) Adolescent and parent experiences with a primary care/internet-based depression prevention intervention (CATCH-IT). Gen Hosp Psychiatry 33(6):543–555

Juarez L, Soto E, Pritchard ME (2012) Drive for muscularity and drive for thinness: the impact of pro-anorexia websites. Eat Disord 20(2):99–112

Kaltenhaler E, Brazier J, De Nigris E, Tumur I, Ferriter M, Beverley C et al (2006) Computerised cognitive behaviour therapy for depression and anxiety update: a systematic review and economic evaluation. Health Technol Assess 10(33):1–186

Kaplan K, Salzer MS, Solomon P, Brusilovskiy E, Cousounis P (2011) Internet peer support for individuals with psychiatric disabilities: a randomized controlled trial. Soc Sci Med 72(1):54–62

Kieling C, Baker-Henningham H, Belfer M, Conti G, Ertem I, Omigbodun O et al (2011) Child and adolescent mental health worldwide: evidence for action. Lancet 378(9801):1515–1525

Kilik M, Avci D, Uzuncakmak T (2016) Internet addiction in high school students in Turkey and multivariate analyses of the underlying factors. J Addict Nurs 27(1):39–46

Kurki M, Koivunen M, Anttila M, Hätönen H, Välimäki M (2011) Usefulness of internet in adolescent mental health outpatient care. J Psychiatr Ment Health Nurs 18(3):265–273

Leigh S, Flatt S (2015) App-based psychological interventions: friend or foe? Evid Based Ment Health 18(4):97–99

Lindberg N (2010) Treatment of adolescents' depression. In: Kaivosoja M, Karlsson L, Ehrling L, Melartin T, Pylkkänen K, Lounamaa R et al (eds) Well-being and malaise among adolescents. Consensus meeting in Espoo. Duodecim, Academy of Finland, Vammala, pp 104–109

Marttunen M, Haravuori H (2015) Situation of the adolescents – why are adolescents becoming marginalized or are they? In: Partanen A, Moring J, Bergman V, Karjalainen J, Kesänen M, Markkula J et al (eds) Plan for mental health and substance abuse work 2009–2015. How to proceed from here? National Institute for Health and Welfare (THL). Working paper 20/2015, Tampere, Suomen Yliopistopaino Oy. pp 83–102. ISBN:978-952-302-538-7. http://www.urn.fi. Accessed 4 May 2016

Marttunen M, Karlsson L (2013) Depression symptoms and depression. In: Marttunen M, Huurre T, Sandström T, Viialainen R (eds) Mental health disorders among adolescents. A guide for adults working with adolescents. National Institute for Health and Welfare. Guide 25. Tampere, Suomen Yliopistopaino Oy. pp 41–58. ISBN:978-952-245-647-2. http://www.urn.fi. Accessed 4 May 2016

Meena PS, Mittal PK, Solanki RK (2012) Problematic use of social networking sites among urban school going teenagers. Ind Psychiatry J 21(2):94–97

Mitchell KJ, Ybarra ML, Korchmaros JD, Kosciw JG (2014) Accessing sexual health information online: use, motivations and consequences for youth with different sexual orientations. Health Educ Res 29(1):147–157

Montanaro E, Fiellin LE, Fakhouri T, Kyriakides TC, Duncan LR (2015) Using videogame apps to assess gains in adolescents' substance use knowledge: new opportunities for evaluating intervention exposure and content mastery. J Med Internet Res 17(10):e245

Moreno MA, Arseniev-Koehler A, Litt D, Christakis D (2016) Evaluating college students' displayed alcohol references on Facebook and Twitter. J Adolesc Health 58(5):527–532

Murphey D, Barry MC, Vaughn BV (2013) Adolescent health highlight: positive mental health-resilience. Child Trends, Publication 2013-3. http://www.childtrends.org/?publications=positive-mental-health-resilience. Accessed 4 May 2016

Nair M, Baltag V, Bose K, Boschi-Pinto C, Lambrechts T, Mathai M (2015) Improving the quality of health care services for adolescents, globally: a standards-driven approach. J Adolesc Health 57(3):288–298

National Health Service (2009) Understanding what matters: a guide to using patient feedback to transform services. Department of Health, London. http://webarchive.nationalarchives.gov.uk/20130107105354/http://www.dh.gov.uk/prod_consum_dh/groups/dh_digitalassets/documents/digitalasset/dh_099779.pdf. Accessed 4 May 2016

Nock MK, Green JG, Hwang I, McLaughlin KA, Sampson NA, Zaslavsky AM et al (2013) Prevalence, correlates, and treatment of lifetime suicidal behavior among adolescents: results from the National Comorbidity Survey Replication Adolescent Supplement. JAMA Psychiat 70(3):300–310

O'Kearney R, Kang K, Christensen H, Griffiths K (2009) A controlled trial of a school-based internet program for reducing depressive symptoms in adolescent girls. Depress Anxiety 26(1):65–72

Official Statistics of Finland (2014) Use of information and communications technology by individuals. Statistics Finland, Helsinki. http://www.stat.fi/til/sutivi/index_en.html. Accessed 4 May 2016

Olesen J, Gustavsson A, Svensson M, Wittchen H, Jönsson B (2012) The economic cost of brain disorders in Europe. Eur J Neurol 19(1):155–162

Pryjmachuk S, Graham T, Haddad M, Tylee A (2011) School nurses' perspectives on managing mental health problems in children and young people. J Clin Nurs 21(5-6):850–859

Rahme E, Low NC, Lamarre S, Turecki G, Bonin JP, Daneau D et al (2015) Attempted suicide among students and young adults in Montreal, Quebec, Canada: a retrospective cross-sectional study of hospitalized and nonhospitalized suicide attempts based on chart review. Prim Care Companion CNS Disord 17(5):10.4088/PCC.15m01806. Published online 2015 Oct 29. doi: 10.4088/PCC.15m01806

Ramos MM, Greenberg C, Sapien R, Bauer-Creegan J, Hine B, Geary C (2013) Behavioral health emergencies managed by school nurses working with adolescents. J Sch Health 83(10):712–717

Renton T, Tang H, Ennis N, Cusimano MD, Bhalerao S, Schweizer TA et al (2014) Web-based intervention programs for depression: a scoping review and evaluation. J Med Internet Res 16(9):50–71

Rice SM, Goodall J, Hetrick SE, Parker AG, Gilbertson T, Amminger GP et al (2014) Online and social networking interventions for the treatment of depression in young people: a systematic review. J Med Internet Res 16(9):e206

Sander L, Rausch L, Baumeister H (2016) Effectiveness of Internet- and mobile-based psychological interventions for the prevention of mental disorders: a systematic review and meta-analysis protocol. Syst Rev 16(5):30

Saulsberry A, Marko-Holguin M, Blomeke K, Hinkle C, Fogel J, Gladstone T et al (2013) Randomized clinical trial of a primary care internet-based intervention to prevent adolescent depression: one-year outcomes. J Can Acad Child Adolesc Psychiatry 22(2):106–117

Slone NC, Reese RJ, McClellan MJ (2012) Telepsychology outcome research with children and adolescents: a review of the literature. Psychol Serv 9(3):271–292

Stasiak K, Hatcher S, Frampton C, Merry SN (2014) A pilot double blind randomized placebo controlled trial of a prototype computer-based cognitive behavioural therapy program for adolescents with symptoms of depression. Behav Cogn Psychother 42(4):385–401

Stengård E, Appelqvist-Schmidlechner K (2010) Mental health promotion in young people – an investment for the future. World Health Organization. http://www.euro.who.int/_data/assets/pdf_file/0013/121135/E94270.pdf. Accessed 4 May 2016

Thapar A, Collishaw S, Pine DS, Thapar AK (2012) Depression in adolescence. Lancet 379(9820):1056–1067

Välimäki M, Kurki M, Hätönen H, Koivunen M, Selander M, Saarijärvi S et al (2012) Developing an internet-based support system for adolescents with depression. JMIR Res Protoc 1(2):e22

van der Zanden R, Galindo-Garre F, Curie K, Kramer J, Cuijpers P (2014) Online cognitive-based intervention for depression: Exploring possible circularity in mechanisms of change. Psychol Med 44(6):1159–1170

Woodgate RL (2006) Living in the shadow of fear: adolescents' lived experience of depression. J Adv Nurs 56(3):261–269

World Health Organization (2012a) Adolescent mental health: mapping actions of nongovernmental organizations and other. http://whqlibdoc.who.int/publications/2012/9789241503648_eng.pdf?ua=1. Accessed 4 May 2016

World Health Organization (2012b) National eHealth strategy toolkit. http://apps.who.int/iris/bitstream/10665/75211/1/9789241548465_eng.pdf?ua=1. Accessed 4 May 2016

World Health Organization (2013) Mental health action plan 2013–2020. http://apps.who.int/iris/bitstream/10665/89966/1/9789241506021_eng.pdf. Accessed 4 May 2016

Wykes T, Haro JM, Belli SM, Obradors-Tarragó C, Arango C, Ayuso-Mateos JL et al (2015) Mental health research priorities for Europe. Lancet Psychiatry 2(11):1036–1042

Part III

Psychiatric/Mental Health Nursing Competencies and Ways of Working

Forming and Maintaining Interpersonal Relationships

19

Manuel José Lopes

19.1 Introduction

From the standpoint of philosophical anthropology, we can say that every human being is constituted of and develops within a relational context (Gevaert 2003). Thus, the relationship with the other is defined as an encounter that materialises in an interpersonal space, where the intersubjectivity constituted by the I-you predominates (Levinas 2011). Accordingly, the relationship with the other assumes a central role in all stages of development. Against this background, if we understand 'disease' and, moreover, mental health problems not only as a pathological process but also as life experiences that are experienced, manifest and expressed throughout the body, and simultaneously as a threat to the integrity of the self, it will then be easy to understand that the relationship takes on added importance. These are the basic assumptions of this text: the whole relationship has therapeutic potential; the relationship is not limited to verbal interaction but is rather a process of sharing that involves the whole person and all forms of communication. In this context, nurses, provided that they are aware of this potential, are in an ideal position to create and develop meaningful interpersonal relationships. Finally, and because nursing is a practical activity or a practical human science (Kim 2010; Meleis 2012; Strasser 1985), it develops from the knowledge generated in the practice itself (Bishop and Scudder 1991; Carper 1978).

M.J. Lopes
São João de Deus School of Nursing, University of Évora, Évora, Portugal
e-mail: mjl@uevora.pt

© Springer International Publishing Switzerland 2018

J.C. Santos, J.R. Cutcliffe (eds.), *European Psychiatric/Mental Health Nursing in the 21st Century*, Principles of Specialty Nursing,
https://doi.org/10.1007/978-3-319-31772-4_19

19.2 The Nurse-Patient Relationship: Some Assumptions

The nurse-patient relationship has, for decades, been considered by many authors as the core of psychiatric/mental health nursing care (Browne et al. 2012; Orlando 1961; Peplau 1990). In fact, it is not possible to provide any nursing care except in the context of a relationship. Arguably, the relationship can be manifest in two forms: the first is the relationship as the context of all care and the second is the relationship as a separate strategy for therapeutic intervention.

In the first case, the relationship is the 'setting' and/or context in which care is provided. This 'setting' is fundamental to the process of care, and its proper use requires mastery of a set of communication techniques and manipulation of the environment to better achieve the therapeutic goals. As such, it requires learning, but it requires, above all, awareness of its importance at all times, and consequently deliberate and judicious use, depending on the therapeutic objectives to be achieved, whenever a relationship of care is established (Lopes 2005, 2006).

In the second case, the relationship is conceptualised as an autonomous intervention strategy, i.e. a *therapeutic relationship*. Against this background, and as a result of the clinical judgement of the nurse, this means that, given the state of health of the person, the relationship is a therapeutic instrument in and of itself. The use of the therapeutic relationship requires that the nurse has a high level of personal and professional development, since such an activity necessitates a high degree of self-awareness and the use of several highly distinctive interpersonal techniques (Lopes 2005, 2006).

While distinctive from one another, both forms of relationship appear to share some fundamental characteristics, among which we highlight the following:

They are dimensions of nursing care and are common to all care given. As mentioned above, the relationship cannot be reduced to a verbal interaction. The relationship is an act of sharing that involves the whole body and all forms of communication (Meleis 2012; Phaneuf 2002; Watson 1985).

They are intentional, i.e. they result from the clinical judgement of the nurse who, faced with a particular health condition, decides to use certain therapeutic tools (Lopes 2006; Meleis 2012; Phaneuf 2002; Watson 2002).

Both are procedural (i.e. *evolve as a process*); however, as we'll see, the therapeutic relationship may become autonomous as a process. In both cases, the diagnostic evaluation and therapeutic intervention occur simultaneously (there isn't a time for evaluation followed by a time for intervention). Thus, diagnostic evaluation and therapeutic intervention change systematically according to the new data collected and incorporated, over time, by the nurse. This procedure gives the process a gradualist, incremental and spiral structure (Carnevali and Thomas 1993; Doenges and Moorhouse 2003; Lopes 2006).

19.3 Therapeutic Relationship: The Process

19.3.1 Basic Components of the Interpersonal Relationship

According to the College of Nurses of Ontario (CNO 2013), there are five basic components in a therapeutic relationship process:

- Trust
- Respect
- Professional intimacy
- Empathy
- Power

To these we may add:

- Caring and the emotional connection or therapeutic alliance

Trust is a central component of the therapeutic relationship and we may define it as:

> The optimistic acceptance of the situation of vulnerability, after careful evaluation, in which the person who trusts believes that the caregiver regards his or her best interests as paramount (Bell and Duffy 2009).

To build trust, nurses must be able to demonstrate clinical competence, promote goodwill in relation to the patient and understand the inherent risks, such as those arising from the imbalance of power in the nurse-patient relationship, which puts the patient in a vulnerable position (Bell and Duffy 2009). Trust needs to be built proactively and gradually and be systematically fed. If trust is broken, it cannot be easily restored (CNO 2013).

Respect: This can be defined as the recognition of the dignity inherent to the value and uniqueness of each individual, regardless of socioeconomic status, personal attributes and the nature of the health problem (CNO 2013). At the same time, it is an ethical duty of nurses at various levels, as the Code of Ethics dictates (Portugal 2009). To treat someone with respect is to treat them as individuals and fellow human beings; it is to avoid labelling people because of their diagnosis or their association with any other group.

Professional intimacy: This is inherent to the type of care and services that the nurses provide and is related to some types of care and the proximity that the patient creates. Psychological, spiritual and social elements may also be involved. Access to the patient's personal information also contributes towards professional intimacy (CNO 2013). This is an increasingly important concept in nursing and is characteristic of the nurse-patient relationship. It is perceived as intrinsic to the therapeutic potential of nursing (Williams 2001). There are two aspects of the nurse-patient relationship that are found in most interactions and which have profound implications for nurses as professionals and as people (Green 2013). The first is *clinical intimacy* which involves nurses touching, massaging, soothing, cleaning, dressing and interacting physically. The other is the *existential crisis*, the possibility of loss, suffering and death that lurks on the horizon in most, if not all, encounters in healthcare (Green 2013).

Empathy: This can be defined as the ability to sensitively understand the emotional world of the other and demonstrate this understanding through communication (Cuff et al. 2014; Goldstein and Michaels 1985). In nursing, empathy includes appropriate emotional distance to ensure objectivity and an appropriate professional response (CNO 2013).

Power: The nurse-patient relationship is an inherently unequal power relationship. Whether or not the nurse is aware of it, he or she has greater power than the patient, because he or she has greater authority and influence within the healthcare system, expertise and access to privileged information (Cutcliffe and Happell 2009). The proper use of power, i.e. according to the interests of the patient, allows the creation of a partnership that meets the patient's needs. The misuse of power is considered abuse.

Caring: This is defined as the moral ideal of nursing, in which the relationship between the totality of the nurse and the totality of the patient protects their vulnerability and preserves humanity and dignity (Watson 1999). The purpose of caring can be reached in the interpersonal relationship through the reciprocity of nonromantic love based on true knowledge of the person, trust and respect reflected in an acceptance and genuine appreciation of the other person (Thomas et al. 2005).

Emotional connection or *therapeutic alliance*: This has been referred to as more important for achieving results than the technique that the therapist uses. Connection in the nurse-patient relationship is the process of recognising and meeting the needs of the spirit (Miner-Williams 2007) and is cultivated by validating the feelings of the patient, asking questions about their main concerns, defining cooperation objectives, pointing out strengths and communicating empathy.

19.4 Structure and Phases of the Therapeutic Relationship

Having identified the basic components of the therapeutic relationship, we will now begin to describe each of the different phases. Therefore, and as we are dealing with a process, the first questions that arise are: How do we handle the 'rapprochement' between the nurse and the patient? How and when does the relationship start? In response to these questions, the relationship begins at the very moment that the person is introduced to us (Lopes 2006) and does not require the person to be present. Therefore, Sapeta (2010) refers to it as 'pre-presence'. In other words, we begin to relate to a person from the moment someone mentions their existence. It is important to be aware of this, because this presentation induces a representation that conditions our first contact with the person (Sapeta 2010).

At the time of the first meeting, the factors favouring rapprochement diverge (Lopes 2006). Nurses are driven by a proactive clinical attitude or by an ethical imperative. They may also be driven by less rational criteria such as similar personal situations and emotional sensitivity. Both involve implicit risks and so require a high degree of self-awareness in order to avoid inappropriate relationships (Lopes 2006). Patients value sympathy, kindness, joy and the personal care demonstrated by nurses (Gomes 2012; Lopes 2006; Oliveira 2011; Sapeta 2010). Interestingly, the concept of *symbiotic kindness* was identified through research conducted with nurses providing end-of-life care (Li 2004).

Upon first meeting, direct diagnostic evaluation also begins as an essential pillar of the care process. In contexts we studied (Lopes 2006), this evaluation begins with the person being asked to give an account through the following three aspects:

- What the patient knows
- What worries the patient
- The patient's strategies/capabilities

These aspects offer us access to the 'history' as the person understands it, providing us with access to three highly relevant levels of information. Realising what the patient knows, we have access to representational dimensions of the disease, which affect the attitudes of the person to them and to the treatments. Understanding what worries the patient allows us to prioritise directing our care towards their concerns, thus giving meaning to the prospect of the co-construction of care (Dunston et al. 2009; McLaughlin 2004). Knowing the patient's strategies and capabilities allows us to focus on that which the person is still able to do and also to assess their adaptability for dealing with the clinical situation.

The next step consists of a comprehensive evaluation, which should include aspects such as:

- Personal and family history
- Appearance and attitude
- Expression of mimicry and motor skills
- Contact and language
- State of consciousness (reflectivity, clarity and orientation)
- Self-consciousness
- Awareness of the body
- Impulses and will
- Mood
- Feelings
- Emotions
- Way of thinking
- Content of thought
- Representation and memory
- Sense-perception
- Physical observation:
  - Functional capacity
  - Physiological data
  - Integrity of the skin and mucous membranes
  - Bowel control

This evaluation aims to understand the impact of changes on self-care, taking into account the family and community relationships of the person (see Fig. 19.1) and contributes to the understanding of transition processes, specifically in terms of self-consciousness, transition conditions and response patterns (Meleis 2010).

As already stated above, the diagnostic evaluation is an ongoing process which evolves towards a greater understanding of the person's situation but also the changes induced by the care given to date (Frias 2010; Lopes 2006; Oliveira 2011; Sapeta 2010).

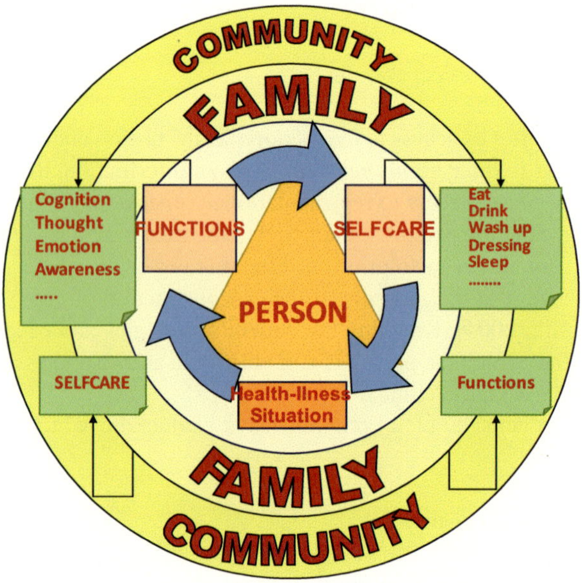

Fig. 19.1 Relationship between the various dimensions in the diagnostic evaluation process

As auxiliary instruments in the diagnostic evaluation process and also as a way to objectify and define forms of measurement, nurses may use various evaluation tools (e.g. scales measuring anxiety, depression, mental state, suicide risk assessment), which can also produce information which may be used later to assess the effectiveness of the interventions. The process of initial diagnostic evaluation necessarily results in a set of diagnostic statements, which should be formulated according to the one of the languages classified. Diagnostic judgements should be validated with the patient. In addition to implementing the co-construction of care and consequently its co-production (Dunston et al. 2009; McLaughlin 2004), this validation has a therapeutic dimension of itself in that it helps in the process of raising awareness and stating problems, a crucial step for beginning to solve them; it contributes to the consolidation of trust and constitutes an unequivocal demonstration of mutual respect of enormous therapeutic potential. It is also clear from what we have just said that the division between the diagnostic phase and the therapeutic intervention phase is merely didactic.

We come now to the so-called therapeutic intervention process. During this phase, it is necessary to identify the structure of this process but also which instruments of intervention are available to the nurse. On the basis of the intervention framework and according to the diagnostic evaluation referred to above and taking into account the capabilities and resources of the person, two levels of intervention are defined (Wheeler 2011). The first and most pressing objective is *stabilisation* and includes more active intervention strategies. People who need this level of intervention usually have had their most basic needs affected, such as the need for food and safety, and feel that they do not have the external and internal resources to respond to the situation. They are people who are facing a severe crisis and who, as such, require the adoption of the case management method and/or hospitalisation.

Although there is no strict connection between the levels of development of an intervention and the techniques to be used, there are recommendations that certain techniques should be preferred at certain stages. At this level, stress management techniques (Marin et al. 2011), relaxation techniques and affective regulation techniques may be useful, among others. We attach a special emphasis to *anxiety management* techniques. Anxiety is a very common reaction and cuts across many health/illness-related and/or life situations, thus taking on a crucial role in any intervention strategy. *Anxiety management* thus becomes very important in order for learning and change to occur. Interestingly, Peplau (1990) considered it a cornerstone of his model and postulated that good interpersonal relationships reduce anxiety, a conclusion that has been supported by recent neurobiological research (Dobbs 2008).

In a study conducted with nurses at a day hospital for patients undergoing a process of cancer chemotherapy, we identified two intervention strategies used by nurses: the management of feelings and information management (Lopes 2006) (see Fig. 19.2) . Although different, they interpenetrate and are mutually reinforcing.

Finally, the use of role supplementation also seems to have potential as an intervention strategy, and this may be defined as the process of raising a patient's awareness to the behaviours, feelings, sensations and goals involved in a certain role (Meleis 2010) in order to thus start the process of change.

These strategies already create a bridge to the level of intervention referred to as *processing* (Wheeler 2011). This is because the goal of this level is to integrate all

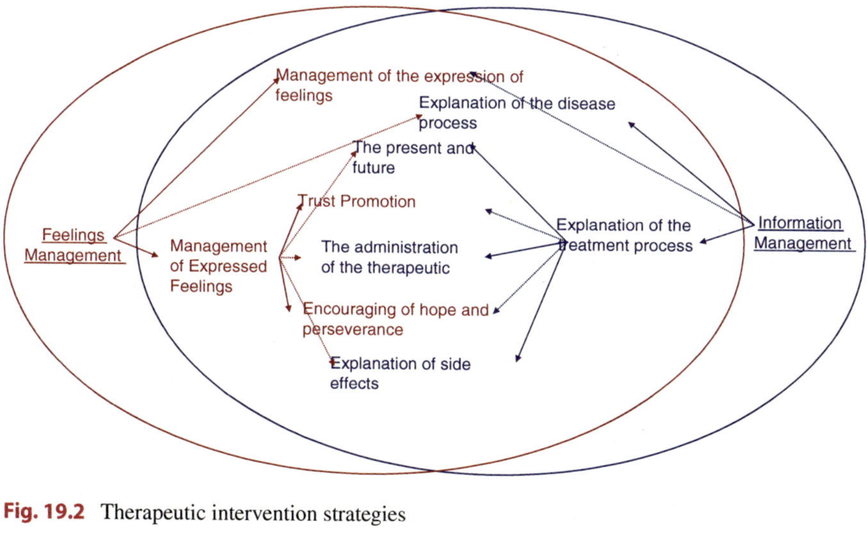

Fig. 19.2 Therapeutic intervention strategies

aspects of fragmented memory in consciousness, allowing access to all dimensions of memory: emotion, sensations, cognitions, beliefs and images associated with the trauma (Shapiro 2001). To achieve these goals, there is a diverse set of intervention techniques, the use of which is at all times dependent on two factors: the characteristics of the patient's clinical situation and the nurse's skills in their use. Among these we highlight cognitive processing therapy, systematic desensitisation, exposure therapy and hypnosis, among others (Wheeler 2011).

With the same objective, we also mention the possibility of using a set of communication techniques (e.g. informing, reassuring, suggesting, clarifying, reflecting, interpreting), which may be understood on a continuum between the two levels of intervention (i.e. stabilisation and processing) and/or as support for expression. At any of the levels, and even during the diagnostic evaluation phase, the use is made of an extremely important therapeutic strategy called the 'narrative strategy'. It consists of making the person narrate to himself or herself their experiences putting words and feelings into the experience as a way to strengthen their ability to regulate their emotions. According to several authors (Pert et al. 1998; Siegel 2006), the identification and expression of feelings has a positive effect on health and serves a regulatory function for the developing brain.

With some similarities to the 'narrative strategy', Meleis (2010) proposes a therapeutic intervention strategy called *debriefing*, which consists of recollecting an experience, thus providing an opportunity to review the difficulties, but also capacities, and to re-examine the reactions and emotions experienced during the same. The objectives of the *debriefing* during critical experiences include helping people to understand, analyse and summarise what they thought, felt and did in a particular situation in order to improve future performance in similar situations.

If we think back to *role supplementation* as a therapeutic intervention strategy, this level will provide the proper context to work on the dimensions that have to do with modelling and role training, i.e. with the development of new skills to deal with the difficulties (Meleis 2010). Finally, we refer to various other therapeutic intervention strategies used by nurses that may be used here. All of them may be incorporated into the group of so-called 'nursing therapeutics', which may be described as interventions performed by nurses in order to modify life processes, living standards, functional health patterns and responses and thus change the course of a person's health/disease. Among these we may highlight the following:

Touch: This may be defined as multidimensional or a gestalt involving voice, posture, affection, intention and meaning within a context, as well as tactile contact (Estabrooks and Morse 1992). In order to be therapeutic, intentionality is assumed and, as such, the creation of the conditions to achieve the therapeutic goals.

Comfort: Although there is no consensus regarding its definition, given that it may be understood as an indicator of outcomes of nursing interventions, as a human need or as a process (Malinowski and Stamler 2002), we may generally define it as the state that nurses desire for their patients. Nevertheless, there is reasonable research regarding this concept as a therapeutic intervention strategy, of which I highlight the work of Oliveira (Oliveira and Lopes 2010; Oliveira 2011).

19.5 Evaluating the Therapeutic Relationship

The use of the term 'evaluating' (i.e. current tense) is intentional because, in a process of this nature, the evaluation has to be undertaken systematically. This will contribute to the achievement of the therapeutic objectives because, as a rule, the process of therapeutic relationship can be lengthy and may require gradual changes in attitudes and behaviours. This can lead to patients becoming fatigued and losing faith, and it is therefore necessary for the person to be systematically made aware of the changes and gains through continuous assessment.

This is also a way to consolidate these changes, raising awareness of them and developing feelings of self-confidence and confidence in the relationship. These criteria generally correspond to the transition process progress indicators, as proposed by Meleis (2010). Additionally, we understand that a considerable effort is required to provide an assessment of the process of therapeutic relationship based on measurable indicators. It is therefore prudent to remember that which we mentioned above, i.e. the importance of using well-validated instruments in the diagnostic evaluation process, which may subsequently be used again to assess progress in these variables.

Conclusion

In conclusion, we can say that forming and maintaining interpersonal relationships in P/MH nursing is a crucial therapeutic intervention and is, also, a fundamental nursing competency. But it's important to understand that therapeutic intervention demands a systematic approach from the P/MH nurses involved and a professional, helping, therapeutic attitude because the nurses are the 'therapeutic instrument' themselves. So, training the therapeutic relationship in nursing (pre- or post-graduate) should not only promote professional competence but also personal development through critical thinking. Finally, we need to promote an alliance between academic and clinical nurses to increase the research about interpersonal relationship as a way to better understand it as a fundamental nursing concept. Essentially we need to demonstrate the contributions of the interpersonal relationship to the health gains of our patients. To do this, we need to systematically measure nursing-sensitive outcomes indicators.

References

Bell L, Duffy A (2009) A concept analysis of nurse–patient trust. Br J Nurs 18(1):46–51

Bishop AH, Scudder JR (1991) Nursing the practice of caring. National League for Nursing, New York

Browne G, Cashin A, Graham I (2012) The therapeutic relationship and mental health nursing: it is time to articulate what we do! J Psychiatr Ment Health Nurs 19(9):839–843. doi:10.1111/j.1365-2850.2012.01944.x

Carnevali D, Thomas M (1993) Diagnostic reasoning and treatment decision making in nursing. Lippincott, Philadelphia

Carper BA (1978) Fundamental patterns of knowing in nursing. Adv Nurs Sci 1(13)
CNO (2013) Therapeutic nurse-client relationship, Revised 2006
Cuff B, Brown S, Taylor L, Howat D (2014) Empathy: a review of the concept. Emot Rev 8(2):144–153
Cutcliffe J, Happell B (2009) Psychiatry, mental health nurses, and invisible power: Exploring a perturbed relationship within contemporary mental health care. Int J Ment Health Nu 18(2):116–125. http://doi.org/10.1111/j.1447-0349.2008.00591.x
Dobbs D (2008) A revealing reflection. Sci Am Mind:22–27
Doenges M, Moorhouse M (2003) Application of nursing process and nursing diagnosis. Philadelphia, F.A. Davis
Dunston R, Lee A, Boud D, Brodie P, Chiarella M (2009) Co-production and health system reform - from re-imagining to re-making. Aust J Public Adm 68(1):39–52. doi:10.1111/j.1467-8500.2008.00608.x
Estabrooks CA, Morse JM (1992) Toward a theory of touch: the touching process and acquiring style. J Adv Nurs 17(4):448–456
Frias C (2010) O processo de construção de cuidados enfermeiro/pessoa em fim de vida: encontro de corpos. Universidade de Lisboa, Lisboa. Retrieved from http://hdl.handle.net/10451/3746
Gevaert J (2003) El Problema del Hombre: Introducción a la Antropología Filosófica. Ediciones Sigueme, Salamanca
Goldstein AP, Michaels GY (1985) Empathy: development, training, and consequences. Lawrence Erlbaum Associates, New Jersey
Gomes L (2012) A presença como cuidado de enfermagem: estudo do processo de desenvolvimento da presença em contexto psiquiátrico. Universidade de Lisboa, Lisboa
Green C (2013) Philosophic reflections on the meaning of touch in nurse–patient interactions. Nurs Philos 14:242–253
Kim HS (2010) The nature of theoretical thinking in nursing. AORN journal (Vol. 73). New York, Springer Publishing Company
Levinas E (2011) Totalidade e infinito. Edições, Lisboa, p 79
Li S (2004) “Symbiotic niceness”: constructing a therapeutic relationship in psychosocial palliative care. Soc Sci Med 58(12):2571–2583. doi:10.1016/j.socscimed.2003.09.006
Lopes MJ (2005) Os clientes e os enfermeiros: construção de uma relação. Rev Esc Enferm U S P 39(2):220–228. doi:10.1590/S0080-62342005000200013
Lopes MJ (2006) A relação enfermeiro-doente como intervenção terapêutica. Proposta de uma teoria de médio alcance. Formasau, Coimbra
Malinowski A, Stamler L (2002) Comfort: exploration of the concept in nursing. J Adv Nurs 39(6):599–606. doi:10.1046/j.1365-2648.2002.02329.x
Marin M-F, Lord C, Andrews J, Juster R-P, Sindi S, Arsenault-Lapierre G, Fiocco AJ, Lupien SJ (2011) Chronic stress, cognitive functioning, and mental health. Neurobiol Learn Mem 96
McLaughlin H (2004) Partnerships: panacea or pretence? J Interprof Care 18(2):103–113. doi:10.1080/13561820410001686873
Meleis AI (2010) Transitions theory. Springer Pub, New York
Meleis AI (2012) Theorical nursing. Development and progress, 5th edn. Wolters Kluwer/Lippincott Williams & Wilkins, Philadelphia
Miner-Williams D (2007) Connectedness in the nurse-patient relationship: a grounded theory study. Issues Ment Health Nurs 28:1215–1234. doi:10.1080/01612840701651462
Oliveira C, Lopes M (2010) Construir Laços de Confiança e Promover o Conforto. Pensar Enfermagem 14(1):67–74
Oliveira C (2011) O cuidado confortador da pessoa idosa hospitalizada: individualizar a intervenção conciliando tenções. Universidade de Lisboa, Lisboa. Retrieved from http://hdl.handle.net/10451/3815
Orlando I (1961) The dynamics nurse-patient relationship. G. P. Putnam’s Sons, New York
Peplau HE (1990) Relaciones interpersonales en enfermería. Salvat Editores, Barcelona
Pert C, Dreher H, Ruff M (1998) The psychosomatic network: foundations of mind-body medicine. Altern Ther 4(4):30–41

Phaneuf M (2002) Comunicação, entrevista, relação de ajuda e validação. Lusociência, Lisboa
Portugal (2009) Procede à primeira alteração ao Estatuto da Ordem dos Enfermeiros, aprovado pelo Decreto -Lei n.º 104/98, de 21 de Abril, Pub. L. No. N.º 180 — 16 de Setembro de 2009. Portugal: Diário da República, 1.ª série
Sapeta P (2010) Cuidar em fim de vida: o processo de interacção enfermeiro-doente. Universidade de Lisboa, Lisboa. Retrieved from http://hdl.handle.net/10451/2043
Shapiro F (2001) Eye movement desensitization and reprocessing (EMDR). Basic Books, New York
Siegel D (2006) An interpersonal neurobiology approach to psychotherapy: awareness, mirror neurons, and neural plasticity in the development of well-being. Psychiatr Ann 36(4):248–256
Strasser S (1985) Understanding and explanation: basic ideas concerning the humanity of the human sciences. Duquesne University Press, Pittsburgh
Thomas JD, Finch LP, Schoenhofer SO, Green A (2005) The caring relationships created by nurse practitioners and the ones nursed: implications for practice. Topics Adv Pract Nurs J 4(4):6
Watson J (1985) Nursing: the philosophy and science of caring. Colorado Associated University Press, Buolder
Watson J (1999) Enfermagem: ciência humana e cuidar - uma teoria de Enfermagem. Lusociência, Loures
Watson J (2002) Intentionality and caring-healing consciousness. Holist Nurs Pract 16(4):12–19
Wheeler K (2011) A relationship-based model for psychiatric nursing practice. Perspect Psychiatr Care 47:151–159. doi:10.1111/j.1744-6163.2010.00285.x
Williams A (2001) A literature review on the concept of intimacy in nursing. J Adv Nurs 33(5):660–667

Psychiatric/Mental Health Nursing Core Competencies: Communication Skills

20

Cândida Loureiro, Helena Quaresma, and José Carlos Santos

20.1 Introduction

As a profession (or discipline) and science, psychiatric/mental health (P/MH) nursing draws on a wide set of knowledge, including nursing models and theories which, in addition to providing theoretical guidance, help systemize practice. Hildegard Peplau's Theory of Interpersonal Relations has became the most significant and widely adapted nursing model for P/MH nurses. Peplau is considered to be the "mother of psychiatric nursing." However, the application of her theory/model extends beyond the specialty area of mental health care. Her major contribution to nursing science was the interpersonal relations theory, which was influenced by Harry Sullivan, Abraham Maslow, and Neal Miller. This theory focuses on the nurse/client relationship and is built on the different stages of personal development. The paradigm shift underlying this theory consists on adopting a perspective of equality, in which the client is a care partner, rather than a mere subject dependent on nursing care (Peplau 1990). Therefore, drawing on knowledge from behavioral science (e.g., the very clear influence of Freud's psychodynamic approach), this theory allows the nurse to depart from a disease-oriented approach and take a different approach through which the psychological meaning of events, feelings, and behaviors can be explored and included in nursing interventions. Taking into account that P/MH nurses have specialized training to identify and meet the client's needs, the nurse must seek to develop a trusting, therapeutic relationship with the client. As this relationship unfolds, the nurse should help the client to identify his/her problems and find solutions.

C. Loureiro (✉) • H. Quaresma
Nursing School of Coimbra, Coimbra, Portugal
e-mail: candida@esenfc.pt

J.C. Santos
Escola Superior de Enfermagem de Coimbra, Nursing School of Coimbra, Coimbra, Portugal

© Springer International Publishing Switzerland 2018

J.C. Santos, J.R. Cutcliffe (eds.), *European Psychiatric/Mental Health Nursing in the 21st Century*, Principles of Specialty Nursing,
https://doi.org/10.1007/978-3-319-31772-4_20

Within this theory, nursing is associated with a dynamic, therapeutic, and interpersonal process in which the actions depend on the participation of two or more individuals. The purpose of nursing is to produce changes in order to achieve positive client health outcomes, emphasizing the notion of personal growth and maturation. Peplau uses the expression "psychodynamic nursing" to describe the dynamic relationship established between the nurse and the person seeking help. The work developed by this author in the 1950s allowed for the interpersonal helping process, based on personal experiences, expectations, beliefs, and values, to be valued and recognized, both in nursing education and practice. Peplau's theoretical perspective was influenced by yet another equally important milestone for nursing—the person-centered approach of Carl Rogers (1902–1987). The Rogerian approach is grounded in a humanist philosophy based on the concept of autonomy in which human beings are able to transform themselves, develop their underlying skills and, above all, gain control over their lives and become autonomous.

20.2 The Skills of Psychiatric/Mental Health Nurses

P/MH nurses have the potential to play a key role in the therapeutic process to the extent that they use themselves as a therapeutic and helpful "tool" and as a model of change. It is therefore essential for nurses to be able to develop their self-awareness/self-knowledge skills so that they can help others grow and identify their own needs. The ability to listen without judging, to decipher silences or what is indirectly said, to believe that people are capable of changing less healthy behaviors and keeping the positive ones, are skills and beliefs that mental health nurses need to develop within their care practice to better understand the clients' health needs and concerns.

Therefore, it is important to explore the communicational skills in mental health, particularly the empathic (or empathy building) skills. Empathy is the act of communicating to another human being that you understand what he/she is feeling and how he/she is feeling it. It is the ability to see the world through the other's eyes and heart. It has been described as both a skill and an attitude (ref) that allows the human species to evolve and that requires a certain dose of mimetics to reach the other as a whole, to see the other side of the issue, thus helping to provide comfort to those in need of support (Pink 2006). It is through empathy that we are transported to the world of the other, without losing ourselves in the process. It is how we communicate understanding.

Within the interpersonal, helping relationship in P/MH nursing, understanding the other and expressing this understanding so as to enable him/her to evolve and develop (if desired) is the ultimate purpose of empathy (Lazure 1999). Being empathic means entering into the other's private perceptual world, temporarily living his/her life, without judging. It includes communicating what you are feeling about the other's world (Rogers 1980). The emphasis is placed on the ability to accurately adopt the other's perspective in terms of thought and feelings without actually experiencing them. There is a genuine interest for the other in terms of experiencing feelings of concern and comfort, and the presence of this emotional component does not necessarily mean that we have to experience the same feelings as the others but rather to understand what the other is feeling.

Empathy provides a penetrating perspective about a given situation, with the purpose of understanding and comforting the other. This allows for an understanding about the other's emotions, his/her way of experiencing difficulties. Establishing an empathic relationship requires certain necessary conditions (Lazure 1999; Rogers 1980), including:

- *Unconditional positive regard*: This acceptance will allow the development of feelings of relief and freedom, since the person feels no need to fight and defend his/her point of view or justify his/her reaction to others. Respecting and accepting the person as a unique being demonstrates a true appreciation for the other with his/her own experiences, feelings, and potential. The P/MH nurse contributes to building self-confidence by not making moral judgments or giving advice.
- *Active listening*: Listening is much more than just hearing; it is an active and voluntary process which, rather than merely implying the use of the stimulated auditory system, means accepting the influence of a set of personal perceptions, both internal and external. Listening is the only way to understand the other. We listen with our ears and our whole body, using visual contact, head nodding, touching, and verbal and nonverbal forms of encouragement. Words do not translate the full reality of the other's experience; they must be associated with facial expressions, tone of voice, gestures, and silence for the true meaning of the other's experience to the deciphered.
- *Empathic understanding*: This understanding requires objective answers, with an accurate and specific verbal reflection, without exaggerating or minimizing what was reported. It is important to try to understand the message as a whole and grasp the essential of the problem so as to actually understand it. The verbal and nonverbal communication of the person providing help should be consistent with the other's emotional status. Empathic understanding and reflection may help the other understand more objectively his/her reactions, because listening to someone reflecting about our own feelings increases awareness, thus expanding our perspective on the situation. Showing understanding contributes to making the other feel rewarded.

20.3 Evidence Concerning the Interpersonal Relationships of Mental Health Professionals from the Users' Perspectives

Eriksen et al. (2012) conducted a study with mental health service users in which "reciprocity" was considered to be the normative basis in the interpersonal relationships with health professionals. In this sense, reciprocity means recognizing the other as a human being, in a relationship in which both parties have the same value and the same right in the promotion of their interests. This aspect is also evident in the results of the study by Grundy et al. (2016) on the service users' perspective about their involvement in the mental health-care planning. The authors believe that a holistic and integrated approach allows for a greater care consolidation while allowing the users to be more informed to choose among the various treatment options. The users desire an increased personalization in the whole process so that the care planning remains tailored to their goals and health needs, as well as an increased focus on recovery, an aspect that remains overlooked. Changes to the professionals' behaviors and communication styles are expected given the need to develop and consolidate explicit and transparent communication protocols at the individual, team, and organization levels, with the purpose of facilitating a more meaningful participation of mental health clients and their carers. The direct involvement in care planning has an impact on service quality and user satisfaction.

In New Zealand, Rydon (2005) conducted a qualitative descriptive study with the purpose of identifying the necessary attitudes, skills, and knowledge of P/MH nurses from the perspective of mental health service users, in a context where governmental and service delivery policy requires that their needs must be effectively met. With regard to the attitudes of P/MH nurses, six categories emerged:

1. Being professional (cultivating positive, nondiscriminatory, and non-stigmatizing attitudes).
2. Conveying hope (believing in recovery and leading the others to believe in it too, without giving unrealistic expectations to the client and family).
3. Working alongside (sharing common goals, working toward the client's independence, in a relationship characterized by honesty, openness, exchange of feedback, appreciation for the family's opinion).
4. Knowing and respecting the person (showing a genuine interest in individuals and families as people with lives beyond the mental disorder, promoting individualized care, creating strong relationships based on mutual respect).
5. Human quality (demonstrating warmth and a willingness and openness to see the person as a person, with dignity).
6. Connection (being available to spend time with the users and their families/carers, being able to recognize subtle behavior changes, allowing nurses to help the client deal with tension and stress in due time and restore the person's wellness in a more effective way). This aspect was also reported by Grundy et al. (2016).

With regard to skills, two categories emerged from the data:

1. Interpersonal skills (being available to listen/active listening, explore the users' problems, and provide counseling, acknowledging the value of the users' family/carers and supporting them, showing empathy and interest)
2. Practical skills (providing follow-up and assistance to cope with a mental disorder, providing support focused on the clients' independence, allowing them to resume their activities of daily living as soon as possible, educating on the health status)

With regard to knowledge, two categories emerged:

1. Personal knowledge (knowing oneself, knowing one's limits, emotional stability, showing a high degree of resilience)
2. Professional knowledge (informing the users about their rights as care consumers, and empowering them to meet their own goals). These results were also reported by Grundy et al. (2016).

Therefore, it is important to identify the barriers/hampering factors and facilitating factors concerning the use of mental health services from the users' perspective. In a study on the community rehabilitation services in Israel, Moran et al. (2015) identified seven categories of indicators for the lack of service use, namely:

1. Lack of knowledge and orientation (lack of understanding about one's rights and the committee's goal to support one's psychiatric rehabilitation, lack of knowledge about the committee procedures and rehabilitation services)
2. Negative perceptions about rehabilitation services (in terms of the promotion of the users' personal goals, services are perceived as hosting people who are too sick and malfunctioning compared to the participant)
3. Lack of users' participation in the decision-making process (users are insufficiently involved as active partners in the decision-making process about their rehabilitation plan and services; lack of concordance between the user's current motivational state for change and the committee members' motives; others deciding for the users)
4. Not feeling heard by the committee (experiencing a disrespectful approach of committee members, seeing the committee as not attuned to the user's needs and goals)
5. Lack of congruence between the user's personal goals and the committee's final decision
6. Lack of skills of the health-care professionals (professionals lack the knowledge about available services, the committee and rehabilitation processes, lack of acquaintance with the user, limiting the professionals' ability to convey the users' interests to members of the committee)
7. Family members' influence on the use of rehabilitation services

Other related studies in this area have produced results that are in line with those reported above (see, e.g., Cutcliffe et al. 2015; Lawn 2015; Rugema et al. 2015), namely, concerning the identification of the benefits of engaging mental health service users, such as:

- A more effective partnership in care
- A more in-depth understanding by the professionals of the mental health experience of both users and their families
- The actual identification of their needs, the recognition of the effectiveness of specific interventions
- The use of empowerment, showing trust, and empathy

The fact that the person feels valued contributes to improving the quality of life (ref). The collaboration between authorities, the organization of mental health services, the existence of a health plan/health insurance, and the increased awareness of mental health issues by the families are other facilitating factors. With regard to the barriers to service use, we highlight the fear of stigma and discrimination, poverty and the lack of family support, insufficient resources and their accessibility, and mental health-related beliefs deeply rooted in certain cultures. Coercion, controlling behavior, lack of interest, and overuse of pharmacological treatments were also highlighted as negative experiences related to the practices of mental health-care professionals (Cutcliffe et al. 2015). Many people with mental health problems choose not to engage or maintain contact with the services due to stigma and discrimination. Negative experiences related to treatment and care also contribute to the lack of user involvement. The mental health reforms and policies should invest in the safety and effectiveness of care, combining the structural reform of the services with the focus on quality, ensuring the provision of safe, effective, and acceptable care by a qualified workforce (WHO 2015).

20.4 The Focus on Recovery in Mental Health

The focus on recovery still poses a major challenge for P/MH nurses and, therefore, it is important to explore this concept and understand its importance for people with a mental disorder to make life changes, as well as for mental health nurses to implement it in their daily practice. The scientific evidence allows guiding mental health professionals toward a practice that can/must be recovery-focused. Leese et al. (2014) conducted a literature review and identified the mental health nurses' key characteristics for a recovery-focused practice.

Three themes emerged from the analysis:

1. Hope (a strong relationship was found between hope and the perceived quality of life and health-related self-efficacy beliefs. Health promotion and encouragement by professionals in moments of greater distress and suffering were perceived as essential for recovery, emphasizing the time spent by nurses in promoting and encouraging hope). This aspect was also evidenced by Rydon (2005).
2. Person-centered care (it is important to identify what matters to each user, for example, his/her personal goals or choice of treatment. Trust and commitment are encouraged through the involvement of the users and their families in care provision, in a decision-making process shared between nurses and service users).
3. Consideration of the service users' opinions on the experience of care (the fact that users were approached by nurses, instead of the opposite, made them feel greatly supported. The nurses' availability is essential to an effective care. It was also highlighted that users are an important source of information and that learning from them improves the care practice, which requires nurses to consider the clients' opinions and expectations).

In the studies reviewed, we found many converging aspects related to facilitating and hampering factors in care settings, regardless of the setting (hospital or community). The studies were conducted in very different countries, such as New Zealand, Rwanda, Australia, Portugal, the United Kingdom, Sweden, Canada, Switzerland, and Germany, which leads us to reflect on the common needs of people with a mental disorder, regardless of their place of residence. We found evidence of the practice of P/MH nursing and the service users' experience related to communication skills, such as:

- The importance of being treated with dignity, respect, as a unique human being who has value exactly as he/she is
- Accepting the person for his/her uniqueness without judging
- Seeing him/her in a positive way and care reciprocity, i.e., not being a mere care receiver but a person capable of collaborating and engaging in his/her own care planning and personalization process
- The importance of knowledge transfer and education of individuals and communities by increasing mental health literacy and reducing stigma, discrimination, fear, and prejudice toward people with a mental disorder, focusing on the client's recovery and resources, using empowerment and being available to provide care, and conveying hope

20.5 Promoting Hope in Mental Health Care: A Skill That Must Be Put into Action

The concept of hope is now, fairly often reported in the literature; hence, it needs to be carefully analyzed. Although hope is a key concept in mental health nursing, it remains insufficiently widespread in the culture of care, education, and research (Cutcliffe 2009). According to Cutcliffe and Herth (2002), hope is considered as an experience of life meaning and purpose, rather than simply an individualized and subjective feeling. It is a healing inner forcer that is essential for the well-being of the person and family. Dufault and Martocchio (1985) believe that hope is a multidimensional and dynamic concept, identifying six dimensions, namely, an affective dimension (sometimes opposite feelings and emotions), a cognitive dimension (realistic processes of perception, desire, interpretation, and judgment), a behavioral dimension (the ability to act), an affiliative dimension (interpersonal relationship, reciprocity, attachment, care, and intimacy), a temporal dimension (a future-oriented hope, taking into account the personal present experience, and influenced by the past experience), and a contextual dimension (related to the individual's circumstances of life).

Hoping is believing that something may happen and change for the best; it is being perseverant and resilient and trusting others, and, in the future, being enthusiastic about life, feeling self-confident, and setting out goals. It is having a realistic perception of the situation, being able to identify possible options and selecting resources, assigning a meaning to life, and even transcending oneself. It allows for an adaptation to illness and an improvement of the individuals' well-being and quality of life (Sachse 2007). According to Cavaco et al. (2010), hope can be seen as a possible escape from the cycle of suffering and experienced as comfort. Therefore, given their privileged position to positively influence the client, nurses must acknowledge the importance of hope in care settings. Hope should be increasingly promoted as an essential component of the nurses' practice.

20.6 Closing Remarks

Having identified and discussed some of the key concepts related to the communication skills of P/MH nurses in this chapter, we can conclude that the use of an ecological model makes increasingly more sense. Care cannot be reduced to include only the person; it should also include the family, the significant persons, the life context, their expectations, and life goals. Above all, we should understand how the person perceives these aspects. Given the fact that human beings are considered systems of interrelated parts, the holistic view confirms that the whole is more than just the sum of its parts. The challenge lies in moving from a disease-centered approach to a more effective person-centered approach. A new understanding of the meaning of mental health problems or so-called mental disorders is also urgent in order to align the professionals' roles and skills with the more effective strategies to help the person's recovery.

A reference should also be made to the time available for care provision, as time was highlighted as an issue in the search the authors conducted. To put into action the previously described skills, P/MH nurses need to plan and manage their time, which should be dedicated to forming and maintaining a relationship of help, respect, empathy, and trust, focusing on listening to the other, promoting hope, guiding, engaging, and assisting. P/MH nurses need time to grow and develop into individual therapeutic agents, to find in themselves ways to maintain and promote hope, time to get to know themselves, their beliefs and emotions, to become more aware of their strengths and weaknesses, to understand the clients' value, to open themselves to others without fear, thus being able to effectively use themselves as therapeutic tools in the interpersonal and communicational context.

References

Cavaco VSJ, José HMG, Louro SPRLP, Ludgero AFA, Martins AFM, Santos MCG (2010) Which is the role of hope in personal health? – systematic review. Referência II Série 12:93–103

Cutcliffe JR (2009) Hope: the eternal paradigm for psychiatric/mental health nursing. J Psychiatr Ment Health Nurs 16:843–847

Cutcliffe JR, Santos JC, Kozel B, Taylor P, Lees D (2015) Raiders of the lost art: a review of published evaluations of inclient mental health care experiences emanating from the United Kingdom, Portugal, Canada, Switzerland, Germany and Australia. Int J Ment Health Nurs 24:375–385

Cutcliffe J, Herth K (2002) The concept of hope in nursing 3: hope and palliative care nursing. Br J Nurs 11(14):977–983

Dufault KJ, Martocchio BC (1985) Symposium on compassionate care and the dying experience. Hope: its spheres and dimensions. Nurs Clin N Am 20(2):379–391
Eriksen KA, Sundfor B, Karlsson B, Raholm M, Arman M (2012) Recognition as a valued human being: perspective of mental health service users. Nurs Ethics 19(3):357–368
Grundy AC, Bee P, Meade O, Callaghan P, Beatty S, Olleveant N, Lovell K (2016) Bringing meaning to user involvement in mental health care planning: a qualitative exploration of service user perspectives. J Psychiatr Ment Health Nurs 23:12–21
Lawn S (2015) Integrating service user participation in mental health care: what will it take? Int J Integr Care 15(4): URN:NBN:NL:UI:10-1-114809
Lazure H (1999) Vivre la relation d'aide: approche théorique et pratique d'un critière de competence de l'infermière. Decarie, Montréal
Leese D, Smithies L, Green J (2014) Recovery-focused practice in mental health. Nurs Pract 110(12):20–22
Moran GS, Baruch Y, Azaiza F, Lachman M (2015) Why do mental health consumers who receive rehabilitation services, are not using them? A qualitative investigation of users' perspectives in Israel. Community Ment Health J. doi:10.1007/s10597-015-9905-1
Peplau HE (1990) Relaciones interpersonales en enfermería: un marco de referencia conceptual para la enfermería psicodinámica. Salvat Editores, Barcelona
Pink DH (2006) A whole new mind: why right-brainers will rule the future. Riverhead Books, New York
Rogers CR (1980) A way of being. Houghton Mifflin Company, New York
Rugema L, Krantz G, Mogren I, Ntaganira J, Persson M (2015) "A constant struggle to receive mental health care": health care professionals' acquired experience of barriers to mental health care services in Rwanda. BMC Psychiatry 15:314. doi:10.1186/s12888-015-0699-z
Rydon SE (2005) The attitudes, knowledge and skills needed in mental health nurses: the perspective of users of mental health services. Int J Ment Health Nurs 14:78–87
Sachse D (2007) Hope: more than a refuge in a storm. A concept analysis using the Wilson method and the Norris method. Int J Psychiatr Nurs Res 13(1):1546–1553
World Health Organization (2015) The European mental health action-plan 2013–2020. World Health Organization Regional Office for Europe, Copenhagen

Group Work in Psychiatric/Mental Health Nursing: The Case for Psychoeducation as a Means to Therapeutic Ends

21

Evelyn Gordon and Maeve Kenny

21.1 Introduction

Over the past two decades, there has been an increase in the provision of psychoeducation in mental health care, coupled with, for some at least, a shift towards promoting pluralistic approaches and challenging the view that there is a single explanatory system for understanding mental health problems. These approaches have evolved from increased recognition of the complexity of mental health problems, acknowledgement of the myriad of interconnecting contributory factors to mental distress and acceptance of the limitations of biomedical illness models. The authors propose that psychiatric/mental health (P/MH) nurses can contribute to this paradigm shift, congruent with their core functions of therapeuctic engagement and person-centred care, through the provision of psychoeducation.

This chapter discusses psychoeducational group work and its relevance and application to contemporary psychiatric/mental health (P/MH) nursing practice. Psychoeducation addresses a range of complex human needs, targeting specific mental health concerns, populations and marginalised communities. These interventions have demonstrated significant psychotherapeutic and psychosocial benefits for service users and carers. There is a significant body of theoretical models and evidence-informed practices within mental health care that the P/MH nurse can draw on to deliver psychoeducational interventions that are complex, flexible and responsive. Much of this literature problematises hierarchical relationships and dispels notions of the P/MH nurse as an expert providing information and imparting

E. Gordon (✉)
School of Nursing and Human Sciences, Dublin City University, Dublin 9, Ireland
e-mail: evelyn.gordon@dcu.ie

M. Kenny
Principal Clinical Psychologist, St Vincent's Hospital, Fairview, Dublin 3, Ireland

© Springer International Publishing Switzerland 2018

J.C. Santos, J.R. Cutcliffe (eds.), *European Psychiatric/Mental Health Nursing in the 21st Century*, Principles of Specialty Nursing,
https://doi.org/10.1007/978-3-319-31772-4_21

advice. P/MH nurses are in a prime position to deliver psychoeducation at multiple levels of service provision, given their easy access to service users and carers.

21.2 Psychoeducation and Groups

Psychoeducation is the fusion and integration of psychological theory and teaching methods resulting in combined psychotherapeutic and educational interventions (Lukens and McFarlane 2004; Reyes 2010). It is designed to engage, inform and educate (Lucksted et al. 2012). Psychoeducation involves provision of information that is clear, accurate, accessible, up-to-date and jargon free and may include components of skills training. Contemporary psychoeducation emphasises the context in which information or skills are offered, privileging a holistic- and strengths-based approach, emphasising health, collaboration, coping, empowerment (Lukens and McFarlane 2004), choice, peer learning and self-responsibility (Thomas and Pender 2008). Shared decision-making is cultivated, combining expertise from personal and professional perspectives. Reyes (2010) views psychoeducation as a cyclical process that helps empower individuals to deal with situations in optimal ways. Enhancing an individual's knowledge broadens their perspective and awareness, which in turn influences their behaviour and emotions leading to greater self-efficacy and self-control (Reyes 2010).

While psychoeducation can be individually tailored, groups have many advantages. They are cost-effective typically having one or two leaders working with up to 15 group members. The power of the group is utilised to foster change and support, as members challenge each other (which they often experience as more effective than leader input), mirror each other, practise reflective listening, help each other reframe key issues, witness the progress of others and receive feedback on their own progress (Substance Abuse and Mental Health Services Administration (SAMHSA) 1999). These processes enhance self-advocacy and counter a sense of defeat (SAMHSA 1999).

21.3 Evidence Base for Psychoeducational Groups

A significant and growing body of evidence indicates that psychoeducational groups can and often do have positive outcomes. Psychoeducational groups for people with mental health problems have demonstrated improved quality of life and reductions in distress and symptoms (Lukens and McFarlane 2004). They have the potential to eliminate the need for more intensive treatments or to reduce waiting times for other interventions when delivered to people presenting for the first time with acute mental distress (Chien et al. 2012). Psychoeducational groups for carers have been found to increase their self-efficacy (Solomon et al. 1996), social connectedness and capacity to cope and decrease burden and psychological stress (Pharoah et al. 2010), while enhancing recovery and reducing relapse rates of relatives (Dixon et al. 2001).

In a systematic review of general and mental health systems, Lukens and McFarlane (2004) reported that psychoeducational groups that are underpinned by an ethos of recovery are associated with psychosocial and psychotherapeutic benefits and service users and carers who are more informed demonstrate better outcomes. They concluded that these interventions are among the most effective of the evidence-based approaches and extend the potential to improve community-based care provision by teaching people with health concerns and their carers how to anticipate and manage periods of crisis and life challenges.

21.4 Theoretical and Practical Issues in Psychoeducational Groups

While psychoeducational groups have been shown to be effective, group leaders need appropriate knowledge and expertise (Brown 2011) to successfully implement these interventions, thereby maximising their benefits and minimising the risk of harm (Lukens and McFarlane 2004; SAMHSA 1999). Selected group work literature and frameworks for best practice are outlined below to assist the P/MH nurse to deliver safe and effective psychoeducational groups.

21.4.1 Therapeutic Factors

Therapeutic or curative factors promote engagement and result in positive outcomes in group work. Eleven such factors have been outlined by Yalom (1970) and Yalom and Leszcz (2005). *Universality* refers to the realisation that one is not alone in their pain or suffering, which brings a sense of relief and belongingness, encourages personal disclosure, builds trust and fosters identification with others and compassion for self and others. *Installation of hope* involves witnessing others overcoming adversity, which can mobilise hope in the intervention and for oneself, and fosters self-advocacy. *Imparting of information* pertains to gaining knowledge and understanding of ones' life situation and oneself and is seen as enhancing progress and self-control. *Altruism* describes the opportunity to be helpful and of benefit to others, typically through sharing or giving advice, increases a sense of usefulness and personal value, fosters positive self-reflection and encourages role versatility between being helped and helping. *The corrective recapitulation of the primary family group* occurs when unresolved response patterns associated with negative experiences in primary relationships are replicated, explored, challenged and resolved within the group. *The development of socialisation techniques* highlights how enhancement of social skills is made possible in the group, explicitly through experiential learning such as skills training and interpersonal feedback or implicitly through development and enforcement of ground rules and modelling. *Imitative behaviour* describes how an adaptive skill used by one group member is imitated by others. *Interpersonal learning* refers to how individual members learn about intimacy and relationships through the supportive group environment, where honest feedback can be given and received. *Cohesiveness* pertains to a sense of belonging and acceptance that being part of a group fosters, generating experiences of being valued and allowing group members to take risks and experiment with change.

Catharsis describes the expression and sharing of emotions that occurs within the group. *The existential factor*, how groups develop to begin to accept rather than avoid their own limitations and the realities of life, is often provoked by significant events in the group, such as a member leaving or the imminent ending of the group. Awareness of these therapeutic factors can enhance opportunities for their development within the group providing the P/MH nurse with framework to use the power of the group to good effect, for example, carefully handling emotional expression so that the emotion is processed in a way that makes sense to the member, or developing imitative behaviours through practical skills teaching and experimentation.

21.4.2 Group Approaches

Theoretical literature often distinguishes between *directive* and *process* groups. Directive groups offer structured goals and leader-directed interventions to assist members to change through sequential activities that facilitate learning, self-discovery and growth (SAMHSA 1999). The leader has a central role in terms of organising and implementing activities and managing participation. Process groups emphasise the importance of the "group-as-a-whole" (Bion 1961); thus relationships within the group are attended to as a means of helping members understand themselves and build relationships that support their learning and recovery. The leader, while not assuming a central role, facilitates the group to become the agent of change. Although there is debate regarding the importance of incorporating a process approach in psychoeducational groups, both approaches can be successfully combined. Achieving and maintaining balance between group relationships and content enhance emotional safety and stimulation, which facilitates achievement of the group's objectives (Champe and Rubel 2012). Attending to process within groups fosters a sense of belonging, cohesion and motivation, factors associated with better outcomes. Combining directive and process approaches can promote the development of the therapeutic factors associated with positive outcomes. The P/MH nurse can use more structured inputs to enhance learning by helping group members to identify and build upon the skills, resources and personal strengths they have utilised to survive and that they continue to use to cope with life challenges and distress. They can support members to share and reflect upon their life experiences and use group relationships to facilitate members to process this material, gain new perspectives and strengthen their resilience.

21.4.3 Group Models

While contemporary psychoeducational groups are underpinned by a recovery ethos, many different therapeutic models and methods can be drawn upon depending on the nature and purpose of the group. The model of the intervention serves to guide the group leader, hold group members and sustain a clear focus. The model incorporates key philosophical concepts (e.g. recovery) and theoretical approaches (e.g. systems, cognitive-behavioural, humanistic/person-centred, psychodynamic,

integrative) underpinning the group, its structure, purpose, content and methods (e.g. experiential learning exercises, didactic teaching). Each of these elements requires consideration and clarification (Thomas and Pender 2008).
The fit between the model and the group leader's values (Brown 2011; Thomas and Pender 2008) and group member's needs (Bohart and Greaves Wade 2013) are important considerations. A clearly defined and explicit model and congruence between this and group leader disposition assist with selection and preparation for the group, guide practical decisions such as the group format (open, closed) and setting (community, clinic, hospital), help anticipate issues that might impact on member access and engagement, facilitate member informed consent, foster a good working alliance between leaders and group members and ensure the approach is clearly understood and adhered to. P/MH nurses have a long tradition of working from models that, at their core, promote person-centred care, interpersonal therapeutic relationships and effective communication (Barker 2001; Pepleau 1991), which form a strong foundation for effective psychoeducational groups.

21.4.4 Group Dynamics

Group dynamics (Lewin 1947) describes the positive and negative forces operating within groups. These forces give rise to the structure, norms, roles and goals that characterise a group and the nature of interpersonal interactions as members negotiate participation and communication patterns (Champe and Rubel 2012). Members take up different roles at various times in groups with constructive or destructive effects. Benne and Sheats (1948) identified three main types of roles: task roles concerned with completing the group's goals, building/maintenance roles concerned with building interpersonal relationships and self-centred roles which disrupt the group and prevent it from reaching its goals. It is important to recognise these roles as they emerge, by noting how members attend to group tasks, how they communicate and how decisions are made. The P/MH nurse can encourage the group to reflect on these issues and address emotions evoked in this process to enhance opportunities for constructive emotional and relational experiences and for new understandings to emerge.

21.4.5 Group Development

The nature and dynamics of a group evolve over its lifetime, and a number of models describe how groups develop (Tuckman 1965; Tuckman and Jensen 1977; Yalom 1970). For example, Tuckman (1965) describes five stages of group development. *Forming* is concerned with orientation to the group, group members and facilitators, and is characterised by testing behaviours and a strong dependence on group leaders, other members and familiar patterns of structure. *Storming* involves a phase of resistance to the task demands and group influence and is characterised by interpersonal conflict and polarisation. *Norming* refers to when resistance has been overcome as in-group cohesiveness develops, new standards evolve, new roles are adopted and personal opinions are more freely expressed. *Performing* refers to the phase wherein issues have been resolved, roles become flexible and functional and group energy is channelled into the task, and *adjourning*, the termination phase of the group, recognises the importance of group separation for members who have been involved in a range of activities and interpersonal exchanges together.

Recognising the developmental stage of the group helps the P/MH nurse to pace the introduction of new and more challenging materials and activities and to be aware of interpersonal challenges that are likely to arise at particular points in the group. The leader's role also changes as the group develops. Typically in the beginning phases, the leader is more active and directive, and as the group develops, their role becomes more consultative (Brown 2011). Awareness and knowledge of group development models assist the P/MH nurse to adjust their leadership style to match evolving group needs and developmental stages.

21.4.6 Group Boundaries

Boundaries refer to "the physical, temporal, emotional, cognitive and /or relational limits that define entities as separate from one another" (Ashforth et al. 2000, p. 474). Healthy boundaries (neither overly fluid/porous nor rigid) allow members to value and express their own views and experiences without compromising those of others and to be aware of their own needs while respecting those of others. Setting boundaries involves establishing ground rules for the acceptable behaviours and attitudes of group members. Ground rules need to be established early in the life of the group as they build security and order in the group and create a sense of relational safety. A collaborative approach actively involves group members and leaders in the development and ongoing review of rules that they consider important for the smooth and efficient running of the group, thereby promoting joint ownership and responsibility. The extent to which rules are defined and how well they are reinforced and adhered to by the leader will determine the ongoing stability and progress of the group.

The role and responsibilities of a leader may differ from their roles and responsibilities in other clinical activities. Thus, there may be a role boundary transition for the P/MH nurse, and it can be helpful to explicitly acknowledge this transition in the group to avoid the confusion caused by role blurring and to maintain security and clarity of focus. This might require a psychological and physical shift, for example, a change in self-presentation (e.g. clothing) and environment.

21.4.7 Group Leaders

The term leader is used to denote the interlinked roles of teaching and facilitation. Brown (2011) highlights that this is a complex role, with varied and multiple responsibilities, and therefore emphasises the need for the effective leader to have a sound knowledge base and to be mentally and physically prepared for the group. She outlines the range of competencies required by leaders to successfully manage their responsibilities, based on the acronym KASST. *Knowledge* means specialised and accurate information about the topic or focus of the group, understanding of group dynamics, stages of development and therapeutic factors. *Art* refers to the capacity to utilise self-awareness, personal development and inner experience to provide sensitive leadership and ensure that personal issues do not impact negatively on the group. *Science* incorporates administrative and executive abilities necessary for the optimal functioning of the group, such as securing resources, planning, organising, directing and developing group materials. *Skills* refer to good communication and interpersonal capabilities and include teaching, facilitating, modelling, conflict management and resolution, and anxiety management. *Techniques* are the means and methods that aid the generation of new ideas, facilitate problem solving, encourage participation and promote and reinforce group learning, including didactic teaching, use of media and experiential exercises (ice-breakers, role play, skills practice).

When planning groups it is wise for leaders to anticipate some challenging behaviours. These may occur, for example, during the storming phase when boundaries are being tested or later when group members know each other better and realise that their beliefs or value systems are being challenged by others giving rise to conflict. Before intervening it is helpful for the leader to consider why the behaviour is perceived as difficult, as this helps them to clarify the purpose and focus of their response. It is beneficial for the leader to demonstrate empathy and understanding by acknowledging the validity of the member's emotional upset, exploring the cause of the challenging behaviour and distinguishing between the emotional experience and the behavioural response. The P/MH nurse has several models for de-escalation to draw on to defuse intense situations (Bowers 2014; Price and Baker 2012) and allow opportunities for modelling and reinforcing prosocial behaviours. When comparing more successful groups with less successful groups, McKenzie et al. (1987), p. 55, found that "the former's leaders were characterized as more caring, charismatic, skillful, and less inhibiting". Group leaders, who can convey genuine belief, who demonstrate interest in and concern for group members and who use their own creativity and take the risk of being authentic and open, can positively influence the group process and outcomes. The reflective capacity of the P/MH nurse can be utilised to develop these skills and enhance therapeutic use of self. This can be facilitated by good mentoring and supervision, which can also aid the leader to reflect on the group dynamic and identify and process personal issues as they arise to prevent negative impact on group functioning, thereby stimulating personal and professional awareness, growth and development.

21.4.8 Group Evaluation

It is helpful to include evaluation structures to ensure the leader and members are on track and the group is progressing towards its objectives. Adherence scales can be designed, if not readily available, that help monitor compliance with the core content and processes of the intervention, and these can be particularly beneficial when delivering an unfamiliar intervention. Reviews can be conducted in-group and between groups helping to consolidate member learning (Thomas and Pender 2008). Outcome data can be gathered prior to, during and following the group intervention, targeting specific objectives, such as well-being, coping skills or progress towards personal goals. Free and accessible outcome measures that track group (Duncan and Miller 2007) and individual member (Miller et al. 2003) progress can highlight problem areas allowing the group leader to intervene early to facilitate constructive engagement and goal achievement. Systematic evaluation helps the P/MH nurse to gather practice-based evidence and monitor the ongoing impact of their psychoeducational group interventions.

21.4.9 Group Members

Yalom (1995) reported that members who were prepared for the group were less anxious, participated more, had less dropout and better attendance rates, demonstrated improved communication skills and expressed emotion more than those who were not adequately prepared. Members need to be ready and motivated; this means being willing to acknowledge and address problematic issues and being prepared to engage in change. The concept of "readiness to change" has been emphasised as an important factor influencing engagement, completion and positive outcomes of treatment (Prochaska and Diclemente 1982; Prochaska et al. 1994). Models of change suggest that people move through five non-linear stages before change is firmly established, with a sixth stage marking the end of the change process. *Precontemplation* refers to resistance to change and denial of a problem, although others may clearly see a difficulty. *Contemplation* describes the phase when the person acknowledges that they have a problem and begins to think about possible solutions, although they may not be ready to take action. *Preparation* is when the person is planning to make change but because they have not resolved their ambivalence they require a clear plan for action. *Action*, when the person overtly modifies their behaviour and their surroundings, requires commitment, time and energy. *Maintenance* describes when the person consolidates the gains made and works to prevent setbacks. *Termination* describes the absence of former problems or when they are no longer viewed as a temptation or threat. Collaboratively assessing a group member's readiness to change helps set appropriate goals. Setting unattainable goals can result in failure; choosing goals that have already been mastered can delay progress, while matching goals to stage of change can maximise the ability to change.

Up to 90% of people seeking treatment for mental distress were exposed to abuse and/or neglect in childhood, and a substantial proportion have experienced trauma (Fruech et al. 2005; Muskett 2014). Many people who have experienced traumatic life events and mental distress lose their sense of purpose and meaning in life, resulting in "existential frustration" (Frankl 2004, p. 106). Consequently, they often feel different, isolated, alone and empty and question their own value and the value of life (Gordon et al. 2014a; Gordon 2016). The group can assist a member who feels lost and alone to reconnect with the self, others and life through sharing their desperation, fears and lost hopes and by identifying with and witnessing their shared human experiences. These processes enhance new understandings about the self and life circumstances, and combat shame, stigma and isolation (Gordon et al. 2014b, 2015). A P/MH nurse who is sensitive to forms of abuse and oppression, including subtle forms of prejudice and discrimination, can help ensure that member's past experiences are acknowledged and resolved within the group and not replicated or left unresolved.

21.5 Contemporary Practice: Examples of Psychoeducational Groups

The authors describe two clinical examples of innovative, well-defined and empirically supported psychoeducational groups from their own practice and research. The first example is a hearing voices group for adults on an acute in-patient unit. The second is a community-based carer group for family and friends of those with mental health problems. Some direct quotations from member-participants are provided to illustrate key aspects of their experiences.

21.5.1 Hearing Voices Group

Hearing voices (HV) groups are based on the work of Romme and colleagues who proposed that HV and other unusual (not typically experienced by others) sensory phenomena are part of a continuum of human diversity and are meaningful in the context of the person's life. This approach highlights the interrelationships between subjective experiences and environmental context, challenging models that view HV as symptoms of mental illness. This view is based on research demonstrating significant causal associations between HV and trauma and/or emotional neglect (Read et al. 2005; Romme and Escher 1989, 1993) and observations that the characteristics of an individual's voices often contain references to their traumas (Romme et al. 2009). The HV approach advocates support, social inclusion, empowerment and justice for voice hearers. HV groups are underpinned by an ethos of *self-help*, whereby expertise by experience is harnessed, *respect* for diverse views and beliefs and *empathy*, fostering a desire to listen to and understand one's own and others' experiences.

The HV psychoeducational group for adults aimed to provide information about the HV approach, share effective coping strategies, highlight stories of recovery, heighten awareness of a local community peer support group and signpost relevant, credible and accessible resources. The group sought to engage with members as partners in the provision of care, which has been shown to be an effective way of preparing individuals to avail of other recovery-oriented community resources and supports (Lukens and McFarlane 2004).

The psychoeducational intervention comprised three brief groups, as it was designed for individuals who typically experienced acute levels of distress and had brief admissions. The groups were structured: the beginning focussed on a brief introduction to the purpose of the group and agreement on the ground rules; the middle of the group focussed on a specific theme, following the structure of the Maastricht Interview (Escher et al. 2000), where the leaders provided relevant written and oral information and ensured time was made available for open dialogue among group members; groups concluded with information about various coping strategies.

The leaders made explicit their positions about confidentiality and clinical note writing, as group members were wary of talking openly about their HV experiences because such information was frequently used to gauge their mental state. Thus, a critical group rule was that information shared within the group was confidential to the group and limitations to confidentiality were addressed and agreed. "I felt comfortable and safe to express myself" (member). This can require a shift in position for P/MH nurses on acute units who may transfer detailed information to other colleagues, a practice inconsistent with the rules and ethos of the group and the HV approach.

In the first group, with the theme "the experience of hearing voices", leaders introduced members to the HV approach, facilitated exploration of the impact of HV on their lives, discussed various ways of understanding HV and provided information about common life situations associated with the onset and progression of HV. Basic distraction-based coping strategies were introduced.

In the second group, the theme "engaging and triggers" involved exploring each person's history of HV, noting changes in their HV experience, identifying associated changes in life circumstances and discussing the meanings of each person's HV experiences. Leaders provided information about recovery in HV and the recovery journeys of experts by experience. Advanced coping strategies were offered, such as voice dialoguing and mapping, which involve drawing a picture of each voice in terms of its message, tone, origins and triggers, so that the individual begins to know their voices and the functions they may serve in their life.

In the third group, the theme, "understanding the experience", focused on the individual's relationship with his/her voices. Information was provided about the three stages of recovery in HV (startling, organisation, stabilisation) (Romme and Escher 1989, 1993), the importance of developing personal and social value and the association between regaining personal power and reductions in distress and improvements in quality of life. Further advanced coping strategies were introduced to support these ideas, behavioural experiments designed to support the regaining of control in ones' life, such as balancing time alone and with others, reorganising daily routines and trying new ways of engaging with the voices, and cognitive strategies to reconstruct ones' relationship with the voices through acceptance and reorganising attention to them. The leaders also provided information on accessing post-discharge community resources and credible sources of information.

Evaluation of these groups indicated members had high levels of satisfaction with the groups, and they found it helpful and liberating to explore their HV experiences. "What I liked best was understanding each other, being able to share…" (member). Members reported increased hope having identified with other experts by experience and having witnessed their stories of recovery, increased awareness of coping strategies and increased interest in their relationship with their voices. Many had ideas about the origins and meaning of their HV experiences but had not previously felt supported to openly discuss such matters. Some group members expressed the desire for more of this kind of intervention. "I would like to learn more about the sources of my voices" (member).

The P/MH nurse can introduce voice hearers to these contemporary ways of understanding and managing their voices and can provide information on community-based peer groups.

21.5.2 Carer Group

Carers play a key role in the recovery and support of relatives struggling with mental health issues (Watkins 2007). Their role is complex and can be stressful, compromising their well-being and ability to provide support for their relative (Higgins et al. 2011; Maurin and Boyd 1990). Despite their key role, carers are frequently excluded from the treatment of their relative due to a variety of issues, such as being viewed as part of the problem (Higgins et al. 2011) or concerns about confidentiality (Kenny et al. 2015). "I don't want to know what secrets my [son] tells his psychiatrist but I do want to know how to care for him…we need to know how to care for them and how to care for ourselves..." (Carer). Despite the known burden associated with caring, support for carers is inadequate, unsuitable or not visible (Higgins et al. 2011; Kenny 2011), and there is growing evidence that carer psychoeducation is effective but persistently underutilised (Lucksted et al. 2012).

The psychoeducational group for carers was embedded within an action research project, which was initiated by a group of carers, clinicians and researchers who sought to increase carer involvement in the planning and delivery of services. The project comprised a focus group with carers designed to explore their experiences of being a carer and being involved with mental health services and two psychoeducational groups. Analysis of the focus group revealed that caring and being involved with services were experienced as "nightmarish and challenging". This theme refers to the psychological, emotional and physical struggles that carers experienced in supporting a relative with mental health problems and engaging with mental health services that were difficult to access and were sometimes hostile (Kenny et al. 2015). "It has been a nightmare because I was thrown totally into a situation I knew nothing about. I found it very difficult to get information" (Carer). The outcomes of the focus group were presented to the clinical teams providing treatment to these carers' relatives, and their responses were recorded.

In the first psychoeducational group, the leaders presented the themes extrapolated by the researchers, along with the responses of the clinical teams. Leaders provided information about the complex and varied role of being a carer, the burden of caring, the need for support, the often neglected role of self-care and some of the dilemmas the teams encountered when dealing with carers. This facilitated carers to reflect upon their experiences from different perspectives and begin to process and make sense of their emotional experiences in a context where they felt heard and safe. The leaders explored carers' perceptions about how clinical teams could respond differently to them, revealing a desire for more information, collaboration and involvement. The group concluded with discussion about the final group and carers identified self-care as their primary need.

In the final group, leaders provided information about local community-based resources, including a local carer support group, common mental health concerns and the clinical teams' plans to promote involvement of carers. Group leaders facilitated experiential exercises designed to support self-care, including mindfulness, guided imagery and relaxation, and led a discussion about prioritising, planning and implementing ongoing self-care activities. "It hasn't been recognised that this has impacted on the families so greatly. It's not just the person [with mental health issues] it's the whole family and the needs of the family" (Carer).

Evaluation indicated that members felt acknowledged and empowered by being able to voice their concerns and needs and by connecting with others who had similar experiences (Kenny et al. 2015). "To be able to talk about what you were experiencing and were heard and understood, the feeling that at last someone cared was good" (Carer).

The P/MH nurse can promote the establishment of psychoeducational groups for carers by facilitating carers to come together, helping them find suitable meeting venues, leading the groups until the members feel ready to take on this role, attending established groups as guest speakers to impart knowledge and teach skills and encouraging their colleagues to involve and support carers. These interventions validate the important role they have as carers, help educate them about the burden of caring and support them to acknowledge and promote self-care. The provision of information early in their involvement with mental health services also helps encourage open dialogue between carers and clinicians and helps to identify and address their emotional and practical needs (Walker and Dewar 2001).

21.6 Conclusions: Psychoedu-Caution

Contrary to a common misperception that psychoeducation is a simplistic form of intervention, the authors have argued that a skilled and knowledgeable group leader can deliver psychoeducational group interventions that result in positive psychotherapeutic and psychosocial outcomes and are cost-effective. Through the promotion of interventions that reflect the diverse, complex and yet to be known aspects of human experiences that intersect with well-being and mental health, the P/MH has opportunities to help reduce stigma, discrimination and social isolation and promote health, resiliency and self-agency among service users, carers and communities. By delivering psychoeducational groups based on emancipatory, recovery-oriented and ecological approaches, the P/MH nurse can contribute to the re-construction of new realities in mental health and mental health nursing. While the clinical examples described demonstrate the versatility and benefits of psychoeducational groups that can be incorporated into contemporary P/MH nursing, caution is advised when considering psychoeducational group interventions. Such interventions also have the potential to reproduce restrictive and oppressive practices and reinforce outdated hierarchical structures and processes when delivered, knowingly or unknowingly, in a poorly informed manner.

References

Ashforth BE, Kreiter GE, Fugate M (2000) All in a day's work: boundaries and micro role transitions. Acad Manag Rev 25(1):472–491

Barker P (2001) The tidal model: developing an empowering, person-centred approach to recovery within psychiatric and mental health nursing. J Psychiatr Ment Health Nurs 8(3):233–240

Benne KD, Sheats P (1948) Functional roles of group members. J Soc Issues 4:41–49

Bion WR (1961) Experiences in group work. Tavistock, London

Bohart AC, Greaves Wade A (2013) The client in psychotherapy. In: Lambert MJ (ed) Bergin and Garfield's handbook of psychotherapy and behavior change, 6th edn. Wiley, New York

Bowers L (2014) A model of de-escalation. Ment Health Pract 17(9):36–37

Brown NW (2011) Psychoeducational groups: process and practice, 3rd edn. Routledge, New York

Champe J, Rubel DJ (2012) Application of focal conflict theory to psychoeducational groups: implications for process, content and leadership. J Spec Group Work 37(1):71–90

Chien WT, Leung SF, Che CS (2012) A nurse-led, needs-based psycho-education intervention for Chinese patients with first-onset mental illness. Contemp Nurse 40(2):194–209

Dixon L, McFarlane WR, Lefley H, Lucksted A, Cohen M, Falloon I, Mueser K, Miklowitz D, Solomon P, Sondheimer D (2001) Evidence-based practices for services to families of people with psychiatric disabilities. Psychiatr Serv 52:903–910

Duncan BL, Miller SD (2007) The group session rating scale. Authors, Jensen Beach

Escher S, Romme M, Hage P (2000) The Maastricht hearing voices interview. In: Romme M, Escher S (eds) Making sense of voices. Mind, London

Frankl VE (2004) Man's search for meaning. Random House, New York

Fruech BC, Knapp RG, Cusack KJ, Grubaugh AL, Sauvageot JA, Cousins VC, Yim E (2005) Patients' reports of traumatic or harmful experiences within the psychiatric setting. Psychiatr Serv 56(9):1123–1133

Gordon E (2016) Transcending suicidality: re-vitalizing worthiness. Lambert Academic Publishing, Saarbrücken

Gordon E, Stevenson C, Cutcliffe JR (2014a) Transcending suicidality: facilitating re-vitalizing worthiness. In: Cutcliffe JR, Santos JC, Links P, Zaheer J et al (eds) Routledge international handbook of clinical suicide research. Routledge, New York

Gordon E, Kenny M, O'Reilly A, Walton T (2014b) Independent evaluation of the SoS eden programme. Dublin City University, Dublin

Gordon E, McElvaney R, MacGabhann L, Farrelly M, Casey B, Pulcherio I (2015) Responding to the suicide bereaved: the mayo model – full report. Dublin City University, Dublin

Higgins A, McGuire G, Watts M, Creaner M, McCann E, Rani S, Alexander J (2011) Service user involvement in mental health practitioner education in Ireland. J Psychiatr Ment Health Nurs 18:519–525

Kenny M (2011) National overview of service user representatives, carers/family representatives and advocacy groups. MHC, Dublin

Kenny M, Gordon E, McCabe C, Clyne A, Walton T, Connolly J (2015) Giving voice to family and friends: report on the family and friends project St Vincent's Hospital and HSE Dublin North City. Authors, Dublin

Lewin K (1947) Frontiers in group dynamics: concept, method and reality in social science; social equilibria and social change. Hum Relat 1:5–41

Lucksted A, McFarlane W, Downing D, Dixon L, Adams C (2012) Recent developments in family psychoeducation as an evidence-based practice. J Marital Fam Ther 38(1):101–121

Lukens EP, McFarlane WR (2004) Psychoeducation as evidence-based practice: considerations for practice, research, and policy. Brief Treat Crisis Intervention 4(3):205–225
Maurin TJ, Boyd CB (1990) Burden of mental illness on the family: a critical review. Arch Psychiatr Nurs 4(2):99–107
McKenzie KR, Dies R, Coché E, Rutan JS, Stone WN (1987) An analysis of AGPA institute groups. Int J Group Psychother 37(1):55–74
Miller SD, Duncan BL, Brown J, Sparks JA, Claud MS (2003) The outcome rating scale: a preliminary study of the reliability, validity, and feasibility of a brief visual analog measure. J Brief Ther 2(2):91–100
Muskett C (2014) Trauma-informed care in inpatient mental health settings: a review of the literature. Int J Ment Health Nurs 23(1):51–59
Pepleau HE (1991) Interpersonal relations in nursing. Springer, New York
Pharoah F, Mari J, Rathbone J, Wong W (2010) Family intervention for schizophrenia. Cochrane Database Syst Rev 12:CD000088. doi:10.1002/14651858.CD000088.pub3
Price O, Baker J (2012) Key components of de-escalation techniques: a thematic synthesis. Int J Ment Health Nurs 21(4):310–319
Prochaska JO, Diclemente CC (1982) Transtheoretical therapy: toward a more integrative model of change. Psychother Theory Res Pract 19(3):276–288
Prochaska JO, Norcross JC, Diclemente CC (1994) Changing for good. Avon Books, New York
Read J, van Os J, Morrison AP, Ross CA (2005) Childhood trauma, psychosis and schizophrenia. Acta Psychiatr Scand 112:330–350
Reyes C (2010). What is psycho-education? http://thepsychoeducationalteacher.blogspot.ie/2010/10/what-is-psycho-education.html
Romme M, Escher S (1989) Hearing voices. Schizophr Bull 15:209–216
Romme M, Escher S (1993) Accepting voices. Mind, London
Romme M, Escher S, Dillon J, Corstens D, Morris M (2009) Living with voices: 50 stories of recovery. PCCS Books, Herefordshire
Solomon P, Draine J, Mannion E, Meisel M (1996) Impact of brief family psychoeducation on self-efficacy. Schizophr Bull 22(1):41–50
Substance Abuse and Mental Health Services Administration (SAMHSA) (1999) Brief interventions and brief therapies for substance abuse, Treatment improvement protocol series, No. 34. SAMHSA, Rockville
Thomas RV, Pender DA (2008) Association for specialists in group work: best practice guidelines 2007 revisions. J Spec Group Work 33(2):111–117
Tuckman BW (1965) Developmental sequence in small groups. Psychol Bull 63(6):384–399
Tuckman BW, Jensen MAC (1977) Stages of small-group development revisited. Group Org Manage 2(4):419–427. doi:10.1177/105960117700200404
Walker E, Dewar BJ (2001) How do we facilitate carer's involvement in decision making? Issues Innovations Nurs Pract 34:320–328
Watkins P (2007) Recovery: a guide for mental health practitioners. Churchill Livingstone, London
Yalom I (1970) The theory and practice of group psychotherapy. Basic Books, New York
Yalom I (1995) The theory and practice of group psychotherapy, 4th edn. Basic Books, New York
Yalom I, Leszcz M (2005) The theory and practice of group psychotherapy, 5th edn. Basic Books, New York

A Family-Focused, Recovery Approach When Working with Families When a Parent Has a History of Mental Health Problems: From Theory to Practice

22

Darryl Maybery and Andrea Reupert

22.1 Introduction

When practitioners work with someone with mental health challenges, typically and historically, there is and has been little consideration of their family. Or when families are considered, they are traditionally regarded as:

> 'causing the mental illness in a family member, as acting to sustain the mental illness or as contributing to relapse'. (Wyder and Bland 2014, p. 180)

In this chapter, we approach families differently, with a particular focus on families where a parent, who cares for children, experiences mental health concerns. The recovery journey for such parents is intimately related to the relationships and interactions within their family and community. As argued below, it is these complex interactions within and outside of families that need to be the focus of mental health services and at least in part, psychiatric/mental health (P/MH) nursing care.

Prevalence estimates indicate that over 50% of people experiencing mental health challenges are parents (Nicholson et al. 2004) while 21–23% of children have at least one parent who experiences mental health concerns (Maybery et al. 2009). The relationship between poor parental mental health and poor outcomes in children has been well substantiated (Hosman et al. 2009) though not all children will

D. Maybery, PhD (✉)
Director School of Rural Health - Monash University, Department of Rural Health and Professor Rural Mental Health Research, PO Box 973, Moe, Victoria, Australia
e-mail: darryl.maybery@monash.edu

A. Reupert, PhD
Director of Professional Psychology Programs in Education, Faculty of Education, Krongold, Monash University, Clayton, Victoria, Australia

© Springer International Publishing Switzerland 2018

J.C. Santos, J.R. Cutcliffe (eds.), *European Psychiatric/Mental Health Nursing in the 21st Century*, Principles of Specialty Nursing,
https://doi.org/10.1007/978-3-319-31772-4_22

be adversely affected. While genetics may very well play an important role in this potential impact, environmental factors are also critical. There is strong evidence that the trans-generational transmission of mental health challenges from parents to children is significantly mediated by parenting and parent-child interactions (Leinonen et al. 2003). Hence, focusing on the parent-child relationship provides an ideal opportunity for early intervention to improve outcomes for children.

Focusing on the parent-child relationship not only contributes to positive outcomes in children but may also facilitate a client's recovery. The successes and failures associated with fulfilling a parenting role can have a profound impact on a client's mood and how they feel about themselves and hence on their overall functioning (Maybery et al. 2015). Thus, having children can provide opportunities for supporting a client's recovery or alternatively undermine recovery, as might occur, for example, when a parent loses custody of his or her children.

Currently there are few recovery interventions and supports developed specifically for families where a parent experiences mental health challenges. In this chapter we bring together concepts around family-focused practice and recovery and translate these into particular practices when supporting such families. We base these discussions on various projects we have conducted over the last 15 years, in partnership with parents, their families, practitioners, policymakers and other researchers in this field.

22.2 Family-Focused Practice

While family-focused practice (FFP) is most commonly employed in the disability and paediatric fields (Dunst et al. 2007), it is only recently being used in association with families in families where a parent experiences mental health challenges. Often used interchangeably with family sensitive, family centred and family focused, we define FFP as '… the involvement of families as part of the usual treatment and care of a parent with a mental illness rather than the delivery of discrete model of family intervention' (Maybery et al. 2014, p. 608).

FFP is a collaborative approach that encompasses both the individual and his or her family (Rosenbaum et al. 1998). The principles of FFP were first developed from a review of the literature by Allen and Petre (1998) and have been expanded since (Dempsey and Keen 2008; Dunst et al. 2007). These principles are summarised as follows:

1. *Family is central to the lives of individuals*. This means identifying the family as a unit of intervention rather than the individual with the presenting 'problem'.
2. *Maximising families' choices and abilities for informed decision-making*, rather than a professional centric model of decision-making. This acknowledges that parents know their children best, know what is best for their children and have ultimate care for their children.
3. *Applying a strengths-based perspective*, as opposed to a deficit or pathological perspective of the family. Rather than 'blame' the family, practitioners need to recognise that all families have strengths that can be further developed and used in problem solving.

4. Recognising that *all families are different* and will require culturally competent services that value diversity and multiple perspectives.

At its heart, FFP provides families with opportunities to be actively involved in decisions and choices, as well as actions to achieve desired goals and outcomes (Dunst et al. 2007).

22.3 Recovery

For many people experiencing mental health challenges, the concept of recovery is about staying in control of their life despite experiencing a mental health problem (Leamy et al. 2011). Deegan (1996, p. 97), defines recovery as:

> '…re-establish[ing] a new and valued sense of integrity and purpose within and beyond the limits of the disability; the aspiration is to live, work and love in a community in which one makes a significant contribution…'

While the medical approach emphasises clinical recovery as a remission of mental health symptoms, the recovery model centres on personal recovery, which is aimed not so much as being symptom-free but instead:

> 'living a satisfying, hopeful, and contributing life, even when there are on-going limitations caused by mental health problems'. (Mental Health Commission of Canada 2012, p. 12)

While often described as an individual journey, recovery is increasingly recognised as a relational concept, where the social environment, in particular one's family, is critical (Reupert et al. 2015a, b). A crucial aspect of any recovery model is support for an individual's choices including his or her choice about being a parent.

There are several links between parenting and recovery that have only recently been documented. For example, Nicholson (2014) found that children may give parents the strength and will to 'keep going' thereby promoting hope, a key recovery component. 'Being a parent' and effectively assuming the parenting role provide parents with meaning and purpose, another element of recovery (Maybery et al. 2015). Parenting may also give opportunities for meaningful interactions and activities and connections into their community (Maybery et al. 2015). Thus, identifying and supporting an individual's parenting role can provide hope, a sense of agency, connectedness, self-determination and meaning, all cognisant with a recovery approach.

Being a member of a family can contribute to recovery in other ways. One's parents, children, partner and others are often critical for supporting a client's recovery journey by providing emotional as well as practical support such as undertaking household chores. Children, for example, might care for their younger siblings when their parent is very unwell, for example, or 'having a bad day' (Riebschleger 2004). The emotional support that families can provide should not be underestimated; Mancini et al. (2005, p. 52) found that families can provide:

'an unwavering and steadfast belief in participants' ability to recover' while Jenkins and Carpenter-Song (2001, p. 394) reported that family members promoted recovery by:

> allowing the individual to be treated as 'just another person rather than being marked as ill and excluded'.

Finally, it is important to note that the behaviour and wellbeing of one family member may impact on others. As outlined earlier we know that children whose parents experience mental health concerns are more likely than their peers to experience a range of adverse psychosocial outcomes, and a child with his or her mental health or behavioural issues will inevitably influence and impact on the mental health and wellbeing of the parent/s. While a vicious cycle can be created between parental and child problems, it is also important to note that a virtuous cycle is possible, i.e. between parental and child recovery, with one re-enforcing the other (Compas et al. 2010). It is this intertwined nature of recovery that is the key to understanding family recovery.

22.4 Family Recovery

There is a paucity of literature that synthesises the concepts of FFP and recovery in relation to families where a parent where a parent experiences mental health challenges. One of the few attempts to do this comes from Nicholson (2014) though her emphasis is on mothers experiencing mental health challenges, with less attention on the recovery journey and needs of different family members. Our framework of family recovery is outlined below. The foundation of this approach is built from the core concepts of FFP (acknowledging that all families are different, a strengths-based perspective, ensuring that family members have choices) along with recovery (including connectedness, hope, identity, meaning and empowerment; Leamy et al. 2011).

1. *Acknowledge the family role of the client.* Family recovery acknowledges, supports and celebrates the family role of clients and in particular their parenting role. This may also involve aspirational family roles in the future (i.e. wanting to be parent in the future) or the grief and loss associated with not fulfilling a role (such as not being a parent or losing custody of children). Men's aspirations and roles in respect to fatherhood are included here (though often neglected by practitioners, Reupert and Maybery 2009).
2. *Families can contribute to recovery.* Family recovery means recognising and valuing the critical role that family's play in the recovery journey of clients, especially children. This means that rehabilitation plans need to incorporate and formally acknowledge families as a source of support and an essential component of a client's recovery journey. Accordingly, families, including children, need to be routinely consulted as part of an individual's treatment team. If we ask (or expect or assume) that families support their ill relative, it only makes sense that the family is then consulted as a part the treatment team.

3. *Families go through their own recovery journey.* Within a recovery paradigm, we need to acknowledge the family's own recovery journey and needs, in parallel with the consumer. This acknowledges the interdependent nature of family relationships, which change over time (e.g. when unwell, family relationships may be one sided and dependent while during the rebuilding phase, families need to 'let go' and move from being a carer to a support person) (Reupert et al. 2015a).

Understanding a family's recovery journey means acknowledging different family members' needs around identity, support, respite and psychoeducation (Wyder and Bland 2014). For family members, recovery may involve developing a life that moves beyond the caring role, learning to better manage their own distress and feeling that they are a valued part of the care team for their relative. In families where a parent experiences mental health challenges, this means that children's needs are identified and addressed.

22.5 From Theory to Practice

There are multiple practices that best embrace the concepts of family recovery for families where parents experience mental health concerns.

22.5.1 For Parents Experiencing Mental Health Challenges

Acknowledge parenting All clients who present for mental health treatment need to be asked about their parenting role, including reproductive goals and hopes for the future. It is also important to acknowledge the parenting role of those who do not actively care for their children, due to custody arrangements or child protection orders, as their parenting role may still be important to their overall wellbeing.

Talking about parenting Family recovery means that ongoing conversations about parenting and caring for children are embedded into treatment discussions and plans.

Initiating discussions about parenting and children within the context of a mental health treatment is not easy however. The stigma associated with mental health issues means that parents and practitioners might be reluctant to discuss mental health issues in the context of family life. Additionally, in some countries, mental health concerns is a legally accepted reason for custody loss (see Kaplan et al. 2009), regardless of the client's parenting ability. Other research has found that many mental health practitioners, including P/MH nurses, do not have the necessary skills and knowledge to work with clients on parenting or their children (Maybery and Reupert 2009). Appropriate training along with supervision and time is necessary for practitioners to practice family recovery (see Reupert et al. 2015b for more information on particular training approaches and models).

Hence it is important to address the reluctance that some parents might have in talking about their children or their parenting. If discussing parenting and children is not a routine part of treatment, such discussions can be surprising or even alarming, particularly if parents are concerned about the involvement of child protection services (Solantaus et al. 2015). Nonetheless, many parents want to talk about their children and are often relieved when given the opportunity to do so (Solantaus et al. 2015). The following is an example script of how a practitioner might 'open the door' to talking about parenting and children in a sensitive manner (adapted from Solantaus et al. 2015).

> 'Many parents who experience mental health issues have questions or concerns about their children. They often worry about things they have noticed or they may have questions about how best to support them. They may also worry about how their illness impacts on their parenting role. Something things go along smoothly, but at other times, thing can be more challenging – and these things can be hard to discuss in families[1]*. Many parents would like to know if there is something they can do for their children… If you are concerned or worried about any of these issues, would you like to discuss them? I might be able to help you in working out what you can do for your children[2]**'.

22.5.2 Children Whose Parent Has a History of Mental Health Problems

Children living in families where parents experience mental health challenges need the same love and security that all children need. Nonetheless, family recovery means that their particular needs are considered and addressed at the same time as their parents.

Giving children a voice It has been said that children whose parents experience mental health challenges are 'invisible' as services predominately attend to their parent (Trondsen 2012) unless there are serious issues around neglect or abuse. Practitioners need to give these children a voice and opportunities to ask questions, consult about their needs and seek their views as to what they think should happen in their family. Their input is especially important when planning for crisis times, for example, deciding where a child might stay when a parent is hospitalised (Reupert et al. 2008).

Opportunities to talk about their parent's illness A common need, articulated by youth themselves, is the opportunity to have conversations about their parents'

[1] *These statements send a message to the client that it is normal to have concerns about their children and that other parents have also been in this situation. The practitioner joins with the parent in their possible concerns and gives the parent permission to talk about any issues they might have. This is different from opening the discussion with, 'How are your children?' which might make the parent feel uncomfortable and defensive.

[2] **It is important to let parents know that they can do things for their children rather having to rely on services, a stance that can be a genuine source of empowerment for the parent.

illness. When child centred and in an age appropriate manner, such conversations may address children's fears about what is happening in the family (Cooklin 2013). Interestingly, many youth want to hear about their parent's illness from the parent themselves (Reupert et al. 2012), and practitioners might work with parents around how they might do this.

Caring role acknowledged Some children whose parent experiences mental health challenges assume a caring role of their siblings and/or parent (Reupert and Maybery 2007). While caregiving has been associated with limiting young people's friendships and schooling, there is growing recognition that the experience of caring can be positive in developing closer family ties and independence (Aldridge and Becker 2003). It is important that this caring role is acknowledged and that children are consulted accordingly. Respite from these caring responsibilities may also be warranted.

22.5.3 The Family as a Whole

A strengths-based approach Rather than focusing on limitations or deficits, a strengths-based approach means practitioners highlight the potentials, strengths, interests, abilities and capacities of parents and their children (Grant and Cadell 2009). This approach is not about denying any problems the parent or child may be experiencing but instead working collaboratively with the parent on mutually agreed goals and drawing on the resources of the family and the community. It is this harnessing a family's resilience that provides the basis for addressing the challenges that they may be facing. Accordingly, parents need to be encouraged to identify strengths for themselves and their children, which in turn may make them feel more positive in their relationships (Nicholson 2014).

Collaborative goal setting typically involves a case management approach in which meetings are held with each family member and the family as a whole to identify short- and long-term goals (Maybery et al. 2012). The practitioner might prompt some key domains around family life and child development and together work out what needs to happen, by when and with whom. For example, goals for children might include wanting to learn more about their parent's illness or having a sleep over at a friend's house. For parents, example goals might involve improving the way they deal with anger or putting aside money for family outings. During this process, the roles and responsibilities of external agencies and informal family networks are negotiated by family members and/or the practitioner. The role of the practitioner is to support each family member to achieve their particular goals over time, drawing on various community and family supports.

Conclusion

Family recovery synthesises two seminal constructs, FFP and recovery, with subsequent practice and organisational implications for how we might work with clients who are parents and their children. At its essence, family recovery means valuing and celebrating the family life of our clients and simultaneously conveying a sense of hope that the lives of these families will be better. It is therefore incumbent on services to provide the necessary organisational and policy initiatives that embed parenting and children as a routine part of treatment.

References

Aldridge J, Becker S (2003) Children caring for parents with mental illness: perspectives of young carers, parents and professionals. Policy Press, Bristol

Allen R, Petre C (1998) Rethinking family-centered practice. Am J Orthopsychiatry 6(1):4–15

Compas BE, Champion JE, Forehand R, Cole DA, Reeslund KL, Fear J et al (2010) Coping and parenting: mediators of 12 month outcomes of a family group cognitive-behavioral preventive intervention with families of depressed parents. J Consult Clin Psychol 78(5):623–634

Cooklin A (2013) Promoting children's resilience to parental mental illness: engaging the child's thinking. Adv Psychiatr Treat 19:229–240

Deegan P (1996) Recovery as a journey of the heart. Psychiatr Rehabil J 19(3):91–97

Dempsey I, Keen D (2008) A review of processes and outcomes in family-centered services for children with a disability. Top Early Child Special Educ 28:42–52

Dunst C, Trivette C, Hamby D (2007) Meta-analysis of family-centred helpgiving practices research. Ment Retard Dev Disabil Res Rev 13:370–378

Grant J, Cadell S (2009) Power, pathological worldviews and the strengths perspective in social work. Fam Soc 90(4):425–430

Hosman C, van Doesum K, van Santvoort F (2009) Prevention of emotional problems and psychiatric risks in children of parents with a mental illness in the Netherlands: I. The scientific basis to a comprehensive approach. Adv Ment Health 8:250–263

Jenkins J, Carpenter-Song E (2001) The new paradigm of recovery from schizophrenia: cultural conundrums of improvement without cure. Cult Med Psychiatry 29:379–413

Kaplan K, Kottsieper P, Scott J et al (2009) Adoption and safe families act state statutes regarding parental mental illnesses: a review and targeted intervention. Psychiatr Rehabil J 33(2):91–94

Leamy M, Bird V, Le Boutillier C, Williams J, Slade M (2011) Conceptual framework for personal recovery in mental health: systematic review and narrative synthesis. Br J Psychiatry 199(6):445–452

Leinonen J, Solantaus T, Runamäki RL (2003) Parental mental health and children's adjustment: the quality of marital interaction and parenting as mediating factors. J Child Psychol Psychiatry 44(2):227–241

Mancini M, Hardiman E, Lawson H (2005) Making sense of it all: consumer providers' theories about factors facilitating and impeding recovery from psychiatric disabilities. Psychiatr Rehabil J 29:48–55

Maybery DJ, Reupert AE (2009) Parental mental illness: a review of barriers and issues for working with families and children. J Psychiatr Ment Health Nurs 16(9):784–791

Maybery D, Reupert A, Patrick K, Goodyear M, Crase L (2009) Prevalence of children whose parents have a mental illness. Psychiatr Bull 33(1):22–26

Maybery D, Goodyear M, Reupert A, Harkness M (2012) Goal setting within family care planning: families with complex needs. Med J Aust 16:37–39

Maybery DJ, Goodyear MJ, O'Hanlon B, Cuff R, Reupert AE (2014) Profession differences in family focused practice in the adult mental health system. Fam Process 53(4):608–617

Maybery DJ, Meadows GN, Clark J, Sutton K, Reupert AE, Nicholson J (2015) A personal recovery model for parents with mental health problems. In: Reupert A, Maybery D, Nicholson J, Gopfert M, Seeman M (eds) Parental psychiatric disorder: distressed parents and their families. Cambridge, Cambridge University Press, pp 312–323

Mental Health Commission of Canada (2012) Changing directions, changing lives: the mental health strategy for Canada. Mental Health Commission of Canada, Calgary

Nicholson J (2014) Supporting mothers living with mental illnesses in recovery. In: Benders-Hadi N, Barber ME (eds) Motherhood, mental illness and recovery. Springer, New York, pp 3–17

Nicholson J, Biebel K, Katz-Leavy J, Williams V (2004) Prevalence of parenthood in adults with mental illness: implications for state and federal policy, programs, and providers. Substance Abuse and Mental Health Services Administration, Rockville, MD

Reupert AE, Maybery D (2007) Families affected by parental mental illness: a multiperspective account of issues and interventions. Am J Orthopsychiatry 77(3):362–369

Reupert A, Maybery D (2009) Fathers' experience of parenting with a mental illness. Fam Soc 90(1):61–68

Reupert A, Green K, Maybery D (2008) Family care plans for families affected by parental mental illness. Fam Soc 89(1):39–43

Reupert A, Goodyear M, Maybery D (2012) Engaging with, and understanding children whose parents have a dual diagnosis. Child Adolesc Mental Health 17(3):153–160

Reupert AE, Maybery DJ, Cox M, Scott Stokes E (2015a) Place of family in recovery models for those with a mental illness. Int J Ment Health Nurs 24(6):495–506

Reupert AE, Maybery DJ, Morgan B (2015b) E-learning professional development resources for families where a parent has a mental illness. In: Reupert A, Maybery D, Nicholson J, Gopfert M, Seeman M (eds) Parental psychiatric disorder: distressed parents and their families. Cambridge, Cambridge University Press, pp 288–300

Riebschleger J (2004) Good days and bad days: the experiences of children with a parent with a psychiatric disability. Psychiatr Rehabil J 28:25–31

Rosenbaum P, King S, Law M, King G, Evans J (1998) Family-centred service: a conceptual framework and research review. Phys Occup Ther Paediatr 18:1–20

Solantaus T, Reupert AE, Maybery DJ (2015) Working with parents who have a psychiatric disorder. In: Reupert A, Maybery D, Nicholson J, Gopfert M, Seeman M (eds) Parental psychiatric disorder: distressed parents and their families. Cambridge, Cambridge University Press, pp 238–247

Trondsen M (2012) Living with a mentally ill parent: exploring adolescents' experiences and perspectives. Qual Health Res 22(2):174–188

Wyder M, Bland R (2014) The recovery framework as a way of understanding families' responses to mental illness: balancing different needs and recovery journeys. Aust Soc Work 67(2):179–196

Psychiatric/Mental Health Nursing and Mental Health Promotion: An Eight Steps Path

23

José Carlos Rodrigues Gomes

23.1 Introduction: Understanding Mental Health

Being of or achieving 'good health' is a value shared by all persons regardless of their geographic, religious, ethnic, socioeconomic or cultural position. Health is a characteristic shared by individuals and society that is built in all policies, in all sectors of society. There is no health without mental health (World Health Organization 2001). Mental health is a broad concept, one that is related to all society elements, and with society itself: how we organize ourselves, how we think, how we relate with ourselves and with each other and how we promote the development of our societal structures and resources. A very common misconception is that mental health cannot be promoted and that mental disorders "are not treatable" and cannot be avoided (Oxley 2012). Consequently, issues related to mental health continue to carry a huge stigma and a deep discrimination, portrayed in negative attitudes toward mental disorders, still too common and with high social, economic and health related costs (World Health Organization 2001; European Commission 2005; Gomes and Loureiro 2013; Organization for Economic Co-operation and Development 2014). In everyday language, the term mental health is used in different ways, and very often has a negative connotation because it is most commonly related to, and talked about in terms of serious and chronic mental health problems or so-called mental illness.

However, the positive aspects of mental health have been increasingly recognized in the scientific community in recent years, but also, to a lesser extent, by the community and policy makers, largely due to actions and reports of various

J.C.R. Gomes
Health Research Unit, School of health Sciences, polytechnic Institute of Leiria, Leiria, Portugal
e-mail: jcrgomes@ipleiria.pt

© Springer International Publishing Switzerland 2018

J.C. Santos, J.R. Cutcliffe (eds.), *European Psychiatric/Mental Health Nursing in the 21st Century*, Principles of Specialty Nursing,
https://doi.org/10.1007/978-3-319-31772-4_23

international organizations. Mental health can be compared to a natural, renewable resource and must be understood as a continuous process that takes place throughout the life cycle. In favourable circumstances, mental health may increase or improve. But mental health can be exploited beyond its natural capacity for renewal, and ultimately, mental health can be challenged, compromised or destroyed by inappropriate actions of society, giving rise to mental health problems (Gomes and Loureiro 2013).

If it is true that mental health is a concept related to the individual, many researchers have expanded the concept including groups (mostly family), organizations (e.g., schools, communities and workplaces) and even the whole society (World Health Organization 2001; Ozamiz et al. 2006; Lethinen 2008; Gomes and Loureiro 2013). Several mental health promotion programmes with this broad approach have been published and evaluated. There is an increasing amount of evidence that mental health promotion is useful and effective, as we can observe in Box 23.1.

Box 23.1 Effectiveness of Some Mental Health Promotion Program

Mental health promotion program (country)	Reference(s) and source(s)	Population and Main results
Midwestern prevention project (USA)	Chou CP, Montgomery S, Pentz MA, Rohrbach LA, Johnson CA, Flay BR, MacKinnon DP. (1998). Effects of a community-based prevention program on decreasing drug use in high-risk adolescents. *American Journal of Public Health,* 88: 944–948. Riggs NR, Pentz MA. (2009). Long-term effects of adolescent marijuana use prevention on adult mental health services utilization: the midwestern prevention project. Substance Use & Misuse. 2009;44(5):616-31. doi: 10.1080/10826080902809691.	Population: Community adolescents 1998: Reduction up to 40% in adolescents' tobacco and marijuana daily use reduction in the consumption of alcohol and other drugs, improvement of constructive communication between parents and children 2009: Findings support the role of early adolescent drug use prevention programs in impacting later mental health problems
Environmental influences on psychological restoration (Sweden)	Hartig T, Evans GW, Jamner LD, Davis DS, Gärling T. (2003). Tracking restoration in natural and urban field settings. *Journal of Environmental Psychology, 23*: 109–123	Population: Healthy adults Psychological restoration, and a subjective experience of relaxation, was significantly faster in those who walked the pedestrian path than those who walked on a city street
Aerobic exercise (USA)	DiLorenzo TM, Bargman EP, Stucky-Ropp R, Brassington GS, Frensch PA, LaFontaine T. (1999). Long-term effects of aerobic exercise on psychological outcomes. *Preventive Medicine, 28:* 75–85.	Population: Healthy adults The participants not only acquired physiological benefits, but also psychological improvements, particularly in situations of depression. After 1 year, significant increase in physical and mental well-being was still present.

Sure start local programs (SSLP) (UK)	The National Evaluation of sure start team. (2007). *National evaluation of Sure Start*. Birkbeck. University of London. http://www.ness.bbk. uk/findings.asp.	Population: Children from 12 to 36 months and their families in deprived urban areas Parents of children under 3 years showed less negative parenting to provide a home and a more favourable learning environment for their children. Children 3 years showed better social development with higher levels of positive social behaviour, and were more independent.
MindMatters (Australia)	Wyn J, Cahill H, Holdsworth R, Rowling L, Carson S. (2000). MindMatters, a whole-school approach promoting mental health and well-being. *Australian and New Zealand Journal of Psychiatry, 34*: 594–601.	Population: Students from secondary school There was an improvement in the identification of students with their school. Identified evidence suggesting that the response of bullying teachers improved. Students who participated in skills development activities felt more confident in their ability to deal with the issues of mental health. Teachers said that the initiative gave them the confidence and skills needed to better support and understand the needs of students.
Developing health promotion in health centre (Finland)	Berkels H et al. (2004). *Mental Health Promotion and Prevention Strategies for Coping with Anxiety, Depression and Stress Related Disorders in Europe. Final Report.* Publications series from the Federal Institute for Occupational Safety and Health, research report Fb 1011, Dortmund: Berlin-Dresden.	Population: Health professionals The impact of the program was shown in (1) improving skills in solving group problems; (2) reduce absenteeism; and (3) increased employee motivation.
The clubhouse model (USA)	McKay C, Johnsen M, Stein R. (2005). Employment outcome in Massachusetts clubhouses. *Psychiatric Rehabilitation Journal, 29:* 25–33.	Population: People with severe mental health problems The evaluation showed that the clubhouse model is effective in reducing hospitalization rates and improve the quality of life as well as in promoting employment, social inclusion, and interpersonal relations.

(continued)

Box 23.1 (continued)

Good neighbour scheme (UK)	Good neighbour scheme. Suffolk ACRE. http://www.suffolkacre.org.uk/main.php.	Population: Older people in community The results have shown an increase in self-esteem and higher positive emotional level. Most users (80%) reported more human company and 52% reported spending more time away from home.
"Pensar saudável, Viver Saudável" [*think healthy. Live healthy*] project (Portugal)	Gomes, J.C.; Cravo, L.; Gaspar, P. (2010). *Projeto "Pensar saudável, Viver Saudável": uma (boa) prática de educação para a saúde baseada na formação pelos pares*. In Pereira, H. e tal (ed.). *Educação para Saúde, Cidadania e desenvolvimento sustentado.* Covilhã. Universidade da Beira Interior.	Population: 9th grade students Recognition of the effectiveness of the project in increasing the school's recognition as a source of health information, improved self-perceived impact of health information, and healthier eating behaviours.
Plano local de Promoção da Saúde mental de Amora [*local mental health promotion plan*] (Portugal)	Gomes, J.C.; Loureiro, I. (2013) O lugar da investigação participada de base comunitária na promoção da saúde mental. *Revista Portuguesa de Saúde Pública, 31 (1)*: 32–48.	Population: An urban community Confirmed the need for an active and effective participation of the community in the development of local health promotion policies

23.2 How Much Can We Save with Effective Mental Health Promotion?

The high prevalence of mental health problems, associated with a chronic and long-term course, imposes a heavy economic burden on society, aggravated by early inaugural frames, often in adolescence or young adult. Data is scarce but it has been pointed out that the burden of providing mental health care, on the gross domestic product (GDP), is 3–4% (International Labour Organization 2000; World Health Organization–Regional Office for Europe 2011; Organization for Economic Co-operation and Development 2014). Higher than the budget deficit limit allowed by the European Commission (3% of GDP) (European Commission 1997). One of the main obstacles to ensure more and better mental health is increasing demands and conflicting allocation of resources (Frewen and Datta 2010). During a recession, like the one experienced recently in Europe, these demands become more intense. In a world that seems more and more worried with finances, money and budgets, economic arguments tend to be highly valued (Van Hilten 2015). While it may be argued that an efficient and effective mental health system should be a priority, others argue that available funds are insufficient to build this structure now. To make budget decision makers understand the merits of investing in mental health promotion rather than other priorities is problematic, mainly because the results or outcomes arising from a mental health promotion intervention is a process that goes far beyond the political calendar or the anxieties of economic markets (Jacka and Reavley 2014). We can observe a similar dynamic in some European countries where, unfortunately, P/MHN are seen as a cost rather than as an investment (Gomes 2015).

Even so, there is a growing body of evidence that shows that the lack of effective resolution of mental health problems results in significant economic repercussions (Organization for Economic Co-operation and Development 2014). To properly assess the costs of mental health, it is not enough to simply consider the costs involved in providing responsive, secondary level, mental health care. The biggest economic impact of mental health problems surges because of their consequences in families, in social life, in urban areas, in labour productivity and in economy. Accordingly, there is a compelling economic case for attempting to prevent the development of debilitating mental health problems in the first place (primary mental health promotion) rather than waiting for mental health problems to occur and then responding to these.

23.3 Building and Promoting Mental Health in an Eight Steps Path

A social/ecological determinants of mental health approach incorporates a deep understanding on how the environment and behaviour affect social processes and the risk of challenges to health ease, and how social and structural conditions increase or decrease persons' and communities' opportunities to be healthy. This approach highlights the importance of cross-cutting interventions that are planned and implemented in various community sectors, with emphasis on the influence of one or more health determinants, rather than focusing on disease determinants. The large body of evidence concerning health determinants is consistent in showing complex interactions among factors and variables across social, environmental, economic and biological dimensions (World Health Organization 2003; Marmot 2005; Gomes and Loureiro 2013). Some of the individual (e.g. age, gender, ethnicity) and genetic factors are not viable targets for mental health promotion activities, although they are important determinants of mental health. So, the challenge for P/MHN is to focus on determinants that can be controlled: on an *eight steps path* (Ozamiz et al. 2006; Lethinen 2008; Gomes and Loureiro 2013).

23.3.1 Step 1: Developing Mental Health Policies

The first step is related to the development of a comprehensive mental health policy. P/MHN should be, though historically they seldom have been, a key contributor to the construction of mental health policy, not least (though certainly not only limited to) in designing mental health plans at regional/local level. A mental health policy on a regional basis should adopt a comprehensive approach and include reference to modern mental health legislation (Lavikainen et al. 2000). This legislation must be based on a mental health policies analysis and on a health impact assessment (WHO 2005) allowing mental health program design (Gomes and Loureiro 2013) that defines how mental health policies will be implemented in practice.

A comprehensive mental health policy is not realized only through the social and health sectors. A deep cooperation between different sectors such as education, employment, housing, environment, economy and justice is vital to success (Loureiro et al. 2011). An active human resources policy (International Council of Nurses 2009) must assure the availability of high quality human resources through adequate provision of mental health training for nurses and other health professionals and for all social and education professionals. In addition, the basic training *curriculum* of many other professions should include training on mental health promotion and other relevant topics related to mental health (employment, justice system and environmental planning). The inclusion of users and carers should be a guiding principle in all social planning and implementation of activities that influence people's well-being, since family has often been considered more as interference, rather than as an effective partner. An information system for comprehensive mental health must be available for effective community mental health level monitoring, planning services, resources allocation, interventions evaluation (Lavikainen et al. 2006) and to design programs to fight stigma that makes it difficult, in many ways, to establish a comprehensive framework for mental health services in society. To fulfil all these requisites, research on mental health promotion and mental health policies should be supported by specific research programs, developed by multidisciplinary teams that include mental health professionals (including P/MHN) and local, regional and national research community to ensure the necessary knowledge about the specific circumstances of each country or region.

Community-based participatory research (Minkler and Wallerstein 2008; Gomes and Loureiro 2013) is a useful methodology to promote changes in the way we organize our societies, empowering individuals and communities. Adequate funding is necessary to ensure sustainability of different mental health interventions. Experience has shown that mental health position, often undervalued compared with other health sectors, easily inhibits the development of the mental health sector (Lethinen 2008). Therefore, it is preferable to have a separate budget for mental health as well as for mental health promotion and mental and behavioural disorders prevention (World Health Organization 2003; European Commission 2005; Gomes and Loureiro 2013).

23.3.2 Step 2: Build Mentally Healthy Communities

Wherever nurses work, their focus is on the individual, his/her family—its health, its ability to grow, care for itself, and contribute to the community (International Council of Nurses 2002). A person's mental health is closely related to the characteristics of the community where he/she lives (Lethinen 2008; WHO 2011; Gomes and Loureiro 2013). The development of mental health promoting communities, e.g., communities that increase social capital (Putnam et al. 1993) requires the proper implementation of policies and mental health programs. Therefore, P/MHN should involve community leaders and stakeholders to support the creation of different types of joint activities and networks that facilitate the participation of all in community development (Lethinen 2008; WHO 2011; Minkler and Wallerstein 2008; Gomes and Loureiro 2013). Empowerment (WHO 1986) is the keyword for this effort. Self-help groups have proved to be cost-effective in helping people deal or cope with the challenges (and mental health risks) associated with different types of stressful life events such as unemployment, divorce, death of a spouse, dependence on drugs or alcohol or family violence issues (Levine, Perkins & Perkins; 2005). Family and friends are commonly support systems but this is certainly not always the case and not all people are able to make use of these support systems, like the elderly, single parents, immigrants and people with mental health problems (Leggatt 2002).

A healthy community coordinates along with religious and volunteer organizations, the necessary social support for these people, through different social support programs types, community work and in facilitating access to different community services (North Mersey Mental Health Improvement Program 2005; McKenzie and Harpham 2006). Respect for diversity and human rights must be these activities basis. An essential healthy community feature is the availability of low-cost community-based mental health services. Services should cover a broad spectrum of activities including the promotion of equity and social justice. No one should be discriminated because of their social status, religion, educational level, ethnicity, age, gender, skills, sexual orientation or political opinion (Okazaki 2009). Equal access to education and employment are basic characteristics of communities with social justice (Cities Environment Report on the Internet 2004). A standard of living adequate for a dignified life should be ensured for all (World Bank 1999).

23.3.3 Step 3: Develop Physical Environment

Since the days of Florence Nightingale, nurses have noted the close relation between physical environment and health (Canadian Nurse Association 2005). This relation is much more complex today. It is therefore important to ensure that mental health aspects are sufficiently considered in urban planning and housing, building mentally healthy living environments (Russell and Killoran 2000). To provide parks and other green spaces in urban areas assure people have a place to walk and enjoy the environment (OECD 1997). Urban environments with high density (CEROI 2004) provide few opportunities for children to play which justify the need to build a network of playgrounds and adventure parks for children of different age levels. Noise and population density are known to be associated with an increased risk of stress and low level of wellness (WHO 1997). All urban areas must have programs to reduce noise and overcrowding of streets and other public places. People should be able to live without fear of violence or harassment in the streets or other public places (Ginot et al. 1997). This can be achieved by assuring public security developing programs to combat bullying, sexual harassment and physical violence.

23.3.4 Step 4: Opportunities to Provide Recreational Activities and Civic Participation

Relaxation, recreation and positive life experiences are important elements in support of a person's mental well-being. P/MHN should work with the community to provide opportunities for education in leisure fostering pleasure, self-fulfilment and new skills development. Subject areas may include foreign languages, crafts, gardening, different artistic activities, or even other hobbies. It has been clearly shown that physical activity positively influences mental health (Hillsdon et al. 2004; Penedo and Dahn 2005). Thus, sports fields, public pools, cycle paths, jogging trails and gymnasiums and other sport facilities should be accessible (Russell & Killoran, 2000). Art in its different forms allows one to relive experiences. This can have a positive influence on mental health, creating opportunities for identification and self-analysis, to a positive emotional experience and for catharsis. Cultural centres, libraries, theatres, art galleries and concert halls not only provide artistic experiences for people, but also provide better health (CEROI 2004). Community networks and civic participation are social capital hallmarks. Participation in youth organizations such as the Scout movement, theatrical youth groups or other similar activities to enhance cooperation and mutual accountability has proved important for adolescents' healthy psychological development (Dibben et al. 2016). Families with young children need special attention. Providing joint activities for parents and children is one of the useful means of support (Allen and Daly 2007).

23.3.5 Step 5: Improving Children's Mental Health in Early Childhood

The basis for mental health in adulthood is built up in childhood. This age group is the most favourable period for the development of activities to promote effective mental health (Gomes 2010). Since the family environment is the natural environment where the child lives and parents are the most important child caregivers, mental health promotion activities should be directed to the whole family. A comprehensive maternal care available for all pregnant women should be organized including regular follow-up visits throughout pregnancy, providing both physical risk and psychosocial risk factors identification. A parental education for both parents (Sonego; Llácer, Galén & Simón; 2013) during pregnancy should be an integral part of public maternal and child health services. A secure early attachment between infant and primary caregiver is a key element for healthy child development (Bowlby, 1969; Ainsworth, 1991). A more generous parental leave after childbirth is associated with better mental health in old age (Avendano et al. 2015). The close relations with both parents are important for the healthy development of the child, and the father should use part of this parental leave (Lethinen 2008). It is important that post-natal care do not look only for the physical development of the child, but also can monitor the child's psychological development, that means that a new understanding of post-natal care is necessary. To support both families and children, it is essential that the community establish a network of well-distributed and high quality kinder gardens with early childhood development interventions (D'Onise et al. 2010). A special emphasis should be directed to parents and families in which there is an increased risk for undesirable child development. Mental health nursing home visits are examples of programs and services to develop effective support (Tamaki 2008).

23.3.6 Step 6: Promoting Mentally Healthy Schools

The school is the place where we find the clear majority of children and adolescents between 6 and 17 years of age (Gomes et al. 2010). Thus, it is both logical and appropriate that most universal activities that promote mental health targeted at these age groups are enacted in schools. Moreover, these activities can be easily integrated into school daily activities. The basis of school mental health promotion focuses on a good pedagogical relationship that promotes respect, autonomy and responsibility (Portugal, Ministério da Educação e Ministério da Saúde, Comissão de Coordenação da Promoção e Educação para a Saúde 2001; Weare 2006). Mental health issues should be integrated throughout the curriculum as a cross-cutting principle covering all school subjects. Education for mental health should continue throughout the school career using a comprehensive approach (Weare 2006) and integrating mental health in school policy and its *curriculum*. A health promoting school offers psychological support to their students, where appropriate. This means that school nurses are an integral part of the school staff and participate in daily school activities so that they can familiarize with the students. Teachers may also need emotional support. The team discussions, individual or group supervision and the possibility of consultation with a mental health specialist (namely a P/MHN) are some ways to help overcome problems. An essential element in the healthy school concept is the active participation of parents in discussions and decision-making concerning their child. A close contact between parents and teachers is a favourable element for all partners involved in the school community. Teamwork strengthens students' sense of solidarity and social skills being one of the compelling keywords in a mentally healthy school daily life. Similarly, cooperation and team work are also important for teachers and staff. The participation of students in all life school levels is also an important element for good mental health. Specific mental health promotion programs have proven effective in improving psychological well-being and safety in schools. Each school must draw the most appropriate programs to their needs and their goals (Wyn et al. 2000; Gomes et al. 2010; Gomes and Loureiro 2013).

23.3.7 Step 7: Promote Mentally Healthy Professional Life

Work is of fundamental importance in human life (Harnois and Gabriel 2000). It is essential for the survival of both society and individual, and satisfies certain basic human needs. It was through work that humanity created both material well-being and abstract culture. Many aspects of the work have a positive impact on mental health worker (Ozamiz et al. 2001). The relationship between work and mental health is complex. Depending on the circumstances work may hinder or promote workers' mental health. Creating a mentally healthy workplace is primarily a responsibility of businesses and employers, together with workers and their representatives. Regular and satisfying work is a cornerstone of the adult population good mental health. Therefore, full employment should be the aim of a comprehensive employment policy. For those whose unemployment shows extension in time, actions should be available to avoid social exclusion and marginalization (Wheaton 1999; Gomes 2004). An important feature of a mentally healthy workplace is that workers have a real and genuine opportunity to contribute to decision making on the strategy, the communication policy and the management of human resources workplace, as well as on the individual working conditions, tasks and objectives. Discrimination, mobbing and sexual harassment are very serious risk factors to workplace mental health level (Freire et al. 2008). Thus, every workplace should have agreed an anti-discrimination action plan on these negative events, involving the whole community.

23.3.8 Step 8: Promoting Mental Health of the Elderly

The number of older people in the community is rapidly increasing in all European countries. Older people face risks in relation to their mental health (Lethinen 2008). Concrete ways to promote mental health in this age group include participation opportunities in community political, economic and cultural decision and learning throughout life, ensuring social participation. Some elderly people live alone and may feel lonely, especially if they have difficulty leaving home. Therefore, programs that seek to help the older person in their everyday life should be organized by the community. Different types of clubs, recreation centres and other social networks can prevent loneliness and isolation (Singh et al. 2016). Feelings of independence and autonomy are also important for older people. These can be strengthened by supporting the creation of "*smart homes*", the provision of equipment to facilitate communication and mobility, and providing employment opportunities in old age or encouraging older employees to stay in the labour market. A poor physical health in older age is a clear risk factor for mental health problems. Therefore, it is important to establish a system of social and health care to provide all elderly primary health services and expertise with high quality, including easy access to psychiatric services, as well as all necessary services and social benefits (Lis et al. 2008). The negative and derogatory attitudes toward aging and older people continue to prevail in our society. We must ensure that human rights are respected about the elderly, fighting against ageism (Butler 1995). One of the possible ways is giving by the *gerotranscendence* theory (Rajani and Jawaid 2015). Tornstam's earlier work (Tornstam 1997) on aging revealed that aging is a natural developmental process towards maturity and wisdom. This advancement in age is accompanied by a gradual shift in meta-paradigm of an aging person, which Tornstam termed as Gerotranscendence: Gero refers to "old" and transcendence means "rising above". Per Tornstam (1997), "It is a shift in meta-perspective from a materialistic and rational view of the world to a more cosmic and transcendent one, normally followed by an increase in life satisfaction" (Tornstam 1997, p. 2).

23.4 Concluding Remarks: Psychiatric/Mental Health Nurse: The Possible Main Mental Health Promoter?

A health promoter is defined as a professional who works to promote health and reduce health inequalities through the practice of different actions (Barry and Jenkins 2007). Despite this broad definition, it is recognized that the combination of knowledge and skills necessary to ensure the practical quality in mental health promotion need specific training—namely in public health, social sciences, epidemiology, education, communication, environment, community, urban or rural development and political science (Barry et al. 2012).

To become a mental health promoter, P/MHN must understand the theory (and apply it in practice), namely, community-based research methodologies, values and health promotion multidisciplinary knowledge base. P/MHN must promote change, empowering individuals, communities and organizations to improve health and reduce health inequalities by performing a variety of health promotion activities, as described on this eight steps path. Furthermore, P/MHN must be skilled in advocating with (and on behalf of) individuals, communities and organizations to improve health and well-being and increase their capacity to carry out health promotion actions. To achieve this, P/MHN must mediate through partnerships and work collaboratively through different areas of knowledge, sectors and partners to improve health promotion actions impact and sustainability. P/MHN must communicate effectively health promotion activities by appropriate methods for different audiences and show leadership, contributing to the development of a shared vision and strategic direction for health promotion action. P/MHN should evaluate the needs and availabilities in environments and systems that lead to political, economic, social, cultural, environmental, behavioural and biological determinants identification and analysis that promote or compromise health. Rooted in this evaluation, P/MHN must plan and develop measurable active health and health promotion goals in response to assessed needs. And then, identify and implement evidence-based strategies to promote effective and efficient culturally sensitive to ethical values health, including human resources and material resources management. Finally, as a mental health promoter, P/MHN must know how to evaluate research and determine health promotion actions scope effectiveness and impact.

Box 23.2 Competences of General Care Nurses

A. Competence to independently diagnose the nursing care required using current theoretical and clinical knowledge as well as to plan, organize and implement nursing care when treating patients based on the knowledge and skills
B. acquired to improve professional practice;
C. Competence to work together effectively with other players in the health sector including participation in the practical training of health personnel based on the knowledge and skills acquired;
D. Competence to empower individuals, families and groups towards healthy lifestyles and self-care based on the knowledge and skills acquired;
E. Competence to independently initiate immediate measures to pre-serve life and to carry out measures in crisis and disaster situations;
F. Competence to independently advise, instruct and support individuals needing care and their attachment figures;
G. Competence to independently ensure the quality of nursing care and assess it;
H. Competence to communicate comprehensively and professionally and to cooperate with members of other professions in the health sector;
I. Competence to analyse the quality of care to improve their own professional practice as general care nurses.

Source: European Federation of Nurses Associations (2015)

Despite the existence of general nursing health promotion competences (EFN, 2015) which are listed in Box 23.2, the proposed *eight steps path* must be executed by P/MHN with advanced training in mental health nursing (including health promotion). The recognition of advanced skills in mental health nursing, both from an academic and from a political and human resources management point of view is important to achieve success in building communities' mental health and make possible for P/MHN to work as effective mental health promoters.

References

Allen S, Daly K (2007) The effects of father involvement: an updated research summary of the evidence. Centre for Families, Work & Well-being, University of Guelph, Guelph, ON

Avendano M, Berkmanb L, Brugiavinid A, Pasinid G (2015) The long-run effect of maternity leave benefits on mental health: evidence from European countries. Soc Sci Med 132:45–53

Ainsworth M (1991) Attachment and other affectional bonds across the life cycle. In: Parkes C, Stevenson-Hinde J, Marris P (eds) Attachment across the life cycle. Routledge, New York, pp 33–51

Barry M, Battel-Kirk B, Dempsey C (2012) The CompHP core competencies framework for health promotion in Europe. Health Educ Behav 39(6):648–662

Barry M, Jenkins R (2007) Implementing mental health promotion. Elsevier, London

Berkels H, Henderson J, Henke N, Kuhn K, Lavikainen J, Lehtinen V, Ozamiz A, Van Den Heede P, Zengiger K (2004) Mental health promotion and prevention strategies for coping with anxiety, depression and stress related disorders in Europe: final report 2001–2003. Publications Series from the Federal Institute for Occupational Safety and Health, Dortmund. 3-86509-118-0

Bowlby J (1969) Attachment and loss: attachment, vol 1. Basic Books, New York

Butler R (1995) Ageism. In: Maddox G (ed) The encyclopedia of aging. Springer, New York

Canadian Nurses Association [CAN] (2005) The ecosystem, the environment, and health and nursing: a summary of the issues. Canadian Nurses Association, Ottawa, ON

CEROI (Cities Environment Report on the Internet) (2004) Available at: www.ceroi.net. Accessed 5 Jan 2010

D'Onise K, Lynch J, Sawyer M, McDermott R (2010) Can preschool improve child health outcomes? A systematic review. Soc Sci Med 70(9):1423–1440

Dibben C, Playford C, Mitchell M (2016) Be(ing) prepared: guide and scout participation, childhood social position and mental health at age 50—a prospective birth cohort study. J Epidemiol Community Health. Published Online First: 10 November 2016

European Commission [EC] (1997) Resolution of the European Council on the Stability and Growth Pact (Amsterdam, 17 June 1997) [Official Journal C 236 of 02.08.1997]. Brussels

European Commission [EC] (2005) Green paper: improving the mental health of the population: towards a strategy on mental health for the European Union. Brussels, Health and Consumer Protection Directorate-General

European Federation of Nurses Associations [EFN] (2015) EFN competency framework. EFN guideline to implement article 31 into national nurses' education programs. European Federation of Nurses Associations, Brussels

Freire P, Novek S, Menec V, Tran T (2008) Assédio moral e saúde mental do trabalhador. Trabalho, Educação e Saúde 6(2):367–380. Rio de Janeiro July/Oct

Frewen N, Datta A (2010) The socio-economic realities of mental health in Ireland. TASK Thinkpieces, Dublin

Ginot L, Ait-Bouali N, Besse M, Chevalier P, Goldberg F, Buisson J (1997) Health and violence as perceived by young people, a study of the parisian region. Sante Publique 9(4):379–396

Gomes J, Loureiro I (2013) O lugar da investigação participada de base comunitária na promoção da saúde mental. Revista Portuguesa de Saúde Pública 31(1):32–48

Gomes J (2004) Desemprego, depressão e sentido de coerência: uma visão do desemprego sob o prisma da saúde pública. Relatório de Investigação para obtenção do Grau de Mestre em Saúde Pública pela Escola nacional de Saúde Pública da Universidade Nova de Lisboa. Lisboa. Escola nacional de Saúde Pública da Universidade Nova de Lisboa. Available at: http://www.ensp.unl.pt/saboga/soc/pulic/04_01_sco_depressao_desemprego.pdf

Gomes J (2010) Saúde mental no ciclo vital. In: Sequeira C, Sá L (eds) Do diagnóstico á Intervenção em Saúde Mental. Sociedade Portuguesa de Enfermagem de Saúde Mental, Porto

Gomes J (2015) Saúde, formação em saúde e desenvolvimento: ousar um novo paradigma. In Cordeiro, R. (Ed.) 35 Anos do SNS … Ideias para o futuro do SNS: o contributo dos enfermeiros. Available at: https://issuu.com/raulcordeiro3/docs/ebookfinal.docx

Gomes J, Cravo L, Gaspar P (2010) Projeto "Pensar saudável, Viver Saudável": uma (boa) prática de educação para a saúde baseada na formação pelos pares. In: Pereira H et al (eds) Educação para Saúde, Cidadania e desenvolvimento sustentado. Universidade da Beira Interior, Covilhã

Harnois G, Gabriel P (2000) Mental health at work: impact, issues and good practices. World Health Organization and International Labour Organisation, Geneva

Hillsdon M, Foster C, Naidoo B, Crombie H (2004) The effectiveness of public health interventions for increasing physical activity among adults: a review of reviews. Yorkshire, Health Development Agency. 1-84279-192-3

International Council of Nurses [ICN] (2002) Nurses always there for you: caring for families. In: International nurses' day 2002. International Council of Nurses, Geneva

International Council of Nurses [ICN] (2009) Guidelines on planning human resources for nursing. International Council of Nurses, Geneva

International Labour Organization [ILO] (2000) Mental health in the workplace. International Labour Organization, Geneva

Jacka F, Reavley N (2014) Prevention of mental disorders: evidence, challenges and opportunities. BMC Med 12:75. Available at: http://www.biomedcentral.com/1741-7015/12/75. First published: May, 9 2014

Lavikainen J, Fryers T, Lehtinen V (eds) (2006) Improving mental health information in Europe. Proposal of the MINDFUL project. National Research and Development Centre for Welfare and Health, Helsinki

Lavikainen J, Lahtinen E, Lehtinen V (eds) (2000) Public health approach on mental health in Europe. National Research and Development Centre for Welfare and Health, Helsinky

Leggatt M (2002) Families and mental health workers: the need for partnership. World Psychiatry 1(1):52–54

Lethinen V (ed) (2008) Building up good mental health. Monitoring mental health environments project, co-funding by the European Union. National Research and Development Centre for Welfare and Health, Helsinki

Lis K, Reichert M, Cosack A, Billings J, Brown P (eds) (2008) Evidence-based guidelines on health promotion for older people. Austrian Red Cross, Vienna

Loureiro I, Gomes J, Dias L, Santos M (2011) A Investigação participada de base comunitária na construção da saúde. Projeto de capacitação em promoção da saúde – PROCAPS: resultados de um estudo exploratório. Instituto Nacional de Saúde Doutor Ricardo Jorge, IP, Lisboa

Marmot M (2005) Social determinants of health inequalities. Lancet 365:1099–1104

McKenzie K, Harpham T (eds) (2006) Social capital and mental health. Jessica Kingsley Publishers, London

Murray L, Perkins D, Perkins D (2005) Principles of community psychology: perspectives and applications, 3rd edn. Oxford University Press, New York

North Mersey Mental Health Improvement Program [NMMHIP] (2005) Building healthy communities. a proposed model for commissioning for health and not just for illness. Available at: http://www.primhe.org/pdf/primhe_healthycommunities.pdf

Okazaki S (2009) Impact of racism on ethnic minority mental health. Perspect Psychol Sci 4(1):103–107

Organization for Economic Co-operation and Development [OECD] (1997) Better understanding our cities: the role of urban indicators. OECD, Paris

Organization for Economic Co-operation and Development [OECD] (2014) Making mental health count: the social and economic cost of neglecting mental health care, OECD health policy studies. OECD Publishing

Oxley L (2012) Mental health: myths and misconceptions: common ways in which mental health issues are misunderstood. Cambridge Psychol J. [Internet]. The Cambridge Student Psychology Journal. Available at: https://cambridgepsychologyjournal.wordpress.com/article/mental-health-myths-and-misconceptions/

Ozamiz J et al (2006) Structural indicators of positive mental health. In: Lavikainen J, Fryers T, Lehtinen V (eds) Improving mental health information in Europe. Proposal of the MINDFUL project. National Research and Development Centre for Welfare and Health, Helsinki

Ozamiz J, Gumplmaier H, Lehtinen V (2001) Unemployment and mental health. University of Deusto, Bilbao

Penedo F, Dahn J (2005) Exercise and well-being: a review of mental and physical health benefits associated with physical activity. Curr Opin Psychiatry 18(2):189–193

Portugal, Ministério da Educação e Ministério da Saúde, Comissão de Coordenação da Promoção e Educação para a Saúde (2001) A Rede Nacional de Escolas Promotoras de Saúde. Editorial do Ministério da Educação, Lisboa

Putnam R, Nanetti N, Leonardi R (1993) Making democracy work: civic tradition in modern Italy. Princeton, Princeton, NJ

Rajani F, Jawaid H (2015) Theory of gerotranscendence: an analysis. Austin Journal of Psychiatry and Behavioral Sciences 2(1):1035. Austin Publishing Group. Published online first: April, 21 2015

Russell H, Killoran A (2000) Public health and regeneration: making the links. Health Education Authority, London. 0-7521-1804-8

Singh L, Singh P, Arokiasamy P (2016) Social network and mental health among older adults in rural Uttar Pradesh, India: a cross-sectional study. J Cross Cult Gerontol 31(2):173–192

Sonego M, Llácer A, Galán I, Simón F (2013) The influence of parental education on child mental health in Spain. Qual Life Res 22(1):203–211

Tamaki A (2008) Effectiveness of home visits by mental health nurses for Japanese women with post-partum depression. Int J Ment Health Nurs 17(6):419–427

Tornstam L (1997) Life crises and gerotranscendence. J Aging Identity 2:117–131

Van Hilten L (2015) Atlas award: to be sustainable, healthcare policy should focus on more than economics. Policymakers need to consider social and political sustainability as well, researchers say. Econ Soc Sci. Posted on May, 21 2015

Weare K (2006) Promoting mental, emotional and social health. A whole school approach. Routledge, New York

Wheaton B (1999) The nature of stressors. In: Horwitz A, Sheid T (eds) A handbook for the study of mental health: social contexts, theories, and systems. Cambridge University Press, Cambridge, UK

World Bank (1999) World development indicators 1999. World development indicators. The World Bank, Washington, DC

World Health Organization–Regional Office for Europe (1997) Twenty steps for developing a healthy cities project, 3rd edn. World Health Organization, Regional Office for Europe, Copenhagen

World Health Organization–Regional Office for Europe (2011) Impact of economic crises on mental health. World Health Organization, Regional Office for Europe, Copenhagen

World Health Organization (1986) The Ottawa charter for health promotion. World Health Organization, Geneva

World Health Organization (2001) Mental health: new understanding, new hope. The world health report. World Health Organization, Geneva

World Health Organization (2003) Investing in mental health. World Health Organization, Geneva

World Health Organization (2005) Mental health: facing the challenges, building solutions. World Health Organization, Regional Office for Europe, Copenhagen

Wyn J, Cahill H, Holdsworth R, Rowling L, Carson S (2000) MindMatters: a whole-school approach promoting mental health and well-being. Aust N Z J Psychiatry 34(4):594–601

Therapeutic Milieu: Utilizing the Environment to Promote Mental Wellness

24

Tyler D. Green

24.1 Introduction

The origins of the therapeutic milieu for the occidental world lay in the examples set forth in the late eighteenth century by the Quakers of York, England, and by Philippe Pinel in France (Cutcliffe et al. 2016). During a time where people with mental health problems were often mistreated and tortured, these progenitors of the therapeutic milieu held to the ideals of human equality. Under the emerging "moral treatment" movement, it was found that many people with mental health problems who were previously deemed "untreatable" were thriving. Chains and isolation were exchanged for fresh air, social interaction, and time spent caring for plants and animals. Members of these communities were empowered through self-government, where rules were set for acceptable behavior. Members not adhering to the rules were placed in a low stimuli environment until the member was able to regain control.

While moral treatment produced good results, arguments were made by leading physicians at the time that even better results could be obtained by combining moral treatment with medical treatment. The downfall of this initial era of moral treatment began in the late nineteenth century as a result of budgetary reductions paired with a reemerging belief that people with mental health problems were physiologically and psychologically inferior. The focus of "treatment" for mental health problems once again shifted to social segregation—sometimes accompanied by psychotropic medication, with additional approaches that included lobotomies, shock therapy, and castration (Scull 2015; Whitaker 2002).

T.D. Green
College of Nursing and Health, Wright State University, Dayton, OH, USA
e-mail: tyler.green@wright.edu

© Springer International Publishing Switzerland 2018

J.C. Santos, J.R. Cutcliffe (eds.), *European Psychiatric/Mental Health Nursing in the 21st Century*, Principles of Specialty Nursing,
https://doi.org/10.1007/978-3-319-31772-4_24

The 1950s saw the rise of a more humanistic movement in mental health care that rediscovered and once again recognized/emphasized client worth (Gournay et al. 1998). This movement was inspired by the likes of Carl Rogers (1951) and Heldegard Peplau (1952), both of whom published works discussing the therapeutic effects of utilizing interpersonal relations and adopted a client-centered approach. Psychiatrist Maxwell Jones (1953) was another influential figure who altered the treatment environment through the incorporation of dramatizations lead by clients. Through what became known as "psychodrama," both clients and health-care providers would act in scripted scenarios to assist clients with working through difficult situations arising in daily life. Accordingly, it can be seen that deliberate and purposeful use (some might say "manipulation") of the environment (both physical and metaphysical aspects) has been a part of the arsenal of interventions available to psychiatric/mental health (P/MH) nurses. As a result, this chapter will examine the purpose and function of a contemporary therapeutic milieu as well as the individuals who exist within it. Specific attention will be given to the nurse-client relationship within the context of the therapeutic milieu, followed by exploring interventions the nurse can utilize to promote client wellness. An overview of Gunderson's (1978) five processes of therapeutic milieu development is also presented in the context of Maslow's hierarchy of needs (Maslow 1943). The chapter concludes with a discussion of the current state of the therapeutic milieu and obstacles to overcome in moving forward.

24.2 Purpose and Function of the Therapeutic Milieu

As a part of a treatment modality, the primary goal of the therapeutic milieu on a mental health hospital unit is the development of an optimal healing environment. This environment can be defined as "one in which the social, psychologic, spiritual, physical, and behavioral components of health care are oriented toward support and stimulation of healing and the achievement of wholeness" (Jonas and Chez 2004, p. S-1). In practice this may translate to interventions such as using the environment to encourage the client to maintain orientation to person, place, time, and situation while simultaneously developing a structured schedule and routine. Clients are able to be provided with education and observed/monitored for evidence of symptoms, improvement/regression, alterations in sleep patterns, interactions with other clients, medication adherence, and completion of independent activities of daily living (ADLs). A controlled or purposefully managed environment can also allow for decreased stimuli, which can be therapeutic in clients who are experiencing altered sensory experiences or excessive heightened fluctuations to their mood (e.g., for some—mania). Many mental health problems are exacerbated by psychosocial stressors, so the psychiatric milieu aims to offer respite from antagonizing situations at home and/or work. Clients are encouraged to experience social interaction with their peers through "groups," which often address a variety of topics that can include exercise, nutrition, stress management, and sleep hygiene. Although client socialization in groups can be beneficial, an emphasis on decreased lengths of hospitalization for clients has interfered with the formation of a strong sense of community (Mahoney et al. 2009).

24.3 Multidisciplinary Team Roles in the Therapeutic Milieu

A variety of professionals/disciplines work on the mental health hospital unit to ensure the milieu maintains therapeutic characteristics. These professionals include nurses, physicians, mid-level practitioners (nurse practitioners and/or physician assistants), social workers, recreational therapists, and patient care technicians (PCT)/nurse aids. The P/MH nurse plays a central role in working with each group to achieve optimal health-care outcomes for the clients. Although not included in the list of professionals, the clients make up the final, but equally important, category of individuals who play a role on the mental health milieu. When viewed as a whole, the group of clients can be therapeutically beneficial to the progress of the individual. The client has the potential to interact with client peers who may have shared experiences, which can allow for the development of a support system as clients strive to achieve their health-care goals. Table 24.1 illustrates these roles and some of their primary functions.

Table 24.1 Roles and Functions of the Multidiciplinary Mental Health Team

Mental health unit roles	Primary function
Nurses	• Form therapeutic relationships with clients • Implement nursing interventions to encourage client safety and recovery • Perform client medication education and administration
Physicians and mid-level practitioners	• Manage client medications • Order safety measures (seclusion and/or restraints) • Manage mental health unit acuity through type and amount of clients admitted (requires communication with nursing team and consideration of staffing)
Social workers	• Consult physician and nursing assessments to determine client progress • Coordinate client family meetings • Oversee client housing and access to mental health resources after discharge
Recreational therapists	• Engage clients through therapeutic groups • Identify overarching themes among client population • Relay client attendance to health-care team
PCT/nurse's aid	• Work closely with the nursing team • Assist with client ADLs • Perform client safety checks and 1:1 safety sits
Clients	• Develop therapeutic relationships with peers and the health-care team • Learn and utilize coping strategies to assist with managing illness • Become educated on the potential benefits and drawbacks of taking psychotropic medication

24.4 Psychiatric/Mental Health Nursing Roles in the Therapeutic Milieu

Hildegard Peplau (1952) was an early proponent of P/MH nursing and popularized her middle-range theory on interpersonal relations. This theory widened the discussion on the idea of using the nurse-client relationship as a vehicle for client healing. Nurses utilizing the "therapeutic self" are able to ideally fill the client's environment with positive, encouraging, and stable relationships. While the analysis and purposeful use of interpersonal interactions in the nurse-client relationship are most commonly found and emphasized in areas of mental health care, it has applications to all areas of nursing.

Before a nurse is able to cultivate and incorporate therapeutic interactions with clients, it is essential for the nurse to first undergo a period of self-reflection and analysis to uncover any beliefs or biases held that may be damaging in client interactions. This self-awareness is the initial step to developing unconditional positive regard (Rogers 1951), which is accepting the client as a fellow human and not as a result of their actions or lifestyle. Another important nursing skill is to develop a familiarity with methods of therapeutic communication, which serve as building blocks for the advancement of a therapeutic client relationship. With appropriate incorporation into practice, therapeutic communication will serve to facilitate the building of trust and the client's expression of feelings. On the other hand, the use of nontherapeutic communication may just as easily tear down or impede the formation of a client relationship. Table 24.2 provides more detail on these types of communication according to Stuart (2013).

When assisting the client through the therapeutic process, Peplau (1952) describes how the nurse takes on a variety of roles in interacting with the client. Potential roles a nurse may fill when working with a client are as a stranger, resource, teacher, counselor, surrogate, and leader.

- *Stranger*: This role usually appears in the beginning of the nurse interaction with the client. The nurse treats the client as they would meet any stranger, with acceptance and respect.
- *Resource*: As a resource the nurse provides and relays information to and on behalf of the client to the rest of the health-care team.
- *Teacher*: As a teacher the nurse provides education to the client, addressing varied topics that may include medications, procedures, and what to expect during hospitalization.
- *Counselor*: As a counselor the nurse seeks to support and encourage the client as they process and find meaning in their experiences.
- *Surrogate*: In this role the nurse can act as the client's advocate. The client may compare the relationship with the nurse to previously experienced relationships or as a frame of reference for future relationships.
- *Leader*: In this role the nurse assists the client to be empowered and responsible for helping to achieve treatment outcomes.

Table 24.2 Therapeutic and Nontherapeutic Communication

Communication type	Description and examples
Active listening	Consists of verbal and nonverbal behaviors by the listener that demonstrate interest in what the client has to say. Good active listening includes giving complete attention to the client interaction, not interrupting, facing the client, utilizing appropriate eye contact, having an open posture, nodding, and using verbal cues
Broad openings	Allows the client to choose the topic after an open-ended prompt Ex. "What is on your mind?"
Restating	Demonstrates listening by repeating main ideas expressed by the client Ex. "I hear you are feeling overwhelmed"
Clarification	An attempt to understand vague communication expressed by the client Ex. "I'm not sure I understand. Would you be able to tell me what you mean when you say…?"
Reflection	Provides validation to the client through repetition or paraphrasing the client's words Ex. "You are saying you are feeling responsible for what happened that day?"
Focusing	Encouraging the client to elaborate on significant topics Ex. "Tell me more about the fight with your parents this morning"
Sharing perceptions	Verification of the listener's understanding of what the client is expressing Ex. "You seem to be very anxious when you talk about your work"
Theme identification	Recognition of a topic that is repeatedly expressed by a client Ex. "I notice you are talking about the different ways you feel betrayed by loved ones"
Silence	Absence of talking allows the client time to process thoughts and can convey acceptance by the nurse Ex. Quietly sitting with the client, employing therapeutic nonverbal behavior
Humor	Making the client laugh can lower tension and can help the client cope with difficult situations. Use carefully to ensure humor is in good taste and cannot be perceived as offensive to client
Informing	Providing information or education to the client Ex. "I would like to tell you about using guided imagery to help manage anxiety"
Suggesting	Presenting alternative options to the client Ex. "If running is hurting your joints, have you considered swimming?"
Close-ended questions	Nontherapeutic and discourages client expression Ex. "Did you enjoy your meal?"
Asking "Why?"	Nontherapeutic and can make client feel judged Ex. "Why do you feel that way?"
Giving advice	Nontherapeutic through disempowerment of the client and focusing on the values and beliefs of the nurse Ex. "You need to end that relationship if you ever want to feel better"

24.5 Psychiatric/Mental Health Nursing Interventions

P/MH nurse is able to utilize a variety of nursing interventions to impact, manage, and influence the milieu.

1. For clients who are struggling with depression and are at risk of self-harm, the nurse is able to influence the milieu through projection of a positive attitude and feelings of hope (Cutcliffe and Stevenson 2008). Management of the milieu may additionally include employing the use of natural daylight and filling the environment with pleasant sights, smells, and sounds (see Cutcliffe and Riahi—Chap. 33 - in this book). The nurse is also able to survey the environment and remove any items that may be used to aid in self-harm. A common example includes the removal of a sheet which can be used for hanging or strangulation.
2. Clients who are at risk of harming others may be placed in a calming room away from others with a potential for seclusion/restraint should the client demonstrate aggressive behaviors. Emphasis should be on seclusion as the use of restraints can be traumatic and degrading to the client, especially to those who have previously experienced physical or sexual abuse. The calming room may engage the senses and promote relaxation through a multifactorial approach that can employ calming colors, aroma therapy, and/or relaxing sounds (see Cutcliffe and Riahi—Chap. 33 in this book). In this circumstance the nurse is also able to influence the environment through utilization of an attitude that communicates respect for the client (Cutcliffe and Stevenson 2008).
3. For clients who are struggling with anger management, the nurse is able to create a permissive environment that encourages coping and is understanding of imperfection. It is important for P/MH nurses to remember that anger is an emotion experienced by all humans and that clients may be ill equipped to cope with their frustration. The permissive environment would not focus on punishment for actions such as verbal outburst but would instead facilitate client catharsis.
4. Client confusion may be addressed through a prominent display of the time, date, and names of the health-care team members providing care. Another intervention to assist with orientation can include having personal objects and items nearby.
5. Clients who are a fall risk will additionally require a night light and be provided with an easily accessible call light or alert bell.
6. Many clients also have difficulty with initiating and maintaining sleep. The milieu may be modified to promote comfort through control of temperature, light, and sound.
7. Clients who are experiencing hallucinations or are in a state of mania often benefit from being placed in an area of decreased environmental stimuli.
8. Conversely, clients who are experiencing loneliness or social isolation may benefit from being placed in an environment of higher environmental stimuli where they may be more likely to talk with a roommate or a peer. (see Lakeman, Chap. 34—on withdrawn/recalcitrant clients).

9. For the client who is at risk of elopement, the nursing team should employ communication with the client as a first line intervention to determine the underlying cause. Brumbles and Meister (2013) describe common reasons for clients wanting to elope from the hospital to include feeling "worried about the security of their home and property" (p. 5), having a need to complete "household responsibilities" (p. 5), or feeling stigmatized and/or "neglected by staff" (p. 5). Communication with the client will provide an opportunity for clients to voice and have their concerns addressed. Should communication not bring resolution to the client's desire for elopement, an alternative intervention might include placing the client in a room away from exits and raising unit awareness through posted signage and communication with other health-care providers.

24.6 Contraband and Client Visitation

In some formal mental health-care systems, management of the therapeutic milieu may include some safety orientated measures including those designed to address the issue of contraband items and client visitations. Upon arrival to the mental health hospital unit, it is important that the client and their belongings be searched for contraband, which includes any item that is not conducive to client safety or recovery. Common items that may be considered contraband could include medications/drugs, clothing with strings and/or wires, weapons, lighters, and/or cellphones/communication devices. During client visitation hours, the visitors must be monitored in a common area to prevent sexual activity and/or the exchange of contraband.

24.7 Medication Education and Administration

The administration of medication should come secondary to the use of therapeutic communication for the P/MH nurse. For some mental health-care systems and for that matter for some P/MH nurses, medication administration plays a central role in maintaining a therapeutic milieu. This role is largely influenced by pharmaceutical companies and an emphasis on the medicalization of illness, by which medications are stressed as the primary approach to provide "treatment." Clients who exhibit behaviors that are aggressive or threatening toward themselves or other clients will often be required to receive an intramuscular injection of a short-term antihistamine, antipsychotic, and/or benzodiazepine class medication. The sedation caused by the administration of these medications is considered a "chemical restraint" and should not be used simply to make the nurse's job easier or for client punishment, as this may be damaging to the therapeutic nurse/client relationship. When the use of medicine is necessary, efforts must be made to communicate with the client that the medicine was administered in the interest of safety. Should the client choose to take a psychotropic medication to help manage their mental health problems, it is important for the nurse to ensure the client is educated on the medication's potential efficacy and side effects.

24.8 Five Processes of Therapeutic Milieu

Gunderson's seminal (Gunderson 1978) paper advanced five processes that are important to the development of a therapeutic milieu. These processes include support, structure, involvement, validation, and containment. The processes support the client's journey toward self-actualization through Abraham Maslow's (1943) "hierarchy of needs," where the individual must first meet physiological, safety, love (belonging), and esteem needs.

- *Support*: Support addresses the areas of love (belonging) and esteem needs. A therapeutic milieu is able to establish a sense of community where clients are able to feel supported by their peers and the hospital staff. The encouragement, sense of belonging experienced by the client, and development of therapeutic relationships may serve to enhance feelings of self-confidence and self-worth.
- *Structure*: The structure of the milieu is therapeutic by working to meet the client's safety and physiological needs. A firm structure assists with client orientation to situation and is able to produce a normalized routine for daily activities. The routine is helpful for limiting behaviors that run contrary to getting optimal rest and nutrition.
- *Involvement*: Involving the client in their own treatment and in therapeutic groups addresses the areas of love (belonging) and esteem needs. In therapeutic groups, clients have the opportunity to develop a sense of community and purpose through collectively supporting other people with overcoming obstacles. Clients are given the opportunity to speak with other clients and offer advice on shared problematic situations. A client's direct involvement in their own plan of care may also help to improve esteem and treatment compliance by allowing the client to be empowered.
- *Validation*: Validation directly works to address the need of self-esteem in clients. Validation can be fostered through nurse-client interactions and allows for the client to be seen as a unique individual who is empowered and able to feel unconditional acceptance.
- *Containment*: The use of containment assists the client with meeting physiological and safety needs. Ideally, hospital containment provides the client with an environment that supports the basic needs of food, water, sleep, and shelter from weather or distressing home environments. An objective of physical containment is also to place the client in an environment free from self- or other-directed harm. To be effective, the area of containment should prevent client elopement but be designed in a manner that does not make the client feel as though they are incarcerated.

24.9 Personal Observations and Experiences of Mental Health Care in the USA: A Wolf in Sheep's Clothing?

There currently exists a major discrepancy between P/MH nursing theory, governmental policy, and clinical practice in many parts of the world. Here, I draw on my own experiences as P/MH nurse, P/MH nurse practitioner, and P/MH nurse educator in the United States of America in order to provide examples and contextualize the educational, policy, and practice schism.

Undergraduate P/MH nursing curricula in the USA commonly include information on the multifactorial cause(s) of mental health problems and a range of responses, interventions, and treatments. The use of self as a therapeutic instrument is detailed as an important, if not vital, component of working with people experiencing mental health problems. Though, it should be noted that even within such curricula, etiological models and treatment paradigms disproportionately emphasize biological causations and a corresponding treatment response headed by psychotropic pharmacology. While medications can certainly have a role in assisting people with managing their mental health problems, not enough stress is placed on utilization of the therapeutic self as a treatment modality. In practice, there remain many physical and emotional barriers between "patients" and the staff. The physical barriers extend to the design of the ward where the nursing station is often walled off from the client living quarters and dayroom. Emotional barriers encompass a widespread societal stigma around mental health problems including a belief that clients need to be changed and made "normal."

The single largest current obstacle to the development of the therapeutic milieu is the medicalization of mental health problems (Szasz 2007; Cutcliffe 2008). This is a result of a number of issues. A full discussion of these factors is beyond the scope of this chapter, although a prominent reason is money. In an effort to save money, insurance companies have pushed for shorter hospital stays and have standardized treatments for the so-called mental illnesses (we prefer the term, mental health problems), according to classification by diagnosis. Despite this standardization many of the clients who are discharged eventually require readmission to the hospital (Kolbasovsky et al. 2010). Staffing is often limited to a minimal nurse to client ratio, and many nurses feel that more time is spent charting than with the patients (Hodgson et al. 2016; Barron and Fleming 2010). In an era of rising health-care costs, this policy of cost containment thwarts, hinders, and arguably discourages the development of therapeutic relationships and can be damaging to clients.

Conclusion

This chapter has examined both the historical and present functions of the therapeutic milieu in the occidental world. The roles of professionals and clients in this setting were addressed; particular emphasis was paid to the role of nurses and interventions that can be incorporated to employ the milieu in promoting client wellness. This chapter also examined Gunderson's (1978) five processes of a therapeutic milieu and medication's overemphasized role in mental health care. Finally, I offer my own observations on the discrepancies between education, policy, and practice affecting the contemporary treatment of those with mental health problems. To realize mental health care that produces best client outcomes, the thoughts and attitudes of health-care professionals need to revert back to the days of "moral treatment." With this mentality, client care will once again be driven by the value of the individual and not by the financial agenda of pharmaceutical and insurance companies.

References

Barron D, Fleming M (2010) How wireless technology can work for service users. Nurs Manag 17(2):18–20

Brumbles D, Meister A (2013) Psychiatric elopement: using evidence to examine causative factors and preventative measures. Arch Psychiatr Nurs 27(1):3–9

Cutcliffe JR (2008) Has the die been cast? Rediscovering the essence of psychiatric/mental health nursing. Br J Nurs 17(2):88–92

Cutcliffe JR, Stevenson C (2008) Feeling our way in the dark: the psychiatric nursing care of suicidal people. Int J Nurs Stud 45:942–953

Cutcliffe JR, Travale RT, Richmond M, Green T (2016) Considering the contemporary issues and unresolved challenges of therapeutic communities for clients with alcohol and substance use problems. Issues Ment Health Nurs 37(9):642–650

Gournay K, Birley J, Bennett D (1998) Therapeutic interventions and milieu in psychiatry in the NHS between 1948 and 1998. J Ment Health 7(3):261–272

Gunderson JG (1978) Defining the therapeutic processes in psychiatric milieus. Psychiatry 41(4):327–335

Hodgson A, Morgan D, Peterson R (2016) Does better nurse staffing improve detection of depression and anxiety as secondary conditions in hospitalized patients with pneumonia? Nurs Econ 34(3):134–143

Jonas WB, Chez RA (2004) Toward optimal healing environments in health care. The Journal of Alternative and Complimentary Medicine 10(Suppl 1):S-1–S-6

Jones M (1953) The therapeutic community: a new treatment method in psychiatry. Basic Books, New York

Kolbasovsky A, Reich L, Myerkopf N (2010) Reducing six-month inpatient psychiatric recidivism and costs through case management. Case Manage J 11(1):1–10

Mahoney JS, Palyo N, Napier G, Giordano J (2009) The therapeutic milieu reconceptualized for the 21st century. Arch Psychiatr Nurs 23(6):423–429

Maslow AH (1943) A theory of human motivation. Psychol Rev 50(4):370–396

Peplau HE (1952) Interpersonal relations in nursing: a conceptual frame of reference for psychodynamic nursing. Putnam, New York

Rogers C (1951) Client-centered therapy: its current practice, implications and theory. Houghton Mifflin, Boston, MA

Scull A (2015) Madness in civilization. Princeton University Press, Princeton, NJ

Stuart GW (2013) Principles and practice of psychiatric nursing, 10th edn. Elsevier, St. Louis, MO

Szasz T (2007) The medicalisation of everyday life – selected essays. Syracuse University Press, Syracuse, NY

Whitaker R (2002) Mad in America: bad science, bad medicine, and the enduring mistreatment of the mentally ill. Perseus Publishing, Cambridge, MA

Psychiatric/Mental Health Nursing Nonphysical Competencies for Managing Violence and Aggression: De-escalation and Defusion

25

Hulya Bilgin and Zeynep Ozaslan

25.1 Introduction

When healthcare systems are examined, the documented increase in the frequency of aggression and violence, all around the world, is difficult to ignore. A recent meta-analysis (Iozzino et al. 2015) which examined 35 published works reports that rates of violent incidents (at least one incident of violence) involving psychiatric patients' were 17%. These, like many other reported results, indicate that psychiatric/mental health (P/MH) staff will, almost inevitably, experience violence during their work life. There are significant individual and substantial economic costs on health services that result, directly and indirectly, from violent and aggressive behavior in mental health system (Price et al. 2015). Such incidents also affect the sense (or perception of safety) and the *actual experience* of safety and security of patients and staff.

For a long time, and in many parts of Europe, P/MH nurses have been using physical methods mostly in order to calm down the patient with aggressive behaviors and manage the violence (Richter 2006, p. 125). Mechanic/physical restraint and seclusion/isolation rooms are the predominant physical methods used by P/MH nurses (Richter 2006, p. 125), and a review of the relevant literature will highlight how these practices appear to be predominant. In some cases, adopting and using physical techniques to help manage (and calm) the aggressive patient might be inevitable; however the evidence appears to indicate that how P/MH nurses respond to violence and aggression is influenced by a number of variables and conditions

H. Bilgin (✉)
Florence Nightingale Nursing Faculty, Psychiatric and Mental Health Nursing, Istanbul University, Istanbul, Turkey
e-mail: hcbilgin@hotmail.com; hulya@istanbul.edu.tr

Z. Ozaslan
Nursing Department, Health Sciences Faculty, Kocaeli University, Kocaeli, Turkey

© Springer International Publishing Switzerland 2018

J.C. Santos, J.R. Cutcliffe (eds.), *European Psychiatric/Mental Health Nursing in the 21st Century*, Principles of Specialty Nursing,
https://doi.org/10.1007/978-3-319-31772-4_25

(Richter 2006, p. 129). Thus responses to violence and aggression appear to be influenced by (a) the overall condition, environment, and situation of the mental health clinic; (b) staff attitudes and values; (c) staff previous exposure to violence and aggression; (d) whether or not P/MH nurses have support systems—such as clinical supervision; (e) psychiatric symptoms of the patient; (f) patient abilities of resolving the conflict and impulsivity; and (g) physiological and pharmacological variables, clinic staff's experiences of resolving the conflict, and their ability and equipment along with the extent of the conflict.

After reporting serious health and security problems including death or posttraumatic stress symptoms resulted from positional asphyxia which is connected with physical techniques, some country policies (the USA and UK) gave priority to nonphysical approaches (e.g., de-escalation techniques) (Price et al. 2015). Other nations have been less forthcoming in advocating for and adopting nonphysical responses to potential violence and aggression, and in some European nations, these techniques are seldom taught (Richter 2006) but do occur spontaneously or "naturally" on some wards/clinics. Accordingly, this chapter will review relevant information about "nonphysical aggression/conflict management (de-escalation)," and it will explore de-escalation/defusion of violent incident interventions.

25.2 Profiles of the Place, People, and Intervention in Conflict Situations

In mental health departments, conflict can and does arise as a result of interpersonal interactions between the staff and the patients and also among/between two or more patients. Some evidence appears to indicate that risk of interpersonal conflict, violence, and aggression is more likely when people are in closer contact with one another (Bilgin 2009; Richter 2006, p. 126). A crucial finding and one that is not always given sufficient acknowledgement in the literature is that attitudes of the mental health personnel, including P/MH nurses, are at least as important in contributing to violence and aggression as the patients' attitude(s) (see, e.g., Cutcliffe and Riahi, in this book). Besides, others' threats, incitement and unfair behaviors, insults regarding personal honor, and misunderstandings which would be a reason for self-defense can cause negative personal attribution. Most of the interpersonal conflicts are based on different views related to what has been said or done (Richter 2006, p. 135).

It is well documented that P/MH nurses are the professional group in mental health care that spends the greatest amount of time in direct contact with patients/clients; they are the only group of mental health professionals who places forming relationships with clients as primary (Cowin et al. 2003; Gleeson and Higgins 2009). This situation perhaps indicates who has the primary responsibility for facing and dealing with aggression and violent behaviors. Attitudes and behaviors of the staff are important points in terms of preventing the aggression/violence in psychiatry clinics. Psychiatric and mental healthcare facilities, wards, and clinics are places where stress levels are often high and the pressure is intense (Richter 2006; Anderson and West 2011). Ideally, P/MH nurses who are experiencing high stress levels would not be the most appropriate staff to approach the aggressive patient. The limited literature in this area seems to suggest that P/MH nurses with unresolved or unprocessed experiences of and reactions to violence/aggression are less effective and less comfortable with dealing with further violent/aggressive incidents (Cutcliffe 1999; Bilgin 2009; Richter 2006, p. 129). Accordingly, given the probability, if not inevitability that P/MH nurses will encounter violence/aggression, then such nurses need to be provided with support and facilities for dealing with their own stress and anger in order to act in appropriate manner.

Once it is remembered that the core of P/MH nursing means developing a relationship with the patient/client, it is perhaps a logical (and "natural") extension of that relationship that P/MH nurses seek to de-escalate and defuse, by means of effective and appropriate use of verbal and nonverbal communication techniques and by therapeutic use of themselves. De-escalation, in terms of its core, is much less coercive in comparison with traditional control techniques. In addition, according to US and European data, isolation and restraint methods are often used on 10–30% of the patients (in adolescence-young and adults range) who stay in acute psychiatry service (Gaynes et al. 2016; Richter 2006; Sailas and Wahlbeck 2005; Sailas and Fenton 2000).

In the published guidelines concerning responding to and managing violence and aggression, (see, e.g., NICE 2015; Holloman and Zeller 2012; APNA 2016), while proactive interventions for preventing aggression and violence are recommended, it has been argued that it is likely not possible to avoid all violence and/or aggression, and consequently there are interventions on different levels to prevent mild violence from turning into serious violence situations. In one of the more recently published set of guidelines, the NICE (2015) document outlines that de-escalation can and should be used in conjunction with PRN medication, under the title of "preventing violence and aggression," and listed the gains of the instructors who work on de-escalation.

25.3 Definition of De-escalation

De-escalation has been used for many years and, in certain facilities (and certain countries), as an approach to responding to aggression and violence, by adopting defusing, negotiation, and conflict-solving methods. Talking down, defusion and diffusion are words used synonymously with de-escalation, and such practices should form the basis of the first response of the healthcare staff when they are faced with aggressive patient. The NICE (2005, p. 9) document describes de-escalation as a complex skill set which can be used to stop the assault cycle during the escalation stage. De-escalation is an approach for managing aggressive and violent behaviors in a more humane manner or way and is arguably more dignified and less coercive than physical interventions. The so-called typical attack cycle (Kaplan and Wheeler 1983 cited in Rao et al. 2012; Leadbetter and Paterson 1995) has been described as triggering, escalation, crisis stage, calming stage, and depression stage (Fig. 25.1).

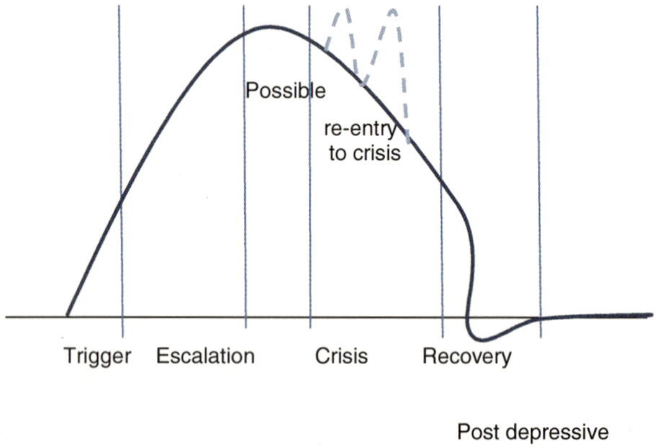

Fig. 25.1 Assault cycle. Kaplan, S. G. & Wheeler, E. G. (1983). Survival skills for working with potentially violent clients. Social Casework

When the aggression of the patient is triggered, using appropriate de-escalation skills might be effective on preventing the assault cycle turning from triggering stage to escalation stage although it becomes quickly (Richter 2006; Spencer and Johnson 2016; Hallett and Dickens 2015).

In NICE (2015), de-escalation was defined as the use of techniques covering verbal and nonverbal communication skills aiming to defuse the anger and stop the aggression. In addition, this guideline highlights how PRN medication can be used as a part of de-escalation strategy, but medication does not constitute de-escalation on its own.

While the authors are advocates for adoption of de-escalation, the approach is not without limitations and critics (Roberton et al. 2012; Richter 2006; Duxbury and Whittington 2005). For example, there remains an absence of any functional definition for de-escalation (and the specific techniques and interventions therein) which has been agreed upon and accepted as the so-called "gold standard." Also there are not any exact guidelines about de-escalation techniques for healthcare personnel to use. Hallett and Dickens (2015) determined on their mixed methodical research, which was made to specify clinic personnel's opinions about de-escalation, that the participants express de-escalation as calming the patient or the condition in terms of its goal and intention, and they define the specific interventions which might be implemented to achieve the goal as verbal communication, relocation, and distraction.

25.4 The Elements of De-escalation and Its Basic Principles

The relationship and interaction between the nurse and the patient are primary in terms of therapeutic care, and it is the first step in case of any de-escalation condition (Richter 2006). As stated above, the de-escalation process can combine nonphysical, verbal, and, to a lesser extent, some physical interventions (NICE 2005, 2015). Basically, non-provocative verbal and nonverbal communication techniques are being used for making the clinician and the patient who might act aggressively get along with each other (Price et al. 2015). Based on the literature (Richter 2006; NICE 2005; Bowers 2014; Price et al. 2015; Dix and Page 2008; Cowin et al. 2003), principles and rationales which must be in de-escalation intervention are presented in the Table 25.1.

Table 25.1 Principles and rationales in de-escalation implementation

Principle	Rationale
Having an attitude with therapeutic intention which includes empathy, interest, respect, mercy, consistency, and unprejudiced approach	It makes the individual feel safe, precious, and open to cooperation
Risk identification, having real expectations about resolving the conflict	Realizing the predictors in advance in terms of individual and environment gives an opportunity to take necessary precautions. If the nonphysical resolution of the conflict is not possible, managing with communication makes the process unnecessarily difficult, extends it, and risks everybody's safety
Establishing control upon the condition, not upon the patient	Even if its nature is an asymmetric relationship, using force toward patients is inconsistently with therapeutic relation
Risk identification, decision-making process, team approach on action, and responsibilities	Colleague's support and observation on the patients and the environment increase the chance of success in one-to-one de-escalation
Starting de-escalation as soon as possible	Before the incidents are escalated, the success rate of nonphysical intervention is high
Saving time to prevent making a fast decision without thinking well dependent on emotional stimulation	Saving time both prevents making fast and incorrect decisions and eases partially the tension between the parties by distracting
Taking spatial precautions/protecting the area	It is necessary both for personal security and personal space which will not result in defensive tactics
Not attempting to show force and be obstinate between the staff and the patients	Unimportant disagreements cause personalization and transformation into big conflicts; the essential point in case of escalation is not to prove that the patient is completely wrong but to prevent violence
Practicing de-escalation with an obvious self-confidence and certainty	A balanced attitude is necessary without negligence which can provoke the opponent and resigned insecurity
Looking out for the security of the environment and other people in the environment (patients, visitors, team members, etc.)	The security of the individuals and other patients in the environment should not be ignored by focusing completely on one-to-one de-escalation
The whole personal view which is offered to the patient (within verbal/nonverbal communication) is important	Nonverbal communication is in the main role when it comes to express the emotions along with the cognitive importance of the language

(continued)

Table 25.1 (continued)

Principle	Rationale
Using de-escalation techniques which are suitable for individual needs and in which realist options are discussed	Instead of automatic, monotype expressions and gesture-movements, communication styles which are suitable for individual's socio-cultural needs both provide flexibility/spontaneity for the carer and make the individual feel that his/her existence/needs are considered important
Isolating the environment from overstimulation	If the environment is crowded and filled with stimulus, communicating in an open and sincere way becomes harder
Approaching to agitation or disturbed behavior in a discreet and restrained manner	Unnecessary show of force and exaggerated authoritative reactions increase the level of the individual's feeling of being controlled instead of calming him/her, and they cause extra risks in terms of security
Being aware of the support resources and response procedures of the crisis	When it gets difficult to handle the situation, it lets fast attempts, makes carer feel that he/she is not alone, and behaves safely
Even while restraining strictly or calling for help, acting very respectfully	Agitated patient is very sensitive to embarrassment and disrespect. Showing respect to the individuals always is in the nature of the occupation
To welcome emotions, not the behaviors, in an emphatic manner	So the negative behavior is not repeated, and the possibly negative emotions are conveyed
Discussing misbehavior without threatening or getting angry	Threat perception triggers the defense stimulation; it means the misuse of the carer's force
Trusting instincts; one should stop when it is felt that de-escalation does not work	Instincts are guiding when it is approached sincerely and when you focus on the individual as a whole; extending the speech increases the risk, jeopardize the security; the motive of individual success should not go beyond the individual's need
Whether it works or not is realized in 2–3 min; help should be sought; crisis management plan should be implemented	

25.5 Models of De-escalation

Models of de-escalation, to a greater or lesser extent, invariably draw upon "communication theory" (Paterson and Leadbetter 1999; Muralidharan and Fenton 2006) in order to inform techniques and interventions to prevent/limit aggression and violence. Several models and/or theories of de-escalation have been advanced, and these are summarized in Table 25.2.

25.6 Effectiveness and Use

De-escalation method is very valuable in terms of calming the patients with less coercive interventions, maintaining therapeutic relationships and providing non-coercive therapeutic environment considering the physical and/or psychological damages of coercive containment methods (restraint, enforced medication,

Table 25.2 Theoretical models and their content

Theoretical models	Content
De-escalation model as a process	Leadbetter and Paterson (1995) de-escalation model
Leadbetter and Paterson (1995)	Consecutive five-step model (trigger, escalation, crisis, healing, and depression after crisis) is based on an assault cycle which branches from basic behavior of the aggressor to the course of the event
McDonnell et al. (2008)	For each stage, dominant emotion of the aggressor is identified, and the intervention's goal and focus which can be made real by staff in terms of skills and tactics are presented
	McDonnell et al. (2008) low arousal model of de-escalation; four principles have been identified
	1. Decreasing staff demands on patients
	2. Abstaining from probable stimulant triggers (direct eye contact, etc.)
	3. Abstaining from probable stimuli nonverbal behavior (aggressive look, etc.)
	4. Struggling with the clinician's belief about aggression management
	It consists of three stages
	1. Pre-crisis interventions
	2. Management of critical incident
	3. Healing after the incident
	For each stage, intervention strategies are recommended
De-escalation model which focuses only on aggressive incident's escalation	Diagnosis (evaluation of the responses of aggression incident, situational variances, and subject) (anger-agitation, etc.), communication (it provides a perpetual approach in a calm and controlled way to the main problem by drawing the attention of the subject, looking out for his/her respectability and cooperation), and tactics (specific tactics such as problem-solving, which decreases the probability of escalation, distraction, offering an option, replacing the patient, and removing the triggers)
Dix and Page (2008)	ACT model asserts cyclical structure (in contradiction with linear) consisting of three independent component. Every element of the perpetual model is discussed by de-escalator
Safewards approach	It focuses on communication strategies and identifies specific de-escalation tactics, requested qualifications, and interpersonal skills. De-escalation process is defined as linear from de-limiting and clarifies stages to conflict resolving
De-escalation model	De-limiting, providing the security in case of acute danger/threat from the side of others and nurse himself/herself
Bowers (2014)	Clarify, it is based on determining what causes patient being agitated or aggressive and helping patient
	Resolve, finding a way of dealing with the problems, offering different actions and opportunity of changing in a kind and flexible manner. It means nurse checking himself/herself, not reflecting anxiety/frustration on communication style. De-escalator qualifications include interpersonal skills such as emotional regulation and empathy/respect. It has been asserted that these qualifications are effective during the process

seclusion, etc.) on both the patient and others (staff, other patients, visitors, etc.) (Lavelle et al. 2016). De-escalation is recommended as an early intervention in the management of aggression in order to prevent escalation to the crisis phase (NICE 2005). It has been implemented in various institutions (except psychiatry hospitals and psychiatry emergency services) such as learning disability services and geriatric services and institutions where police intervention is necessary (NHS Project 2013). Here it must be taken in consideration that de-escalation techniques change according to the population and its extent.

In order to make de-escalation techniques effective, the relationship focused on mutual trust and understanding should be strengthened (Richter 2006; Price and Baker 2012). Interpersonal relationship and communication skills are essential elements of this intervention's effectiveness.

De-escalation, where possible, should also try and make room for listening to and considering patients and carers as part of decision-making process. Alternative views and approaches to dealing with violence, such as the biomedical model, see aggressive behaviors as a part of the illness spectrum, and some develop the idea that the behavior cannot be prevented (Lee 2001). On the other hand, the dominant controlling attitude to "calm the patient" in traditional, biomedical views and understanding should be turned into a collaborative endeavor, where "the individual is encouraged to help himself/herself calm down by using his/her own power" (Richmond et al. 2012). In this context, practicing de-escalation for calming the psychiatric patient may also serve as an experiential learning opportunity for the client (and the nurse).

In their systematic examination of various interventions for controlling the acute psychiatry patient in case of crisis, Muralidharan and Fenton (2006) asserted that de-escalation was found to be the least coercive (intrusive) intervention and more humane. Similarly, Lee (2001) asserts that with therapeutic and especially verbal de-escalation, it is possible to change and break the aggression cycle in a more therapeutic and simpler way. It is argued and well documented that aggressive incidents are rarely spontaneous, random acts (Stevenson cited in Lee 2001). Much more commonly, violent and aggressive incidents have a context and antecedence (or more likely antecedents) and are often the end point in a progressive process (see Cutcliffe and Riahi, in this book); in such models, there then become multiple opportunities and possibilities where the P/MH nurse might intervene and interrupt the escalation of aggression to violence. In some cases, particularly those where more is known about the particular patient and his/her history of responses/incidents, it then becomes more possible to make accurate predictions in terms of the de-escalation intervention(s) that is likely to be most effective and predictions in terms of the particular antecedence that seems to preface violent/aggressive behavior. In such situations, positive proactive interventions can be implemented.

Though de-escalation has an intuitive logic to it, given the literature and theory on explanations of violence and the therapeutic value of being heard/listened to (Richter 2006), and despite the fact that de-escalation is identified as the first step to manage violence or aggression in published guidelines (e.g., NICE 2015), there is, however, a distinct lack of robust empirical evaluation of this practice (Richter 2006;

Bowers et al. 2006; Roberton et al. 2012; Richmond et al. 2012; Bowers 2014; Hallett and Dickens 2015; Rao et al. 2012). There are many methodological, theoretical, and conceptual problems (Duxbury and Whittington 2005) associated with determining the effectiveness of de-escalation; these have been identified as:

- Lack of clear incidence
- Lack of clear, operational definition
- Complexity of staff views on skills
- The role of interpersonal conflicts on aggressive behavior

P/MH nurses have the tendency to use the familiar techniques (i.e., physical restraint or de-escalation method, etc.) in spite of the necessities of the condition. In fact, while it is stated that interventions which include physical contact are the last resort to be used, both anecdotal and some empirical literature exist which speaks to how often de-escalation techniques are not used at all and the first "option" is physical restraint/seclusion (Richter 2006).

In addition, it is unlikely that any one particular approach to de-escalation will be successful or effective in all situations and for all clients; it may even be the case that from time to time, the attempt at de-escalation could be unsuccessful (for a range of reasons). Richmond et al. (2012) state that de-escalation has the aim to overcome the immediate aggressive behavior and it does not have long-lasting effectiveness. It is determined that for agitated individual to become calm, effective de-escalation should take approximately 5–10 min (Stowell et al. 2012). Price and Baker (2012) emphasized that the effectiveness of de-escalation is related to identify the reasons in the source of patient's aggressive behavior and empathy. Also they stated that in order to develop nurse's empathy skill, attention should be focused on psychological tendencies beneath the patient's aggressive behavior in de-escalation education and training.

An important point which should be remembered is that staff behavior can foreshadow or contribute to the violence just as patient behavior can. Thus training and education in de-escalation should include material and exercises for increasing the awareness of the staff about their attribution style and behaviors. While everyone agrees that trust is the most important of the key elements in patient-nurse relationship, one may ignore that distrust is one of the cognitive beliefs that causes aggression to reach destructiveness. Useful points of de-escalation intervention to each part involved in are presented in Table 25.3 (Nau et al. 2009; Cowin et al. 2003; Paterson and Leadbetter 1999; Roberton et al. 2012).

25.7 Implementation

P/MH nurses are, frequently, at the center of aggressive incidents. A successful de-escalation is highly dependent on the principles of existent therapeutic relationship. Considering that nurses work under a heavy workload, institutional pressure and threats toward work safety in almost all psychiatry services, experiencing tension in

Table 25.3 De-escalation to each part; its advantages

On the nurse side	On the patient side
• Advantages of using de-escalation as an early intervention are more than the use of determination and isolation from nurses' perspective	• Verbal and nonverbal communication skills help individual pass to a calmer personal space
• It can be a basis for the realization of therapeutic relationship with the patient	• It strengthens health and goodness condition
• It provides a progress within the personnel's morale and trust; even during the de-escalation education, personnel's level of morale and trust increases	• It develops the communication with the healthcare personnel and enables cooperation
• It can make the nurse feel more comfortable and safe	
• Self-respect and self-efficacy become factors that increase job satisfaction and provide change	
• Since de-escalation use requires cognitive demands from the nurse, it causes the nurse to question his/her actions, to gain insight and awareness, and to take more responsibilities	
• One may feel that using control and identification interventions as soon as the condition occurs is an administrative inadequacy	

the interactions built with the patients, are distinctly possible. And this is an aspect that can interrupt or interfere with successful de-escalation interventions. National Health Services (UK) (2015) states that verbal de-escalation and solution-oriented approach should be implemented in a calm manner as secondary protective intervention within the frame of individualized care plan by keeping the patient in the communal area when disturbed/agitated behavior occurs for the first time.

As stated earlier, there is currently an absence of a "standardized" approach for effective de-escalation, and some would argue that a standardized approach (i.e., automaton-like, non-individualized) is not necessary or indicative of best practice. Nevertheless, there do appear to be some skills, techniques, attitudes, and interventions that are shared across different approaches to de-escalation. Table 25.4 provides a summary of the communication skills that appear to be consistent across different models (Bowers 2014; Skolnik-Acker 2008; Stowell et al. 2012).

25.8 Skills Required for De-escalation

Being competent in de-escalation, essentially, is a sophisticated activity which requires more than understanding of the aggression that based on the theoretical basis. In fact, calming people who are very angry or agitated is not something magical but rather involves the communication of real, genuine feelings of interests and understanding to the individual. De-escalation techniques, as a therapeutic interaction way with the patient, emphasize the therapeutic use of nurse's own personality

Table 25.4 Communication skills for de-escalation

Verbal communication (Aim: to reduce the emotional stress and gain the confidence of patient who has problems)	*Nonverbal communication* (Aim: to give a sense of confidence and comfort to the individual having tension)
Body language and verbal communication should reflect the same message	
• Active and empathic listening is the basis	• Physical stance
• Use of soft, low tone, simple language	• A tense facial expression without anxiety
• Not criticizing the patient, avoiding discussion	• Open, non-defensive body language
• Speaking short but to the point	• Slow and gentle movements
• Explanation of the restrictions and rules in an authoritarian but respectful tone	• Breathing in and out deeply
• Offering options and optimism, paying attention to whether the options that are offered include patient safety	• Acting quietly and safely/sure
• Trying not to persuade, avoiding provocative acts	• Concentrating on the situation rather than observing oneself and thinking he/she might be unsuccessful
• Whenever possible, getting to the individual's way of thinking; saying "help me understand what you are saying" instead of asking "how do you feel"	• Not taking the situation personally, not feeling like defending and justifying oneself to the patient
• Not pushing the individual's feelings or not interpreting their emotions analytically	• Performing a plain emotional response against all kinds of humiliation-insult that are directed by the patient
• Consenting to agree or disagree	• Avoiding every kind of sign that can be meant as disrespect (making suggestions, sorting demands, behaviors which are beneficent, imitative, and seeing them like children)
• Where appropriate, suggesting performing behaviors, "Do you want to take some fresh air?"	• If there is time, before going next to the patient, removing the religious, political accessories and jewels
• Remembering that, in de-escalation, there is no other extent other than dealing with trying to turn anger into a safer level	• Being always on the same eye level
	• Respecting the personal distance
	• Not turning back for any reason on the patient
	• Encouraging the individuals to sit and if they want to stand, letting them stand
	• Leaving extra physical space with the individual (up to four times of the usual distance)
	• Not standing still completely in front of the individual, if necessary, standing by creating an angle that enables to move sideways
	• Not making eye contact continuously/constantly—letting them turn their glances to another direction
	• Not pointing or shaking finger
	• Not laughing (may seem like imitation or anxiety)
	• Not touching (even if it is culturally appropriate)
	• Not keeping hands in pockets, keeping them above

and its relationship with the individual (Paterson and Leadbetter 1999). The limited evaluatory evidence in this area seems to suggest that training and education in de-escalation theory and techniques are needed; effective de-escalation appears to need more than reading printed materials. In other words, transferring of the owned knowledge to the level of consciousness and its implementation is needed. In addition, individual factors (unprejudiced, sensitive approach to the different, making empathy, listening, effective use of verbal/nonverbal communication, positive personality traits, etc.) are effective on individual's meeting of conflict management and individual's being successful in de-escalation.

De-escalation requires the P/MH nurse to draw upon and apply his/her range of knowledge, attitudes, and skills and acknowledges that their reactions or responses to agitated clients are pivotal to the success/failure of the de-escalation. Possessing this awareness, P/MH nurses understand not only that the responsibility for de-escalation resides primarily with them but also that a range of factors—some associated with the healthcare system/organization and some with the P/MH nurses themselves—may have contributed to the rise of aggression and violence in the client (see Cutcliffe and Riahi, in this book). Thus, patient-nurse interactions, which may have inadvertently contributed to the aggression/violence, may be allowed to become a means of solving the problem instead of the position of being the source of the problem.

25.8.1 Requirements to Implement Effective De-escalation

The first and only aim of the de-escalation is to decrease the anger level as possible as debate level. De-escalation techniques are not innate predispositions become in naturalistic ways. In other words, there are a few necessities to implement efficient and qualified de-escalation. As a carer tries to de-escalate patients, basic drives such as fight-flight should not be applied. Table 25.5 presents requirements for effective de-escalation based on literature (Richter 2006; Inglis and Clifton 2013) and personal attributions.

Table 25.5 Requirements for effective de-escalation

• Self-awareness (to recognize and to be able to manage individual emotions and the way of living/expression styles of emotions, to be aware of transference and counter-transference points)
• Role flexibility (when needed, to soften the rules-obligations that are connected to professional role, to look outside from the professional role, to understand the condition of being a human)
• Empathy (especially in difficult meetings including conflict)
• Acceptance of diversities/uncertainties (positive approach to different perspectives, to remain calm against hostile behavior, not to make exaggerated sense outpouring)
• To protect the patient's autonomy and dignity
• Making an early attempt is very important to prevent the cycle of escalation, detection, and isolation
• In the hospitalization process, discussing the ways of restrictive containment methods with the patient is really a valuable exercise
• Education

25.8.2 Guidelines for Good Implementation

It was recommended in violence prevention and management courses by NICE (2005, 2015) (National Institute for Health and Care Excellence 2005–2015) that an important part of the training period should be separated for these issues. The International Society of Psychiatric-Mental Health Nurses (ISPN) (2007) suggested that, in escalating situations, conflict resolution, problem-solving, and de-escalation are the response tools, and also detection and isolation should be used as a last resort. Holloman and Zeller (2012) (Best Practices in Evaluation and Treatment of Agitation) (Stowell et al. 2012) represents step-by-step guidelines for clinicians and nurses with a flowchart and easy-to-follow recommendations for managing agitation in emergency department. APNA (2016) tells that P/MH nurses can demonstrate care and advocacy through active listening and respectful, therapeutic interactions and provide counseling and education to prevent violence in all community settings.

25.8.3 Implications for Practice

Both motivation and progress of aggressive behaviors in psychiatry services are not different from the conflict situations in other parts of the public. What is ironic is that although de-escalation/nonphysical/non-touch interventions are the main study area of the interpersonal interaction and relationship process and they rank first in primary education programs of different professions toward healthcare, controller interventions mostly based on the use of physical force precluded them. Practice of safe and positive action includes real support for the patients and others in the prevention of violence and managing it in a therapeutic way. In psychiatric services, de-escalation, when aggression unfortunately could not be prevented, is an inseparable part of the system of hierarchical responses, and all the personnel should act properly in accordance with this hierarchy.

Conclusion

First of all, in aggression management, there is a need for evidence-based research and systematic reviews, which are emphasized as the first option, that are based on the effectiveness of de-escalation. Two Cochrane researches (Spencer and Johnson 2016; Rao et al. 2012) are being prepared which are about de-escalation effectiveness on aggression management of the individuals who have learning difficulties and psychosis due to aggression.

References

American Psychiatric Nurses Association (APNA) (2016) APNA position statement: violence prevention. https://www.apna.org/files/public/Resources/APNA%20Position%20Paper%20-%20Violence%20Prevention.pdf

Anderson A, West SG (2011) Violence against mental health professionals: when the treater becomes the victim. Innov Clin Neurosci 8(3):34

Bilgin H (2009) An evaluation of nurses' interpersonal styles and their experiences of violence. Issues Ment Health Nurs 30(4):252–259

Bowers L, Brennan G, Flood C, LiPang M, Oladapo P (2006) Preliminary outcomes of a trial to reduce conflict and containment on acute psychiatric wards: city nurses. J Psychiatr Ment Health Nurs 13(2):165–172

Bowers L (2014) A model of de-escalation. Ment Health Pract 17(9):36–37

Cowin L, Davies R, Estall G, Berlin T, Fitzgerald M, Hoot S (2003) De-escalating aggression and violence in the mental health setting. Int J Ment Health Nurs 12(1):64–73

Cutcliffe JR (1999) Qualified nurses' lived experience of violence perpetrated by individuals suffering from enduring mental health problems: a hermeneutic study. Int J Nurs Stud 36(2):105–116

Dix R, Page MJ (2008) De-escalation. Psychiatr Intensive care:24–31

Duxbury JA, Whittington R (2005) Causes and management of patient aggression and violence: staff and patient perspectives. J Adv Nurs 50:469–478

Gaynes BN, Brown C, Lux LJ, Brownley K, Van Dorn R, Edlund M, Viswanathan M (2016) Strategies to de-escalate aggressive behavior in psychiatric patients???

Gleeson M, Higgins A (2009) Touch in mental health nursing: an exploratory study of nurses' views and perceptions. J Psychiatr Ment Health Nurs 16(4):382–389

Hallett N, Dickens GL (2015) De-escalation: a survey of clinical staff in a secure mental health inpatient service. Int J Ment Health Nurs 24(4):324–333

Holloman GH, Zeller SL (2012) Overview of project BETA: best practices in evaluation and treatment of agitation. West J Emerg Med 13(1):1–2

Inglis P, Clifton A (2013) De-escalation: the evidence, policy and practice. J Intellect Disabil Offending Behav 4(3/4):100–108

International Society of Psychiatric-Mental Health Nurses (2007) Scope and standards of psychiatric mental health nursing practice

Iozzino L, Ferrari C, Large M, Nielssen O, de Girolamo G (2015) Prevalence and risk factors of violence by psychiatric acute inpatients: a systematic review and meta-analysis. PLoS One 10(6):e0128536

Kaplan SG, Wheeler EG (1983) Survival skills for working with potentially violent clients. Social Casework

Lavelle M, Stewart D, James K, Richardson M, Renwick L, Brennan G, Bowers L (2016) Predictors of effective de-escalation in acute inpatient psychiatric settings. J Clin Nurs 25(15–16):2180–2188

Leadbetter D, Paterson B (1995) De-escalating aggressive behaviour. Management of violence and aggression in health care, 49–84

Lee F (2001) Violence in A&E: the role of training and self-efficacy. Nurs Stand 15(46):33–38

McDonnell AA, Gould A, Sturmey P (2008) Staff training in physical interventions: a systematic literature review. Unpublished manuscript, available from first author

Muralidharan S, Fenton M (2006) Containment strategies for people with serious mental illness. Cochrane Libr

National Health Services (NHS) Project (2013) Conflict resolution training: implementing the learning aims and outcomes. http://www.nhsbsa.nhs.uk/Documents/SecurityManagement/Conflict_resolution_training_guidance_July_2013.pdf

National Health Services (NHS) (2015) Proactive care policy including de-escalation and seclusion. http://www.sompar.nhs.uk/media/1232/proactive-care-policy-v5aug-2015.pdf

National Institute for Health and Clinical Excellence (2005) Violence: the short-term management of disturbed/violent behaviour in in-patient psychiatric settings and emergency departments. NICE, London

National Institute for Health and Care Excellence (NICE) (2015) Violence and aggression: Short-term management in mental health, health and community settings. NICE Guideline NG10

Nau J, Halfens R, Needham I, Dassen T (2009) The de-escalating aggressive behaviour scale: development and psychometric testing. J Adv Nurs 65(9):1956–1964

Paterson B, Leadbetter D (1999) De-escalation in the management of aggression and violence: towards evidence-based practice. In: Aggression and violence. Macmillan Education, London, pp 95–123

Price O, Baker J (2012) Key components of de-escalation techniques: a thematic synthesis. Int J Ment Health Nurs 21(4):310–319

Price O, Baker J, Bee P, Lovell K (2015) Learning and performance outcomes of mental health staff training in de-escalation techniques for the management of violence and aggression. Br J Psychiatry 206(6):447–455

Rao H, Yeung WL, Jayaram MB (2012) De-escalation techniques for psychosis-induced aggression or agitation. Cochrane Libr

Richmond JS, Berlin JS, Fishkind AB, Holloman GH, Zeller SL, Wilson MP, Ng AT (2012) Verbal de-escalation of the agitated patient: consensus statement of the American Association for Emergency Psychiatry Project BETA de-escalation workgroup. West J Emerg Med 13(1):17

Richter D (2006) Nonphysical conflict management and deescalation. In: Violence in mental health settings. Springer, New York, pp 125–144

Roberton T, Daffern M, Thomas S, Martin T (2012) De-escalation and limit-setting in forensic mental health units. J Forensic Nurs 8(2):94–101

Sailas E, Wahlbeck K (2005) Restraint and seclusion in psychiatric inpatient wards. Curr Opin in Psych 18:555–559

Sailas EES, Fenton M (2000) Seclusion and restraint for people with serious mental illnesses. Cochrane Database of Systematic Reviews 1:CD001163

Skolnik-Acker E (2008) Verbal de-escalation techniques for defusing or talking down an explosive situation. National Association of Social Workers, Massachusetts Chapter, committee for the study and prevention of violence against social workers. Retrieved May, 31, 2011

Spencer S, Johnson P (2016) De-escalation techniques for managing aggression. Cochrane Libr

Stowell KR, Florence P, Harman HJ, Glick RL (2012) Psychiatric evaluation of the agitated patient: consensus statement of the American Association for Emergency Psychiatry Project BETA psychiatric evaluation workgroup. West J Emerg Med 13(1):11

Part IV

Human Experiences of Mental Health Problems and Psychiatric/Mental Health Nursing Responses

Problems Affecting a Person's Mood 26

German López-Cortacans, Carme Ferré-Grau, and José Carlos Santos

26.1 Introduction

The so-called 'mood disorders,' also known as or referred to as 'affective disorders,' are commonplace, and current epidemiological evidence suggests that depression is the most common affective "disorder,"[1] with around 350 million people suffering from depression. It is one of the most common mental health problems worldwide, with a significant social, family, and economic impact. 'Major depressive disorder' is the third cause of global disability (WHO 2016). According to the World Mental Health Survey Initiative, in 61,392 community adults in 11 countries in the Americas, Europe, and Asia, the aggregate lifetime prevalence for BP-I disorder was 0.6%, 0.4% for BP-II, 1.4% for subthreshold BP, and 2.4% for Bipolar Spectrum (Merikangas et al. 2011). In Europe, the prevalence is approximately 1% (Pini et al. 2005).

The so-called 'depressive disorders' have different classifications, but the most common symptoms are depressed mood, loss of interest and enjoyment, and reduced energy leading to diminished activity for at least 2 weeks. Many

[1] For the remainder of the chapter, the authors/editors will use the term "disorder"—in single inverted commas, to communicate the contested nature of this term.

G. López-Cortacans
Primary Care Center, Catalan Institute of Health, Barcelona, Spain

C. Ferré-Grau (✉)
Department of Nursing, Rovira i Virgili University, Tarragona, Spain
e-mail: carme.ferre@urv.cat

J.C. Santos
Escola Superior de Enfermagem de Coimbra, Nursing School of Coimbra, Coimbra, Portugal
e-mail: jcsantos@esenfc.pt

© Springer International Publishing Switzerland 2018

J.C. Santos, J.R. Cutcliffe (eds.), *European Psychiatric/Mental Health Nursing in the 21st Century*, Principles of Specialty Nursing,
https://doi.org/10.1007/978-3-319-31772-4_26

people with depression also suffer from anxiety symptoms and disturbed sleep and appetite and may have feelings of guilt or low self-worth, poor concentration, and even medically unexplained symptoms (WHO 2016). A manic episode is characterized by a distinct period during which there is an abnormally and persistently elevated, expansive, or irritable mood and abnormally and persistently increased goal-directed activity or energy (American Psychiatric Association 2013).

Although sometimes manifesting the same symptoms, these 'disorders' differ according to the intensity/severity of the symptoms and their persistence or recurrence. In clinical depression, these symptoms affect significantly the lives of people suffering from this 'disorder' and their relationships with the social and family environment (Gonzalez et al. 2010). According to the Diagnostic and Statistical Manual of Mental Disorders (American Psychiatric Association 2013) and the International Classification of Diseases (WHO 2010), the so-called 'mental disorders' can be unipolar and bipolar:

1. Unipolar 'disorders': They include the 'major depressive disorder' (MDD) and are classified as mild, moderate, or severe depending on the severity of the symptoms, if it is a single or recurrent episode, and the frequency of occurrence of the depressive symptoms over time. The so-called dysthymic 'disorder' and 'persistent affective disorder' are depressive 'disorders' with less intense symptoms, but prolonged in time and with a significant impact on the family, social, and professional life of the person suffering from it. However, "instead of focusing on the end-point diagnosis of 'depression', therapists might seek idiosyncratic formulations of the antecedent and current conditions (including the patient's individual attributed meanings) which have shaped the patient's expression of this misery" (Pilgrim and Bentall 1999:272) and focus on their narratives (Grant 2015).
2. Bipolar 'disorders': They are characterized by sudden mood changes, alternating between manic episodes (happiness) characterized by unmotivated euphoria, fast thinking, agitation, delusions of grandeur, verbiage, dispersed attention, disinhibition, and increased activity and other episodes with clear depressive symptoms (sadness), such as inhibition, sadness, pessimism, and unhappiness, among others. These changes can be very acute in manic-depressive psychoses and/or less intense as in cyclothymic 'disorders.'

Patients feel overwhelmed and flawed and a loss of autonomy. P/MH nurses can help facilitate a sense of personal control for people with 'bipolar disorder' by exploring the meaning of the symptoms for that person, implementing symptom management strategies, addressing social stigma, and facilitating active involvement in treatment (Crowe et al. 2012). The so-called bipolar disorder is associated with the highest risk of suicide among all so-called major 'psychiatric illnesses' (Schaffer et al. 2015). Despite this, the impact of bipolar disorder is generally poorly understood by P/MH nurses as evidenced by the sparse literature available in this field (Crowe et al. 2012).

The most recent treatment guidelines recommend combining pharmacological with psychoeducation interventions (Goodwin et al. 2016). Crowe et al. (2012) identified psychosocial interventions and all incorporated some features of a psychoeducation, including developing an acceptance of the disorder, awareness of its prodromes and signs of relapse, and communication with others, and several emphasized regular sleep and activity habits. The most apparently successful interventions have delivered input over many sessions in a group or family-focused setting (Bilderbeck et al. 2016), and there is a need for Psychiatric/Mental Health (P/MH) nurse to conduct high-quality trials on the clinical effectiveness of these interventions (Crowe et al. 2012). In the Netherlands, Goossens et al. (2008) identified the most common five interventions among nurses: nurse accessibility, information and education, support and counseling, action plans, and monitoring of medication use. However, they concluded that a systematic approach to the nursing process is simply lacking.

Unipolar depressive 'disorders' are ten times more frequent than 'bipolar disorders' and are associated with a higher comorbidity rate than other physical and psychological conditions. Some psychiatric/mental health nurses emphasize the use of psychotropic medication (Simon 2002) for "treating" people diagnosed as suffering from depression, but the authors of this chapter argue that patients and families should also receive treatment based on an integral care, with nursing care playing a key role in their care and development.

26.2 Prevalence of Depression and Mania: Health and Social Impact

According to the European Study of the Epidemiology of Mental Disorders (ESEMeD), lifetime prevalence rates of major depressive 'disorder' (MDD) are 8.9% for men and 16.5% for women, and their incidence has been increasing over the past few decades (Nutt et al. 2007). In a study conducted in primary health-care centers in the province of Tarragona, Spain, the authors found that one out of every seven consecutive patients treated in primary care consultations suffered from MDD, most of them having a comorbid form together with other psychiatric problems such as anxiety and substance abuse (Aragonès et al. 2004). MDD is characterized by psychological, behavioral, and somatic alterations that are often recurrent and become chronic in 25% of the cases (Ayuso-Mateos et al. 2006). Due to its clinical evolution, MDD has a 13% probability of recurrence in the first months, increasing to 85% in the following 15 years (Mueller et al. 1999), with a 50% risk of a second episode in the 2 years after the first episode, and a 80–90% risk of a third episode after the second episode (Kanai et al. 2003). A meta-analysis of 41 studies conducted in different countries found that the overall prevalence of depression in primary care was 19.5% (Mitchell et al. 2009). In Europe, the results of the prediction of depression in European general practice attendees (PREDICT) study carried out in six different countries showed a prevalence of depression in primary care consultations of 12.2% (8.5% for men and 13.9% for women) (King et al. 2008).

Studies in Spain with adult populations found a prevalence of depression ranging from 9.6% to 20.2% (Cano et al. 2012).

A mania cumulative incidence rate of 2.9% for manic and 4.0% for hypomanic episodes was found in Germany (Beesdo et al. 2009). In older psychiatric patients, the overall prevalence of late-life mania was estimated to be 6.0% in the reported 1519 older psychiatric inpatients. In elderly inpatients with bipolar disorder, the mean prevalence of late-onset mania was 44.2% (Dols et al. 2014). Age of first onset of bipolar disorder is most frequently reported in late adolescence and early adulthood (Pini et al. 2005) and decreases with age, from 1.4% in individuals aged 18–44 years to 0.1–0.4% in those aged 65 years and over (Brieger and Marneros 2005).

26.3 Interventions

According to WHO ((2015):7), the best practices for the management of moderate-severe depressive disorder are: "As first-line therapy, health care providers may select psychological treatments (such as behavioral activation [BA], cognitive behavioral therapy [CBT], or interpersonal psychotherapy [IPT]) or antidepressant medication (such as selective serotonin reuptake inhibitors [SSRIs] and tricyclic antidepressants [TCAs]). They should keep in mind the possible adverse effects associated with antidepressant medications, the ability to deliver either intervention (in terms of expertise, and/or treatment availability), and individual preferences."

According to Geddes and Miklowitz (2013), although advances in drug treatment for 'bipolar disorder' remain quite modest, antipsychotic drugs are effective in the acute treatment of mania. Lithium has the strongest evidence for long-term relapse prevention, and substantial progress has been made in the development and assessment of adjunctive psychosocial interventions. In a systematic review, Miziou et al. (2005:1) confirm "the usefulness only of psychoeducation for the relapse prevention of mood episodes and only in a selected subgroup of patients at an early stage of the disease who have very good, if not complete remission, of the acute episode. Cognitive-behavioral therapy and interpersonal and social rhythms therapy could have some beneficial effect during the acute phase, but more data are needed. Mindfulness interventions could only decrease anxiety, while interventions to improve neurocognition seem to be rather ineffective. Family intervention seems to have benefits mainly for caregivers, but it is uncertain whether they have an effect on patient outcomes" (REF).

26.3.1 The Interpersonal Approach

Given that CBT has a specific chapter and that psychopharmacology is not the focus of this book, we will only address interpersonal psychotherapy (IPT). IPT is an evidence-based therapy, which was originally developed to treat major depression (Law 2011), but can be used in other mood disorders. IPT is a time-limited, interpersonally focused, psychodynamically informed psychotherapy that has the goals of symptom relief and improving interpersonal functioning. IPT is concerned with the *interpersonal context*—the relational factors that predispose, precipitate, and perpetuate the patient's distress (Robertson et al. 2008). There are usually five distinct phases in the IPT approach: assessment, the initial sessions, middle sessions, termination sessions or conclusion of acute treatment, and maintenance sessions. According to WHO (2016), IPT identifies four categories associated with onset and persistence of depression: grief, disputes, life changes, and loneliness/social isolation. In this case, the intervention focuses on four problem areas and has eight weekly 90 min group sessions plus one initial session for each individual.

In a meta-analysis by Cuijpers et al. (2011), IPT proved to be efficient in the treatment of depression, both as an independent treatment and in combination with pharmacotherapy.

26.3.2 Identification of Major Depressive "Disorder" and Current Approaches in Primary Care

Given the high prevalence, the trend toward chronicity, and the high social health costs of MDD, new therapeutic strategies are needed to reduce disability and its social health costs. This trend toward the chronicity of depression has led some authors to propose that MDD should be addressed as a chronic disease (Holm and Severinsson 2012). Different collaborative programs between primary care and mental health services have emerged in the last two decades. These programs share the common goal of better managing chronic mental health problems through strategies to improve health-care interventions, including strategies for people suffering from depression, and adjust the care organization to these patients' needs. Primary health care gains even more importance since no significant differences were found in interpersonal functioning between treatment-seekers and nontreatment-seekers, suggesting that, even though depressed individuals do not request professional help for their mental difficulties, they still suffer a degree of impairment in their interpersonal relationships.

26.3.3 The Chronic Care Model Applied to Depression

The Chronic Care Model, which was developed by the MacColl Institute for Healthcare Innovation in Seattle, USA (Wagner et al. 1996), is the main framework for innovative care models. This model proposes a reorganization of care and profound changes in the organization and management of health-care services, incorporating a new relationship with the patient and greater integration of services and continuity of care (Reiss-Brennan et al. 2006) (Fig. 26.1).

This model results from various care and organizational proposals to improve the management of chronic diseases within integrated systems of suppliers. It was developed based on systematic reviews of medical literature and the contributions of a national panel of experts, with special attention to the importance of rethinking and redesigning the professionals' clinical practice in primary health care (Coleman

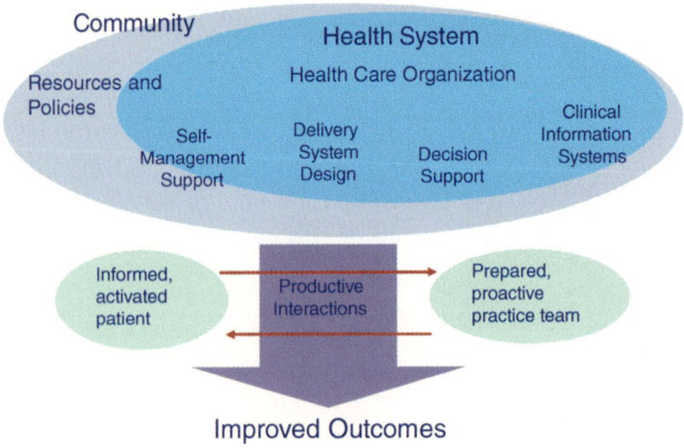

Fig. 26.1 Chronic care model (Wagner et al. 1999)

et al. 2009). The structural axis of the Chronic Care Model is based on a professional-patient relationship that enhances self-care, promotes a standardized adaptation, and establishes the objectives of a collaborative care plan, thus aiming to provide a continuous follow-up. To improve health outcomes, clinical practice was redesigned to encompass initiatives in the following areas (Coleman et al. 2009):

- Organization of the health-care system
- Relationship with the community
- Redesign of the health-care system
- Support to self-care
- Support to decision-making
- Clinical information systems
- Self-management support
- Decision support
- Delivery system design
- Clinical information systems
- Health-care organization
- Community resources

This model has also been adapted to improve multidisciplinary management and the approach to depressive "disorders" in the community.

26.3.4 Effectiveness of Collaborative Care

The Collaborative Care Model enhances the intervention of care managers, who are usually nurses with the following competencies:

– Patient clinical follow-up
– Promotion of medication adherence

- The use of psychoeducational resources to plan nursing care based on the patient's specific needs
- Integration and coordination of interventions from different professionals (family doctors, psychiatrists, psychologists, social workers, and other health professionals) to provide a better assistance and quality care for the patients

In a recent meta-analysis of 37 studies comparing the approach to depression using the Collaborative Care Model and usual care, the results showed solid evidence on the effectiveness of this model, namely, improved depressive symptoms, adherence to treatment, response to treatment, remission and recovery of symptoms, quality of life/functional status, and satisfaction with care (Thota et al. 2012). All effect estimates in the study were significant.

26.3.5 The Interventions for Depression Improvement (INDI) Model

In Tarragona, Spain, a program was designed to address depression in primary health care: the Interventions for Depression Improvement (INDI) model, which included clinical, training, and organizational measures. The INDI model is a program based on the Collaborative Care Model, whose main objective is to improve the management of depression in primary care. To this end, it is designed as a feasible tool, easy to apply in the public health system (Aragonès et al. 2007). The study protocol has already been published (Aragonès et al. 2007) and registered in http://isrctn.org (ISRCTN16384353). This was a randomized controlled trial with two study groups: the intervention group, which received this depression management intervention, and the control group, in which patients with depression received usual care.

26.3.6 The Role of Nursing in the INDI Program

One of the key differences between the intervention group and the control group is the P/MH nurse's key role in the development of the program in the intervention group (INDI), whereas the P/MH nurse does not actively intervene in depression management in the control group (usual care). The nurse is responsible for the assessment and planning of nursing care, the psychoeducational support of patients and families in the development of their self-management skills, the proactive and systematic clinical follow-up of patients with depression, and the monitoring and promotion of therapeutic compliance.

26.3.7 Organizational Aspects of the Nursing Intervention

26.3.7.1 Design of a Timetable for Follow-Up Visits

The program of approach to MDD included a recommended timetable for follow-up visits. During the acute phase of depression, three clinical follow-up visits were recommended: the first visit would take place between the second and the fourth week after the beginning of treatment, or earlier depending on the suicide risk, followed by visits every 2 or 4 weeks during the first 3 months, and, subsequently, at longer intervals, depending on the patient's evolution and the clinical data provided by the nurse in the monitoring sheet (López-Cortacans et al. 2012). The visits were scheduled by the nurse in charge of the consultation, so as to ensure the patient's assistance in the consultations and avoid discontinuity or withdrawal of the clinical follow-up and the treatment. The visits should last at least 30 minutes to improve the quality of care and achieve a better approach. If the patient missed the visit, he/she would be contacted by phone to try to reschedule (Aragonès et al. 2008).

26.3.7.2 Contents of the Follow-Up Visits

In the follow-up visit, the P/MH nurse implemented the psychoeducational interventions designed according to the patient's needs. Therapeutic adherence was systematically assessed by identifying the adverse effects and the obstacles and providing tools to overcome them. During the follow-up visits, the patient's clinical evolution was quantitatively assessed using PHQ-9, which also allowed the P/MH nurse to assess suicidal ideation. Both the information recorded and the PHQ-9 score were shared with the family doctor to facilitate decision-making regarding the therapeutic plan (changes in treatment, management of side effects, reassessment, interconsultation, referral). The consultations also facilitated the collaboration among different care providers (family doctors, psychiatrists, and nurses) and between the patients and these services.

26.3.7.3 Coordination with Mental Health Services

When primary care and mental health services share the responsibility for care delivery, the responsibilities for monitoring and treating patients and disclosing the therapeutic plan to patients and, if necessary, to families and caregivers should be clearly defined. The specialized psychiatric intervention was integrated into the care process and coordinated with the other professionals (family doctor and nurse). The existing resources, such as consultation, interconsultation, and referral, were optimized, and flexible communication mechanisms were established (via computer and telephone) so as to allow psychiatrists, family doctors, and nurses to share clinical information on the patients. When patients with depressive symptoms needed specialized care, the family doctor always informed them of the reason for and the purpose of referral, with the previous consent of the patient and/or family (Aragonès et al. 2007).

26.3.8 The Psychiatric/Mental Health Nurse's Psychoeducational Intervention in the INDI Program

Depression education has proven to be an effective tool in helping depressed patients to know more about their 'condition,' take responsibility for their treatment, and start playing an active role in the therapeutic process. According to the UK National

Institute for Health and Care Excellence (NICE 2009) clinical guidelines, psychoeducation should be one of the first interventions to be performed when patients present some type of depressive symptom. It is also useful for their families, since it helps them to understand how depression affects their relatives and, consequently, empowers them to treat their relatives in the best way possible (López-Cortacans et al. 2012). The term psychoeducation encompasses interventions aimed to inform patients and their families about the disease and its treatment, facilitating the understanding and the responsible management of their condition. Although psychoeducation can be performed by any health-care professional, in the collaborative care model, it is the P/MH nurse who often educates depressive patients and their families (Ekers et al. 2013).

In the INDI model, the nurse designs care plans based on the psychoeducation of the patients and their families. The psychoeducational contents are adjusted to the patients' needs and demands, and that is why the nurse should conduct a clinical interview in the first appointment to evaluate the patient and establish an effective communication based on the therapeutic relationship. Education in chronic diseases, such as depression, aims to empower the patient for disease self-management with a view to acquiring greater control over the decisions and actions affecting his/her health. The specific objectives of psychoeducation in the INDI model are presented below (López-Cortacans et al. 2012; Aragonès et al. 2008).

26.4 Information About Depression and/or Mania

Conveying accurate and clear information about depression and/or mania to the patients helps ensure their right to be duly informed about their 'condition' and consequently, participate in the decisions concerning their health. It also helps them fight against the stigma and prejudice associated with mental 'disorders' in general and depression in particular, as well as clarifies their doubts concerning depression. Patients usually have doubts about the definition of depression itself, since, in most cases, depression is commonly used in everyday language, leading to a confusion between clinical depression and feelings related to life difficulties, such as sadness, stress, or distress, rather than 'disorders' (Aragonès et al. 2012a, b).

The attribution of certain characteristics, such as weakness of character, lack of willingness, or inability to deal with adversity and problems, is another important component of social prejudice about depression (Aragonès et al. 2012a, b). Therefore, patients' uncertainties should be addressed, and they should be explained that although feeling occasionally sad is part of daily life, in some people, these feelings are more intense, persistent, and accompanied by other depression-related symptoms that lead to distress and have a negative impact on activities of daily living. For this reason, professionals should intervene whenever there is a potential diagnosis of depressive 'disorder.'

In this context of terminological confusion, nurses should design strategies to replace the sense of guilt felt by many patients regarding their own condition and offer an explanation for depression and/or mania that includes the biological, social, and psychological components (Aragonès et al. 2012a, b). Patients need to be aware of the clinical characteristics of depression and/or mania in order to be able to identify, using a clear language, and discuss the symptoms with more impact on their feelings and thoughts, such as sadness, weakness, sense of inability to address daily activities and challenges, loss of interest in previously pleasant activities, or an abnormally and persistently elevated, expansive, or irritable mood and abnormally and persistently increased goal-directed activity or energy in the case of mania.

P/MH nurses should also consider offering information (if it is the client's wish), about the impact of depression and/or mania on functioning and skills: lack of energy and initiative, fatigue, and difficulty in making decisions, concentrating, or thinking clearly. Patients should be informed that their difficulty in performing activities of daily living is probably a manifestation of their mental health problem and that it is not related to their lack of will or decreased motivation (Aragonès et al. 2012a, b).

Another obstacle is associated with the relatives and friends' perception of the patient's depressive symptoms as a mere state of sadness or bad mood that should be resolved in the short term. In other cases, depressive symptoms are associated with intentional disinhibition, so as to avoid the responsibilities for activities of daily living. This lack of understanding can increase the sense of guilt and decrease self-esteem, which is usually associated with depression, and increase the tendency to social isolation and, consequently, their wish to die. So, the lack of communication between patients and their families can deteriorate, hampering their recovery. The social stigma toward depression should also be highlighted since it can prevent depressed individuals from seeking help and advice and hamper treatment adherence, compliance, and social reintegration. The fight against prejudice implies changing the beliefs about depression and the way society looks at people with depression (Aragonès et al. 2012a, b).

With regard to bipolar disease, individuals who experience the condition as highly stigmatizing feel the stigma internally, but also within their social circles, health-care settings, workplaces, or schools. Stigma is associated with shame, withdrawal from social networks, concealment of the diagnosis, and reduced quality of life (Hawke et al. 2013).

26.5 Education About Treatments and the Need for Treatment Adherence

When a patient is diagnosed with depression and/or mania, his/her understanding of depression and/or mania, unlike that of the professional, is usually surrounded by mistaken beliefs and ideas. Therefore, the professional should evaluate the patient's knowledge and the resources available for coping with these conditions (Aragonès et al. 2008). Patients should also be provided with understandable information concerning the role, efficacy, mechanism of action, and adverse side effects of any medication prescribed or considered. Their questions should be clarified and answered, and misconceptions must be undone.

26.6 Education About the Benefits of Physical Exercise

A recent meta-analysis found that regular moderate-intensity exercise improves the quality of life and has a positive impact on physical and psychological health. In depressive patients, exercise has beneficial neurochemical and psychological effects (self-esteem, efficacy, socialization) (Stanton and Reaburn 2014). In addition, there is a broad consensus on the potential of physical exercise for socialization as it can promote the acquisition of social roles and rules and strengthen self-esteem, self-concept, sense of identity, and solidarity. In patients with MDD, particularly mild-to-moderate MDD, a structured and supervised 10–12-week exercise program, of moderate intensity, with 40–45 min sessions, 2–3 times per week, could improve depressive symptoms (Cooney et al. 2013). With regard to bipolar "disorder," there is no consensus about these benefits, and exercise can be a double-edged sword for patients (Thomson et al. 2015). In fact, Wright et al. (2012) found that exercise could be beneficial in helping to direct excess energy, but potentially detrimental in exacerbating maniac symptoms and potentially putting patients at risk for a spiraling of maniac and hypomanic symptoms. On the other hand, Suto et al. (2010) found that exercise is among the most helpful factors in managing bipolar "disorder."

26.7 Inclusion of the Family in Patient Care

In this psychoeducational model, emotional suffering takes place within a relational context where the person interacts with his/her surroundings (family, work, social networks). From this perspective, having a family member with depression and/or mania affects the family functioning. Therefore, P/MH nurses must identify the potential negative impact of depression and/or mania on the family and plan interventions for its reduction. They should also help the families in their relationship with the patients, highlighting what they can do to help, but also the more harmful behaviors or attitudes that they should avoid (Aragonès et al. 2008). A qualitative observational study with relatives of depressed patients found that care is mainly provided by the family, leading to a significant emotional burden (Ferré-Grau 2008). With regard to burden-related aspects, the central idea is that the contact with a depressed relative, regardless of the type of relationship, age, or gender, is a difficult experience that is hard to understand. In addition, most family members believe that both patients and caregivers find it difficult to understand depression, and this generates conflicts in the family relationships and social rejection (Ferré-Grau 2008).

26.7.1 Effectiveness of the INDI Program

This new care program has a similar effectiveness to that of similar interventions found in the literature: the response (Fig. 26.2) and remission (Fig. 26.3) rates of

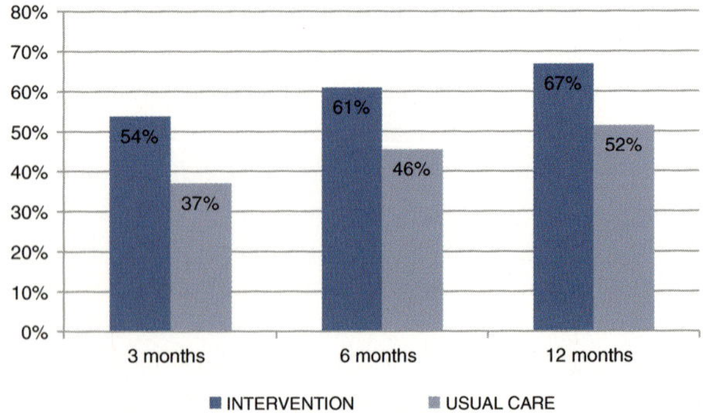

Fig. 26.2 Response rate (PHQ-9 ≤ 50% from baseline) (Aragonès et al. 2012b)

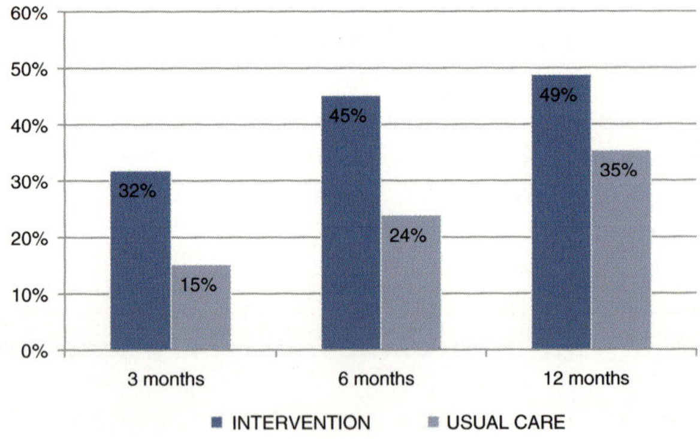

Fig. 26.3 Remission rate (PHQ-9 < 5 points) (Aragonès et al. 2012b)

depression are about 15–20% higher in patients receiving the INDI model after 3 months and at the 12 months follow-up.

Another relevant effect is the significant decrease of suicidal ideation in the intervention group when compared to the control group, which was 67% at the 12 months follow-up.

This may be very significant for public health care considering the high prevalence of depression in primary care and its massive impact on health and quality of life. The potential benefits of the generalization of the INDI model are, therefore, substantial (Aragonès et al. 2012a, b). An economic evaluation of the impact of the model on the health-care system (health costs) and society (health costs and costs related to lost productivity) in terms of cost-effectiveness (clinical effects) and cost-utility (effects on functioning and quality of life) was also conducted. The INDI program leads to better health outcomes than usual care, both in terms of cost-utility (QALY) and clinical effectiveness (depression-free days). These positive outcomes have been achieved with a moderate increase in costs, which results in favorable cost-effectiveness and cost-utility ratios (Aragonès et al. 2014).

The INDI program has been implemented in primary care settings, the level of care that offers greater accessibility and where the most common mental health problems in the population can be more equally and efficiently managed. In addition, it is an intervention adjusted to the current priorities and strategies established in the Spanish National Health System for an approach to chronicity, both in terms of objectives and implementation (López-Cortacans 2015). Nurses should acquire competencies and skills to intervene in mental health conditions, namely, in MDD, thus providing advanced direct care to depressive patients and their families (Ferré-Grau 2005).

From this perspective, the active involvement of P/MH nurses in the design, participation in, and development of research on collaborative care programs for depression management provides a new framework for improving their professional skills. For this reason, nursing professionals should be able to access the best evidence-based training/education on health care and its delivery. In order to meet the needs of patients and their families and ensure an effective health-care system, it is necessary to promote research on quality care, namely, on health conditions that require continuous care, such as depression.

26.8 Concluding Remarks

The so-called mood disorders are one of the most prevalent mental health 'disorders' worldwide, associated with high burden of disability. Increased accessibility and fight against stigma are essential to cope with depression and mania and promote well-being. For this reason, an early recognition and intervention could be the best answer for individuals, families, and society. Primary care settings play a key role in prevention and recovery with different approaches and interventions; however, further studies are needed to find the best available evidence on this topic. The Collaborative Care Model and the INDI Model (in Spain) proved to be efficient in treating these conditions. In addition, a person-centered approach with a focus on patients' narratives and meanings, rather than on diagnosis and a medicalized language, could be an important basis for future nursing interventions. P/MH nurses can implement several interventions and approaches which, despite their differences, have in common the fact that relational skills and the establishment of a productive therapeutic alliance is more important than any technique.

References

American Psychiatric Association (2013) Diagnostic and statistical manual of mental disorders, 5th edn. American Psychiatric Publishing, Arlington, VA

Aragonès E, López-Cortacans G, Sánchez-Iriso E, Piñol JL, Caballero A, Salvador-Carulla L, Cabasés J (2014) Cost-effectiveness analysis of a collaborative care programme for depression in primary care. J Affect Disord 159(13):85–93

Aragonès E, Caballero A, Piñol JL, López-Cortacans G, Badia W, Hernández JM, Casaus P (2007) Assessment of an enhanced program for depression management in primary care: a cluster randomized controlled trial. The INDI project (interventions for depression improvement). BMC Public Health 7:253

Aragonès E, Cardoner N, Colom F, López-Cortacans G, Gilaberte I (2012a) Guia de buena práctica clínica. Psicoeducación en pacientes con depresión. Organización Médica Colegial, Madrid

Aragonès E, López-Cortacans G, Badia W, Hernández JM, Caballero A, Labad A (2008) Improving the role of nursing in the treatment of depression in primary care in Spain. Perspect Psychiatr Care 44(4):248–258

Aragonès E, Piñol JL, Labad A, Masdéu RM, Pino M, Cervera J (2004) Prevalence and determinants of depressive 'disorders' in primary care practice in Spain. Int J Psychiatry Med 34(1):21–35

Aragonès E, Piñol JLL, Caballero A, López-Cortacans G, Casaus P, Hernández JM, Badia W (2012b) Effectiveness of a multi-component programme for managing depression in primary care: a cluster randomized trial. The INDI project. J Affect Disord 142(1–3):297–305

Ayuso-Mateos J, Nieto-Moreno M, Sánchez-Moreno J, Vázquez-Barquero JL (2006) Clasificación Internacional del Funcionamiento, la Discapacidad y la Salud (CIF): aplicabilidad y utilidad en la práctica clínica. Med Clin 126(12):461–466

Beesdo K, Hofler M, Leibenluft E, Lieb R, Bauer M, Pfennig A (2009) Mood episodes and mood disorders: patterns of incidence and conversion in the first three decades of life. Bipolar Disord 11:637–649

Bilderbeck AC et al (2016) Psychoeducation and online mood tracking for patients with bipolar disorder: a randomised controlled trial. J Affect Disord 205(2016):245–251

Brieger P, Marneros A (2005) Bipolar disorders in late life. In: Kasper S, Hirschfeld RMA (eds) Handbook of bipolar disorder: diagnosis and therapeutic approaches. Taylor & Francis Group, LLC, Boca Raton, FL, pp 83–93

Cano A, Salguero JM, Mae C, Dongil E, Latorre JM (2012) La depresión en atención primaria: prevalencia, diagnóstico y tratamiento. Papeles del Psicólogo 33(1):2–11

Coleman K, Austin BT, Brach C, Wagner EH (2009) Evidence on the chronic care model in the new millennium. Health Aff 28(1):75–85

Cooney GM, Dwan K, Greig CA, Lawlor DA, Rimer J, Waugh FR, McMurdo M, Mead G (2013) Exercise for depression. Cochrane Database Syst Rev 9

Crowe M, Inder M, Carlyle D, Wilson L, Whitehead L, Panckhurst A, O'Brien A, Joyce P (2012) Feeling out of control: a qualitative analysis of the bipolar disorder. J Psychiatr Ment Health Nurs 19(4):294–302

Cuijpers P, Geraedts A, Oppen P, Andersson G, Markowitz J, van Straten A (2011) Interpersonal psychotherapy for depression: a meta-analysis. Am J Psychiatry 168:581–592

Dols A, Kupka RW, van Lammeren A, Beekman AT, Sajatovic M, Stek ML (2014) The prevalence of late-life mania: a review. Bipolar Disord 16:113–118

Ekers D, Murphy R, Archer J, Ebenezer C, Kemp D, Gilbody S (2013) Nurse-delivered collaborative care for depression and long-term physical conditions: a systematic review and meta-analysis. J Affect Disord 149(1–3):14–22

Ferré-Grau C (2005) Depressió pacients i familiars. Cossetània, Valls

Ferré-Grau C (2008) Dimensiones del cuidado familiar en la depresión: Un estudio etnográfico. Índex Enfermería 17(3):178–182

Geddes J, Miklowitz D (2013) Treatment of bipolar disorder. Lancet 381(9878):1672–1682

Gonzalez L et al (2010) Vivencia de los cuidadores familiares de adultos mayores que sufren depresión. Rev esc enferm 44(1):32–39. doi:10.1590/S0080-62342010000100005

Goodwin G et al (2016) Evidence-based guidelines for treating bipolar disorder: revised third edition recommendations from the British Association for Psychopharmacology. J Psychopharmacol 30:495–553

Goossens P, Beentjes T, Leeuw J, Klein E, Achterberg T (2008) The nursing of outpatients with a bipolar disorder: what nurses actually do. Arch Psychiatr Nurs 22(1):3–11

Grant A (2015) Demedicalising misery: welcoming the human paradigm in mental health nurse education. Nurse Educ Today 35:e50–e53

Hawke L, Parikh S, Michalak E (2013) Stigma and bipolar disorder: a review of the literature. J Affect Disord 150:181–191

Holm AL, Severinsson E (2012) Chronic care model for the management of depression: synthesis of barriers and facilitators of success. Int J Ment Health Nurs 21(6):513–523

Kanai T, Takeuchi H, Furukawa TA, Yoshimura R, Imaizumi T, Kitamura T, Takahashi K (2003) Time to recurrence after recovery from major depressive episodes and its predictors. Psychol Med 33(5):839–845
King M, Nazareth I, Levy G, Walker C, Morris R, Weich S, Bellón-Saameño JA et al (2008) Prevalence of common mental 'disorder's in general practice attendees across Europe. Br J Psychiatry 192(5):362–367
Law R (2011) Interpersonal psychotherapy for depression. Adv Psychiatr Treat 17(1):23–31
López-Cortacans G (2015) Propuesta de mejora para la sostenibilidad del sistema sanitario público desde el marco competencial enfermero. Enferm Clin 25(3):149–150
López-Cortacans G, Badia W, Caballero A, Casaus P, Piñol JL, Aragonès E (2012) Efectividad de un programa para el abordaje multidisciplinar de la depresión que potencia el rol enfermero en Atención Primaria. Metas de Enfermería 15(2):28–32
Merikangas K et al (2011) Prevalence and correlates of bipolar spectrum disorder in the world mental health survey initiative. Arch Gen Psychiatry 68(3):241–251
Mitchell AJ, Vaze A, Rao S (2009) Clinical diagnosis of depression in primary care: a meta-analysis. Lancet 374(9690):609–619
Miziou S, Tsitsipa E, Moysidou S, Karavelas V, Dimelis D, Polyzoidou V, Fountoulakis K (2005) Psychosocial treatment and interventions for bipolar disorder: a systematic review. Ann General Psychiatry 14:19
Mueller TI, Leon AC, Keller MB, Solomon DA, Endicott J, Coryell W (1999) Impact of bipolar disorder. J Psychiatr Ment Health Nurs 19:294–302
NICE (2009) Depression in adults with a chronic physical health problem: treatment and management. In: NICE clinical guideline 91. NICE, London
Nutt DJ, Kessler RC, Alonso J, Benbow A, Lecrubier Y, Lépine JP et al (2007) Consensus statement on the benefit to the community of ESEMeD (European study of the epidemiology of mental 'disorder's) survey data on depression and anxiety. J Clin Psychiatry 68(2):42–48
Pilgrim D, Bentall R (1999) The medicalization of misery: a critical realistic analysis of the concept of depression. J Ment Health 8(3):261–274
Pini S, Queiroz V, Pagnin D, Pezawas L, Angst J, Cassano G, Wittchen H (2005) Prevalence and burden of bipolar disorders in European countries. Eur Neuropsychopharmacol 15(4): 425–434
Reiss-Brennan B, Briot P, Cannon W, James B (2006) Mental health integration: rethinking practitioner roles in the treatment of depression: the specialist, primary care physicians, and the practice nurse. Ethn Dis 16(2):37–43
Robertson M, Rushton P, Wurm C (2008) Interpersonal psychotherapy: an overview. Psychother Australia 14(3):46–54
Schaffer A, Isometsä ET, Tondo L, Moreno DH, Sinyor M, Kessing LV, Turecki G, Weizman A, Azorin J-M, Ha K, Reis C, Cassidy F, Goldstein T, Rihmer Z, Beautrais A, Chou Y-H, Diazgranados N, Levitt AJ, Zarate CA, Yatham L (2015) Epidemiology, neurobiology and pharmacological interventions related to suicide deaths and suicide attempts in bipolar disorder: part I of a report of the International Society for Bipolar Disorders Task Force on suicide in bipolar disorder. Aust NZ J Psychiatry 49(9):785–802
Simon G (2002) Evidence review: efficacy and effectiveness of antidepressant treatment in primary care. Gen Hosp Psychiatry 24(4):213–224
Stanton R, Reaburn P (2014) Exercise and the treatment of depression: a review of the exercise program variables. Aust J Sci Med Sport 17(2):177–182
Suto M, Murray G, Hale S, Amari E, Michalak EE (2010) What works for people with bipolar disorder? Tips from the experts. J Affect Disord 124:76–84. doi:10.1016/j.jad.2009.11.004
Thomson D, Turner A, Lauder S, Gigler M, Berk L, Singh A, Pasco J, Berk M, Sylvia L (2015) A brief review of exercise, bipolar disorder, and mechanistic pathways. Front Psychol 6:147
Thota AB, Sipe TA, Byard GJ, Zometa CS, Hahn RA, McKnight-Eily LR, Chapman DP et al (2012) Collaborative care to improve the management of depressive 'disorder's: a community guide systematic review and meta-analysis. Am J Prev Med 42(5):525–538

Wagner E, Austin B, Von Korff M (1996) Organizing care for patients with chronic illness. Milbank Q 74(4):511–554

Wagner EH, Davis C, Schaefer J, Von Korff M, Austin B (1999) A survey of leading chronic disease management programs: are they consistent with the literature? Manag Core Q 7(3):56–66

WHO (2010) International statistical classification of diseases and related health problems. 10th revision

WHO (2015) Update of the mental health gap action programme (mhGAP) guideline for mental, neurological and substance use disorders WHO mhGAP guideline update May 2015

WHO (2016) Depression. Fact sheet, http://www.who.int/mediacentre/factsheets/fs369/en/ Retrieved Apr 2016

Wright K, Armstrong T, Taylor A, Dean S (2012) "It's a double edged sword": a qualitative analysis of the experiences of exercise amongst people with bipolar disorder. J Affect Disord 136:634–642. doi:10.1016/j.jad.2011.10.017

The Person Experiencing Anxiety 27

Columba McLaughlin

27.1 Introduction

According to the European Regional Office of the World Health Organization (WHO 2015), anxiety is a mental health problem and currently is one of the main causes of disability and early retirement (Shear 2012; WHO 2015). They affirm that anxiety is a major burden on European economies, and this in turn has demanded policy action from health-care authorities. Furthermore, given the ubiquitous nature of anxiety in humans, it may be of little surprise that the reported incidence of anxiety-related mental health problems is high; according to Baxter et al. (2014) and their Global Burden of Disease study, the so-called anxiety disorders were the sixth leading cause of disability, in terms of years of life lived with disability (YLDs), in both high-income and low- and middle-income countries.

Indeed, the experience of anxiety is very much a normal part of everyday life for humans, especially when we are facing situations that are perceived to be dangerous or difficult. Human life is full of challenges, and for many, experiencing challenges is stressful and creates anxiety in some people. The human experience of anxiety is usually initiated by the perception of a negative cognitive stimulus (Lupien et al. 2007). The holistic response to the perceived threat initiated by a person's sympathetic nervous system can, if unchecked, impact profoundly on a person's physical and mental health. However, relevant to the person's story, the negative effects of anxiety are preventable, manageable and ultimately treatable (Mental Health Foundation 2014). In caring for people experiencing anxiety, psychiatric/mental health (P/MH) nurses are likely to need to help the person address both psychological and behavioural issues. As a result, this chapter will: (1) explore the aetiology and theoretical origins of anxiety—in so doing, it is necessary to draw upon seminal

C. McLaughlin
Ulster University, Derry, BT48 7JL, UK
e-mail: c.mclaughlin@ulster.ac.uk

© Springer International Publishing Switzerland 2018

J.C. Santos, J.R. Cutcliffe (eds.), *European Psychiatric/Mental Health Nursing in the 21st Century*, Principles of Specialty Nursing,
https://doi.org/10.1007/978-3-319-31772-4_27

and classic works and thus some of the references will be of a recognized vintage, (2) differentiate between the closely related concepts of stress and anxiety, (3) explore the common holistic manifestations of anxiety in the individual—for some this might be considered as signs and symptoms, (4) explore the potential impacts of anxiety on a person's physical and mental health and (5) explore how P/MH nurses can respond to and help the individual learn to manage their experience of anxiety.

27.2 Understanding the Human Experience of Stress

It is difficult to discuss anxiety without discussing the concept of stress. The manifestation of anxiety is imbedded in the person's experience of what they perceive to be stressful situations. While unchecked stress and pernicious anxiety are clearly linked with the development of mental health problems, the presence of stress or anxiety in a person's lived experiences does not necessarily indicate that the person has a mental health problem (mental illness for some). Indeed, the experience of anxiety is reported in both those who have been termed 'mentally ill' and those that have not (Achim et al. 2011; Young et al. 2013). Further, there are substantive differences between stress and anxiety. For instance, stress is caused by life events that put a person under physical and mental pressure (Sandi 2013). Also, the experience of managing a stressful event is educational and developmentally valuable, from an experiential point of view at least (Joëls et al. 2006). Whereas, the experience of anxiety can include all the physiological and psychological symptoms of stress, but its symptoms appear as a result of unrealistic and excessive worry (Shear 2012). In addition, while stress can have a positive effect on the person's psyche and help them to achieve personal goals, anxiety is characterised with apprehension and thoughts of impending doom about life events that are real or imagined. Thus, while stress and anxiety have similar symptoms, the aetiology and progress of both is somewhat different.

[1]Selye's three-phase model of the human body's response to stress (Selye 1956, 1978) is a 'classic' theoretical model. The *1st phase (Alarm Reaction)* occurs immediately when the stressor is sensed. For instance, a sudden unexpected loud noise will elicit an ultra-fast autonomic nervous system response. In this 1st phase, the physiological response is mediated by the sympathetic-adrenomedullary axis (SAM). Also, the SAM can be activated through an implied threat where a person perceives the event as being novel, uncontrollable and unpredictable (Lupien et al. 2007). In brief, upon sensing the stressor, the hypothalamus immediately activates the sympathetic branch of the autonomic nervous system. This then stimulates the adrenal medulla to release adrenaline and noradrenaline. These neurotransmitters create the physiological responses noticeable in stress situations (e.g. increased

[1]For a more comprehensive description and explanation of these processes, the reader is referred to any of the major and for many seminal texts on stress and anxiety.

heart rate, increased blood pressure, trembling, muscle tension, nausea and sweatiness). This is called the 'fight or flight' response (Cannon 1929).

Should the stressor persist, then *Phase 2 (Stage of Resistance)* will commence within a few minutes of the initial stress event. In this phase the physiological response is maintained by the hypothalamic-pituitary-adrenocortical axis (HPA) (Smith and Vale 2006). The person remains in a state of high alert, and physiological arousal also remains high. Furthermore, everyday life events that impact on a person's physical, mental and emotional well-being are known as stressors, and they can result in HPA activation (Smith and Vale 2006). For example, normal events, such as meeting work deadlines, driving safely through the early morning traffic and paying household bills each month have the potential to create stress in a person. However, any stressful everyday life event, if not successfully dealt with, has the potential to create *distress* in a person (Selye 1956, 1978). Distress is a negative form of stress, and, by activating the HPA axis, it produces very unpleasant physical effects such as increased cardiovascular activity and emotional effects such as worry and rumination. If the person does not resolve the issue causing them distress, then the continued HPA activity could become detrimental to their physical and mental health and their well-being (Smith and Vale 2006).

Unfortunately, not all stressful events are easily resolved. People can and do experience distress with real-life events that they consider a threat to them. In such situations, the resistance phase is prolonged, and the endocrine response ensures that the major organs of the body are mobilised to respond to any demand that the stressor makes. For example, the release of the hormone 'cortisol' will stimulate the liver to release glucose and give the body energy (Kalat 2014). Furthermore, as the body becomes used to the stressor, the presence of neurotransmitters and hormones in the body is maintained at a lower level. While being so prepared may seem like a positive defensive strategy, the reality is that the muscular tension, sweatiness, trembling and the mental alertness felt by the person as a result of the HPA activity can begin to have a negative effect on the body's defence systems. If the person is experiencing distress and it is prolonged and not dealt with, then *Phase 3 (Stage of Exhaustion)* is possible. This prolonged defence response may result in damage to the immune system (Kalat 2014) leading to illness or increased susceptibility to illness, an increased risk of high blood pressure and heart disease (Smith and Vale 2006).

What a person thinks about a stressor is highly relevant to how they respond to it (Selye 1978). For example, a person may have previous experience of successfully dealing with a particular stressor. If the person experiences this stressor again, they will still experience the HPA response. However, their previous 'learned' success can help mitigate the unpleasant physiological effects, and the HPA response would help them to remain focused and physically prepared to meet the challenge of the stressor (Smith and Vale 2006). This type of stress is known as *eustress* (Selye 1978). It is a positive reaction to any impending life event that creates a need within the person to achieve success and overcome the challenge that the stressor presents with. Furthermore, if the person has the correct coping skills and has had previous success in dealing with a particular stressor, there is a good chance that they will successfully deal with the stressor again (Bandura 1982). Having successfully dealt with a stressful life experience, a person's feeling of self-efficacy is enhanced (Bandura 1982). This learning can be a buffer in preventing the person from experiencing *distress* when meeting future challenges. Thus, it is the person's perception of the stressor's threat level and their ability to overcome it that will determine whether they will experience *eustress* or *distress.*

27.3 Understanding the Human Experience of Anxiety

Everyone experiences anxiety at some time in their lives. *For example, before confronting challenges in their lives, such as going to interviews of when university examinations are scheduled, most people will become mentally and physically aroused and, to some degree, apprehensive. These emotional responses are justified and categorised as normal emotions to these life events.* However, anxiety really becomes a problem when it interferes with a person's day-to-day life. People react differently to novel situations and a person's cognitive appraisal of each situation in terms of their coping ability is key in determining how anxious they will feel (Martin 2016). Thus, depending on a person's appraisal of their ability to successfully confront a challenge, *one person may experience mild anxiety, while another person might experience a more severe form of anxiety that is overwhelming and debilitating*. A person may see anxiety as a mental health problem only when they are unable to sleep at night and are worrying about things that are not likely to happen.

Some anxiety is normal, healthy, enhances performance and helps a person to focus on a task but only up to a point (Royal College of Psychiatrists 2017). For instance, according to the Yerkes-Dodsón law, there is an empirical relationship between arousal and performance (Yerkes and Dodson 1908). This law proposes that performance will increase with physiological or mental arousal. However, when levels of arousal become too high, as in anxiety, performance will decrease and can render the person unable to perform everyday activities. Yerkes and Dodson (1908) demonstrated this in their bell-shaped curve which increases and then decreases with higher levels of arousal. The body's response to anxiety is very much similar to the body's response to stress. In terms of physiological symptoms, anxiety mimics the 'resistance' phase of Selye (1978) model. However, the difference between both is that most stressful life events will eventually reach a climax when the stressor has been successfully challenged. Whereas in anxiety, the person's cognitive appraisal is distorted, the outcome is uncertain and the person might remain in continuous fear of a catastrophic event happening to them. In brief, when a person's thoughts become preoccupied with unnecessary worry over a number of days and they feel that they need to avoid everyday events, there is a possibility that they are experiencing anxiety. As in the body's response to stress, when a person experiences anxiety, their hypothalamic-pituitary-adrenocortical (HPA) axis will be activated. As a result of this activation, the person will experience some of the physiological, behavioural and cognitive symptoms that are shown in Table 27.1.

Table 27.1 Symptoms associated with the experience of anxiety

Physiological symptoms
• Tachycardia, increased blood pressure, chest pain, flushed face, dizziness and faintness
• Hyperventilation, shortness of breath
• Nausea, vomiting
• Muscle tension, trembling, balance difficulties, fidgeting, rigidity
• Sweating
Behavioural symptoms
• Increased alcohol intake, drug taking, smoking
• Avoiding social events
• Speech difficulties
• Nail biting
• Sleeping difficulties
Cognitive symptoms
• Reduced concentration
• Selective attention to potential danger and safety
• Sense of impending doom
• Fear
• Worry
• Rumination
• Apprehension
• Forgetfulness
• Poor memory

27.4 The Aetiology of Anxiety

A number of theoretical perspectives, such as cognitive (Freeman and DiTomasso 1994) and biological (Jacofsky et al. 2013), suggest how anxiety arises in a person. Cognitive theory suggests that some people overestimate the threat level to them and underestimate their ability to cope with such threat. According to the cognitive theory, it is these misinterpretations that create anxiety in a person. In effect the person can feel overwhelmed and threatened at the thought of an imminent negative life event. Alternatively, biological theories, advanced by Jacofsky et al. (2013) suggest that anxiety is created within a person as a result of an imbalance in specific neurotransmitters. For instance, in anxiety there is a reduction in gamma-aminobutyric acid (GABA) and serotonin and an increase in norepinephrine (Sinha et al. 2004). The emphasis here is on the imbalance of these neurotransmitters rather than any impactful life event or experience. Nonetheless, irrespective of differing theoretical perspectives, the person will exhibit some of the aforementioned physiological, behavioural and cognitive symptoms (Table 27.1).

27.5 Anxiety Disorders

High levels of anxiety can be very disabling and can interfere with a person's interpersonal, occupational and social functioning (Freeman and DiTomasso 1994). In anxiety disorders, a person will experience exaggerated worry, apprehension, muscular tension and tachycardia that are not in keeping with the stressor. There are a number of different specific (so-called) anxiety disorders that seriously affect a person's physical and mental health. These are post-traumatic stress disorder (PTSD), generalised anxiety disorder (GAD), phobia, obsessive-compulsive disorder (OCD) and panic disorder (PD) (Wolman and Stricker 1994). When activated each of these anxiety disorders will activate the sympathetic nervous system (SNS) and create a high state of anxiety in a person. Thus, the person will experience a wide range of physiological, cognitive and behavioural symptoms. The person with the anxiety disorder is the expert in how it affects them. P/MH nurses, in their assessment, planning and delivery of care, must at all times include the client as active participants in all aspects of their care (NICE 2011).

A major key to the reduction of the excessive activities of the SNS is the activation of the parasympathetic nervous system (PSNS). The PSNS counteracts the SNS and slows down breathing and heart rate and decreases muscle tension. In order to activate the PSNS, nurses have a variety of care interventions at their disposal. However, deciding the chosen care intervention must include the person and be tailored towards the person's needs (NICE 2011). Furthermore, supportive family members are important in care delivery, and any information given to them should be culturally appropriate.

27.6 Post-traumatic Stress Disorder (PTSD)

Post-traumatic stress disorder is defined in the ICD-10 (World Health Organization (WHO) 1992) under code F43.1. PTSD is very different to other anxiety disorders because it is related to a devastating life event that has a real origin in the person's life experience (WHO 1992). In brief, the person re-experiences a previous extremely catastrophic event such as violent personal assault, natural disaster, military combat or some other event that was life threatening at the time (American Psychological Association (APA 2016a) (recovered 4 January 2017). Thus, while the event has occurred in the past, it has left the person with an aftermath of distressing memories. However, it is important to know that (1) not everyone, who experiences a devastating life event, will experience PTSD (NIMH 2016a) and (2) some people learn and develop post-traumatic growth following such an experience (Calhoun and Tedeschi 2014; Joëls et al. 2006).(*For a more in-depth discussion on post-traumatic growth, please see* Chap. 12.) Nonetheless, for a person experiencing PTSD, any sensory, social or environmental reminders of the traumatic event will arouse intense distress in the person. The person will experience symptoms such as flashbacks and nightmares (Parson 1994; SAMHSA 2014). They frequently struggle with obsessive thoughts about what happened, what they should have done and the possibility of revenge. Also, they frequently have difficulty sleeping, and they may be irritable an exhibit anger (NICE 2005a). These disturbing cognitive activities will activate the HPA axis, and the person will experience severe physical symptoms as well. As a result of these reactions, the person may also take behavioural action in avoiding people or situations associated with the event.

27.6.1 P/MH Nursing Responses to Clients Experiencing PTSD

In assessing a client's needs, nurses should be knowledgeable about traumas that predispose to PTSD. These include domestic violence, road traffic accidents, childhood sexual abuse, bullying, rape and other violent assaults. P/MH nurses have a role to play in helping people suffering from PTSD. SAMHSA (2014) advocates that nurses should approach the person in a matter-of-fact yet supportive manner because this helps build trust between the person and the nurse. Initially, it might be very difficult for a PTSD sufferer to discuss details of the trauma. Therefore, nurses should spend time with the client establishing a trusting therapeutic relationship before addressing the traumatic event. The nurse-client therapeutic relationship is key, and developing such relationships will promote trust and help the person grow towards recovery from their traumatic experiences (Cronin et al. 2014; Ferencik and Ramirez-Hammond, (recovered 3rd January 2017). However, P/MH nurses must ensure that time is spent with clients in developing this relationship (Peplau 1994; Whittington and McLaughlin 2000) and engaging therapeutically with the person (Cutcliffe and Barker 2002).

The National Center for PTSD (recovered 8 December 2016) declares that psychological debriefing is not always an appropriate mental health intervention, and in some instances, it may increase traumatic stress or complicate recovery. However, CBT that focuses on the trauma is the recommended main treatment intervention for PTSD (Parson 1994; NICE 2005a). Therefore, non-trauma-focused interventions, such as relaxation or non-directive counselling, should not be seen as primary treatment interventions with people suffering PTSD symptoms (NICE 2005a). More recently, SAMHSA (recovered 23rd December 2016) recommends cognitive restructuring through CBT, where the person is helped to make sense of their bad memories and their negative thinking. Furthermore, SAMHSA (Recovered 23rd December 2016) also recommends exposure therapy, where the person is exposed in a safe way to the trauma they experienced. Additionally, NICE (2005a) recommends that therapy should be held at least once each week for between 8 and 12 sessions delivered by the same nurse specially trained in post-trauma psychotherapy. What's more, while the transient nature of PTSD precludes the use of benzodiazepines in the management of PTSD (Bernardy 2013), antidepressants may be prescribed if the person shows clinical signs of depression (NIMH 2016a).

27.7 Generalised Anxiety Disorder (GAD)

Generalised anxiety disorder (GAD) is defined in the ICD-10 (World Health Organization 1992) under code F41.1. GAD is one of the most prevalent mental health problems seen in primary care (Achim et al. 2011). It is a chronic debilitating so-called disorder where the person persistently and excessively worries about non-specific life events or objects (Mental Health Foundation 2014). The person living with GAD is often worried about health, money, work or family even when these worries are unrealistic. Also, they will frequently have difficulty in identifying the specific cause of their worry. According to the DSM-IV criteria, a diagnosis can be made if the person has suffered this type of worry for 6 months (Shear 2012). We have to bear in mind that long-term anxiety such as this will involve long-term HPA activation, and this will, as previously described, impact on the person's physical and mental health. However, GAD varies in its severity, and this has implications for treatment.

27.7.1 P/MH Nursing Responses to Clients Experiencing GAD

In their comprehensive and holistic assessment, the P/MH nurse needs to consider symptom severity, duration, degree of distress, functional impairment, personal history and any comorbidities such as depression (NICE 2011). There are a number of guidelines where P/MH nurses can draw from that are useful in helping people experiencing anxiety. For instance, the Substance Abuse and Mental Health Services Administration (SAMHSA) guidelines (SAMHSA 2014) offer best practice guidelines for the prevention and treatment of mental disorders. These guidelines come in the form of specific Treatment Improvement Protocols (TIPs) that strive to convey frontline information to relevant health-care authorities. In addition, NICE (2011) guidelines recommend a stepped care model to guide therapeutic interventions (Table 27.2).

This stepped care model shows that interventions are based on the severity of the symptoms. For instance, depending on the severity of the GAD presentation, P/MH nurses will decide the level of intervention required. The higher the step, the more intense is the intervention.

Step 1, a person will present with low anxiety, and the nursing interventions would include education about the disorder and monitoring of their cognitive and behavioural symptoms.

Step 2, the person will be experiencing mild anxiety, and prescribed interventions would consist of guided self-help which would include the use of

Table 27.2 NICE (2011, p. 13) stepped care model for generalised anxiety disorder

Focus of the intervention	Nature of the intervention
Step 4: Complex treatment-refractory GAD and very marked functional impairment, such as self-neglect or a high risk of self-harm	Highly specialist treatment, such as complex drug and/or psychological treatment regimens, input from multi-agency teams, crisis services, day hospitals or inpatient care
Step 3:GAD with an inadequate response to step 2 interventions or marked functional impairment	Choice of a high-intensity psychological intervention (CBT/applied relaxation) or a drug treatment
Step 2: Diagnosed GAD that has not improved after education and active monitoring in primary care	Low-intensity psychological interventions: individual non-facilitated self-help, individual guided self-help and psychoeducational groups
Step 1: All known and suspected presentations of GAD	Identification and assessment, education about GAD and treatment options, active monitoring

computerised cognitive behavioural therapy programmes such as 'FearFighter™', 'Beating the Blues™' or 'MoodGYM™' they may be referred to group therapy.

Step 3, the person will present with moderate-to-severe anxiety and will require supportive help from P/MH nurses. In this step the person will also require help from specialist qualified P/MH nurses in delivering high-intensity psychological therapy such as one-to-one cognitive behavioural therapy (CBT), eye movement desensitisation and reprocessing (EMDR) or applied relaxation therapy. Also, in this step the person may be prescribed a suitable medication.

Step 4, the person will present with severe anxiety and marked functional impairment and possibly at risk of self-harm. This is a very serious step and more intense interventions such as cognitive behaviour therapy (CBT), medications or even hospitalisation may be required (NICE 2011).

27.8 Phobias

Phobias are defined in the ICD-10 (World Health Organization 1992) under code F40. A phobia is an irrational fear of a situation or object or living creature (Mental Health Foundation 2014). This is a specific anxiety (so-called) disorder, and it has a fear response that is identified with a specific cause, despite the person being aware that their fear is irrational and/or disproportionate to the perceived threat. There are two types of phobia and these are real phobias and psychological phobias (Allaboutcounselling recovered 21 December 2016). A real phobia is where a person has had previous direct contact with an entity that resulted in them experiencing severe anxiety. For example, a young person may have climbed a tree and got stuck requiring rescuing. In later life this has potential to create a fear of heights in the person. Furthermore, a person may have a medical condition such as an allergy towards skin care products. Both of these fears are not unreasonable, and the phobias are not psychological.

However, there are psychological phobias which are manifested in the absence of any direct contact with an entity. Examples of commonly known phobias are public speaking, spiders and open spaces (MIND 2014). While the person has such a specific fear, the exact cause of this fear is frequently unknown. Such phobias are psychological, and they usually begin when a person believes there is a possible threat of danger to them from an entity. According to Marks et al. (1991), with this distorted thinking, the person increasingly tries to avoid the anxiety provoking entity. However, in so doing they reinforce the phobia and maintain the pattern of behaviour (SAMHSA 2014; APA 2016b).

Irrespective of the aetiology of the phobia, the person will try to avoid any situation involving their specific phobia. However, if they cannot avoid such a specific situation, then they will experience anxiety. While a fear of spiders might minimally interfere with a person's quality of life, some phobias such agoraphobia or social phobia could impact heavily on a person's ability to socialise in shopping malls, sports stadiums and in work places (MIND 2014).

27.8.1 P/MH Nursing Responses to Clients Experiencing a Phobia

When phobia interferes with a person's lifestyle to a degree of incapacity, current evidence suggests that the most effective responses should include CBT (SAMHSA 2014; MIND 2014). The specialist trained P/MH nurse will use CBT to help the person explore their understanding of the phobia and help them to create new thinking within them. In some severe cases, the treatment may include desensitisation therapy, and CBT will help the person to prepare for this. Desensitisation therapy is combined with positive reinforcement through a process of graduated exposure to the phobic entity as described by the seminal works of Jones (1924) and Wanderer (1972).

27.9 Obsessive-Compulsive Disorder (OCD)

Obsessive-compulsive disorder is defined in the ICD-10 (World Health Organization 1992) under code F42. It is characterised by recurrent thoughts (obsessions) and behaviours (compulsions) that are intrusive (MIND 2014), and the person wants to repeat them over and over again (NIMH 2016b). The person usually understands that their actions are irrational, but they struggle to avoid doing so. In brief, a person will have an intrusive thought or sudden impulse that urges them to perform a behaviour. If the behaviour is not carried, it would result in the person experiencing anxiety and becoming distressed until such time as the behaviour is performed. Many behaviours associated with the compulsion are ritualistic, and the person is compelled to complete the ritual in a specified way in order to get relief. Some common examples of OCD are where the person may wash their hands constantly or clean obsessively in a ritualistic way. It seems that the performance of the ritual reduces the person's distress.

27.9.1 P/MH Nursing Responses to Clients Experiencing OCD

The compulsion only becomes incapacitating when it interferes with a person's daily activities and psychotherapy, therefore, focuses on changing the behaviour and neutralising negative thoughts (NIMH recovered 22nd December 2016c). Furthermore, NICE (2013) updated the core interventions recommended for the treatment of obsessive-compulsive disorder. This then has influenced the six-step pathway for the treatment of people with OCD as recommended by National Institute for Health and Care Excellence (NICE 2005b). Depending on the severity of the OCD, the six-step pathway recommends interventions at each step. P/MH nurses are well placed, as part of the multidisciplinary team, to deliver care to clients with OCD in each of the steps.

27.9.1.1 Step 1: Awareness and Recognition

The National Institute for Health and Care Excellence (NICE 2005b) recommends that health-care authorities should have a mental health multidisciplinary team

Table 27.3 Exploring the possibility of comorbid OCD

(From NICE 2005b, p.12)
• Do you wash or clean a lot?
• Do you check things a lot?
• Is there any thought that keeps bothering you that you would like to get rid of but cannot?
• Do your daily activities take a long time to finish?
• Are you concerned about putting things in a special order, or are you very upset by mess?
• Do these problems trouble you?

(MHMDT) offering age-appropriate (adult and children) client care. The MHMDT should be specialist trained in OCD assessment and evidence-based treatment of people with OCD. The team should provide high-quality information and professional advice to clients with OCD and to their carers. Also, the MHMDT should collaborate with family/carers, voluntary agencies and members of the public to increase awareness and understanding of OCD.

27.9.1.2 Step 2: Recognition and Assessment

In this step the person may or may not be diagnosed with OCD. However, they may have come to the attention of the MHMDT as a result of other mental health concerns such as anxiety, depression or substance abuse. In this step, the P/MH should explore the possibility of comorbid OCD and will need to ask very direct and specific questions (Table 27.3) and explore the answers:

The P/MH nurse should carry out a risk assessment to ascertain the impact of the person's compulsive behaviours on themselves or others. Also, the risk of self-harm or suicide must be included in this assessment.

27.9.1.3 Steps 3–5: Treatment Options for People with OCD

Initial treatment might be best provided in primary care settings. However, a person who has more impaired functioning, who has not responded to the initial treatment or who has a higher level of comorbidity will require care from team members who have higher levels of expertise and have more experience in the management of people with OCD. Treatment options should be age specific and offered separately for adults and for children. These treatment options are well outlined in NICE (2005b). In brief, treatment options would range from low-intensity treatments such as brief one-to-one CBT using self-help materials or telephone support or group therapy to intensive CBT by specially trained P/MH nurses. In addition, the client and the MHMDT should consider if a pharmacological intervention is required. If after ten therapist hours (one-to-one CBT) or after 12 weeks' pharmacological interventions, NICE (2005b) recommend that the MHMDT review the person's progress and, if necessary, implement additional treatment options.

27.9.1.4 Step 6: Intensive Treatment and Inpatient Services for People with OCD

A small number of people with severe OCD might not respond effectively to treatments offered in Steps 3–5. In such cases, inpatient services, with P/MH and other staff who specifically qualified in the treatment of people with OCD, would be appropriate. Importantly, inpatient services should be specifically considered when:

- There is risk to life.
- There is severe self-neglect.
- There is extreme distress or functional impairment.
- There has been no response to adequate trials of pharmacological/psychological/combined treatments over long periods of time in other settings.
- The compulsions and avoidance behaviour are so severe or habitual that they cannot undertake normal activities of daily living.

(NICE 2005b, p. 29–30).

27.10 Panic Attacks

Panic disorder is defined in the ICD-10 (World Health Organization 1992) under code F41.0. According to the Mental Health Foundation (MHF), panic attacks strike abruptly and peak rapidly and are characterised by a pounding heart, feeling faint, chest pains and the person thinks they are going to die (Ballenger 2007; MHF 2014; NIMH 2016d). While Johnson et al. (2010) suggest that the neuropeptide orexin (hypocretin), which regulates arousal, wakefulness and appetite, is implicated in the development of panic disorder, Copeland et al. (2013) suggested that distressing childhood experiences, such as bullying, can contribute to the risk for developing panic disorder in a person. Furthermore, while bullies themselves were not prone to developing panic disorder in adult life, both victims of bullying and those bullies who themselves were bullied (bullies/victims) had a high risk of developing panic disorder in adult life (Copeland et al. 2013). In addition, SAMHSA (2015) suggests that anxiety disorders, including panic disorder, usually develop in childhood and can last into adulthood.

There are some well-known triggers for panic attack such as: too many stressful events, phobias and emotional worries. Nonetheless, panic attacks can occur without warning in the absence of any obvious threat of harm to the person (APA 2016b). There is an overwhelming sense of fear, and with the almost instantaneous activation of the sympathetic-adrenomedullary (SAM) axis, the person may think that they are having a heart attack (NIMH 2016d). Most panic attacks can last for a few minutes but repeated attacks can recur for several hours (APA 2016b). Furthermore, Ballenger (2007 p. 95) makes the point that because panic attacks are so frightening, the person will often develop a fear of their reoccurrence. Experiences of panic attacks, particularly when they have a history of occurring in public spaces, can lead the person experiencing the attacks to avoid venturing into public places, adding a further dimension of complexity (avoidance, personal isolation) to the problem (Ballenger 2007; APA 2016b).

27.10.1 P/MH Nursing Responses to Clients Experiencing a Panic Attack

NICE (2011) provides a very detailed five-stepped care guidance for people with panic disorder. At some stage people with panic disorder will come into contact with P/MH nurses. Thus, P/MH nurses will need a firm understanding of the severity of panic disorder and its potential consequences on the person's mental health and their social interaction. Most specialists would agree that a cognitive behavioural therapy is the best treatment for panic disorder; however, in some severe cases, the person may be prescribed a suitable medication. (APA 2016b). Also, the therapeutic alliance has an important role in achieving successful treatment outcomes in people with anxiety disorders (Cronin et al. 2014), and P/MH nurses will have a role to play in helping people suffering with panic disorder. However, it will depend on the severity of the anxiety being experienced as to what P/MH nurses can do to help a person experiencing a panic attack. Let us consider a four-stage model with the aim of guiding P/MH nurses in helping the person prevent, cope with and reduce the number of panic attacks occurring.

27.10.1.1 Pre-panic Attack Interventions

In this 1st stage, the person may present as calm, but they will be feeling uncomfortable but don't feel overly threatened. P/MH nurses in their daily engagement with clients are in prime position to notice any changes in a client's normal behaviour and take steps to prevent the exacerbation of any perceived anxiety provoking issue. If something has triggered their feelings that something dreadful is going to happen, then it must be dealt with. For example, the environment might be the actual trigger for an attack. If a person feels an attack coming on, then changing the environment might prevent the attack. However, a complication of this solution might be the development of 'avoidance' and by not addressing the issue; it could reinforce the person's thinking that the threat of something dreadful happening is real. By avoiding the issue and by not testing the validity of the threat could lead to the development of phobias in later life (SAMHSA 2014; APA 2016b). Nonetheless, avoidance may be the only option available at that time, and the P/MH nurse should note that, in future therapy, the trigger, its validity and appropriate interventions will need exploration.

However, in the absence of any obvious triggers, the P/MH nurse can help the client using grounding techniques to refocus them on the here and now. By being calm, the P/MH nurse can induce calmness in the client by using expressions such as: '*I can see that you are scared at the moment but you are in a safe place now*'; and '*Relax your shoulders and take a slow deep breath*' (SAMHSA 2014). Helping the person to take deep slow breaths is useful in settling both mind and body reactions (Benson and Procotr 2011). Particularly, exhalation should be longer than the inhalation. Controlling one's breathing aids in relaxation by stimulating the vagus nerve and in turn activating the parasympathetic nervous system (PSNS). Once the PSNS has been activated, it will induce a reduction in sympathetic nervous system activity, and the person's breathing will slow, their heart rate decrease, the blood vessels relax and the blood pressure will lower. The PSNS puts the body into a state of calm (Boore et al. 2016).

27.10.1.2 During Panic Attack Interventions

If a comprehensive risk assessment indicates no risk of aggression on the client's part, then P/MH nurses can assist the client through a panic attack with a number of interventions. The therapeutic alliance (genuineness, flexibility and the ability to truly listen to a client is effective in helping clients (Laska et al. 2013; Cronin et al. 2014). While a person is having a panic attack, the P/MH can help greatly by:

(a) Staying with the client
(b) Maintaining a calm supportive presence
(c) Offering verbal reassurance such as: '*you will not leave them alone*'
(d) Saying to him or her that the symptoms are not a sign of anything harmful happening and will pass (Salkovskis 2014)

In addition, the P/MH nurse can distract the client's thoughts by gently saying '*Calm down, you're are in a safe place*' or '*Take slow deep breaths*', and P/MH nurses can also breath with the client. Words and supportive actions like these interfere with the activation of the client's SAM and by focusing on breathing can activate the parasympathetic nervous system (Benson and Procotr 2011) and so stop the panic attack.

27.10.1.3 Post-Panic Attack Interventions

A one-off experience of panic attack does mean there is an underlying mental health issue (Salkovskis 2014). Nonetheless, following a panic attack, the P/MH nurse should be supportive and can help the person by allowing them time to express their thoughts and feelings about their experience. They should identify any stressors that the client has been under and also, identify any other triggers for the panic attack. In addition, P/MH nurses can help the client develop a number of anxiety-reducing techniques such as:

(a) *Deep breathing exercises*: As previously outlined.
(b) *Developing a mantra*: Using a word that distracts their thoughts such as 'safe', 'peace' and 'relax'. The person can choose their own word that interferes with the SAM or HPA activity and induces PSNS activity.
(c) *Muscular relaxation*: Induces PSNS activity.
(d) *Aromatherapy*: Induces relaxation and PSNS activity.
(e) *Mindfulness*: This is the process of learning to be present in this moment and observing (1) *internal experiences* such as thoughts and internal body activities and (2) *external experiences* such as interactions with others. It helps a person to stay grounded in the present rather than focus on traumas in the past or worrying about the future (SAMHSA 2014).

The above techniques can help a person 'ride out the storm' and minimise the impact of the sympathetic nervous system. However, while they make living with anxiety easier, they are not curative. The most effective treatment for panic disorder is cognitive behavioural therapy. This allows the person to understand their thinking, behaviours and thoughts and question why they feel the way they do (Salkovskis 2014; RCP 2017). For effectiveness, there should be between 7 and 14 CBT sessions (NICE 2011). During therapy the client and the specialist qualified P/MH nurse could explore a range of relevant issues including the validity of any identifiable triggers. Talking therapy such as CBT should be delivered only by suitably trained and supervised professionals (NICE 2011).

In addition, some clients may be prescribed antidepressants for any accompanying depression but these can also help to relieve anxiety (RCP 2017). They have to be taken regularly, and they usually take 2–4 weeks to work effectively. Usually, one of the SSRI antidepressants will be tried initially, and if that is not effective, then the client may be prescribed a tricyclic antidepressant. It is recommended that antidepressant drug therapy be continued for at least a year and then gradually reduced (NICE 2011; Salkovskis 2014). In deciding whether to avail of CBT or medications or a combination of both, the client might consider that CBT has no known side effects and is effective, whereas antidepressant medication is effective but has numerous side effects.

27.10.1.4 Educational Interventions

The therapeutic alliance contributes to better treatment outcomes (Cronin et al. 2014), and P/MH nurses can use their therapeutic alliance with the person experiencing panic disorder to help them:

(a) Identify any triggers as prewarning can prevent a full attack.
(b) Understand that the frightening physical symptoms experienced are linked to anxiety and are not indications of any medical pathology.
(c) Practice their breathing and relaxation exercises each day.
(d) Explore online CBT programmes such as the NICE approved *FearFighter*™, *MoodGYM*™ or *Beating the Blues*™ to ascertain which is best suited to their needs.
(e) Explore the possibility of joining a support group for those experiencing anxiety or panic attacks.

Conclusion

Human experiences of anxiety, while ubiquitous and varied, can become a disabling mental health issue for clients, and responding appropriately and effectively to these issues can be challenging for nurses. However, even a cursory review of the relevant literature and evidence will show that there are a number of effective and tested theories and responses to anxiety-related mental health problems (SAMHSA 2014; NICE 2014; MIND 2014). Indeed, for many of these issues, a range of responses can be located in the literature. Further, while there appears to be little or no argument in the substantive literature that anxiety can manifest a range of mental health problems for the individual, it is also the case that anxiety appears to be synonymous with or irreducible from the human experience per se *(see suffering chapter).* Indeed, the absence of any anxiety in an individual, even when faced with extreme threats, might be a cause for concern in and of itself. Anxiety and stress responses in the person involve the activation of the SNS; the body in effect mobilizes certain resources in order to defend itself and to prepare itself for 'fight or flight'. Conversely, this 'survival' reaction can also lead to unpleasant cognitive, physiological and behavioural responses that impact on the person's mental and physical health. When a person's daily activities are impacted by their anxiety levels, current guidelines recommend that care intervention is planned in conjunction with the person and is tailored towards their specific needs. Anxiety appears to be amenable to treatment with CBT. Mindfulness and other supportive psychotherapies and suitably qualified/trained P/MH nurses are in a key position to provide some (all) of this interpersonal help. Lastly, given the frequency that P/MH nurses are likely to encounter clients with anxiety-related problems, it would seem logical and necessary to ensure that P/MH nurses are equipped with the relevant knowledge, attitudes and skills, either pre- and/or postgraduate, to enable them to offer such interventions.

References

Achim AM, Maziade M, Raymond E, Olivier D, Mérette C, Roy MA (2011) How prevalent are anxiety disorders in schizophrenia? A meta-analysis and critical review on a significant association. Schizophr Bull 37(4):811–821

Allaboutcounselling (Recovered December 2016) Psychological phobias: understanding unreasonable fear

American Psychological Association (2016a) Trauma. http://www.apa.org/topics/trauma/ (recovered 4th January 2017)

American Psychological Association (2016b) Panic disorder. http://apa.org/topics/anxiety/panic-disorder.aspx (recovered 4th January 2017)

Ballenger J (2007) Panic disorder and agoraphobia. In: Fink G (ed) Stress consequences: mental, neuropsychological and socioeconomic. Elsevier, New York, pp 95–99

Bandura A (1982) Self-efficacy mechanism in human agency. Am Psychol 37(2):122–147

Baxter AJ, Vos T, Scott KM, Ferrari AJ, Whiteford HA (2014) The global burden of anxiety disorders in 2010. Psychol Med 44(11):2363–2374

Bernardy N (2013) The role of benzodiazepines in the treatment of posttraumatic stress disorder (PTSD). PTSD Res Q 23(4):1–3. (Recovered December 20th 2016)

Benson H, Procotr W (2011) Relaxation revolution: the science and genetics of mind body healing. Scribner, New York

Boore J, Cook N, Shephard A (2016) Essentials of anatomy and physiology for nursing practice. Sage, London

Calhoun L, Tedeschi R (eds) (2014) Handbook of posttraumatic growth: research and practice, 2nd edn. Psychology Press, New York

Cannon W (1929) Bodily changes in pain, hunger, fear and rage, 2nd edn. Appleton and Co., New York

Copeland W, Wolke D, Angold A (2013) Adult psychiatric outcomes of bullying and being bullied by peers in childhood and adolescence. JAMA 70:419–426

Cronin C, Brand B, Mattanah J (2014) The impact of the therapeutic alliance on treatment outcome in patients with dissociative disorders. Eur J Psychotraumatol 5:22676. doi:10.3402/ejpt.v5.22676
Cutcliffe J, Barker P (2002) Considering the care of the suicidal client and the case for 'engagement and inspiring hope' or 'observations'. J Psychiatr Ment Health Nurs 9:611–621
Ferencik SD, Ramirez-Hammond R (Recovered 3rd January 2017) Trauma-informed care best practices and protocols doe Ohio's domestic violence programs. Ohio Domestic Violence Network. http://www.ncdsv.org/images/ODVN_Trauma-InformedCareBestPracticesAndProtocols.pdf
Freeman A, DiTomasso R (1994) The cognitive theory of anxiety. In: Wolman B, Stricker G (eds) Anxiety and related disorders: a handbook. Chapter 5. John Wiley and Sons, New York, pp 141–169
Joëls M, Pu Z, Weigert O, Oitzl M, Krugers H (2006) Learning under stress: how does it work? Trends Cogn Sci 10(4):152–158
Jacofsky M, Santos M, Khemlani-Patel S, Neziroglu F (2013) Biological explanations of anxiety disorders. https://www.mentalhelp.net/articles/biological-explanations-of-anxiety-disorders/ (Accessed 22nd December 2016)
Johnson P, Truitt W, Fitz S, Minick P, Dietrich A, Sanghani S, Träskman-Bendz L, Goddard A, Brundin L, Shekhar A (2010) A key role for Orexin in panic anxiety. Nat Med 16(1):111–115
Jones MC (1924) A laboratory study of fear: the case of Peter. The Pedagogical Seminary 31:308–315
Kalat J (2014) Biological psychology, 11th edn. Wadsworth, Belmont
Laska K, Smith T, Wislocki A, Minami T, Wampold B (2013) Uniformity of evidence-based treatments in practice? Therapist effects in the delivery of cognitive processing therapy for PTSD. J Couns Psychol 60(1):31–41
Lupien S, Maheu F, Tu M, Fiocco A, Schramek T (2007) The effects of stress and stress hormones on human cognition: implications for the field of brain and cognition. Brain Cogn 65:209–237
Marks M, Basoglu M, Alkubaisy T, Sengun S, Marks I (1991) Are anxiety symptoms and catastrophic cognitions directly related? J Anxiety Disord 5:247–254
Martin B (2016) Stress and personality. http://psychcentral.com/lib/stress-and-personality/ (Recovered 21st December 2016)
Mental Health Foundation (2014) Living with anxiety: understanding the role and impact of anxiety in our lives. Mental Health Foundation, London
MIND (2014) Understanding phobias. National Association of Mental Health, London
National Center for PTSD (Recovered 8th December 2016) Types of debriefing following disasters. http://www.ptsd.va.gov/professional/trauma/disaster-terrorism/debriefing-after-disasters.asp
National Institute for Health and Care Excellence (2005a) Post-traumatic stress disorder: management. NICE, Manchester
National Institute for Health and Care Excellence (2005b) Obsessive-compulsive disorder and body dysmorphic disorder: treatment – clinical guideline. Manchester, NICE
National Institute for Health and Care Excellence (2011) Generalised anxiety disorder and panic disorder in adults: management. NICE, Manchester
National Institute for Health and Care Excellence (2013) Obsessive-compulsive disorder: evidence update 47. NICE, Manchester
National Institute for Health and Care Excellence (2014) Obsessive-compulsive disorder and body dysmorphic disorder overview. https://pathways.nice.org.uk/pathways/obsessive-compulsive-disorder (accessed Dec. 22nd 2016)
National Institute for Mental Health (2016a) Post-traumatic stress disorder. https://www.nimh.nih.gov/health/topics/post-traumatic-stress-disorder-ptsd/index.shtml (recovered 3rd January 2017)
National Institute for Mental Health (2016b) Obsessive-compulsive disorder. https://www.nimh.nih.gov/health/topics/obsessive-compulsive-disorder-ocd/index.shtml#part_145345 (recovered 22nd December 2016)
National Institute for Mental Health (2016c) Anxiety Disorders. https://www.nimh.nih.gov/health/topics/anxiety-disorders/index.shtml (recovered 22nd December 2016)

National Institute for Mental Health (2016d) Panic disorder: when fear overwhelms. https://www.nimh.nih.gov/health/publications/panic-disorder-when-fear-overwhelms/index.shtml (recovered 9th January 2017)
Parson E (1994) Post-traumatic stress disorder (PTSD): its Biopsychobehavioral aspects and management. In: Wolman B, Stricker G (eds) Anxiety and related disorders: a handbook. Chapter 13. John Wiley and Sons, New York, pp 404–514
Peplau H (1994) Psychiatric and mental health nursing: challenge and change. J Psychiatr Ment Health Nurs 1:3–7
Royal College of Psychiatrists (2017) Anxiety, panic and phobias. http://www.rcpsych.ac.uk/expertadvice/problemsdisorders/anxiety,panic,phobias.aspx (recovered 4th January 2017)
Salkovskis P (2014) Panic disorder. http://www.nhs.uk/conditions/panic-disorder/pages/introduction.aspx (recovered 8th January 2017)
Sandi C (2013) Stress and cognition. WIREs Cognit Sci 2013(4):245–261. doi:10.1002/wcs.1222 9. (recovered 20th Dec 2016)
Sinha S, Mohlman J, Gorman J (2004) Neurobiology. In: Heimberg R et al (eds) Generalized anxiety disorder: advances in research and practice. Chapter 8. Guilford Press, New York, pp 187–216
Selye H (1956) The stress of life. McGraw-Hill, New York
Selye H (1978) The stress of life. McGraw-Hill Education, New York
Shear K (2012) Generalized anxiety disorder in ICD-11. In: Mario M, Reed G (eds) The ICD-11 classification of mood and anxiety disorders: background and options, 11(Supplement 1). World Psychiatry, pp 82–88
Smith S, Vale W (2006) The role of the hypothalamic-pituitary-adrenal axis in neuroendocrine responses to stress. Dialogues Clin Neurosci 8(4):383–395
Substance Abuse and Mental Health Services Administration (SAMHSA) (2014) A treatment improvement protocol: trauma-informed care in behavioural services: TIP 57. U.S. Department of Health and Human Services, Rockville
Substance Abuse and Mental Health Services Administration (SAMHSA) (2015) Mental disorders. https://www.samhsa.gov/disorders/mental (recovered 23rd December 2016)
Substance Abuse and Mental Health Services Administration (SAMHSA) (2016) Treatment for post-traumatic stress disorder. (Recovered December 22nd 2016)
Wanderer Z (1972) Existential depression treated by desensitization of phobias: strategy and transcript. J Behav Ther Exp Psychiatry 3(2):111–116
Whittington R, McLaughlin C (2000) Finding time for patients: an exploration of nurses' time allocation in an acute psychiatric setting. J Psychaitr Ment Health Nurs 7:259–268
Wolman B, Stricker G (1994) Anxiety and related disorders: a handbook. John Wiley and Sons, New York
World Health Organization (1992) International statistical classification of diseases and related health problems (ICD-10). WHO, Geneva
World Health Organisation Regional Office for Europe (2015) The European mental health action plan 2013 – 2020. WHO, Copenhagen
Yerkes RM, Dodson JD (1908) The relation of strength of stimulus to rapidity of habit-formation. J Comp Neurol Psychol 18:459–482. doi:10.1002/cne.920180503
Young S, Pfaff D, Lewandowski K, Ravichandran C, Cohen B, Őngűr D (2013) Anxiety disorder comorbidity in bipolar disorder, schizophrenia and schizoaffective disorder. Psychopathology 46(3):176–185

28 Integrated Care – 'Schizophrenia': A Challenge for Psychiatric/Mental Health Nursing

David González-Pando and Fernando Alonso-Pérez

28.1 Introduction

For many years, schizophrenia was considered to be a chronic biological disorder, only treatable by means of providing medication and basic care. This vision that guided the mental health system was not person centred. Fortunately, the relationship between service users and professionals has notably changed in the last decades, including the response to and understanding of psychotic symptoms. Nowadays, psychiatric/mental health (P/MH) nursing and other professionals involved in mental health care recognize the important role of contextual factors in the development and response to 'schizophrenia', and they know that psychosocial interventions have been found to help facilitate recovery in a significative way (Lemos et al. 2015). Thus, P/MH nurses provide integral, humanistic and person-centred attention/responses in which interpersonal therapeutic relationships form the basis for all their interventions and care. The authors here are referring to a special and genuine relationship in which the patient can be himself, have his/her own feelings and express them freely, knowing that nurses shall not make value judgements or manifest disapproval (Peplau 1991).

Mental health is a complex field, with many different approaches possible but one common underlying interest: the person behind the so-called mental health disorders. Seeing the client first and foremost as a 'unique, human person' helps P/MH nurses hold onto conceptualizations of 'schizophrenia' other than that of a 'psychiatric diagnosis or syndrome', and it can lead to a better understanding of the role played by non-biological factors in the aetiology and development of psychotic symptoms (García-Montes and Pérez-Alvarez 2003). However, this approach

D. González-Pando (✉) • F. Alonso-Pérez
University of Oviedo, Asturias, Gijón, Spain, UK
e-mail: gonzalezpdavid@uniovi.es

© Springer International Publishing Switzerland 2018

J.C. Santos, J.R. Cutcliffe (eds.), *European Psychiatric/Mental Health Nursing in the 21st Century*, Principles of Specialty Nursing,
https://doi.org/10.1007/978-3-319-31772-4_28

collides with the dominant trend in much of contemporary psychiatric care: biologically oriented psychiatry, underpinned by the biomedical illness model. Nowadays, psychiatry has been described as a project of clinical neuroscience (Insel and Quirion 2005) or an 'applied neuroscience' strongly situated in a technological paradigm. But following Bracken et al. (2012, p. 3):

> Psychiatry is not neurology; it is not a medicine of the brain.

Accordingly, the authors of this chapter defend a pluralistic and non-reductionist view of the so-called mental disorders, including schizophrenia. It means keeping one's attention beyond biological conditions; it means being aware of the psychosocial and cultural factors involved in its origin (see John Read's work here on traumatic backgrounds in schizophrenic clients). That is not to suggest that we ignore or completely abandon/reject neurobiological findings because, ultimately, behaviour is inextricably linked with the brain; rather we incorporate such thinking and explanations vis-à-vis schizophrenia into a new perspective, for example, in a socio-developmental model (Morgan and Hutchinson 2010). This approach integrates social aspects (trauma, life adversities, urbanicity, family dysfunction), neurobiological functioning (dopaminergic system) and psychological experiences (psychotic symptoms), but the dopaminergic hyperactivity is considered an effect of the social cause, not the aetiology of schizophrenia, which could explain high rates of psychosis in migrant population and ethnic minorities (Coid et al. 2008; Tortelli et al. 2015). This model incorporates (integrates) the findings from studies of brain neuroplasticity (e.g. Pajonk et al. 2010) and epigenetic mechanisms related to psychopathology (Gónzalez-Pardo and Pérez-Álvarez 2013), and also this model sees the human brain (and a genome function) as influenced by and responsive to variables of experience and behaviour, instead of offering the usual views of brains or genes as autonomous agents.

Thus, within this approach the idea that the environment, particularly life adversities, produces a special hypersensitivity of the mesolimbic system, increasing dopaminergic activity and consequently the risk of psychosis, in a circular loop that begins in life circumstances and ends in the abnormal behaviour through the brain function, in which epigenetic modifications are involved (Pérez-Álvarez 2012). According to Villagrán (2003), a central problem of biological psychiatry is that it adopts a unidirectional aetiological model for the so-called mental illness in which an altered brain produces an altered function, causing behavioural disturbance and then social maladjustment. In our opinion, this offers an unsatisfactory vision of psychopathology like an epiphenomenon produced by molecular changes in the brain. This simplistic and linear scheme should be overtaken and replaced by a circular, holistic model where successive and continuous reciprocal influences between different factors lead to psychosis, and also it provides a guide in order to avoid reductionisms and ensure an integral (biopsychosocial) and comprehensive care. The conceptual and clinical implications of embracing such a model are significant, particularly given that understanding schizophrenia as an alteration of ipseity (a disorder of the self) rather than schizophrenia as a brain disease (Pérez-Álvarez et al. 2010) is very different conceptualizations and results in very different approaches to practice. Read et al. (2006) who sought to assess the effectiveness of anti-stigma programmes in relation to schizophrenia found that biogenetic causal theories and diagnostic labelling as 'illness' were both positively related to perceptions of dangerousness and unpredictability and to fear and desire for social distance. According to these findings, presenting schizophrenia as a so-called mental illness, 'an illness like any other', serves to increase stigma – not reduce it.

28.2 Multiple Perspectives

Schizophrenia can be approached from at least two different points of view and two general models. The two perspectives, broadly speaking, are the categorical (or clinical) view, used more in medicine, based in symptoms and the fulfilment of diagnostic criteria as a dichotomic decision, and the dimensional view, with more tradition in psychology. The dimensional model is based, for example, on the apparent absence of precise boundaries between delusions and other beliefs firmly maintained, which may suggest that there is a continuum from the normal belief until delusional (Strauss 1969). It means that psychosis appears at the end of a continuum and not abruptly across a dividing line between 'psychotic' and 'normal' (Claridge 1980; Linscott and van Os 2010). This approach is consistent with a dimensional evaluation of psychotic symptoms in DSM-5 (Barch et al. 2013). In fact, attenuated psychotic symptoms are a very common phenomenon in adolescence: magical thinking, reference ideas and/or delusion or hallucination experiences (e.g. see Lemos-Giráldez et al. 2011). Moreover, hearing voices is not only a very common phenomenon in general population; it is a natural part of the human experience, and in this sense the practice and philosophy of the Hearing Voices Movement (HVM) introduced by Romme and Escher (1989) have shown an alternative to the biomedical understanding of auditory verbal hallucinations for over 25 years. In fact, HVM has allowed a better understanding of these experiences with important implications for research and practice (Corstens et al. 2014).

In 1994, it was acknowledged and documented in the DSM-IV (American Psychiatric Association) that the categorical approach has significant limitations, noting that sometimes there are no clear boundaries between different disorders or between normality and abnormality. Currently, DSM-5 (APA 2013) presents a mixed model, although the dimensional model is basically complementary, including five basic dimensions for schizophrenia: delusions, hallucinations, disorganized thoughts/speech, abnormal psychomotor behaviour and negative symptoms. Therefore, a dimensional perspective could be more appropriate to describe the phenomena like schizophrenia, a disorder without precise limits for diagnosis. Not in vain, DSM-5 (APA 2013) defines schizophrenia by exclusion (in terms of what it is not). The assumption that most people can have some degree of abnormality at some point of their lives could be beneficious in fighting stigma and offers the possibility of considering psychiatry not as a discipline related to madness if not related with normality (Horwitz 2002), providing a less negative image.

Schizophrenia and the so-called schizophrenic spectrum disorders represent a first-order public health problem: 26 million people have been diagnosed as suffering from schizophrenia, and every year 1.5 million (new) people receive the diagnosis, making schizophrenia one of the ten leading causes of disability (World Health Organization 2001). The cost of care is very high, 2–3% of the total in health services (Carr et al. 2004), without regard to the indirect costs in lost productivity of patients and caregivers or family costs. If that was not enough, the suffering is unquantifiable, and up to 5–10% of our patients die prematurely by suicide (Lemos et al. 2015).

Given that it is not uncommon for some people diagnosed with schizophrenia to follow a chronic course and that antipsychotic medication is only moderately effective on so-called positive symptoms (nothing or minimally on negatives), and these drugs do not reduce the frequency of psychosis in schizophrenia after the first few years (Harrow et al. 2014), psychosocial interventions and specialized mental health care are essential to achieve improvement, recovery and a higher quality of life. Moreover, we should note that medication does not improve the insight of problems nor social skills and abilities to cope with stress of everyday life.

28.3 The 'Slippery' Nature of Schizophrenia and Its Implications for P/MH Nursing: The Need for Recovery-Focused Care

Schizophrenia, the sublime object of psychiatry (Woods 2011), is the most representative of so-called functional psychosis, a paradigm example of so-called severe mental disorder and, according to its heterogeneous symptoms, a whole compendium of psychopathology. However, in addition to the conceptual difficulties (Lemos et al. 2015) and absence of pathognomonic symptoms or biomarkers that are required for an unequivocal diagnosis, we have to add that there is no single symptom in schizophrenia that may not be present in other disorders. Thus, heterogeneity of symptoms (between individuals and within the same subject over time) has been explained by clinical subtypes (paranoid, hebephrenic "disorganized", catatonic, etc.) and maintained by clinical tradition in spite of its low diagnostic validity and reliability. Consequently, it is not surprising for the elimination of subtypes in DSM-5 and probably in the future ICD-11.

The multiple and diverse aetiological hypotheses introduced to explain schizophrenia show its enigmatic and puzzling character. Considering only the overabundance of pathophysiological findings (different neurotransmitters, many neuronal circuits, etc.), Maj (2011) stated that these findings are less indicator of an increase of knowledge and understanding of schizophrenia; rather they are a sign and add to the sense of uncertainty and confusion. The essential problem for P/MH nursing is that conceptual confusion may also manifest or promote uncertainty in our nursing interventions and practices and, the most important thing, in the relationships we establish with service users. The problem is that a satisfactory understanding of schizophrenia may be impossible without a phenomenological approach, in the line of Blueler (the introducer of the term 'schizophrenia' in 1908) continued by Minkowski (the introducer of the notion of 'loss of vital contact with reality') and others (Jaspers, Conrad, etc.). Actually, phenomenology is recovering the psychopathological tradition, conceiving schizophrenia as an ipseity disorder (Sass and Parnas 2007), characterized by an intensified awareness of things which are normally implicit or pre-reflexive, by a diminished sense of oneself as the subject of experience and action and by alteration of perceptive articulation with the world (Pérez-Álvarez et al. 2010).

The implications for P/MH nursing are crucial. They indicate the clear need to treat people who are diagnosed as 'schizophrenic' as individuals, paying attention to them and supporting their first-person experiences (hyper-reflexivity, diminished self-affection and loss of vital contact with reality), with openness and acceptance. Our role could be essential to provide security and confidence especially in the loss of vital contact with reality, when the person experiences an alteration of familiarity with the world (feeling strangeness and perplexity). As Peplau (1991) said, the simple presence of nurse provides security. Accordingly, P/MH nursing can adopt a phenomenological attitude to provide a better support (trusting and empathic) and accompany genuinely these anomalous subjective experiences in which patients feel recognized in terms of ipseity. It links with the 'narrative of recovery' of the sense of self, instead of usual 'narrative of illness', often as a chronic disease at the expense of lifetime medication. Thus, beyond the traditional treatment of symptoms, it is given increasing importance to the process of recovery as something broader than simply reducing symptoms (Andresen et al. 2011).

'Recovery' focuses on the patient's social ability to perform rewarding activities in order to achieve meaningful objectives which make worth life living. It is a way of living a satisfying and hopeful life even with the limitations caused by schizophrenia. 'Recovery' involves an increase of psychosocial functioning and received support, a decrease of the perceived stress and a raise or promotion of the person's quality of life, by the full incorporation of all resources available from the community (Anthony 1993). According to Jacobson and Greenley (2001), recovery is also the process of 'recovering' the self by re-conceptualizing the so-called illness as only a part of the self, not as a definition of the whole. Our service users could begin to experience a sense of self-esteem and self-respect that allows them to confront and overcome the stigma, allowing further connection with the self. It is the patient who must become an active agent in his own life and who should take control, because regaining control is a determining factor for empowerment. Empowerment may be seen as an attempt to correct the dependency that many people develop after long-term interactions with the mental health system, and it has three components to consider: autonomy, courage and responsibility (Jacobson and Greenley 2001). In this regard, the aim of recovery is to have more and more responsible people making their own choices and plans for reaching goals assuming its consequences.

28.4 Key Principles of Care

In this context, providing listening and accepting the symptoms is essential. The psychotic symptoms could be seen as attempts to express or make sense of certain overwhelming circumstances, hence the importance of personal narratives in the recovery process of psychotic experiences (Pérez-Álvarez 2011). But narratives can have a single author or could be co-created with others, among the participants involved in the experience. With this in mind, the open dialogue approach (Seikkula et al. 2006), a variant of the Finnish model of Alanen and colleagues, is a person-centred and network-based approach to mental health care that could put mental health care and P/MH nursing, at least in the view of the authors of this chapter, on the right track (and the service user's needs first), because it attaches great importance to the narrative in the recovery process. The central idea is the provision of psychotherapeutic treatment for all patients within their own personal support systems. The seven key principles are:

(a) Provision of immediate help within the first 24 h, if it is possible at home.
(b) A social network perspective of the service user's presenting difficulties is sought through a meeting involving the family and any other key members of the service user's network (friends, employers or neighbours as potential partners in the process).
(c) Flexibility and mobility in the care provided from the professional team.
(d) Responsibility (a person responsible for organizing meetings and care).
(e) Psychological continuity by the team, as involved as possible, constructing new meanings for symptoms and sharing experiences.
(f) Tolerance of uncertainty (e.g. not introducing diagnosis or pharmacological treatments straight away).
(g) And finally, dialogism, which is the idea of promoting an open dialogue to reach changes in the patient or in the family, thus fostering a sense of agency in service users and their family (Seikkula et al. 2006).

The aim is to develop a dialogical communication in which the participants become co-creators of the shared reality (constructing words for the experiences that occur when psychotic symptoms are present) between the patient and their support system as an intervention directed to empower the family and social network. These seven key principles are endorsed highly by both staff and users (Razzaque and Wood 2015) indicating that it may be an acceptable approach and an alternative to the often unsatisfactory usual clinical practice. Open dialogue has an encouraging emerging evidence base for people with psychosis, improving indicators of clinical evolution and reducing significantly the hospitalization need and the pharmaceutical costs. For example, in the Seikkula et al. (2006) 5-year follow-up study on first-episode psychosis, 82% of participants did not have any residual psychotic symptom, and 86% had returned to their studies or a full-time job, while 'only' 29% of patients used neuroleptic medication at some stage of the treatment. The results are better than those found commonly in 'treatment as usual' studies, not only in terms of symptom reduction but also in recovering of significant personal activities. Psychosocial approaches can help patients to recover faster from their psychosis, and it does not have to be merely a secondary element in mental health care.

However, in the dominant biomedical context, although the limitations of medication-centred treatments have been showed (Harrow et al. 2014), the focus is still on (and almost reduced to) medication, which can make the destiny of schizophrenia as a chronic illness. Medication and the patient's response to it is then the essential question to observe (to increase, reduce or change it). As Pérez-Álvarez (2011) said, the current model is an institutional question more than a clinic question. From many years we know the paradox that patients from developing countries show a clearly better outcome than the patients from developed countries, where we have the most 'developed and advanced' biomedical treatments. Therefore, since the current panorama of mental health care is complex and confusing, we need radical approaches to reach the root of the problems and the facts we try to understand.

28.5 Positive and Negative Symptoms: New Psychotherapeutic Perspectives for P/MH Nurses

Nowadays, a complex so-called disorder such as schizophrenia needs an integrated approach based in evidence, as it offers the cognitive-behavioural therapy (CBT). CBT has been found to be an effective approach in managing/treating psychosis, especially with regard to its efficacy in addressing positive symptoms, and many therapeutic resources based in this approach are present in nursing interventions (cognitive restructuring, behaviour modification, reality tests, etc.). We cannot forget that P/MH nursing is the professional group (or discipline) who spend most time in direct contact with patients, sharing multiple experiences in a therapeutic context. Consequently, our role is crucial, and, always in coordination with other professionals, our work could represent the difference between achieving or not achieving the common goals that the interdisciplinary staff has established with the patient.

28.6 Delusion Management

For a normalizing attitude, it is interesting to see that delusions are not always absolutely irreducible ideas, because they do not always remain unshakable (unchangeable). In fact, the degree of conviction can be variable, and patients often seek new alternative explanations for what happens. According to it, P/MH nurses can realize very important work, providing support and continuity of care under certain basic assumptions:

- Appear available, accessible and establish a collaborative relationship.
- Never confront delusions directly. Doing so would increase its strength (according to the psychological reactance theory).
- Accept the patient's belief initially but avoiding reinforcement.
- Listening attentively without showing alarm contextualizing the experience in the continuous normality disorder.
- Not require the abandonment of delusion, just ask to be open to the possibility of alternative explanations.

- If a debate is established, focus it on the data that belief is based, instead of on delusion content. We better start talking about less important beliefs or peripheral aspects of it.
- Provide positive reinforcement to attempts of the patient to reach alternative explanations.
- Never put on risk our good established therapeutic relationship (if is threatened, it is better a tactical retreat, until a more propitious moment).
- Adapt interventions to the opening margin showed by the patient.
- Consider the distortion in contact with reality produced by psychosis and the possibility that establishes the therapeutic relationship takes a long time.

28.7 Psychiatric/Mental Health Nurses: Talking About Delusions

There are no universal correct responses for all cases possible, but guidance to enhance nursing interventions can be offered. Box 28.1 (see below) illustrates one approach to responding to delusional thinking through open questions, from the perspective of a cognitive restructuring intervention. The aim is to explore the scope of delusions, reconsidering the facts underlying, including possible alternative explanations, even encouraging the patient to argue against their own beliefs.

Sometimes the patient may appear upset or angry; in such cases it is important to show empathy, understand and help create and respond from a 'place' of serenity; e.g. 'Excuse me, I didn't want to bother you; it's just that I can't fully understand what you are telling me'. The intention of this intervention is that the patient takes a different perspective, rising to the position of a trusted person (Lemos et al. 2015). Moreover, we can introduce a model of explanation informing that what is happening is a psychotic experience, an experience that many people have under great stress, that leads us to explanations or ideas that other persons cannot share because these beliefs are not based on objective data. But, once again, according to Peplau (1991), the information is useful when it is offered in a caring, responsive and comfortable interpersonal relationship.

Box 28.1 Open Questions and Cognitive ReStructuring Verbal Interventions

Let's see. Explain to me these things; I will try to understand you.

What do you mean with…?
How do you explain these things that are happening?
Why do you think others (family or friends) can't share your explanations?
Do you believe that there may be alternative explanations?
Would you be less distressed with an alternative explanation?

Additionally, simple behavioural experiments can be introduced to test the validity of patient's beliefs. With our support, patients could begin to regard delusions like hypotheses that could be tested. The aim is not to show that he/she was wrong but achieve a less anxiogenic alternative explanation in order to weaken delusion. These procedures are usually conducted with great care and prudence. An example cited by Lemos et al. (2015, p. 180) shows a patient who believed that all people could hear his thoughts. The experiment introduced consisted in asking the patient for reading in silence while a sound recording was on. As only the therapist's voice appears in the recording, the patient could think 'people cannot hear my thoughts, perhaps it could be just my imagination'. Our practice of taste (and test) in the patient's food or drink when poisoning ideas are present (a common delusion in paranoid schizophrenia) shares the same principles in the context of weaken delusions. The question is that even under intensive positive symptoms, our patients can learn and adapt behaviour because they remain sensitive to the influence of environment (González-Pando et al. 2016). For additional suggestions, interventions and activities involved in delusion management, the reader is referred to Bulechek et al. (2013, p. 142).

28.8 Hallucination Management

Hallucinations are perceptions of phenomena, for which there is no external, verifiable objective evidence and for which the person (client) ascribes an external attribution in its origin, representing a significant distortion and an additional difficulty in the contact with reality (Lemos et al. 2015). This experience has been explained as the external attribution of self-generated events. It usually appears with more intensity during periods of stress or threatening experiences, and some environmental conditions increase it: social isolation, sensory or sleep deprivation, drugs, ambiguous stimuli, etc. Hallucinations normally reflect concerns, threats, beliefs or memories (hence the importance of exploring its meaning through narratives) and are often intrusive and unpleasant (Lemos et al. 2015). Auditory hallucinations, the hallucination most frequently experienced in schizophrenia, tend to weaken with verbal concurrent tasks (talking, singing) and activities such as physical exercise, keeping busy or listening to music. It is very important to introduce appropriate interventions: providing correct lighting, ensuring adequate sleeping and promoting social relationships. However, we must consider that hallucinations are a problem only if they create emotional and behavioural problems (something especially evident in the imperative voices). The problem is not the hallucination (like hearing voices) but the reaction to and relation established with this experience and how the person responds to it (as something horrible to avoid). In this sense, our serenity is crucial when hallucinations are present. Psychiatry has often reinforced the idea that for achieving happiness, it is essential to be free of psychotic experiences, while the key is to relate to them in a different way (Chadwick 2009). Currently, new psychotherapeutic perspectives are being introduced to change the patient's pathogenic relationship with psychotic experiences, such as mindfulness (therapies based on) and ACT (acceptance and commitment therapy). The aim, in phenomenological terms, is to attenuate hyper-reflexivity and recovery of the sense of self, including immersion in significant activities to life, grounded in values, because, once again, reducing symptoms is not enough to regain a normal life (Pérez-Álvarez et al. 2010). About auditory hallucinations, a person can say 'I hear voices, they are a part of me and I accept its presence'. Additional options and activities/interventions related to the hallucination management can be seen in Bulechek et al. (2013, p. 208).

28.9 Management of Negative Symptoms

As is the case with hallucinations and delusions, negative symptoms could be seen as interrelated phenomena in feedback or even as members of a same functional class of behaviour. They include a decreased emotional expression (affective flattening and alogia) and an amotivational syndrome (apathy, anhedonia and social isolation) which can be observed until by up to 50% of service users some years after diagnosis.

Deficit symptoms are the main cause of functional impairment in the so-called schizophrenia and the first concern in families, so it should be considered as a priority focus of attention and care. In the 1950s, Skinner saw that the essential problem about psychotic inpatients was not about what they do but about what they do not do, being the basic question how to case behaviour missing (Skinner 1979).

Families suffer emotional overload providing care (Gomes and Mello 2012), and often they show critical and hostile attitudes which we know as expressed emotion (Leff and Vaughn 1984), strongly associated with an increased risk of relapse. Psychoeducation is here very important because carers can see the behaviour in terms of irresponsible attitude or simple laziness. As negative symptoms could be understood as 'protection mechanisms' against certain situations that increase

Key Principles for Reacting to and Managing Negative Symptoms:

- Identify personal goals to achieve and commit to actions that lead to it.
- Generate an atmosphere of hope (realistic optimism).
- Adapt procedures to cognitive deterioration and slow patient functioning.
- Consider the crucial role of environment (behavioural poverty may be a reflection of environmental poverty).
- Ensure that the patient maintains a sufficient degree of control over environmental events that affect them.
- Instil a feeling of self-control and ability to organize one's life.
- Stimulate social interaction and reinforce communication and emotional expression.
- Encourage recreational activities and art therapies.

positive symptoms, we have to be especially cautious with the basic interventions proposed. It can also be useful to improve depressive symptoms in schizophrenia (often difficult to differentiate from negative symptoms).

28.10 Final Considerations

Psychopathology is not a provisional language; it is something necessary for understanding the experiences of the people we try to help. In this sense, phenomenology allows us to capture the essential phenomena and particular lived experiences of schizophrenia. Under the principles of acceptance, membership and reciprocity, interpersonal relationships represent the most adequate approach, recovering the sense of self and understanding the psychotic experiences in a biographical context. In this track, P/MH nursing can also recover its best humanistic tradition. Therefore, P/MH nursing must be formed in a psychosocial perspective, to comprehend what is happening to their service users, responding with interpersonal skills and covering needs from the base of a therapeutic person-centred relationship.

Our working model must be also community based, remembering that patients have more power at home than in the hospital (Peplau 1991). In this sense, the assertive community treatment (Bond et al. 2001) is a recommended and cost-effective approach for people with schizophrenia, based in an interdisciplinary work, a low staff-to-client ratio and the delivery of a comprehensive package of services to clients in the community (Lemos et al. 2015). We must work collaboratively on different factors: families, environment, habits, health care, personal relationships, stigma and self-stigma. If everything fails, we should still keep contact with the families, reinforce relationships, reach agreements, establish goals with the patient, improve motivation and work with enthusiasm on recovery, despite of the symptoms. Recovery is a deeply human experience facilitated by the deeply human responses of others, but professionals do not hold the key to recovery; consumers do (Anthony 1993). In this sense, the final consideration for us could be 'the probability of recovery is based on the simple but profound idea that people who have been diagnosed with schizophrenia are persons and remain being' (Pérez-Álvarez 2011, p. 103).

References

American Psychiatric Association (1994) Diagnostic and statistical manual of mental disorders, 4th edn. Author, Washington

American Psychiatric Association (2013) Diagnostic and statistical manual of mental disorders, 5th edn. American Psychiatric Publishing, Washington

Andresen R, Oades LG, Caputi P (2011) Psychological recovery: beyond mental illness. Wiley-Blackwell, New York

Anthony WA (1993) Recovery for mental illness. The guiding vision of the mental health service system in the 1990s. Psychosoc Rehabil J 16:11–23

Barch DM, Bustillo J, Gaebel W, Gur R, Heckers S, Malaspina D et al (2013) Logic and justification for dimensional assessment of symptoms and related clinical phenomena in psychosis: relevance to DSM-5. Schizophr Res 150(1):15–20

Bond GR, Drake RE, Mueser KT, Latimer E (2001) Assertive community treatment for people with severe mental illness. Dis Manag Health Out 9(3):141–159

Bracken P, Thomas P, Timimi S, Asen E, Behr G, Beuster C et al (2012) Psychiatry beyond the current paradigm. Br J Psychiatry 201:430–434

Bulechek GM, Butcher HK, Dochterman JMM, Wagner C (2013) Nursing interventions classification (NIC). Elsevier Health Sciences, Amsterdam

Carr VJ, Lewin TJ, Neil AL, Halpin SA, Holmes S (2004) Premorbid, psychosocial and clinical predictors of the costs of schizophrenia and other psychoses. Br J Psychiatry 184(6):517–525

Chadwick P (2009) Terapia cognitiva basada en la persona para la psicosisperturbadora. Paradox, Madrid

Claridge G (1980) Acercamiento dimensional a la esquizofrenia. Análisis y Modificación de Conducta 6:445–478

Coid JW, Kirkbride JB, Barker D, Cowden F, Stamps R, Yang M et al (2008) Raised incidence rates of all psychoses among migrant groups: findings from the East London first episode psychosis study. Arch Gen Psychiatry 65(11):1250–1258

Corstens D, Longden E, McCarthy-Jones S, Waddingham R, Thomas N (2014) Emerging perspectives from the hearing voices movement: implications for research and practice. Schizophr Bull 40(Suppl 4):S285–S294

García-Montes JM, Pérez-Alvarez M (2003) Reivindicación de la persona en esquizofrenia. Int J Clin Health Psychol 3(1):107–122

Gomes MS, Mello R (2012) Overload generated by the interaction with schizophrenia patients: nursing building family care. SMAD Rev Elec Salud Mental Alcohol Drogas 8(1)

González-Pando D, Beltrán-García P, Martínez-Suárez P (2016) Exploring learning potential in schizophrenic inpatients in different psychopathological conditions. Clin Health 27(2):81–88

Gónzalez-Pardo H, Pérez Álvarez M (2013) Epigenetic and its implications for psychology. Psicothema 25(1):3–12

Harrow M, Jobea TH, Faulla RN (2014) Does treatment of schizophrenia with antipsychotic medications eliminate or reduce psychosis? A 20-year multi-follow-up study. Psychol Med 42:10

Horwitz A (2002) Creating mental illness. University of Chicago Press, Chicago

Insel TR, Quirion R (2005) Psychiatry as a clinical neuroscience discipline. JAMA 294(17):2221–2224

Jacobson N, Greenley D (2001) A conceptual model of recovery. Psychiatr Serv 52(5):688

Leff J, Vaughn C (1984) Expressed emotion in families: its significance for mental illness. Guilford Press, New York

Lemos S, Fonseca E, Paino M, Vallina O (2015) Esquizofrenia y otros trastornos psicóticos. Síntesis, Madrid

Lemos-Giráldez S, Paino M, Sierra-Baigrie S, Muñiz J (2011) Síntomas psicóticos subclínicos en población general adolescente. Actas Esp Psiquiatr 39(3):155–162

Linscott RJ, van Os J (2010) Systematic reviews of categorical versus continuum models in psychosis: evidence for discontinuous subpopulations underlying a psychometric continuum. Implications for DSM-5, DSM-VI, and DSM-VII. Annu Rev Clin Psychol 6:391–419

Maj M (2011) Understanding the pathophysiology of schizophrenia: are we on the wrong or on the right track? Schizophr Res 127:20–21

Morgan C, Hutchinson G (2010) The sociodevelopmental origins of psychosis. In: Morgan C, Bhugra D (eds) Principles of social psychiatry. Wiley, Oxford, pp 193–214

Peplau HE (1991/1952) Interpersonal relations in nursing: a conceptual frame of reference for psychodynamic nursing. Springer Publishing Company, New York

Pajonk FG, Wobrock T, Gruber O, Scherk H, Berner D, Kaizl I et al (2010) Hippocampal plasticity in response to exercise in schizophrenia. Arch Gen Psychiatry 67:133–143

Pérez-Álvarez M (2011) Esquizofrenia y cultura moderna. Ediuno, Oviedo

Pérez-Álvarez M (2012) Esquizofrenia y cultura moderna: razones de la locura. Psicothema 24(1):1–9

Pérez-Álvarez M, García-Montes JM, Sass L (2010) La hora de la fenomenología en la esquizofrenia. Clin Health 21(3):221–233

Razzaque R, Wood L (2015) Open dialogue and its relevance to the NHS: opinions of NHS staff and service users. Community Ment Health J 51(8):931–938
Read J, Haslam N, Davies E (2006) Prejudice and schizophrenia: a review of the mental ilness is a illness like any other approach. Acta Psychiatr Scand 114:303–318
Romme MA, Escher AD (1989) Hearing voices. Schizophr Bull 15(2):209
Sass LA, Parnas J (2007) Explaining schizophrenia: the relevance of phenomenology. In: Chung MC, (Bill)Fulford KWM, Graham G (eds) Recovering schizophrenia. Oxford University Press, New York, pp 63–95
Seikkula J, Aaltonen J, Alakare B, Haarakangas K, Keranen J, Lehtinen K (2006) Five year experience of first episode nonaffective psychosis in open-dialogue approach: treatment principles, follow-up outcomes, and two case studies. Psychother Res 16(02):214–228
Skinner BF (1979) Contingencias de reforzamiento. Un análisis teórico. Trillas, México
Strauss JS (1969) Hallucinations and delusions as points on continua function. Arch Gen Psychiatry 21:581–586
Tortelli A, Errazuriz A, Croudace T, Morgan C, Murray RM, Jones PB et al (2015) Schizophrenia and other psychotic disorders in Caribbean-born migrants and their descendants in England: systematic review and meta-analysis of incidence rates, 1950–2013. Soc Psychiatry Psychiatr Epidemiol 50(7):1039–1055
Villagrán JM (2003) Hacia una psiquiatría biológica no reduccionista: los modelos interdisciplinares. In: Baca E, Lázaro J (eds) Hechos y valores en psiquiatría. Triacastella, Madrid, pp 485–513
World Health Organization (2001). The World Health Report 2001: Mental health: new understanding, new hope. World Health Organization. Geneve
Woods A (2011) The sublime object of psychiatry: schizophrenia in clinical and cultural theory. Oxford University Press, Oxford

Human Experiences of and Psychiatric/ Mental Health Nurses' Responses to Problems Related to Dementias and Cognitive Impairment

29

Helena Quaresma, Cândida Loureiro, and José Carlos Santos

29.1 Introduction

The rise in life expectancy for the population of the occidental world has increased the number of people aged over 65 years who live in developed countries, a fact that is corroborated by the analysis of some demographic indicators. By 2045–2050, people can expect to live to (on average) 83 years of age in developed regions and 74 years in developing regions (UNPF 2012, p. 3), and the world's older adult population is expected to reach 2 billion. Consequently, by 2050, it is estimated that people aged over 60 years will represent 10% of the population in Africa, 24% in Asia, 24% in Oceania, 25% in Latin America and the Caribbean, 27% in Northern America, and 34% in Europe (Idem, 2012). Population aging, which is directly related to greater longevity, is associated not only with a set of biological, psychological, and social changes that can gradually lead to significant losses of autonomy in the performance of activities of daily living but also with a higher incidence of neurodegenerative disorders, which may not result from a normal aging process (Alzheimer's Australia 2012; WHO 2012). According to EU Joint Programme – Neurodegenerative Disease Research (JPND), these disorders involve the progressive degeneration and/or death of nerve cells, causing dementia (EU Joint Programme–Neurodegenerative Disease Research n.d.). Accordingly, this chapter is intended to discuss the definition and provides a general overview of the basic elements related to dementia, intervention, psychoeducation, and person-centered psychiatric/mental health nursing care of older adults living with dementia, their families, and caregivers.

H. Quaresma (✉) • C. Loureiro
Nursing School of Coimbra, Coimbra, Portugal
e-mail: quaresma@esenfc.pt

J.C. Santos
Escola Superior de Enfermagem de Coimbra, Nursing School of Coimbra, Coimbra, Portugal

© Springer International Publishing Switzerland 2018
J.C. Santos, J.R. Cutcliffe (eds.), *European Psychiatric/Mental Health Nursing in the 21st Century*, Principles of Specialty Nursing,
https://doi.org/10.1007/978-3-319-31772-4_29

29.2 Definition and Overview of Basic Elements

Dementia is a generic term that refers to a syndrome of different etiologies, all of which are disease(s) of the brain,

> usually of a chronic or progressive nature, in which there is disturbance of multiple higher cortical functions, including memory, thinking, orientation, comprehension, calculation, learning capacity, language and judgement. (WHO 1993, p. 45)

The main characteristic of dementia is the progression of cognitive deficits, such as memory loss, aphasia, apraxia, agnosia, and disturbance of executive function that progressively lead to a decrease and, subsequently, impairment in occupational or social functioning (WHO 2012). The DSM-5 (2014) includes the term dementia under the newly named and broader entity, *major neurocognitive disorder*, although the term dementia is not precluded from use in the etiological subtypes in which that term is standard. The DSM-5 abandons the previous diagnostic criterion which required memory to be one of the affected cognitive areas and comes closer to the ICD-10, in which cognitive changes must be severe enough to interfere with the activities of daily living.

According to the World Health Organization (WHO), 35.6 million people worldwide suffer from dementia, and this number is expected to double by 2030 (65.7 million) and triple by 2050 (115.4 million) (OECD 2013). The majority of people suffering from dementia live in Asia (35%) and in Europe (28%) (European Parliament 2010). The overall prevalence of dementia is estimated to be 1–2% at the age of 65, reaching up to 30% at the age of 85 (American Psychiatric Association 2014). Due to the magnitude of this problem, the WHO declared dementia as a public health problem with consequences for individuals, families, caregivers, and health-care systems (World Health Organization 2012; European Parliament 2010).

Types of dementia can be found in neurodegenerative diseases such as Alzheimer's disease, frontotemporal lobar degeneration, Lewy body dementia, Parkinson's disease dementia, Huntington's disease, Pick's disease, and Creutzfeldt-Jakob disease, as well as in non-neurodegenerative diseases such as vascular dementia, hydrocephalus, post-traumatic dementia, systemic diseases, viral infections, toxicity-related diseases, or even malnutrition (World Health Organization 2012). In many cases, the progression of dementia can be delayed through disease management. However, most dementias are caused by neurodegenerative diseases, particularly Alzheimer's disease, which, despite the advances in medical knowledge, are still progressive and irreversible diseases.

Alzheimer's disease is characterized by an abnormal accumulation of the beta-amyloid protein, which leads to the formation of several plaques between neurons and, consequently, of fibrillary tangles due to an abnormal aggregation of the tau protein. These changes damage the connections between neurons (synapses), ultimately causing them to die. These brain changes occur gradually and begin several years before the first warning signs (Alzheimer's Australia 2012). However, both the cholinergic hypothesis and the amyloid cascade hypothesis have proved to be insufficient for understanding Alzheimer's disease. New lines of research on Alzheimer's disease and dementias in general have led to the multifactorial hypothesis, i.e., the combination of several risk factors divided into two different groups. One of these groups includes the non-modifiable factors such as genetics and age, which is a key factor since the prevalence of Alzheimer's disease doubles every 5 years after the age of 65. Hereditary forms of dementia are extremely rare in the general population, such as Huntington's disease, some forms of frontotemporal dementia, and familial Alzheimer's disease (FAD). Although the most studied gene in FAD – APOE-e4 (Farrow 2010) – can be found in significantly younger individuals (it usually appears around 50 years of age), it has a lower prevalence (Alzheimer's Australia 2012).

Through the identification of modifiable risk factors, the multifactorial hypothesis enables the preventive approach (Eustache et al. 2015). These modifiable risk factors include obesity, diabetes, high blood pressure, high cholesterol, depression, social isolation, intellectual and physical inactivity, smoking, and brain damage induced by heavy alcohol intake (Farrow 2010). Finally, another important evidence-based risk factor is institutionalization. It is therefore important for individuals to remain in their family environment as long as possible, which requires changing the organization of health-care services so as to meet the populations' new needs and support relative or nonrelative caregivers (Direção-Geral da Saúde 2016).

Diagnosing dementias is a complex process that requires a differential diagnosis (Direção-Geral da Saúde 2011). The early symptoms of the disease can often be ignored or undervalued by the patients themselves and their relatives, since they fail to distinguish between the changes resulting from normal aging and the first signs of maladjustment. Sequeira (2007) believes that the diagnosis can be further complicated by age, education, sociocultural level, comorbidity, and even behavioral/functional changes caused by other problems. Assessment tools should be used to achieve an accurate and early diagnosis (Sheehan 2012). These tools include the Mini-Mental State Examination (MMSE), a cognitive assessment tool widely used in elderly dementia patients since it enables screening for cognitive impairment by educational level (Folstein et al. 1975); the Global Deterioration Scale (GDS), which assesses dementia in seven stages (Reisberg et al. 1982); and the Clinical Dementia Rating (CDR), which assesses dementia in five stages (Hughes et al. 1982; Morris 1993). The three instruments have been translated and validated for several countries, including Portugal.

29.3 Interventions

According to the European Collaboration on Dementia (EuroCoDe) project, which is conducted by Alzheimer Europe and funded by the European Commission (2014), treatment should reconcile pharmacological interventions, always taking into account the relevance of non-pharmacological measures. Pharmacological strategies are aimed at delaying disease progression and controlling some behavioral symptoms (restlessness, anxiety, etc.), and special attention should be given to the use of psychotropic drugs. In turn, the non-pharmacological treatment includes a set of nonchemical interventions aimed, for example, at maximizing the patient's cognitive functioning, delaying disease progression and the consequent loss of abilities, helping in the process of disease adaptation, and minimizing the caregiver's distress and burden (Gitlin et al. 2012).

Regardless of the techniques used, non-pharmacological interventions are based on principles of rehabilitation in order to reduce the impact of the disease, develop or maintain autonomy, improve cognitive function or prevent its sudden deterioration, improve the general health status, stimulate cognitive skills, promote personal identity and self-esteem, and minimize stress (Álvarez et al. 2014; Sequeira 2010). They include the establishment of specific routines, environmental changes (such as signposting), mild physical activity programs, animal-assisted interventions, music therapy, art therapy, aromatherapy, and specific techniques used to delay cognitive deterioration (Fleta and León 2011). The following techniques can be particularly useful:

1. Music therapy can be used to promote interpersonal interaction and cognitive activation motor rehabilitation, when associated with dance, and decrease anxiety (Sung et al. 2012).
2. Reality orientation (RO) therapy is a social therapy based on the repetition of current information and attitudes of (re)socialization directed to memory and executive functions. It was initially developed in 1968 by James Folson as a formal or informal technique that must adapt to the patient's preferences. It aims to understand and develop the patient's knowledge of the surrounding environment and locate him/her both temporally and spatially. It includes activities oriented to everyday tasks; guided walking exercises to help identify important locations in the surrounding area and identify the colors of the walls, floor, stairs, and layout of surrounding environments; and continuous cognition and memory stimulation exercises integrated in the patients' daily activities, with situational guidance (Douglas et al. 2004).
3. Reminiscence therapy aims to stimulate the patient's remote memory, with significant facts of his/her lives. The reactivation of past experiences helps to preserve the identity and contributes to update the patient's episodic memory. This technique should take into account the patient's personal reality; should be adapted to age, culture, profession, lifestyle, and experience; and should only develop the aspects related to his/her biography. Some of the techniques that can be used include face-name association, which implies creating visual images as a strategy to remember names, or verbal semantic association, in which the patient recalls words related to the name of objects, by associating as many ideas as possible with a given object (Afonso 2011).
4. Cognitive stimulation is mainly directed to the mnesic function and consists of training memory, attention, and information processing with the purpose of improving the patient's performance, environmental adaptation, and social integration (Knowles 2010).

29.4 Psychoeducation

Psychoeducation is a direct intervention process used to help family members to adopt methods that enable the mutual expression of needs and desires, as well as to help families to solve their daily problems when suffering from or caring for a person with a mental disorder (Falloon et al. 1993). The two key objectives of psychoeducational interventions are to provide patients and their relatives with knowledge on dementia and on ways to cope with the associated problems on a daily basis and decrease family stress and the caregivers' emotional and occupational burden, providing them with emotional and social support (Chien et al. 2011). This support should promote the caregivers' well-being by giving access to information, developing care-related skills, and raising awareness on the need to engage in other activities. It must be implemented in the initial phase and included in the treatment and therapeutic planning.

The WHO and Alzheimer's Disease International (2012) believe that psychoeducational programs for family caregivers are an important resource to ensure treatment effectiveness to the extent that they allow delaying the institutionalization of the person with dementia, thus reducing health-care-related costs. In turn, in a meta-analysis study, Chien et al. (2011) concluded that individuals in a psychoeducational group show higher levels of psychological well-being and a lower incidence of depression.

29.5 Person-Centered Psychiatric/Mental Health Nursing Care of the Older Adult Living with Dementia

P/MH nursing care directed to dementia patients aims at promoting their independence in the 14 basic human needs and physical safety, improving communication, reducing anxiety and restlessness, managing the therapeutic regimen, and providing support to caregivers. (Ordem dos Enfermeiros 2010; Sequeira 2010). With regard to basic human needs, people with dementia should be encouraged to make decisions and to participate in self-care activities, by exploring their potential and respecting their limitations. According to Sidani (2011), self-care is considered as an integral component of chronic disease management and the maintenance of an acceptable level of functionality.

Caring for people with dementia and their families or caregivers implies focusing on their needs and abilities, going beyond the valorization of the symptoms. Their experiences and the meaning assigned to them must be taken into account in order to understand reality from the patient's perspective. This will serve as basis for a personalized intervention plan, within an individualized approach that takes into account the social and family contexts.

The provision of a person-centered care to the person with dementia aims at maintaining individuality, promoting the patients and their caregivers' well-being, and appreciating the person regardless of his/her age or cognitive ability (Brooker 2007). The perspective of dementia patients and their relative or nonrelative caregivers is at the center of care, favoring their relationships with the others so as to promote a social supportive environment. Taking into account the individuals' own culture and knowing their personal experience are essential to understand their behaviors and develop a plan adjusted to their needs, strengths, abilities, interests, and preferences (Love and Pinkowitz 2013). According to Edvardsson et al. (2008), the provision of high-quality person-centered care to people with dementia promotes their well-being, allows identifying their needs, offers shared decision-making opportunities, and involves both formal and informal caregivers, taking into account their family and social contexts.

Communication is one of the key aspects in caring for people with dementia (Egan et al. 2010). The use of multiple communication strategies allows extending the interaction between the person with dementia and the others, allowing him/her to exercise his/her individuality. Some facilitating strategies consist of adapting the style of language and voice tone, using short and easy-to-understand sentences, and using nonverbal communication. Therefore, the use of communication strategies requires creativity (use of notes, photos, pictures) to ensure that the families and the close social network can use their content. Allan and Killick (2008) argue that the families and the close social network, by sharing memories and identities, are more likely to have the necessary resources to communicate in a more stimulating way. The use of adequate and perceptible stimuli can improve the communication between dementia patients and their caregivers, thus reducing social isolation and contributing to the well-being and dignity of people with dementia. However, in order to mitigate stress, confusion, and restlessness, excessive stimulation should be avoided (Timlin and Rysenbry 2010).

The management of the activities of daily living according to one's culture and previous habits is another key aspect for maintaining the skills and perception of well-being of dementia patients (Smit et al. 2014). However, due to the gradual loss of abilities, participating in activities becomes increasingly difficult for him/her. People with dementia can remain active for a longer period of time if the rooms are decorated with personal and recognizable objects, making them more familiar (Zeisel 2013), as well as if signs are used to help people to identify and find what they are looking for. However, in most situations, the level of dependence and the health-care needs increase progressively, and informal caregivers become central to the care process. Caregivers constantly face increasing difficulties related to the progressive cognitive decline, the functional deterioration, and the behavioral changes.

29.6 Family and Caregivers

According to Meleis (2010), the experience of a chronic disease within the family demands a change of roles and adjustments in family functioning, requiring a transition to the role of informal caregivers. This author argues that role supplementation is an intervention that can be used to avoid or mitigate role insufficiency and reduce stress, through strategies of role clarification, education, counseling, and psychoeducation. Informal caregivers of dementia patients report physical, psychological, emotional, social, and financial difficulties resulting from the continuous care provision. This situation of overload is referred to as the caregiver's burden, i.e., the psychological state resulting from the combination of physical effort, emotional pressure/emotional stress, social constraints, and economic demands (Carvalho 2013).

Zarit et al. (2008) believe that caregivers are often both mentally and physically exhausted, experiencing periods of major stress, which causes well-known health problems, such as depression, anxiety (Garcia 2010), psychosomatic disorders, immunological changes, and cardiovascular changes (Yee and Schulz 2000). Therefore, care must focus not only on the patients but also on the informal caregivers, and the assessment of their burden should be a major concern. One of the most commonly used instruments to assess burden is the Burden Interview Scale (Zarit et al. 2008). Psychiatric/mental health nurses (P/MHN) are adequately trained and have the necessary skills to meet the needs of dementia patients and their caregivers. The *Ordem dos Enfermeiros* (Portuguese Nurses' Association) (2010a, p. 1) states that:

> the interventions of the P/MHN aim to help adapting the patient and family's responses to better cope with specific mental disorder-related problems, with the purpose of preventing the worsening of the situation and the patient's social isolation, promoting the recovery and quality of life for the whole family.

The P/MHN should intervene immediately after the diagnosis, so as to facilitate the transition processes of the person with dementia, the caregiver, and the family by providing adequate care to their needs and avoid a situation of burden and stress for informal caregivers (Sequeira 2007). The challenge is to understand the experiences of informal caregivers, so as to develop interventions based on their needs, seeing them as care partners and involving them in the planning and development of services from which they can benefit.

> The relatives of people with mental disorders should be considered as key partners in the provision of care, and encouraged to participate in this care provision and to receive the necessary training and education. (DGS 2008, p. 14)

The interventions of the PMHN should empower the informal caregiver to better understand the disease and use strategies to facilitate care provision. Caregivers should receive guidance on the importance of cognitive stimulation, adequate management of the therapeutic regimen, use of effective coping strategies, negotiation of ways to request help, and encouragement to participate in social and leisure activities (Sequeira 2010).

We believe that nursing visits in mental health facilitate the contact with the patients and their families, allowing the PMHN to understand the family dynamics and the relatives' involvement in the treatment and identify any difficulties, introducing the necessary changes to the care plan. According to Meleis (2010), nursing visits provide the patient/informal caregiver with the necessary support to continue treatment. Despite the difficulty in quantifying the outcomes of the proposed interventions, these can be observed in the dementia patients' quality of life, well-being, behavior, and performance, as well as in the caregivers' quality of life and well-being (Álvarez et al. 2014). The diversity and complexity of the aspects related to the support and training of dementia patient's caregivers, who must be considered as care partners, should be acknowledged. We must not forget that the well-being of informal caregivers is essential to the well-being of people with dementia and their maintenance at home.

References

Afonso RMLBM (2011) Reminiscência: Como técnica de intervenção psicológica em pessoas idosas, 1ª edn. Fundação Calouste Gulbenkian, Lisboa

Allan K, Killick J (2008) Communication and relationships: an inclusive social world. In: Downs M, Bowers B (eds) Excellence in *dementia care: research into practice*. Open University Press, Maidenhead, pp 212–229

Álvarez PM-L, Bellver R, Carruesco GT (2014) KNOW alzheimer: Respuestas concretas a dudas reales: manual de consulta para cuidadores y familiares. Profármaco, Barcelona, Espanha. Retrieved from http://envejecimiento.csic.es/documentos/documentos/KAManualCuidadoresAlzheimer-08-2014.pdf

Alzheimer's Australia (2012) What is dementia?. Retrieved from https://fightdementia.org.au/sites/default/files/helpsheets/Helpsheet-AboutDementia01-WhatIsDementia_english.pdf

American Psychiatric Association (2014) Manual de diagnóstico e estatística das perturbações mentais, 5ª edn. Climepsi, Lisboa

Brooker D (2007) Person-centred dementia care-making services better. Jessica Kingsley Publishers, Londres e Filadélfia

Carvalho LIC (2013) *Cuidador informal da pessoa com demência: Avaliação do cuidado informal e maneiras como o prestador de cuidados enfrenta as dificuldades*. Master's dissertation, Coimbra, Portugal: Escola Superior de Enfermagem de Coimbra

Chien LY, Chu H, Guo JL, Lião YM, Chang LI, Chen CH, Chou KR (2011) Caregiver support groups in patients with dementia: a meta-analysis. *Int J Geriatr Psychiatry* 26(10):1089–1098. doi:10.1002/gps.2660

Direção Geral de Saúde (2008) Plano nacional de saúde mental 2007–2016: Resumo executivo. Direção Geral de Saúde, Lisboa

Direção-Geral da Saúde (2011) Abordagem terapêutica das alterações cognitivas. Direção Geral de Saúde, Lisboa

Direção Geral de Saúde (2016) Saúde mental em números. Direção Geral de Saúde, Lisboa

Douglas S, James I, Ballard C (2004) Non-pharmacological interventions in dementia. Adv Psychiatr Treatment 10(3):171–177. doi:10.1192/apt.10.3.171

Edvardsson D, Winblad B, Sandman P (2008) Person-centered care of people with severe Alzheimer's disease: current status and ways forward. Lancet Neurol 7:362–367

Egan M, Bérubé D, Racine G, Leonard C, Rochon E (2010) Methods to enhance verbal communication between individuals with Alzheimer's disease and their formal and informal caregivers: a systematic review. Int J Alzheimers Dis 2010:1–12. doi:10.4061/2010/906818

EU Joint Programme–Neurodegenerative Disease Research (n.d.) What is neurodegenerative disease? Recuperado de http://www.neurodegenerationresearch.eu/about/what/

European Commission (2014) Implementation report on the commission communication on a European initiative on Alzheimer's disease and other dementias. European Commission, Brussels. Retrieved from http://ec.europa.eu/health/major_chronic_diseases/docs/2014_implreport_alzheimer_dementias_en.pdf

European Parliament (2010) Report on a European initiative on Alzheimer's disease and other dementias (2010/2084(INI)).Retrieved from http://www.europarl.europa.eu/sides/getDoc.do?pubRef=-//EP//TEXT+REPORT+A7-2010-0366+0+DOC+XML+V0//EN

Eustache F, Chételat G, Desgranges B, de La Sayette V (2015) Alzheimer: Fatalité ou espoir? Le muscadier, Paris

Falloon IRH, Laporta M, Fadden G, Graham-Hole V (1993) Managing stress in families. Routledge, London, England

Farrow M (2010) Towards a dementia prevention policy for Australia: implications of the current evidence. Alzheimer's Australia. Retrieved from http://yourbrainmatters.org.au/sites/default/files/Towards%20Dementia%20Prevention%20Policy.pdf

Fleta J, León M (2011) Manual de actuación en la enfermedad de Alzheimer y otras demencias. In: Gobierno de Canarias. Retrieved from http://documents.mx/documents/manual-de-actuacion-en-la-enfermedad-de-alzheimer-y-otras-demencias-2011pdf.html#

Folstein MF, Folstein SE, McHugh PR (1975) Mini-mental state: a practical method for grading the cognitive state of patients for the clinician. J Psychiatr Res 12(3):189–198. doi:10.1016/0022-3956(75)90026-6

Fundación Reina Sofia (2012) Guía práctica para profesionales que trabajan con enfermos de Alzheimer.Retrieved from http://www.fundacionreinasofia.es/Lists/Documentacion/Attachments/15/Guia%20profesionales_Alzheimer_final.pdf

Garcia J (2010) Los tiempos del cuidador: el impacto de la dependencia de los mayores en la vida cotidiana de sus cuidadores. IMSERSO, Madrid, Espanha

Gitlin LN, Kales HC, Lyketsos CG (2012) Managing behavioral symptoms in dementia ssing non-pharmacologic approaches: an overview. J Am Med Assoc 21(308):2020–2029. doi:10.1001/jama.2012.36918

Hughes CP, Berg L, Danzinger LW, Coben LA, Martin RL (1982) A new clinical scale for the staging of dementia. Br J Psychiatry 140:566–572. doi:10.1192/bjp.140.6.566

Knowles J (2010) Cognitive stimulation therapy. Working with older people: community care. Policy Pract 14(1):22–25. doi:10.5042/wwop.2010.0075

Love K, Pinkowitz J (2013) Person-centered care for people with dementia: a theoretical and conceptual framework. Generations 37(3):23–29. Retrieved from http://www.asaging.org/blog/person-centered-care-people-dementia-theoretical-and-conceptual-framework

Meleis AI (2010) Transitions theory. Springer, New York

Morris J (1993) The CDR: current version and scoring rules. Neurology 43:2412–2413

OECDE (2013) Health at a glance 2013: OECD indicators. Autor Retrieved from.doi: 10.1787/health_glance-2013-en

Ordem dos enfermeiros (2010) Regulamento das competências comuns do enfermeiro especialista em saúde mental. Ordem dos Enfermeiros, Lisboa. Retrieved from http://www.ordemenfermeiros.pt/legislacao/Paginas/RegulamentoCompetenciasComunsEspecificas.aspx

Ordem dos enfermeiros, Mesa do colégio de especialidade de Enfermagem de Saúde Mental e Psiquiátrica (2010) Adequação técnico-científica da admissão das pessoas com demência nas unidades de dia e promoção da autonomia da RNCCI (art.° 21 do Dec. Lei. 101/2006 de 6 de Junho) (Parecer n° 2/2010). Recuperado de http://www.ordemenfermeiros.pt/documentos/Documents/Parecer02_MCEESMP_Adequacaotec_cientifica_adm_pessoas%20com%20demencia.pdf

Reisberg B, Ferris SH, Leon MJ, Crook T (1982) Global deterioration scale (GDS) for assessment of primary degenerative dementia. Am J Psychiatr 139:1136–1139. Retrieved from http://www.fhca.org/members/qi/clinadmin/global.pdf

Sequeira CAC (2007) Cuidar de idosos dependentes: diagnósticos e intervenções. Quarteto, Coimbra

Sequeira CAC (2010) Cuidar de idosos com dependência física e mental. Lidel, Lisboa

Sidani S (2011) Self-care. In: Doran D (ed) Nursing outcomes: the state of science, 2ª edn. Jones & Bartlett, Burlington, MA, pp 131–200

Sheehan B (2012) Assessment scales in dementia. Ther Adv Neurol Disord 5(6):349–358. doi:10.1177/1756285612455733

Smit D, Willemse B, de Lange J, Pot AM (2014) Wellbeing-enhancing occupation and organizational and environmental contributors in long-term dementia care facilities: an explorative study. Int Psychogeriatr 26:1–12. doi:10.1017/S1041610213001397

Sung HC, Lee W, Li TL, Watson R (2012) A group music intervention using percussion instruments with familiar music to reduce anxiety and agitation of institutionalized older adults with dementia. Int J Geriatr Psychiatry 27(6):621–627

Timlin G, Rysenbry N (2010) Design for dementia: improving dining and bedroom environments in care homes. Royal College of Arts, London, England

United Nations Population Fund, HalpAge International (UNPF) (2012) Ageing in the twenty-first century: a celebration and a challenge? UNPF, New York

World Health Organization (1993) The ICD-10 classification of mental and behavioural disorders: diagnostic criteria for research. WHO, Geneva

World Health Organization, Alzheimer's Disease International (2012) Dementia: a public health priority. World Health Organization, Alzheimers Disease International, Geneva

Yee JL, Schulz R (2000) Gender differences in psychiatric morbidity among family caregivers: a review and analysis. Gerontologist 2:147–164

Zarit SH, Charles D, Irene L (2008) Diagnosis and management of caregiver burden in dementia. Handb Clin Neurol 89:101–106

Zeisel J (2013) Improving person-centered care through effective design. Generations, J Am Soc Aging 37(3):45–52. Retrieved from http://www.thehearth.org/articlesimages/Generations%20 Article.pdf

Problems Related to Substance and Alcohol Misuse

30

Fatma Yasemin Kutlu and Gul Dikec

30.1 Introduction: Substance-Related "Disorders"

30.1.1 Substance Use "Disorders"

The essential feature of a substance use disorder is a cluster of cognitive, behavioral, and physiological symptoms indicating that the individual continues using the substance despite significant substance-related problems (American Psychiatric Association 2013, p. 483). When the use of substance affects impinges or impacts upon the individuals' ability to fulfill their roles at work, at school, or at home, it is categorized as a (so-called) substance use disorder. The individual expresses a desire to stop using the substance or wants to control his/her usage, but it's a waste of effort, and the use of substance continues to increase (Hicdurmaz and Öz 2016).

30.1.2 Substance-Induced "Disorders"

Substance-induced disorders are categorized as "intoxication, withdrawal, other substance-induced disorders and unspecified other (unknown) substance-related disorder" (American Psychiatric Association 2013, p. 485).

Substance intoxication: "The essential feature is the development of a reversible substance-specific syndrome due to the recent ingestion of a substance. Substance

F.Y. Kutlu (✉)
Mental Health and Psychiatric Nursing Department, Florence Nightingale Nursing Faculty, Istanbul University, 34452 İstanbul, Turkey
e-mail: ykutlu@gmail.com

G. Dikec
Nursing Department, Health Science Faculty, Istinye University, Istanbul, Turkey

© Springer International Publishing Switzerland 2018

J.C. Santos, J.R. Cutcliffe (eds.), *European Psychiatric/Mental Health Nursing in the 21st Century*, Principles of Specialty Nursing,
https://doi.org/10.1007/978-3-319-31772-4_30

intoxication is common among those with a substance use disorder but also occurs frequently in individuals without a substance use disorder" (American Psychiatric Association 2013, p. 485).

Substance withdrawal: The essential feature is the development of a substance-specific problematic behavioral change, with physiological and cognitive concomitants, that is due to the cessation of, or reduction in, heavy and prolonged substance use (American Psychiatric Association 2013, p. 485).

Other substance-induced disorders: Other substance-induced disorders are discussed in the related mental disorder part of DSM-V (American Psychiatric Association 2013, p. 487).

Unspecified other (unknown) substance-related disorders: This diagnosis is used when substance use causes clinically significant distress or impairment but does not meet the full criteria for a specific substance-related disorder (American Psychiatric Association 2013, p. 585).

30.2 Etiological Factors in Substance and Alcohol Misuse Problems

Addiction to a substance is a holistic problem that manifests in symptoms or problems in each of the different dimensions of the person (e.g., biological, psychological, cultural, spiritual, and social factors play a role) (Ulug and Ozturk 2015).

30.2.1 Biological Factors

Substances' effect on the brain: A common feature of substances which cause addiction is that they directly activate the reward system of the brain. In various studies (Chiara 1995; Gardner 2005), findings repeatedly indicate that addictive substances affect the behavior in a common way by increasing synaptic dopamine, which is a main component of NAc of ventral striatum. This increase is asserted as a necessary way to reinforce the use of substance and develop the addiction (Halter 2014).

Heredity: Heredity has a big role in alcohol addiction. The children of people who have a history of alcohol misuse are three times more likely to develop addiction than the children of parents who do not have a history of substance misuse. Having a strong resistance power against alcohol is an important risk factor of developing alcohol addiction (Ulug and Ozturk 2015).

30.2.2 Psychological Factors

Psychodynamic theoretical explanations of substance misuse include the view that substance misuse problems are related to the fixation to oral stage of punitive superego and psychosexual development. Sadock and Sadock (2007) assert that alcohol is used for controlling "panic," opioids for reducing "anger," and amphetamines for moderating depression. Some researchers believe that decreased self-esteem, depression, passiveness, and incompetence in communication are seen among the individuals who misuse substances (Halter 2014).

30.2.3 Sociocultural Factors

Social and environmental factors also appear to be important and relevant to both the development of and continuation of one's addiction (Hicdurmaz and Öz 2016). . Many psychotropic substances create a pleasurable experience which can "encourage" the individual to seek, to recreate or repeat the "high," or to use a phrase from "street culture"; users are described as "chasing the dragon".[1] Besides, family dynamics and conditions can serve as either protective or risk factors (Yuncu and Aydin 2012). It's reported that environmental factors are responsible for misusing substances at the early ages (Yuncu and Aydin 2012). Delaying a young person's first encounter with a psychoactive substance and growing up in a positive, familial environment appears to reduce the possibility of developing substance addiction (Yuncu and Aydin 2012). The risk of meeting the substance for the first time is independent from genetic effect. However, people who have genetic susceptibility are open to the risks after meeting the substance for the first time (Yuncu and Aydin 2012). Further evidence regarding sociocultural impacts and influences on substance misuse behavior include the mimicking or copying the behavior of cultural role models; identifying with such individuals and the values/behaviors they display (Hicdurmaz and Öz 2016). Cultural factors too are effective upon substance use and its addiction. In an environment, where the standards of judgment don't accept and don't support substance use, the rate of use is low; on the other hand, if the use of substance has social value, the rate might be high (Ulug and Ozturk 2015).

30.3 Commonly Encountered Substances and Their Features

The use or misuse of alcohol and/or substances is a problem which has social, physical, and psychiatric outcomes and impacts. Substances are commonly separated into legal and illegal groups. Ironically, the rates of mortality and morbidity associated with many legalized substances (e.g., tobacco, alcohol) are significantly higher than rates associated with substances that are currently illegal (Lingford-Hughes and Clementi 2008, see Cutcliffe and Saadeh 2014 for a recent comparison). That is not to suggest that the use of currently illegal substances does not lead to (holistic)

[1] While the phrase "Chasing the Dragon" originally referred to inhaling the vapor from an opiate, the meaning has morphed somewhat from the original, opiate-specific reference, and in contemporary parlance, it is used more a generic metaphor for an addict's constant pursuit of the feelings of their first high. The "dragon" being mythical represents a goal that can never be achieved, because it does not exist.

health problems but more to stress the counterintuitive relationship between degree of harm associated with the substance and current legal/illegal status of the substance (Cutcliffe and Saadeh 2014). The most recent version of the American Psychiatric Association 2013 DSM-V, under the title of substance use and addiction disorders, includes the following substances: alcohol, caffeine, cannabis, hallucinogens, inhalant, opioid, sedative-hypnotic or anxiolytic, stimulant, tobacco, and other substances (p. 481). All substance and their features was shown in Table 30.1.

30.3.1 **Alcohol** (American Psychiatric Association 2013, p. 490)

Alcohol is a substance that has been used in many cultures for centuries; it is also an addictive substance (Ulug and Ozturk 2015). Alcohol can cause behavior and mood changes resulting from its effect on the central nervous system. When blood alcohol level is 100–200 mg/dl, intoxication occurs, and when the level is 400–700 mg/dl, death occurs. With individuals who are experiencing alcohol addiction, withdrawal commonly develops after withdrawing or reducing alcohol for 4–12 h; delirium tremens develop in on people who have been drinking for a long time on the following second or third day after withdrawing alcohol.

Despite the prevalence of worldwide alcohol consumption, the majority of the world's adult population abstained from drinking alcohol in the past 12 months (WHO 2014). These individuals may be lifetime abstainers or former drinkers. Absolute worldwide alcohol consumption is estimated at 6.2 liters per person over the age of 15, and this equals to 13.5 g alcohol per person daily. 24.8% of this consumption is unrecorded (WHO 2014). Almost 16% of drinkers who are 15 years old or above the age of 15 consume alcohol in a heavy episodically way (WHO 2014).

Alcohol consumption is described as an important component in the causation of more than 200 diseases, injuries, and state of health on ICD-10 (International Classification of Diseases) (WHO 2014; Rehm et al. 2010; Shield et al. 2013). A positive correlation between consumption of alcohol and the development of tuberculosis and infectious diseases such as pneumonia has been reported (Rehm et al. 2009). A similar correlation has been discovered between alcohol consumption and the development of HIV positive status and sexually transmissible diseases (Baliunas et al. 2010; Hahn et al. 2011). In addition, there is a clear causal effect of alcohol consumption on HIV/AIDS patients' adherence to antiretroviral treatment, which can be quantified, as well as on the course of HIV/AIDS among patients who are not yet on antiretroviral therapy (Hendershot et al. 2009; Azar et al. 2010; Gmel et al. 2011). 5.9% of all deaths worldwide are related to or associated with alcohol consumption (WHO 2014). According to WHO 2014 data, 139 million DALYs (disability-adjusted life years) or 5.1% of global disease burden is related to or associated with alcohol consumption. The rate of deaths based on alcohol consumption and the highest rate of DALYs have been reported in the Europe region of WHO (WHO 2015).

The particular pattern of alcohol misuse has been reported to be significant and meaningful (WHO 2015). For instance, excessive consumption of alcohol during

Table 30.1 Human experiences to problems related to substance and alcohol misuse (Austin and Boyd 2008; Boyd 2008; Moyer et al. 2013; Ulug and Ozturk 2015; Townsend 2014)

Substance	The experience during the substance use	Intoxication experience	Withdrawal experience	Long-term or regular use experience
Alcohol	CNS depressant, relaxation, reduction in inhibition, lack of concentration, apathy, sleep	Increase in sexual or aggression stimulation, fluctuation in emotions, disruptions of judging, speech coordination, nystagmus, and flushing	Tremor, nausea-vomiting, joylessness, tachycardia, sweating, increase in blood pressure, anxiety, depressive mood, temporary hallucinations or illusions, headache, insomnia, delirium tremens (for people who drink too much alcohol and for a long time)	Tolerance, addiction, peripheral neuropathy, alcoholic myopathy, Wernicke encephalopathy, Korsakoff psychosis, alcoholic cardiomyopathy, esophagitis, gastritis, pancreatitis, alcoholic hepatitis, liver cirrhosis, leukopenia, thrombocytopenia, sexual function disorder
Caffeine	CNS stimulant, wakefulness, happiness, joy	Vasoconstriction, uneasiness, irritability, excitement, insomnia, flushing, diuresis, gastrointestinal disorder, muscle contractions, thought and speech disorder, tachycardia or arrhythmia, psychomotor agitation	Headache, exhaustion, dysphoric mood, agitation, difficulty in focusing, nausea, vomiting, pain, or stiffness in muscles	Physical and psychological addiction
Cannabis	Increased awareness for external stimulus, change in perception, euphoria, disappearance of inhibition, sound sensitivity	Motor coordination disorder, euphoria, anxiety, the sensation of slowdown of time, judging disorder, isolation, blood in conjunctivitis, increase in appetite, cottonmouth, tachycardia	Irritability, rage, aggression, anxiety, insomnia, decrease in appetite or losing weight, uneasiness, depressed mood, stomachache, tremors, sweating, fever, tremble, headache	Psychological addiction (physiological addiction is contradictive)

(continued)

Table 30.1 (continued)

Substance	The experience during the substance use	Intoxication experience	Withdrawal experience	Long-term or regular use experience
Hallucinogens	Deterioration of the skill of perception, visual hallucination	Significant nausea and depression, reference ideas, the fear of becoming insane, paranoid thoughts, judging disorder, perceptual changes, mydriasis, tachycardia, sweating, tremor, vision opacity, shivers, coordination disorder		Tolerance, psychological addiction, panic, bad trip, flashback
Inhalant	Uncontrolled behavior, euphoria	Aggression, apathy, judging disorder, euphoria, dizziness, nystagmus, coordination disorder, speech disorder, fatigue, lethargy, decrease in reflexes, psychomotor retardation, trembling, muscle weakness, vision opacity, double vision, stupor, or coma		Irresponsible behaviors, skipping school, leaving the house, words or behaviors that concealing the volatile substance use, respiratory infections, lung cancer
Opioid	Analgesic and sedative effect, decrease in the sensitiveness for psychological and physiological pain, euphoria	Initially euphoria and then apathy, dysphoria, psychomotor agitation or retardation, deterioration in judging, extreme decrement or dilatation in pupils, numbness, coma, deterioration in speech, attention and memory	Dysphoric mood, nausea and vomiting, muscle aches, shedding tear, nasal drainage, dilation in pupils, piloerection or sweating, diarrhea, yawning, fever, insomnia	Tolerance, addiction
Sedative, hypnotics, anxiolytics	CNS depressant, calming the anxiety, anesthesia, coma, and even death	Speech disorder, coordination disruption, fatigue, nystagmus, cognitive disorder, stupor, or coma	Hyperactivity, athetosis, insomnia, nausea and vomiting, hallucinations or illusions, psychomotor agitation, anxiety, grand mal episodes	Physiological and psychological addiction, cross tolerance, and addiction

Stimulant	CNS stimulant, increase in joy, enthusiasm, cheer, attention, and performance	Euphoria or emotional blunting, changes in sociability, hyper alertness, interpersonal sensitiveness, anxiety, tension or rage, stereotypical behaviors, deterioration in perception, tachycardia or bradycardia, dilatation in pupils, increased or decreased blood pressure, sweating or chilling, nausea, vomiting, loss of weight, respiration depression, chest pain, arrhythmia, confusion, episode, dyskinesia, dystonia, or coma	Dysphoric mood, exhaustion, vivid, unpleasant dreams, insomnia or hypersomnia, increase in appetite, psychomotor retardation, or agitation	
Nicotine	Loss of appetite, increase in blood pressure		Irritability, tenseness, rage, insomnia, dizziness, tremor, decrease in blood pressure, muscle contraction	Addiction, embolism, coronary heart disease, obstructive lung disease, cerebrovascular diseases, and peripheral vascular diseases

one short period of time (i.e., commonly referred to as "binge drinking") is associated with higher risks (WHO 2015). It's been estimated that 23 million Europeans will misuse alcohol in the upcoming years (Anderson and Baumberg 2006). This situation results in alcohol being ranked third out of a list of 26 risk factors which are associated with causing diseases in Europe (WHO 2015). In all the cultures that are being investigated, with the increase in differences of risky behaviors, men consume more amount of alcohol, and they do it more frequently than women (WHO 2015). Although many pregnant women withdraw alcohol, significant numbers of women continue to drink alcohol on dangerous levels during this period (WHO 2015).

30.3.2 **Caffeine** (American Psychiatric Association 2013, p. 503)

Caffeine as a stimulant found in many drinks (coffee, tea), chocolate, and over-the-counter medications including analgesics. Doses of less than 200 mg stimulate the cerebral cortex and increase mental activity (Boyd 2008). At a dose of 300 mg, caffeine can cause tremors, poor motor performance, and insomnia (Bonte et al., as cited in Boyd 2008, pg. 549). Doses of 500 mg increase the heart rate; stimulate respiratory, vasomotor, and vagal centers and cardiac muscles, resulting in increased force of cardiac contraction; dilate pulmonary and coronary blood vessels; and constrict blood flow to the cerebral vascular system (Boyd 2008). Psychiatric symptoms can be exacerbated (APA as cited in Boyd 2008, pg. 549).

The essential feature of caffeine intoxication is recent consumption of caffeine and five or more signs or symptoms that develop during or shortly after caffeine use. Symptoms include restlessness, nervousness, excitement, insomnia, flushed face, diuresis, and gastrointestinal complaints, which can occur with low doses (e.g., 200 mg) in vulnerable individuals such as children, the elderly, or individuals who have not been exposed to caffeine previously. Symptoms that generally appear at levels of more than 1 g/day include muscle twitching, rambling flow of thought and speech, tachycardia or cardiac arrhythmia, periods of inexhaustibility, and psychomotor agitation (American Psychiatric Association 2013, p. 504).

Caffeine withdrawal syndrome can include headache; marked fatigue or drowsiness; dysphoric mood, depressed mood, or irritability; difficulty concentrating; and flu-like symptoms (nausea, vomiting, or muscle pain/stiffness) (American Psychiatric Association 2013, p. 506).

30.3.3 **Cannabis** (American Psychiatric Association 2013, p. 509)

Cannabis's psychoactive substance is tetrahydrocannabinol (THC). While dependent on the concentration (percentage) of THC in the cannabis and the person's degree of tolerance to the substance, concentrations do differ widely and inhalation of cannabis results in an effect, on average, that continues for 2–4 h, whereas the effect appears to last longer if ingested orally (Ulug and Ozturk 2015).

Intoxication and withdrawal develop related to THC. Throughout the historical process, THC had been used as antiseptic and analgesic. Afterwards it was prohibited because of its misuse. Currently, there are people who claim that THC have therapeutically features and defend that they should be legal. It may also be an attempt to decriminalize/legalize the marijuana in the west world and parts of Europe (Cutcliffe and Saadeh 2014). Therefore, new studies are needed to explain treatment value and side effects of cannabis and the others' the therapeutic effect mechanism according to evidence-based practice. While these studies are conducted, on the other hand, it should educate the public about the addictive potential of cannabis and other important hazards to prevent misunderstandings that marijuana is a "harmless herbal medicine" (Tellioglu and Tellioglu 2012).

According to EMCDDA (2015a, b) annual report EDR, it's indicated that 75.1 million people consume cannabis in Europe. Being the most commonly used drug, it's also reported as the substance which is the reason for people, who applied for consultancy for the first time, to start a treatment. Approximately 14.6 million young Europeans or 11.7% of this group consumed hashish previous year, and 8.8 million of them are between the ages of 15 and 24. Lifetime consumption levels of cannabis differ prominently from country to country: while it is 1/3 of adults in Denmark, France, and the United Kingdom, it is 8% or less than 1/10 in Bulgaria, Romania, and Turkey. It's been emphasized in the report that in Nordic countries, the cannabis consumption increases.

30.3.4 **Hallucinogens** (American Psychiatric Association 2013, p. 520)

Hallucinogen term refers to drugs that produce euphoria or dysphoria, altered body image, distorted or sharpened visual and auditory perception, confusion, incoordination, and impaired judgment and memory. Severe reactions may cause paranoia, fear of losing one's mind, depersonalization, illusions, delusions, and hallucinations (Boyd 2008). There are more than 100 different hallucinogens with substantially different molecular structures (Boyd 2008). Hallucinogens occur both in "natural" forms (e.g., mescaline) and as synthetic forms (i.e., lysergic acid diethylamide-LSD, phencyclidine-PCP, 3,4-methylenedioxyamphetamine-MDMA).

Evidence indicates that certain hallucinogens can be addictive or that people can develop a tolerance to them. Use of some hallucinogens also produces tolerance to other similar drugs. For example, LSD is not considered an addictive drug because it doesn't cause uncontrollable drug-seeking behavior. However, LSD does produce tolerance, so some users who take the drug repeatedly must take higher doses to achieve the same effect. This is an extremely dangerous practice, given the unpredictability of the drug. In addition, LSD produces tolerance to other hallucinogens, including psilocybin. On the other hand, PCP is a hallucinogen that can be addictive. People who stop repeated use of PCP experience drug cravings, headaches, and sweating as common withdrawal symptoms. Scientists need more research into the tolerance or addiction potential of hallucinogens.

It has been estimated that approximately 1.8 million young adults will have used MDMA in 2014 (EMCDDA 2015a, b). The level of hallucinogenic mushroom and LSD consumption in Europe has been generally low and stable for a few years (EMCDDA 2015a, b). It's been detected that the rate is 25 times more among the people who go to the night clubs comparing to general population (EMCDDA 2015a, b).

30.3.5 **Inhalants** (American Psychiatric Association 2013, p. 533)

Inhalants are volatile substances that produce chemical vapors that can be inhaled to induce a psychoactive, or mind-altering, effect. Although other abused substances can be inhaled, the term "inhalants" is used to describe a variety of substances whose main common characteristic is that they are rarely, if ever, taken by any route other than inhalation. Inhalants can be breathed in through the nose or the mouth. Inhaled chemicals are absorbed rapidly into the bloodstream through the lungs and are quickly distributed to the brain and other organs. Inhaled chemicals are absorbed rapidly into the bloodstream through the lungs and are quickly distributed to the brain and other organs. Within seconds of inhalation, the user experiences intoxication along with other effects similar to those produced by alcohol. High-dose consumption of volatile substances causes intoxication symptoms in a brief time. According to the 2010 National Survey on Drug Use and Health (NSDUH), there were 793,000 persons aged 12 or older who had used inhalants for the first time within the past 12 months; 68.4% were under the age of 18 (NIDA 2012).

Inhalants are easily absorbed through the lungs and are widely disturbed in the body. The person experiences a sense of euphoria, but as the dose increases, confusion, perceptual distortions, and severe CNS depression appear. Inhalant users are also at risk for sudden sniffing death. Long-term inhalant use can cause brain damage and cognitive impairment (Boyd 2008). A withdrawal syndrome is reported, similar to alcohol withdrawal but milder (WU et al, as cited in Boyd 2008, pg. 555).

30.3.6 **Opioids** (American Psychiatric Association 2013, p. 540)

The term opioid is used generally to include a number of related substances including opium, opium derivatives, heroin, and synthetic opium like methadone (Ulug and Ozturk 2015). Methods of administration include imbibing the substance via one's mouth and nose and subcutaneous, intramuscular, and intravenous injection. The effects of such substances are likely to be experienced shortly after imbibing and depending on dosage and tolerance; the effect continues for 4–6 h. That's why it might be necessary to use it at least twice or three times in a day. Opioid tolerance develops quickly (Ulug and Ozturk 2015). As a result of regular use for a week or 2 weeks, addiction develops (Ulug and Ozturk 2015). It is predicted that the yearly average extensity of opium derivatives consumption among adults is 0.4%, and this rate means in 2013, there were 1.3 million problematic opium derivative consumers in Europe. The ones who consume opium derivatives represent 41% of all drug addicts who started a special treatment in Europe in 2013, and approximately 20% of them started a treatment for the first time. The mostly used opium derivative in Europe is heroin (EMCDDA 2015a, b).

While patterns of opioid use do vary considerably in different parts of the world, in Europe in general, there is evidence to suggest that the number of new users, people who use heroin for the first time, is decreasing (EMCDDA 2015a, b), whereas in the United States, the number of new users appears to be growing (at least in part as a result of the massive growth in prescription, opiate dependency) (National Institute of Health 2014). The epidemiological evidence, such as it is, suggests that there is a positive correlation between habitual use of opioids (in Europe) and the age of the user where as the number of habitual users decreases and the average age increases (EMCDDA 2015a, b). Significant numbers of problematic opium derivative users in Europe who have a long polydrug addiction history are now in their mid-forties and mid-fifties (EMCDDA 2015a, b). Even though deaths of very young population are worrying, only 8% of reported deaths caused by overdose are under the age of 25. Intravenous injection is generally linked with opium derivative use. According to the results of 14 countries in EMCDDA 2015, in the group between the ages 15 and 64, intravenous injection is seen less than one in a thousand or more than nine. The level of intravenous injection among heroin users varies from 8% in Netherlands to 100% in Lithuania. Out of the people who used three main drugs intravenously, intravenous injection choice of the individuals who started a treatment for the first time in Europe has decreased from 28% in 2006 to 20% in 2013.

30.3.7 **Sedatives, Hypnotics, and Anxiolytics** (American Psychiatric Association 2013, p. 550)

Sedative, hypnotics, or anxiolytics are medications with different chemical structures which cause central nervous system (CNS) depression (Ulug and Ozturk 2015). The psychoactive effect of these substances appears to be enhanced when they are taken together or with alcohol. They cause physiological and psychological addiction, and they may develop tolerance and addiction (Ulug and Ozturk 2015).

30.3.8 **Stimulants** (American Psychiatric Association 2013, p. 561)

Substances from this group stimulate by increasing norepinephrine, epinephrine, or dopamine levels (Ulug and Ozturk 2015). Amphetamine, synthetic stimulants, stimulants which are not amphetamine, and cocaine are the strongest stimulants because of their physiological addiction feature (Ulug and Ozturk 2015). According to EMCDDA 2015, cocaine is the most common illegal stimulant in Europe. It's predicted that 2.3 million young adults between the ages 15 and 34 used cocaine during

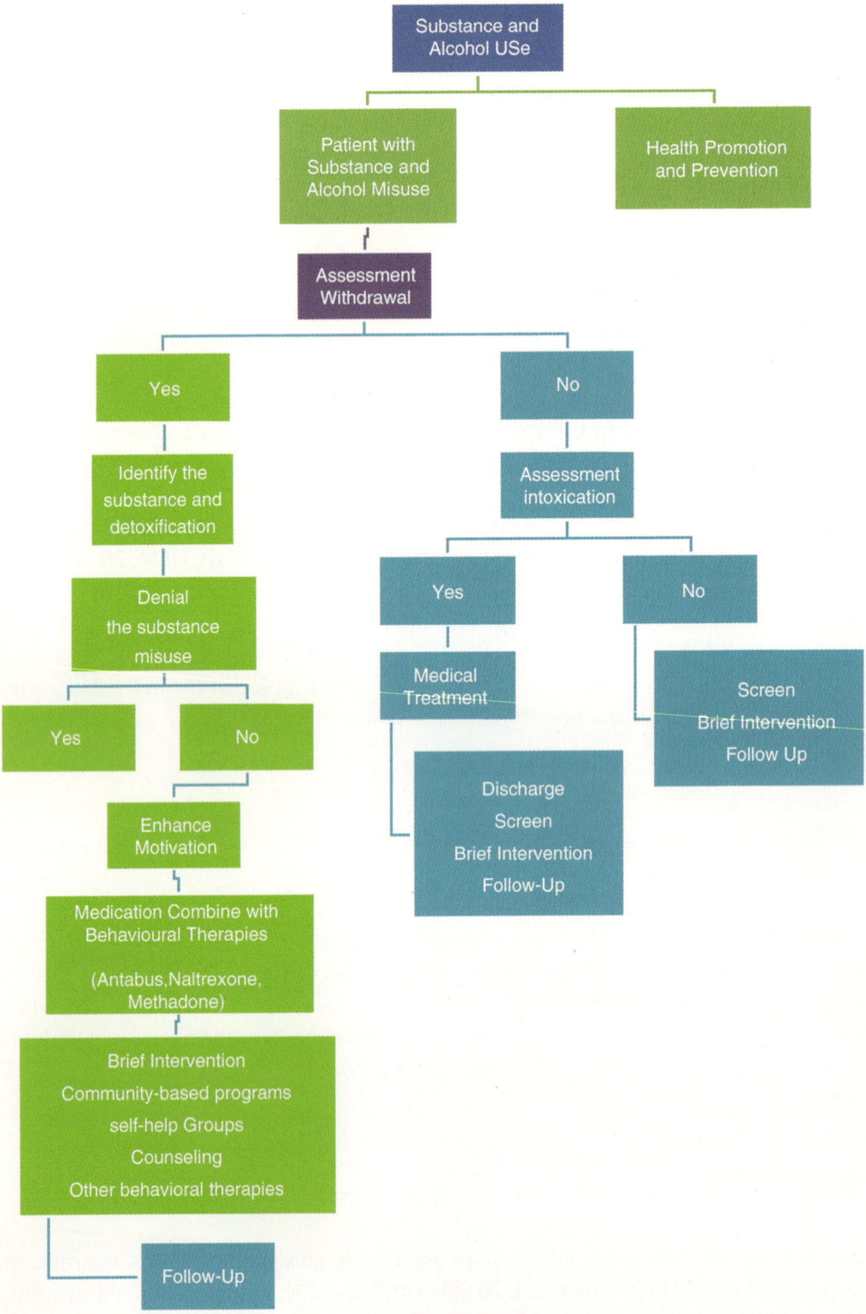

Fig. 30.1 Prevention and treatment algorithm in problems related to substance and alcohol misuse

the previous year. Eight hundred deaths have been reported due to cocaine use in Europe. It's estimated that in 2014, 1.3 million (1%) young adults used amphetamine. The latest estimations of use indicate differences in national rates of use, reportedly differing between 0.1% and 1.8%. It's been observed that many European countries' rates of amphetamine have been stable since 2000 when you take a look at the present data. Only in Spain and the United Kingdom, the rates of amphetamine use have decreased.

30.3.9 Tobacco (American Psychiatric Association 2013, p. 571)

One of the substances that is used most commonly is cigarette tobacco. Smoking is more prevalent among people who have substance abuse and psychiatric patients (Breslau, Novak and Kesler 2004 cited Boyd 2008, p. 549). Specific substance of tobacco is dark brown liquid, and it is called nicotine (Ogel 2010). Nicotine stimulates the central, peripheral, and autonomic nervous system (Boyd 2008). Repeated use of nicotine produces both tolerance and dependence (Boyd 2008). Nicotine addiction is extremely powerful and is at least as strong as addictions to other drugs such as heroin and cocaine; 70% of those who quit relapse within a year (NIDA 2000 cited Boyd 2008, p. 549). Nicotine withdrawal is marked by mood changes and physiologic changes (Boyd 2008).

30.4 Psychiatric/Mental Health Nurses Responses to Problems Related to Substance and Alcohol Misuse

P/MH have a long history of providing care and playing an active role in preventing substance addictions, or/and in minimizing the harm associated with using, and in treatment and each step of rehabilitation (Çoskun 2010). The clear consensus within the relevant literature is that treatment for and responses to substance misuse and addiction require a multidimensional, multi-perspective, and multidisciplinary "teamwork" approach (Çoskun 2010). Moreover, recent, significant, and compelling evidence indicates the significant majority of people with substance misuse problems will have a personal history of trauma (see Chap. 39) (Fig. 30.1).

30.5 Health Promotion and Substance Misuse Prevention Efforts and Approaches

Substance use is one of the most important worldwide health problems. Therefore it's essential to place great importance to societal prevention. It is important preventing an individual from using alcohol/substance in hazardous or harmful ways. Successful primary prevention helps avoid the suffering, cost, and burden associated with ill-health. Effective screening and brief interventions in primary health care are central to the public health effort to reduce the prevalence of hazardous and harmful use of psychoactive substances (Watson et al. 2010).

Environmental prevention uses policy interventions to create environment that supports healthy and safe behavior. For example:

- Increasing alcohol taxes and reducing discount drink specials substantially reduce heavy and hazardous drinking among college and high school students.
- Decreasing the number of alcohol outlets in a community is closely associated with reduction in rates of alcohol-related youth violence.
- Holding retailers liable for damage inflicted on others by intoxicated and underage patrons promotes responsible server practices and reduces alcohol-related traffic crashes.
- Increasing the minimum legal drinking age to 21 substantially reduces youth alcohol-related motor vehicle crashes; and increasing enforcement of laws prohibiting sales to underage drinkers reduces youth access to alcohol.
- Reducing noncommercial forms of youth access to alcohol shows promise in reducing youth drinking problems.
- Reducing the amount of youth exposure to alcohol advertising and increasing the number of alcohol counter-ads have a positive impact on youth beliefs and intentions regarding alcohol use and may influence drinking decisions.
- Combining environmental strategies such as those listed above and implementing them in a comprehensive community program result in substantial reduction in underage drinking and alcohol-related problem rates (American Medical Association 2002).

Also, although the availability of school-based education programs is relatively high, the effects of these programs on society are limited and low. Suggestions about the development of school-based education programs should be made. On the other hand, there are significant effects of media programs with regard to form a basis for special interferences and raise awareness about problems of alcohol use. There exists some evidence about the activities of primary health-care professionals in terms of the reduction of harmful alcohol use. It's been estimated that as a result of practicing the modeling based on the first stage directed to 25% of the society which is being improved by WHO and under risk in European Union member countries, 480,000 illnesses and premature death year can be prevented, and its cost is 740 million euros per year (Chisholm et al., as cited in WHO 2012, pg. 40).

30.6 Screening and Brief Interventions

Nurses can make a significant impact on the prevalence of hazardous and harmful use of psychoactive substances by engaging in screening and brief interventions (Watson et al. 2010). The general features of brief interventions are raising the awareness and focusing on advice for the change (Babor et al. 2010; Watson et al. 2010; Moyer and Finney 2015). The success of brief intervention for people who are under the risk of substance use and substance abuse is reasonably high. Brief interventions are brief and low cost and shorten the waiting period for long-term treatments; training or/and educating P/MH nurses in how to use brief interventions is also relatively quick and inexpensive. Such interventions are also used in general health-care and routine applications. Brief intervention is an approach/method that first seeks to examine the problem and then motivates people who have substance addiction to do something (Watson et al. 2010).

Screening for substance use and evaluatory studies of the same, in addition to evaluatory studies about brief interventions, between the dates of 1994 and 2008 appear quite frequently in international literature. These studies were undertaken in Australia, Canada, Denmark, Finland, Hong Kong, South Africa, Sweden, Taiwan, the United Kingdom, and the United States, and various scales of screening and brief interventions were used. In a study of college students having potentially dangerous alcohol use, it was found after 6 weeks of observation that in comparison with the control group, there is a considerable decrease in the alcohol consumption rate, private problems, and the frequency of intensive use periods of the group on which brief interventions were applied (Kypri et al. 2004).

In a study where cognitive behavioral therapy (CBT) and brief interventions were compared, there were no statistically significant differences detected after 6 months follow-up. It's reported that the cost/benefit calculation of brief intervention is better than cognitive behavioral therapy. When the satisfaction levels of the participants were analyzed, there was no difference between CBT and brief intervention (Shakeshaft et al. 2002 cited Ogel 2010, p. 87). It has been shown that the economic advantages of the applications of alcohol screening and brief interventions are much better than other conventional medical services. Studies generally reveal that it's more profitable to use the methods of alcohol screening and brief intervention in health-care organizations (Kraemer as cited in Ogel 2010, pp. 87-88). The brief interventions of a nurse were found to be effective in a randomized controlled trial of individuals who visited a primary health-care center in Stockholm for a health check (Tomson as cited in WHO 2010, pp.16). Fleming et al. (2002) Conducted a randomized controlled trial and economic evaluation of a brief intervention for hazardous and harmful alcohol users. The participants in the treatment group reported significant reductions in alcohol use, and the economic evaluation suggested that substantial savings in health-care costs could be achieved as a result of early intervention. Lock et al as cited in WHO 2010 also conducted a randomized controlled trial and economic evaluation of a brief intervention for hazardous and harmful alcohol use. Most of the patients in both groups reported reduced alcohol use between baseline and 6 months follow-up, but no significant effects were found (cited Watson et al. 2010).

> Brief interventions are an appropriate response to clients presenting at a general health or community setting and who are unlikely to need, seek, or attend specialist treatment. It may be all the client may want to be given clear concise information by a professional. It is important part of the overall approach of harm reduction. (Boyd 2008, p. 565)

Brief intervention is most successful when working with people who are experiencing few problems with alcohol/drug use, have low levels of dependence, have a short history of alcohol/drug use, and have stable backgrounds. Also, it is successful people who are unsure or ambivalent about changing their alcohol/drug use (Boyd 2008).

30.7 Treatment and Care

Substance and alcohol misuse treatment can include medications, behavioral therapies, or their combination. No single treatment is appropriate for all individuals. Treatment needs to be readily available. Effective treatment should meet the multiple needs of the individual. An individual's treatment and care must be assessed continually and modified according to the person's changing needs. Remaining in treatment is critical for treatment effectiveness. Counseling or other behavioral therapies are critical components of effective treatment. Medications are an important element of treatment, especially when combined with counseling or other behavioral therapies. Medical detoxification is only the first stage of addiction treatment, and it manages the acute physical symptoms of withdrawal associated with stopping substance use. Strong motivation can facilitate the treatment process. Possible drug use during treatment must be monitored, because lapses can occur. Treatment programs should provide assessment and counseling for HIV/AIDS, hepatitis B and C, tuberculosis, and other infectious diseases. Recovery from addiction can be a long-term process and frequently requires multiple episodes treatment (NIDA 2012).

30.7.1 Acute Intoxication

Acute intoxication occurs when high-level alcohol or substance is used. In case of acute alcohol intoxication, the respiratory passage should be kept open, and aspiration should be prevented. Gastric lavage isn't helpful as alcohol mixes with the blood in a brief time. On severe conditions, hemodialysis might be necessary. If hypoglycemia is developed, glucose solution can be given. Apart from that, in order to prevent Wernicke's encephalopathy, vitamin B1, agitation, and if there is aggressive behavior brief-acting benzodiazepine or haloperidol can be given (Townsend 2012). Vital signs are evaluated and create safe environment. The family is informed and guided for addiction treatment when the patient is conscious (Çoskun 2010; Cam and Engin 2014).

In case of opioid intoxication, the patient is generally in coma. That's why respiratory passage should be kept open and the patient should be intubated if it's needed or tracheotomy should be opened, and fluid treatment should be administered. Naloxone, naltrexone, and nalmefene can be lifesaving during the opioid intoxication treatment (Townsend 2012). Vital signs are watched, creating safe environment and assessment risk of infection comorbid mental or physical illness and story of trauma. The family is informed and guided for addiction treatment when the patient is conscious (Çoskun 2010; Cam and Engin 2014).

30.7.2 Withdrawal Treatment

The control of the withdrawal symptoms is the first stage of the treatment (Austin and Boyd 2008). It's quite important for preparing the individual for treatment and establishing therapeutic relation (Jones et al. 2012). It need to observation the patient with withdrawal of alcohol or substance and inform to the reaction of body are temporary because of withdrawal of alcohol or substance. If the patient is agitated or confused, the level of consciousness should be assessed and vital signs controlled every 15 min until the patient becomes conscious. Stimuli such as light, noise, and motion should be reduced. If the patient could not eat or drink and signs of dehydration are observed, IV solution should be given and takeoff followed. If the patient lose her/his control or has potential to harm himself/herself or others, the patient should be restricted and secluded. Ordered treatment needs to be implemented (Çoskun 2010; Fortinash and Worret 2011).

Benzodiazepines are the most frequently used pharmacological agents during alcohol withdrawal treatment (Townsend d). Progress in withdrawal is usually measured (or more accurately—estimated) by P/MH nursing assessment of symptoms of withdrawal—perhaps including the use of standardized instrumentation or not (Devos-Comby and Lange 2008). Some specialists use anticonvulsants in order to reduce withdrawal and alcohol craving. In addition to this, giving multivitamin and thiamine are frequently practiced protocols (Townsend 2012). Methadone is used during the opioid withdrawal treatment. The withdrawal treatment of amphetamine and cocaine is alike, but a beneficial evidence-based agent isn't found (Austin and Boyd 2008).

Patients who are intoxicated or in withdrawal are assessed with standardized measurements such as Alcohol Use Disorders Identification Test (AUDIT) (Babor et al. 2001), Michigan Alcohol Screening Test (MAST) (Selzer 1971; Selzer et al. 1975), and CAGE (Ewing 1984) and referred to pharmacotherapy, behavioral therapies, or their combination.

30.7.3 Pharmacotherapy Combined with Behavioral Therapies

The individuals who have alcohol and substance misuse might start using the substance again after the substance withdrawal. That's why it's necessary to prevent relapses during rehabilitation process. For preventing relapses during rehabilitation, using medication is possible for alcohol, cigarette, and opiate dependence. Disulfiram, naltrexone, and acamprosate are used for alcohol addiction, bupropion and varenicline for nicotine addiction, and methadone and buprenorphine for opioid addiction treatment (Townsend 2012).

The researches on alcohol addiction state that naltrexone treatment gives good results together with cognitive behavioral therapy. It blocks intoxication effects of opioids and the search for substance during opioid addiction treatment. It's been found that naltrexone is effective on patients with high motivation and good social support. Before the start of its use, opioid consume should be cut, or else withdrawal symptoms start to occur. Besides, some various results are found like antidepressants from SSRI group reduce the desire for alcohol consumes (Townsend 2014). Methadone is given to opiate users on low dose and under control. With simultaneous rehabilitation activities, reducing strong desires and withdrawal symptoms and overcoming addiction behaviors are aimed (Dilbaz 2012).

Pharmacotherapy for alcohol dependence is most effective when combined with some behavioral support, but this doesn't need to be specialized, intensive counseling. Nurses as well as counselors can offer brief but effective behavioral support that promotes recovery. Applying this medication management approach in such settings would greatly expand access to effective treatment, given that many patients with addiction either don't have access to specialty treatment or refuse a referral (NIH 2016).

30.7.4 Community-Based Environmental Prevention Programs

One approach for reducing problems related to substance and alcohol misuse and preventing the laps is community-based prevention programs. Community-based environmental prevention programs as described focus not so much on changing the behavior of the individual drinker but on changing the environment in which a person consumes alcohol (Treno and Lee 2002). Environmental approaches focus on the community in numerous components, including the following:

- Individual drinkers
- Vendors of alcohol, including both places where alcohol is consumed and places where alcohol is sold
- Social events where alcoholic beverages are sold and consumed
- Local laws, regulations, and enforcement agencies
- Local medical clinics and treatment facilities
- Social organizations that may support and promote public health campaigns, including schools, churches, business organizations, and social club (Treno and Lee 2002)

On the other hand, less obvious components of the community system affecting and affected by alcohol problems include the social networks and family connections through which people "learn" drinking attitudes and behaviors. These social networks may play a particularly important role with underage drinkers, who most likely obtain alcohol through friends and family networks (Treno and Lee 2002).

30.7.5 Alcoholic Anonymous (AA), Narcotics Anonymous, and Twelve-Step Programs

Is self-help groups established for solving the similar problems of alcohol misusing and healing. It's been accepted as an approach for long soberness. The most important feature of AA is that it practices principles called twelve-step program and actualize them (Boyd 2008).

Twelve-step programs are the effective treatment modality for all addictions. These programs offer the behavioral, cognitive, and dynamic structure needed in recovery (Varcoralis and Halter 2009).

In systematic review, Ferri et al. (2006) reported "no experimental studies unequivocally demonstrated the effectiveness of AA or TSF approaches for reducing alcohol dependence or problems. One large study focused on the prognostic factors associated with interventions that were assumed to be successful rather than on the effectiveness of interventions themselves, so more efficacy studies are needed" (Ferri et al. 2006).

Narcotic Anonymous is self-help groups established for substance addiction apart from alcohol (Boyd 2008).

30.8 Counseling Approaches

30.8.1 Person-Centered Counseling

Person-centered counseling is a common and effective approach in addiction treatment. Person-centered counseling is also referred to as client-centered therapy, person-centered therapy, and Rogerian psychotherapy after its founder, psychologist Carl Rogers (Fleck 2013). The focal spot is to strengthen the ego states. The P/MH should be warm, kind, and nonjudgmental, and he/she should draw the lines (Boyd 2008; Ogel and Evren 2012). They make the patient see the results of substance use during counseling, and the patients say that they want to make changes. A plan is made in order to keep the individual away from substance after the problem is identified and soberness is succeeded. Practices about reactions of the patient are made when the desire for substance is strong. The counseling should include the family. The consultant helps each family member see how he or she affects the substance misuse.

In study Heather et al. (2009), which they did for finding out the counseling's activity on individuals with heavy alcohol consumption who stayed in hospital's general service, it's been stated that individuals who received counseling reduced alcohol consumption after 6 months of discharging (Heather et al. 2009).

A further thought as yet under-explored element of psychotherapeutic, interpersonal works with this client group is that of instilling, inspiring, promoting, and maintaining the person's hope. For instance, Koehn and Cutcliffe (2012) reported on their study, titled "The Inspiration of Hope in Substance Abuse Counseling" (2012), that they discovered a three-stage process of hope inspiration in clients with substance misuse problems. First stage is to evaluate the patient without judging. It's believed that it won't be able to improve when the layer of the hope instilling process is therapeutic cooperation. The second step includes three major psychosocial processes. And these are helping the individual during the decision process, making the patient hopeful about future and extending personal or interpersonal network along with the communication. The last stage includes the review of hope instilling process and the ending of it (Koehn and Cutcliffe 2012).

30.8.2 Motivational Interviewing (MI)

Motivational interviewing is an approach to working with clients with substance misuse issues fields that has gained importance in recent years (Ogel 2010). One of the most effective aspects of MI is that it is short termed and can have long-lasting effects on withdrawal (Ogel 2010). MI is a direct and client-centered approach which is used for changing the behavior by helping the client discover and analyze the ambivalence. On the other hand, MI is a specific way of helping the individual understand the problems and go into action for the change. It's a useful method especially for the people who are unwilling to change or ambivalent. It's been showed by researches that MI is effective on changing the behaviors of the clients.

Motivational interviewing in a scientific setting out performs traditional advice giving in the treatment of a broad range of behavioral problems and diseases. The motivational interviewing techniques (MIT) have recently attracted the attention. This technique has been increasingly used for changing behaviors that may be placing patients at risk of developing health problems or may be preventing management of chronic conditions. Studies showed that ethanol levels of patients who received MI found lower (Rubak et al. 2005). While Navidian et al. (2015) were making MI with individuals who received 100 methadone maintaining treatment, they found that the substance desire of individuals who joined the research during 12 months of follow-up was reduced and the soberness span was considerably long in comparison with the control group (Navidian et al. 2015). The meta-analytic review of 15 randomized controlled trials reveals that brief MI is an efficacious strategy for reducing alcohol consumption (Vasilaki et al. 2006).

30.8.3 Cognitive Behavioral Therapy

Cognitive behavioral therapy (CBT) is an important choice for addiction treatment (Ogel 2010). It is an individualized, collaborative approach to psychotherapy that emphasizes the importance of thoughts, feelings, and expectancies. CBT is based on social learning theory. Learning process plays an important role in the development and continuation substance and alcohol misuse. The same learning processes can be used to help individuals reduce their substance and alcohol misuse. CBT also is based on stress and coping theory. These theories promote that life stressors are likely to trigger the use of avoidance- or emotion-focused coping strategies such as substance use individuals who have low self-efficacy and poor problem-solving coping skills in an attempt to avoid experiencing distress. CBY focuses on challenging individuals' positive expectancies about substance use, enhancing their self-confidence and self-efficacy to resist substance misuse, and improving their overall and specific skills for coping with life stress (Penberthy et al. 2011).

CBT for substance use disorders focuses on helping clients in two major behavioral ways. The first is to help reduce the intensity and frequency of their urges to use, by underlying beliefs and cognitions about using. The second is to teach the patients' specific techniques for controlling and managing their urges to use. In other words, the basic goals are to reduce the pressure to use and increase control (Penberthy et al. 2011).

Evidence from meta-analytic reviews supports the efficacy of CBT for alcohol and drug use disorders (Dutra et al. 2008; Magil and Ray as cited in McHugh et al. 2010).

> "Regarding alcohol treatment, the strongest evidence was reported for behavioral skill training and pharmacotherapy interventions (Miller and Wilbourne, 2002 Cited WHO 2012, p. 40). Areas with less impact were 12- steps facilitation, group psychotherapy, educational lectures and films, mandatory attendance at Alcoholics Anonymous meetings and general alcoholism counseling."

30.9 Person-Centered Psychiatric/Mental Health Nursing Process

P/MH nurses may encounter patients with addiction problems in outpatient clinics, daily hospitalizations, acute services, or community mental health services. Also some patients may have co-occurring problems: a mental health and a substance misuse problem (see Chap. 39). Alcohol and substance misuse, commonly, cause physical problems—especially in cases of longer-term use. For these reasons, such patients may be found in general and emergency services. P/MH nurses should focus on their patients' experiences. When data is being collected, a trusting relationship should be built; communication should be based on cooperation and needs to be perpetual and patient centered.

30.9.1 Assessment

Assessment is crucial to understanding level of use, abuse, or dependence and to determining the patient's denial or acceptance of treatment (Boyd 2008). Assessment is the beginning of the process, and it is important for individuals with substance use disorders or substance use risks. When the manner of substance use and physical and mental assessments of the individual are being made, evidence-based, individual-centered, and recovery-oriented path should be taken. The nurse should be cognizant of and observe the verbal and nonverbal reactions of the patient and also be aware of their own attitude for the substance using patient. In the first examination, therapeutic boundaries should be formed, and the patient should be evaluated without any judgments (Jones et al. 2012).

For the assessment of the patient, standardized measurements such as Alcohol Use Disorders Identification Test (AUDIT) (Babor et al. 2001), Michigan Alcohol Screening Test (MAST) (Selzer 1971; Selzer et al. 1975), and CAGE (Ewing 1984) can be used. In the evaluation of the patient related to the substance use, tolerance and withdrawal symptoms, reason for wanting to quit, prior alcohol or substance use history, reason to start substance use, and family and social support should be specified. During physical evaluation, questions about the patient's way of life should be asked too. Individuals who have substance misuse may also have psychiatric diagnoses; for this reason, these should be treated together (Babor et al. 2010; Jones et al. 2012).

Denial is an important problem at the beginning of treatment. Denial can be expressed in a variety of behaviors. They say "I didn't have any problems," I don't get drunk all the time," and "I don't have withdrawal symptoms, so I can't be an alcoholic." Also, countertransference is the total emotional reaction of the treatment provider to the patient. Patients can generate strong feelings and reactions in nurses and other health-care providers (Boyd 2008).

Motivation is a key predictor of whether individuals will change their substance use behavior (Boyd 2008). Attention should be paid whether the individual is ready for a change or not (Halter 2014). Transtheoretical model (TTM) can be used to decide if the individual is ready for change. TTM of change, a theoretical model of behavior change, was originally explained by Prochaska and DiClemente (1983). The TTM is a model of intentional change that focuses on the decision-making abilities of the individual rather than the social and biological influences on behavior as other approaches tried (Velicer et al. 1998). The stages of the TTM are the precontemplation, contemplation, decision, action, maintenance, and relapse. The model has been applied to a wide variety of problem behaviors like smoking cessation, alcohol abuse, and drug abuse. Motivational enhancement therapy (MET) is based on the Prochaska and DiClemente's stages of change model, which is applicable in smoking cessation and alcohol abuse (Prochaska et al. 1992; Velicer et al. 1998).

30.9.2 Outcome Criteria

Outcome criteria of every problem should be asserted in every treatment plan goals. Outcome criteria for the substance abuser may involve decrease in withdrawal symptoms, maintaining soberness, maintaining treatment motivation and commitment, getting used to the new lifestyle, and maintaining it after discharge from the hospital. In person-centered care, the patient is expected to set his or her own goals. For this reason, the nurse and the patient should be in cooperation (Fortinash and Worret 2011).

30.9.3 Planning

Planning requires attention to the patient's gender, age, social status, income, substance use history, and current condition. Planning must also address the patient's major psychological, social, and medical problems. Involvement of appropriate family members is essential (Varcorolis and Halter 2009).

The strengths of the individual and the sides of whom that needs to be improved should be identified, and treatment priorities should be specified. At this stage, the nurses should maintain their professional role and should show flexibility according to the needs of the patient. Planning is, focusing on the problems identified, specifying the attempts within goals. This treatment plan will be shaped based on assessment and diagnosis stages. Planning should consist of providing patient security, reducing the frequency and acuteness of symptoms, motivation and preparation for the change, and determining support systems, strengths, and sociocultural needs.

30.9.4 Implementation

At all levels of practice, the nurse can play an important role in the intervention process. A standardized treatment and care plan for a substance abuser is nonexistent; various combined and extensive attempts according to the reason of illness, severity, present state of the patient, and their needs can be applied. Although addicts share some characteristics and dynamics, they have significant differences. These differences influence the recovery processes either positively or negatively.

P/MH nurses should assess the patient's readiness for the change at every stage. A therapeutic relationship is an effective way to promote positive change in people. A variety of nursing interventions are used in the care of patients with substance and alcohol misuse. It is critical that the nurse establish a therapeutic relationship with these patients. (Boyd 2008).

Communication strategies are designed to address behaviors that almost all substance abusers. The nurse's ability to develop a warm, accepting relationship with an addicted patient can help the patient feel safe enough to start looking problems with some degree of openness and honesty. It is important to communicate in culturally appropriate ways. The role of the nurse is to provide support, education, and nonjudgmental confrontation. The nurse must establish good rapport with the patient.

30.9.5 Evaluation

Evaluation involves the effectiveness of the treatment plan: patient's symptoms, behavioral changes since the first examination until now, and their goals. Though it is known that in every period there will be relapses, nonuse of substance or taking part in self-help groups in order to keep sober should be supported. Because of the differences in male and female relapses, setting personal goals and evaluation of these goals should be done. Evaluation should be a long-term and an ongoing process.

Conclusion

The use or misuse of alcohol and/or substances is a problem that has social, physical, and psychiatric outcomes and impacts in Europe and worldwide. In the DSM-V (2013), under the title of substance use and addiction disorders, includes the following substances: alcohol, caffeine, cannabis, hallucinogens, inhalant, opioid, sedative-hypnotic or anxiolytic, stimulant, tobacco and other substances, and substance-induced disorders are categorized as intoxication, withdrawal, other substance-induced disorders and unspecified substance-related disorder.

Firstly, it is important to prevent an individual from using alcohol/substance in hazardous or harmful ways. Screening and brief interventions are an appropriate response to clients presenting at a general health or community setting and who are unlikely to need, seek, or attend specialist treatment. In addictive individuals, several treatment modalities are used. These are acute intoxication treatment, withdrawal treatment, and counseling and behavioral approaches, which can include person-centered counseling, motivational interviewing, and cognitive behavioral therapy, e.g. But, there is no one best treatment method for all people.

P/MH nurses may encounter patients with addiction problems in outpatient clinics, daily hospitalizations, acute services, or community mental health services. Also some patients may have co-occurring problems. P/MH nurses should focus on their patients' experiences and whether the individual is ready for a change or not. A therapeutic relationship is an effective way to promote positive change in people.

References

American Medical Association (2002) Environmental prevention: the environmental approach to prevention: implementing alcohol policies. http://www.alcoholpolicymd.com/alcohol_policy/effects_ep.htm. Accessed 20 Dec 2016

American Psychiatric Association (2013) Desk reference to the diagnostic criteria form DSM-5. American Psychiatric Association, Arlington VA, pp 481–591

Anderson P, Baumberg B (2006) Alcohol in Europe a public health perspective: a report for European Commission. Institute of Alcohol Studies, London

Austin W, Boyd MA (2008) Psychiatric and mental health nursing for Canadian practice, 2nd edn. Walters Kluwer, Alphen aan den Rijn, pp 564–573

Azar MM, Springer SA, Meyer JP, Altice FL (2010) A systematic review of the impact of alcohol use disorders on HIV treatment outcomes, adherence to antiretroviral therapy and health care utilization. Drug Alcohol Depend 112:178–193

Babor T, Caetona R, Casswell S, Edwards G, Giesbrecht N, Garaham K et al (2010) Alcohol no ordinary: commodity: research and public policy, 2nd edn. Oxford University Press, New York

Babor TF, Higgins-Biddle JC, Saunders JB, Monteiro MG (2001) AUDIT: the alcohol use disorders identification test. Guidelines for use in primary care, 2nd edn. World Health Organization, Department of Mental Health and Substance Dependence, Geneva, pp 5–38

Baliunas D, Rehm J, Irving H, Shuper P (2010) Alcohol consumption and risk of incident human immunodeficiency virus infection: a metaanalysis. Int J Public Health 55:159–166

Boyd MA (2008) Psychiatric nursing contemporary practice, 4th edn. Lippincott, New York, NY, pp 537–570

Cam O, Engin E (2014) Madde Bağımlılığı (substance addiction). In: Çam O, Engin E (eds) Ruh Sağlığı ve Hastalıkları Hemşireliği; Bakım Sanatı (Mental health and illness: care art), 1st edn. Istanbul Tıp Kitapevi, Istanbul. (In Turkish)

Chiara D (1995) The role of dopamine in drug abuse viewed from the perspective of its role in motivation. Drug Alcohol Depend 38(2):95–137

Çoskun S (2010) Bağımlılık Tedavisinde Hemşirelik (Nursing in addiction treatment). In: Ogel K (ed) Sigara, Alkol ve Madde Kullanım Bozuklukları: Tanı, Tedavi ve Önleme (Tobacco, alcohol and substance disorders: diagnosis, treatment and prevention). Istanbul, Yeniden Yayınları. (In Turkish)

Cutcliffe JR, Saadeh B (2014) Grounded in evidence or a puritanical legacy: a critique of United States of America twenty-first century drug policy. Subs Use Mental Health 7(3):195–206. https://doi.org/10.1080/17523281.2013.826271
Devos-Comby L, Lange JE (2008) Standardized measures of alcohol-related problems: a review of their use among college students. Psychol Addict Behav 22(3):349–361
Dilbaz N (2012) Opioid intoksikasyonu ve yoksunluğu tedavisi (opioid intoxication and withdrawal treatment). In: Evren C, Ogel K, Uluğ B (eds) Alkol Madde Bağımlılığı Tanı ve Tedavi el Kitabı (manual of diagnosis and treatment for alcohol-substance addiction), 1st edn. Tuna Matbaacılık, Ankara, pp 91–107. (In Turkish)
Dutra L, Stathopoulou G, Basden S, Leyro T, Powers M, Otto M (2008) A meta-analytic review of psychosocial interventions for substance use disorders. Am J Psychiatry 165(2):179–187
Engin E, Kutlu Y (2014) Bağımlılıklarda Bakımın İncelikleri (The subtleties of care in addiction). Türkiye Klinikleri Psikiyatri Hemşireliği Özel Sayısı 1:73–79. (In Turkish)
European Monitoring Center for Drug and Drug Addiction (2015) European drug report 2015: trends and developments. Publications Office of the European Union, Luxembourg
Ewing JA (1984) Detecting alcoholism. The CAGE questionnaire. JAMA 252(14):1905–1907
Ferri M, Amato L, Davoli M (2006) Alcoholics anonymous and other 12-step programmes for alcohol dependence. Cochrane Database Syst Rev 3:CD005032. https://doi.org/10.1002/14651858.CD005032.pub2
Fleck JR (2013) A person-centred approach to addiction treatment. In: Cooper M, O'Hara M, Schmid P, Bohart A (eds) The handbook of person-centred psychotherapy and counselling, 2nd edn. Palgrave McMillan, Basingstoke, Hampshire
Fortinash KM, Worret H (2011) Psychiatric nursing care plans, 5th edn. Mosby, Maryland Heights, MO, pp 283–301
Gardner EL (2005) In: Lowinson JH, Ruiz P, Milmann RB, Langrod JG (eds) Brain-reward mechanisms, pp 19–33. (In Turkish)
Gmel G, Shield K, Rehm J (2011) Developing a methodology to derive alcohol-attributable fractions for HIV/AIDS mortality based on alcohol's impact on adherence to antiretroviral medication. Popul Health Metr 9:5
Hahn JA, Woolf-King SE, Muyindike W (2011) Adding fuel to the fire: alcohol's effect on the HIV epidemic in Sub-Saharan Africa. Curr HIV/AIDS Rep 8:172–180
Halter MJ (2014) Foundation of psychiatric mental health nursing a clinical approach, 7th edn. Elsevier, New York, pp 418–428
Heather N, Rollnick S, Bell A, Richmond R (2009) Effects of brief counselling among male heavy drinkers identified on general hospital wards. Drug Alcohol Rev 15(1):29–38
Hendershot CS, Stoner SA, Pantalone DW, Simoni JM (2009) Alcohol use and antiretroviral adherence review and meta-analysis. J Acquir Immune Defic Syndr 52:180–202
Hicdurmaz D, Öz F (2016) Interpersonal sensitivity, coping ways and automatic thoughts of nursing students before and after a cognitive-behavioral group counseling program. Nurse Educ Today 36:152–158
Jones JS, Fitzpatrick JJ, Rogers VL (2012) Psychiatric-mental health nursing an interpersonal approach, 2nd edn. Springer, New York, pp 318–331
Koehn C, Cutcliffe J (2012) The inspiration of hope in substance abuse counselling. J Humanist Couns 51:78–98
Kypri K, Saunders JB, Williams SM, RO MG, Langley JD, Cashell-Smith ML, Gallaghe SJ (2004) Web-based screening and brief intervention for hazardous drinking: a double-blind randomized controlled trial. Addiction 99(11):1410–1417
Lingford-Hughes A, Clementi N (2008) Addiction and substance misuse. Medicine 36(8):422–429
McHugh RK, Hearon BA, Otto MW (2010) Cognitive-behavioral therapy for substance use disorders. Psychiatr Clin North Am 33(3):511–525. https://doi.org/10.1016/j.psc.2010.04.012
Moyer A, Finney J (2015) Brief interventions for alcohol misuse. CMAJ 187(7):502–506
National Institutes of Health (2014) America's addiction to opioids: heroin and prescription drug abuse. https://www.drugabuse.gov/about-nida/legislative-activities/testimony-to-congress/2016/americas-addiction-to-opioids-heroin-prescription-drug-abuse

National Institutes of Health (2016) Helping patients who drink too much: a clinician's guide Updated 2005 Edition. https://pubs.niaaa.nih.gov/publications/Practitioner/CliniciansGuide2005/guide.pdf. Accessed 20 Dec 2016

Navidian A, Kermansarayi F, Tabas EE, Saeedinezhad F (2015) Efficacy of group motivational interviewing in the degree of drug craving in the addicts under the Methadone Maintenance Treatment (MMT) in South East of Iran. Arch Psychiatr Nurs 30:144–149

NIDA (2012) Principles of drug addiction treatment: a research-based guide, 3rd edn. NIH Publication, Bethesda, pp 2–5. https://www.drugabuse.gov/publications/principles-drug-addiction-treatment-research-based-guide-third-edition. Accessed 3 Jan 2017

Ogel K (2010) Sigara, Alkol ve Madde Kullanımın Bozuklukları: Tanı, Tedavi ve Önleme (Tabocco, alcohol and substance disorders: diagnosis, treatment and prevention). Yeniden Yayınları, Istanbul, pp 179–296. (In Turkish)

Ogel K, Evren C (2012) Alkol Madde Kullanım Bozukluğu Olan Hastaya Yaklaşım (approach to patient who alcohol-substance use disorders). In: Evren C, Ogel K, Uluğ B (eds) Alkol Madde Bağımlılığı Tanı ve Tedavi el Kitabı (manual of diagnosis and treatment for alcohol-substance addiction), 1st edn. Tuna Matbaacılık, Ankara, pp 91–107. (In Turkish)

Penberthy JK, Wartella JA, Waughan M (2011) Cognitive behavioural therapy for addiction. In: Johnson BA (ed) Addiction medicine. Springer, New York, pp 729–750

Prochaska JO, Diclemente CC (1983) Stages and processes of self-change of smoking: toward an integrative model of change. J Consult Clin Psychol 51(3):390–395

Prochaska JO, DiClemente CC, Norcross JC (1992) In search of how people change. Applications to addictive behaviours. Am Psychol 47:1102

Rehm J, Samokhvalov AV, Neuman MG, Room R, Parry CD, Lönnroth K et al (2009) The association between alcohol use, alcohol use disorders and tuberculosis (TB). A systematic review. BMC Public Health 9:450

Rehm J, Baliunas D, Borges GL, Graham K, Irving H, Kehoe T et al (2010) The relation between different dimensions of alcohol consumption and burden of disease – an overview. Addiction 105:817–843

Rubak S, Sandbaek A, Lauritzen T, Christensen B (2005) Motivational interviewing: a systematic review and meta-analysis. Br J Gen Pract 55(513):305–312

Sadock BJ, Sadock VA (2007) Synopsis of psychiatry: behavioral sciences/clinical psychiatry, 10th edn. Wolter Kluwer/Lippincott Williams & Wilkins, Philadelphia

Selzer ML (1971) The Michigan alcoholism screening test (MAST): the quest for a new diagnostic instrument. Am J Psychiatry 3:176–181

Selzer ML, Vinokur A, van Rooijen L (1975) A self-administered short version of the Michigan Alcoholism Screening Test (SMAST). J Stud Alcohol 36:117–126

Shakeshaft AP, Bowman JA, Burrows S, Doran CM, Sanson-Fısher RW (2002) Community-based alcohol counselling: a randomized clinical trial. Addiction 97:1449–1463

Shield KD, Parry C, Rehm J (2013) Chronic diseases and conditions related to alcohol use. Alcohol Res 35:155–171

Tellioglu T, Tellioglu Z (2012) Tıbbi Esrar Psikiyatrik Bozuklukların Tedavisinde Kullanılabilir mi? (Can medical marijuana be used in the treatment of psychiatric disorders?). Bull Clin Psychopharmacol 22(1):98–109. (In Turkish)

Towsend MC (2012) Psychiatric mental health nursing, concepts of care in evidence-based practice, 7th edn. Davis Company, Philadelphia, PA, pp 466–487

Towsend MC (2014) Essentials of psychiatric mental health nursing, concept of care in evidence-based practice, 6th edn. Davis Company, Philadelphia, pp 302–329

Treno A, Lee J (2002) Approaching alcohol problems through local environmental interventions. https://pubs.niaaa.nih.gov/publications/arh26-1/35-41.htm. Accessed 20 Dec 2016

Ulug B, Ozturk O (2015) Psikoaktif madde kullanımına bağlı ruhsal bozukluklar (Psychiatric disorders related psychoactive substance use). In: Öztürk O, Uluşahin A (eds) Ruh Sağlığı ve Bozuklukları (Mental health and disorders), 13th edn. Nobel Tıp Kitapevi, Ankara, pp 511–554. (In Turkish)

Varcorolis EM, Halter MJ (2009) Essentials of psychiatric mental health nursing: a communication approach to evidence-based care. Saunders Elsevier, St. Louis, pp 328–359
Vasilaki EI, Hosier SG, Cox VM (2006) The efficacy of motivational interviewing as a brief Intervention for excessive drinking: a meta-analytic review. Alcohol Alcohol 41(3):328–335
Velicer WF, Prochaska JO, Fava JL, Norman GJ, Redding CA (1998) Smoking cessation and stress management: applications of the transtheoretical model of behavior change. Homeostasis 38:216–233
Watson H, Munro A, Wilson M, Kerr S, Godwin J (2010) The involvement of nurses and midwives in screening and brief interventions for hazardous and harmful use of alcohol and other psychoactive substances. World Health Organization, Geneva
World Health Organization (2014) Global status reports on alcohol and health. WHO Library Cataloguing-in-Publication Data, Luxembourg
World Health Organization (2015) The European health report 2015: Targets and beyond – reaching new frontiers in evidence. WHO Library Cataloguing-in-Publication Data, Copenhagen
Yuncu Z, Aydin C (2012) Alkol Madde Kullanım Bozukluklarında Etyoloji (Aetiology in alcohol-substance use disorders). In: Evren C, Ogel K, Ulug B (eds) Alkol-Madde Bağımlılığı Tanı ve Tedavi El Kitabı (Manual of diagnosis and treatment for alcohol-substance addiction), 1st edn. Tuna Matbaacılık, Ankara, pp 19–33. (In Turkish)

Part V

Specific Challenges

Problems Related to Eating, Nutrition, and Body Image

31

Christopher Modica

31.1 Introduction

Eating concerns often emerge out of a complex interplay of biological, psychological, and social forces. Research shows that family dynamics (Kluck 2010), perceived pressure to conform to appearance ideals (Cafri et al. 2005), dissatisfaction with one's appearance (Stice and Shaw 2002), pubertal timing and development (Klump 2013), genetics (Wade et al. 2013), and a host of personality characteristics such as perfectionism (Vohs et al. 1999) and obsessionality (Roberts et al. 2011) can be related to eating behaviors. Therefore, even with meaningful advancements in treatment (Stice et al. 2012) and prevention (Stice et al. 2013a), those charged with caring for, supporting, and treating individuals with eating concerns are obliged to consider multiple facets of an individual's inner experience and outer world. This task is a grand undertaking.

The unique role of the psychiatric/mental health (P/MH) nurse can be integral to the unified front of clinicians who seek to assist those struggling with eating concerns. As with all mental health matters, the treatment of eating concerns should be guided by prudent clinical judgment rooted in prevailing treatment research and theory. This edict touches the clinical work of the psychiatrist, physician, psychologist, and the nurse. However, treatment is not a sterile matter; the relationship between struggling individuals and those who endeavor to assist them is consequential (Horvath et al. 2011). Previously described as engaging in a journey alongside patients (Carson and Arnold 1996), nurses are in a unique position to build working relationships with individuals with eating concerns that are grounded in a thoughtful understanding of culture, as well as compassion, respect, empathy, and trust. This relationship allows room for a struggling individual to give voice to his/her

C. Modica
Wright State University, Dayton, Ohio, USA
e-mail: chris.modica@ymail.com

© Springer International Publishing Switzerland 2018
J.C. Santos, J.R. Cutcliffe (eds.), *European Psychiatric/Mental Health Nursing in the 21st Century*, Principles of Specialty Nursing,
https://doi.org/10.1007/978-3-319-31772-4_31

inner experience, needs, and values, which often constitute the sinews of their pain. Another outgrowth is a deep sense of honor for an individual's life journey and a respect for the experience of his/her suffering. With this spirit in mind, the goal of this chapter is to arm the psychiatric/mental health (P/MH) nurse with knowledge to provide sound and empathic care by offering an empirically based review of diagnoses, epidemiology, theories of development, and common eating disorder treatments that are most often found in adults and adolescents.

31.2 Eating "Disorder" Diagnoses

The current edition of the Diagnostic and Statistical Manual of Mental Disorders (American Psychiatric Association 2013; DSM-5) outlines several eating disorders which are most common in adults: anorexia nervosa (AN), bulimia nervosa (BN), and binge eating disorder (BED). Additionally, the DSM-5 includes two diagnoses (i.e., Other Specified Feeding or Eating Disorder and Unspecified Feeding or Eating Disorder) that can be used to denote disordered eating that is clinically significant, but does not meet full diagnostic criteria of one of the other previously mentioned disorders. These latter diagnoses were formerly diagnosed as Eating Disorder Not Otherwise Specified (ED-NOS) in the DSM-IV-TR (American Psychiatric Association 2000).

In general, AN is characterized by restricted eating which leads to significantly low body weight, coupled with an intense fear of gaining weight (American Psychiatric Association 2013). Additionally, AN includes a significantly disrupted body image and/or an "undue influence of body weight and shape on self-evaluation" (American Psychiatric Association 2013, p. 339). Bulimia nervosa is defined as the presence of recurrent episodes of binge eating combined with recurrent episodes of compensatory behaviors intended to avert weight gain (e.g., vomiting, laxatives, excessive exercise). Binge eating is further specified as eating significantly larger amounts of food than what is typical and a sense of lack of control over eating (American Psychiatric Association 2013). Like AN, BN also includes a criterion that one's "self-evaluation is unduly influenced by body shape and weight" (American Psychiatric Association 2013, p. 345). Unlike the DSM-IV-TR (American Psychiatric Association 2000), the DSM-5 codified BED and defined it as recurrent episodes of binge eating that are associated with other subjective phenomenon, for example, engaging in binge eating when not hungry or feeling disgusted or guilty after binge eating (American Psychiatric Association 2013). Unlike BN, the DSM-5 indicates that individuals with BED do not engage in recurrent compensatory behaviors following episodes of binge eating.

31.3 Prevalence, Incidence, and Course

Much of the corpus of research concerning the prevalence of eating disorders predates the DSM-5 publication and therefore may not fully reflect the current diagnostic taxonomy. Research studies also display significant methodological heterogeneity (e.g., sample size, country of origin, diagnostic criteria). Thus, direct comparisons between studies can be problematic. Since comprehensive reviews of prevalence and incidence rates of eating disorders have been provided elsewhere (e.g., Smink et al. 2014), this chapter will provide a brief overview.

31.3.1 Prevalence

Table 31.1 provides a summary of overall prevalence rates from large-scale studies spanning various countries.

Two important themes can be gleaned. First, rates of eating disorders in women and girls appear to be higher than in men and boys. Second, when loosening criteria to include sub-threshold disorders (i.e., broad diagnoses), rates of each disorder generally increase. While not reported in Table 31.1, it should be noted that lifetime prevalence rates of any eating disorder have been found to be 5.7% for women and 1.2% for men (Smink et al. 2014). Research also suggests that White women have higher rates of disordered eating (Wildes et al. 2001), as well as higher rates of weight concerns (Rakhkovskaya and Warren 2014), compared with non-White women.

Many individuals struggle with eating concerns that do not meet full criteria for AN, BN, or BED (Smink et al. 2014). For example, Hudson et al. (2007) found that lifetime prevalence rates of binge eating in general were 4.5% for men and women in the USA. Further, in a large study of adolescents and adults in the USA, Le

Table 31.1 Prevalence rates for eating disorders in various countries (% overall (% female, % male))

Country	Sample	AN	Broad AN	BN	Broad BN	BED
United States[a]	Adolescents	0.3 (0.3, 0.3)		0.9 (1.3, 0.5)		1.6 (2.3, 0.8)
United States[b]	Adults	0.6 (0.9, 0.3)		1.0 (1.5, 0.5)		2.8 (3.5, 2.0)
Netherlands[c]	Adolescents	(1.7, 0.1)		– (0.8, 0.1)		– (2.3, 0.7)
Finland[d]	Adults	– (2.2, –)	– (4.2, –)			
Finland[e]	Adults			– (1.7, –)	– (2.3, –)	
Sweden[f]	Adults	– (0.6, 0.07)	– (1.2, 0.07)			
Australia[g]	Adults	– (1.9, –)	– (2.4, –)	– (2.9, –)		– (2.9, –)
Multinational[h]	Adults	– (0.9, 0.0)		– (0.9, 0.1)		– (1.9, 0.3)

Note: (–) denotes no data presented or gathered; *AN*, *BN*, and *BED* represent strict/full diagnostic criteria; Broad AN and Broad BN represent subclinical presentations/diagnostic criteria
[a]Swanson et al. (2011)
[b]Hudson et al. (2007)
[c]Smink et al. (2014)
[d]Keski-Rahkonen et al. (2007)
[e]Keski-Rahkonen et al. (2008)
[f]Bulik et al. (2006)
[g]Wade et al. (2006)
[h]Preti et al. (2009) (Belgium, France, Germany, Italy, Spain, and the Netherlands)

Grange et al. (2012) found 81.0% and 75.1%, respectively, were diagnosed as otherwise specified, corresponding to a lifetime prevalence rate for ED-NOS in adolescents and adults of 4.8% and 4.6%, respectively. Similar results have been observed in a study from Portugal (Machado et al. 2007).

While rates of eating disorders in boys and men appear to be higher than previously thought (Darcy 2011; Striegel-Moore et al. 2009), Maine and Bunnell (2010) state that gender represents the clearest risk factor. Rates of AN, BN, and BED have been shown to be roughly 1.75–3 times higher for women than men (Hudson et al. 2007). Hoek and van Hoeken (2006) reported an even greater female-to-male ratio of 10:1 for AN and BN, though sex ratios have been found to be considerably lower when studying younger populations (Madden et al. 2009). Interestingly, the gendered ratio in binge eating is altered. For example, Hudson et al. (2007) discovered that rates of sub-threshold BED were three times higher for men than women. What is more, Grilo (2006) noted a 3:2 male-to-female ratio of BED.

31.3.2 Onset and Incidence

Both AN and BN appear to emerge in adolescence (Keski-Rahkonen et al. 2007, 2008). However, research shows some variability. In a review, Hoek and van Hoeken (2006) observed that across various countries, incidence rates for AN in women and girls appear to be the highest between the ages of 15 and 19, whereas women aged 20–24 appear to have the highest incidence rates for BN.

Incidence rates also show variability depending on methodology and country. In a review of published studies, Hoek and van Hoeken (2003) reported average incidence rates of 8/100,000 for AN and 12/100,000 for BN (in person years). Much higher rates have been observed in individual community-based studies in Finland (Keski-Rahkonen et al. 2007, 2008) potentially due to small sample sizes and broad diagnostic definitions (Smink et al. 2006). Hoek and van Hoeken (2003) noted that incidence rates of AN and BN for males are below 1/100,000. As reviewed by Smink et al. (2006), incidence rates for BED have been found to be 1010/100,000 for females and 660/100,000 for males.

31.4 Theories of Development

Effective treatment of eating concerns should be grounded in an understanding of etiological models. Stice (2001b) has summarized various etiological theories including the spiral model (Heatherton and Polivy 1992); a model of perfectionism, weight status, and self-esteem (Vohs et al. 1999); and a cumulative stressor model that incorporates development through puberty (Levine and Smolak 1992). Other models have conceptualized eating disorders as an addiction (Davis and Claridge 1998). The array of existing causative models attests to the multifaceted nature of eating concerns.

31.4.1 Sociocultural Theories

Some time ago Streigel-Moore et al. (1986) discussed how sociocultural appearance-related pressures faced by women can be axiomatic to eating concerns. Their conceptualization drew attention to insidiousness and pervasiveness of appearance-related pressures embedded in Western society and also the psychological processes by which pressures and cultural beauty ideals can result in eating concerns.

Subsequently, sociocultural models of eating disorders, such as the dual pathway model (Stice 1994) and tripartite influence model (Thompson et al. 1999), have received considerable attention and are critical to understanding the development of disordered eating.

The dual pathway model posits that at a foundational level, the importance and centrality of appearance and thinness for women in Western cultures are embedded in the sociocultural landscape (Stice 1994). Resultant are sociocultural pressures to conform to these standards, which are transmitted through the media, peers, and family (Stice 1994). Because the standards and beauty ideals transmitted are generally unattainable, the aforementioned pressures can lead many women to experience dissatisfaction with their body. However, a critical factor in this model is that pressures are thought to influence body dissatisfaction through thin ideal internalization. Thin ideal internalization refers to the degree to which an individual accepts and adopts the cultural ideal regarding thinness as a determinant of beauty (Thompson and Stice 2001). Thus, while sociocultural pressures may directly lead to body dissatisfaction, the theory suggests that the degree to which an individual internalizes those ideals plays a consequential role.

Theoretically, body dissatisfaction is linked to disordered eating through two pathways, dietary restraint and negative affect, both of which have psychological and physiological underpinnings. Dietary restraint can lead to the initiation of clinical levels of disordered eating directly. Additionally, prolonged dietary restraint may naturally lead to rebounding episodes of disinhibited eating and binge episodes (Stice 2001a). Negative affect is thought to lead to disordered eating because eating can assuage emotional distress and negative affect may impair interoceptive eating cues of fullness (Stice and Bearman2001a; van Strien et al. 2005).

Research has provided support for both sociocultural models. Higher appearance-related pressures from the media (Grabe et al. 2008), peers (Johnson et al. 2015), and family (Menzel et al. 2010) are associated with greater thin ideal internalization and body image concerns in nonclinical adolescents and young adults (Cafri et al. 2005; Cattarin and Thompson 1994; Wertheim et al. 2002). Higher levels of thin ideal internalization are also associated with greater body image concerns (Cafri et al 2005; Stice and Bearman 2001). More recently, research has shown that increases in social media use (e.g., Facebook) are associated with greater body image concerns (Fardouly and Vartanian 2015). The tripartite influence model shares similar features to the dual pathway model but adds the variable of appearance comparison, which has been shown to lead to greater thin ideal internalization and body image concerns (Keery et al. 2004). Research has also provided support for the dual pathway model and tripartite influence model when multiple variables in each theory are modeled or examined together (Halliwell and Harvey 2006; Nouri et al. 2011; Rogers et al. 2009; van den Berg et al. 2002).

Sociocultural ideals regarding beauty can be culture specific in regard to race, age, or gender (Algars et al. 2009; Frisbey 2004). For example, it has been suggested that in the USA, Black women, compared with White women, may not consider weight as strongly in their overall body image (Breitkopf et al. 2007). Thus, it is important to note the potential moderating influence that race, age, and gender may have in sociocultural models. In the USA, there exists a more muscular ideal for men (Labre 2005), compared to a thin ideal for women (Field et al. 1999). Body image concerns may decrease also with age (Algars et al. 2009). Additionally, compared to Black and Hispanic women, White women report higher thin ideal internalization (Rakhkovskaya and Warren 2014), higher appearance comparisons (Schaefer et al. 2015), higher body shame (Breitkopf et al. 2007), and higher body dissatisfaction and dietary restraint (Wildes et al. 2001) and may be more likely to consider themselves overweight compared to Black women (Breitkopf et al. 2007).

31.5 Treatment Models and Effectiveness

Treatment of eating concerns can be delivered in inpatient, residential, day treatment, intensive outpatient, and outpatient settings (Birmingham and Beumont 2004; Mehler and Anderson 2010). Treatment can include a combination of individual therapy, group therapy, nutritional counseling, family therapy, psychoeducation, psychiatric medication, and, in severe cases, refeeding protocols as a last resort (National Institute for Health and Clinical Excellence 2004). What follows is a concise review of major types of treatments and support for their effectiveness.

31.5.1 Cognitive Behavioral Psychotherapy

Cognitive behavioral therapy (CBT) for eating concerns has received significant research attention (see Galsworthy-Francis and Allan 2014 for a review). This structured treatment includes weekly self-monitoring of eating and weight, exploring and challenging cognitive distortions, between-session behavioral experiments aimed at challenging cognitions and eating habits, and preventing relapse (Pike et al. 2010). CBT for BN is similar but with a narrowed focus on the factors that maintain binging and purging behaviors. After the original formulations, Fairburn (2008) has augmented his treatment model to include a focus on self-esteem, mood intolerance, perfectionism, and interpersonal problems in an updated treatment model termed enhanced CBT (i.e., CBT-E).

Research on the effectiveness of CBT for AN has spanned several countries such as New Zealand (McIntosh et al. 2005), England (Gowers et al. 2007), and Italy (Brambilla et al. 2010). Given significant methodological heterogeneity, in general, research has shown that CBT is an effective treatment for AN when it is delivered in inpatient settings (Dalle-Grave et al. 2013) and outpatient settings (Touyz et al. 2013) and combined with family therapy (Gowers et al. 2007) or nutritional counseling (Bowers and Ansher 2008). While CBT appears to be an effective treatment, large-scale reviews of existing research (Galsworthy-Francis and Allan 2014) have posited that the variations in treatment protocols as well as lack of clear superiority over alternative treatments do not fully demonstrate that it is the treatment of choice.

Manualized CBT is regarded as the treatment of choice for BN and BED (Chakraborty and Basu 2010; National Institute for Health and Clinical Excellence 2004). Studies have shown that CBT is effective for reducing binging and purging behaviors in adults (Knott et al. 2015; Vocks et al. 2010; Wilfley et al. 2002) and normal-weight adolescents (Dalle-Grave et al. 2015) and more effective than other treatments such as psychoanalysis (Poulsen et al. 2014) and medication (i.e., fluoxetine) alone (Grilo et al. 2012). However, not all individuals benefit from CBT for BN with reports of complete elimination of binge eating and purging in roughly 30–50% of individuals treated (Wilson 1996).

31.5.2 Interpersonal Psychotherapy

Interpersonal psychotherapy (IPT) is also an effective treatment for eating concerns. IPT treatment is rooted in the interpersonal theory of psychological distress, which was originally formulated to treat depression (Markowitz and Weissman 2012). In general, treatment focuses on how a client's interpersonal relationships contribute to eating pathology. Treatment seeks to identify one of four areas of concern: role transitions, interpersonal role disputes, grief, and interpersonal deficits (Gilles 2001). Concerns in these areas may serve as triggers for eating problems or may cause other mental health concerns such as depression, which may link to eating concerns (MacFarlane et al. 2008). In several ways, IPT has been shown to be as effective as CBT for AN at posttreatment (McIntosh et al. 2005) and long-term follow-up (Carter et al. 2011). Similarly, IPT has been shown to be effective in reducing binge eating in BED (Wilfley et al. 2002), as effective as CBT in reducing binge eating in BN (Wilson et al. 2010), and effective at reducing binge eating in individuals with disordered eating in general (Fairburn et al. 2015).

31.5.3 Family Psychotherapy

The connection between family of origin and eating concerns has been a topic of interest for some time (Minuchin et al. 1978). Family-based treatment is rooted in the rich theoretical underpinnings of systemic models of distress, which suggest that individual behavior and distress can be embedded within as well as an outgrowth of the family system (Stanton 2013). Thus, while not ignoring the individual factors, distress can be understood as emanating from the structures, roles, and/or dynamics of the family system as a whole (Colapinto 1991).

The Maudsley approach is generally regarded as the family's treatment of choice for AN. Treatment initially focuses on assisting parents as a unified front to enable their child to restore eating and weight (Le Grange and Eisler 2009). This is followed by empowering children to regain personal control of eating, fostering autonomy, and helping the child form his/her own identity. Orchestrated interventions are done with an agnostic stance toward the genesis of the eating disorder. In general this family-based approach has been shown to be effective for AN (Le Grange and Eisler 2009; Lock et al. 2010) and BN (Dodge et al. 1995; Le Grange et al. 2007, 2015).

31.5.4 Medication

The treatment of eating disorders can also be approached through pharmacological avenues, often in conjunction with other therapeutic treatments and under close monitoring of side effects (National Institute for Health and Clinical Excellence 2004). Due to the implication of serotonin dysfunction, and associated obsessional thinking, anxiety, and depression that often accompany AN, the use of antidepressants is common with AN. However, reviews have found that the effectiveness of antidepressant medication in treating AN is either inconclusive (Bulik et al. 2007) or unsupported (Hay and Claudino 2012). Second-generation antipsychotic mediation can also be used with AN based on neurological models that implicate dopamine and serotonin in eating disorder etiology (Kaye 2008). However, a recent meta-analysis (Dold et al. 2015) found no significant differences between second-generation antipsychotic medication and control conditions on weight gain, dropout, or secondary measures of eating disorder-specific symptomology.

The use of antidepressant medication in the treatment of BN and BED is more widely accepted, with fluoxetine being described as the drug of choice (Birmingham and Beumont 2004). In their review, Hay and Claudino (2012) found that though attrition is high in many studies, the use of antidepressant medication is associated with reduced binging, reduced purging, and improvements in anxiety and mood symptomology. Similarly, in a meta-analysis, Reas and Grilo (2008) suggested that the use of medication to treat BED is superior to placebo and is associated with cessation from binge eating (47.8% vs. 27.5%), respectively, in the short term. The long-term effectiveness of medication to treat BED was not supported by the available studies.

31.6 Nutritional Counseling

Often individuals with eating concerns have developed attitudes or schemas regarding food, nutrition, and healthy eating that necessitate specialized attention. Thus, while nutritional counseling should not be considered a stand-alone intervention (National Institute for Health and Clinical Excellence 2004), it can play a vital role in the treatment of eating concerns whether concurrent with treatment or after.

Nutritional counseling may include meal planning, education about caloric intake and nutrients, weight maintenance, or exercise parameters. These may be integrated with homework assignments, goal setting, parental involvement, and reading (Hsu et al. 1992; Mittnacht and Bulik 2015). Though nutritional counseling for weight loss has received research attention (Molenaar et al. 2010), the effectiveness of nutritional counseling has not received significant research attention in the context of eating disorders. One study with a small sample size (O'Connor et al. 1988) reported significant decreases in binge eating and vomiting when nutritional counseling was administered independent of other treatments. Given the lack of research attention, it is still suggested that dieticians and nutritionists can play an active and crucial role in a treatment team at various stages of recovery and treatment.

31.7 Other Treatments

While a detailed review of all treatment approaches is beyond the scope of this chapter, it is important to note other established, validated, and promising treatments for eating concerns. For example, dialectical behavior therapy (Fischer and Peterson 2015), motivational interviewing (Cassin et al. 2008), cognitive remediation therapy (Dingemans et al. 2014), and integrative cognitive affective therapy (Wonderlich et al. 2014) have been shown to be effective for treating symptoms of eating concerns. Additionally, group CBT for eating disorders has also been shown to be effective for BN (Jones and Clausen 2013) and BED (Chen et al. 2003). Developments in eating disorder prevention have also shown considerable progress, in particular the dissonance-based prevention program (i.e., the Body Project) (Stice et al. 2008a). Research shows that at 3-year follow-up, the Body Project is associated with reductions in body dissatisfaction, thin ideal internalization, and eating disorder symptoms and is associated with a 60% reduction in eating pathology compared with an assessment-only control condition (Stice et al. 2008a).

31.8 Current Developments and Future Directions

There are also promising future directions for treatment, theory, and prevention. Researchers are exploring the application of acceptance and commitment therapy (Katter 2010), mindfulness interventions (Godfrey et al. 2015), and the impact of spirituality (Berrett et al. 2007) on eating disorder treatment. Research has also begun to explore the impact of caloric deprivation on brain reward systems (Stice et al. 2013a, b) as well as the association between eating disorders and trauma (Tagay et al. 2014). A fruitful area of exploration continues to be the treatments targeting neuropsychological functioning (i.e., increasing cognitive flexibility) in individuals with eating disorders (van Noort et al. 2016) as well as Internet-based treatments (Aardom et al. 2014).

Conclusion

This chapter sought to illuminate the inner fabric that can often underlie clinical eating concerns. Behind the scenes, eating concerns often represent more than a struggle with eating, but potentially a complex interweaving of internalized cultural ideals, attitudes toward one's body, and insidious pressures related to appearance. These forces can culminate into debilitating cycles of dietary restriction and dietary disinhibition that the psychological field recognizes as eating disorders. Whether in momentary interactions or prolonged connections, mental health nurses are in a position to foster healing through empathic and respectful care that is rooted in an understanding of culture, theory, and treatments.

References

Aardom JJ, Dingemans AE, Boogaard LH, van Furth EF (2014) Internet and patient empowerment in individuals with symptoms of an eating disorder: a cross-sectional investigation of a pro-recovery focused e-community. Eat Behav 15:350–356

Algars M, Santtila P, Varjonen M, Witting K, Johansson A, Jern P (2009) The adult body: how age, gender, and body mass index are related to body image. J Aging Health 21:1112–1132

American Psychiatric Association (2000) Diagnostic and statistical manual of mental disorders, 4th edn. American Psychiatric Association, Washington, DC

American Psychiatric Association (2013) Diagnostic and statistical manual of mental disorders, 5th edn. American Psychiatric Publishing, Arlington

Berrett ME, Hardman RK, O'Grady KA, Richards PS (2007) The role of spirituality in the treatment of trauma and eating disorders: recommendations for clinical practice. Eat Disord 15:373–389

Birmingham CL, Beumont P (2004) Medical management of eating disorders. Cambridge University Press, Cambridge

Bowers WA, Ansher LS (2008) The effectiveness of cognitive behavioral therapy on changing eating disorder symptoms and psychopathology of 32 anorexia nervosa patients at hospital discharge and one year follow-up. Ann Clin Psychiatry 20:79–86

Brambilla F, Dalle Grave R, Calugi S, Marchesini G, Baroni S, Marazziti D (2010) Effects of cognitive-behavioral therapy on eating disorders: neurotransmitter secretory response to treatment. Psychoneuroendocrinology 35:729–737

Breitkopf CR, Littleton H, Berenson A (2007) Body image: a study in a tri-ethnic sample of low income women. Sex Roles 56:373–380

Bulik CM, Berkman ND, Brownley KA, Sedway JA, Lohr KN (2007) Anorexia nervosa treatment: a systematic review of randomized controlled trials. Int J Eat Disord 40:310–320

Bulik CM, Sullivan PF, Tozzi F, Furberg H, Lichtenstein P, Pedersen NL (2006) Prevalence, Heritability, and Prospective Risk Factors for Anorexia Nervosa. Arch Gen Psychiatry 63 (3):305

Cafri G, Yamamiya Y, Brannick M, Thompson JK (2005) The influence of sociocultural factors on body image: a meta-analytic review. Clin Psychol Sci Pract 12:421–433

Carson VB, Arnold EN (1996) Mental health nursing: the nurse-patient journey. W. B. Saunders & Co, Philadelphia

Carter FA, Jordan J, McIntosh VW, Luty SE, McKenzie JM, Frampton CMA, Joyce PR (2011) The long-term efficacy of three psychotherapies for anorexia nervosa: a randomized controlled trial. Int J Eat Disord 44:647–654

Cassin SE, von Ranson KM, Heng K, Brar J, Wojtowicz AE (2008) Adapted motivational interviewing for women with binge eating disorder: a randomized controlled trial. Psychol Addict Behav 22:417–425

Cattarin J, Thompson JK (1994) A three-year longitudinal study of body image and eating disturbance in adolescent females. Eat Disord 2:114–125
Chakraborty K, Basu D (2010) Management of anorexia and bulimia nervosa: an evidence-based review. Indian J Psychiatry 52:174–186
Chen E, Touyz SW, Beumont PJV, Fairburn CG, Griffiths R, Butow P, Basten C (2003) Comparison of group and individual cognitive–behavioral therapy for patients with bulimia nervosa. Int J Eat Disord 33:241–254
Colapinto J (1991) Structural family therapy. In: Horne A, Passmore JL (eds) Family counseling and therapy, 2nd edn. F. E. Peacock Publishers Inc., Itasca, pp 77–106
Dalle-Grave R, Calugi S, Sartirana M, Fairburn CG (2015) Transdiagnostic cognitive behaviour therapy for adolescents with an eating disorder who are not underweight. Behav Res Ther 73:79–82
Dalle-Grave RD, Calugi S, Conti M, Doll H, Fairburn CG (2013) Inpatient cognitive behaviour therapy for anorexia nervosa: a randomized controlled trial. Psychother Psychosom 82:390–398
Darcy AM (2011) Eating disorders in adolescent males: a critical examination of five common assumptions. Adolesc Psychiatry 1:307–312
Davis C, Claridge G (1998) The eating disorders as addiction: a psychobiological perspective. Addict Behav 23:465–475
Dingemans AE, Danner UN, Donker JM, Aardoom JJ, van Meer F, Tobias K, van Elburg AA, van Furth EF (2014) The effectiveness of cognitive remediation therapy in patients with a severe or enduring eating disorder: a randomized controlled trial. Psychother Psychosom 83:29–36
Dodge E, Hodes M, Eisler I, Dare C (1995) Family therapy for bulimia nervosa in adolescents: an exploratory study. J Fam Ther 17:59–77
Dold M, Aigner M, Klabunde M, Treasure J, Kasper S (2015) Second-generation antipsychotic drugs in anorexia nervosa: a meta-analysis of randomized controlled trials. Psychother Psychosom 84:110–116
Fairburn CG (2008) Cognitive behavior therapy and eating disorders. Guilford, New York
Fairburn CG, Cooper A (2007) Thinking afresh about the classification of eating disorders. Int J Eat Disord 40:107–110
Fairburn CG, Bailey-Staebler S, Basden S, Doll HA, Jones R, Murphy R, Cooper Z (2015) A transdiagnostic comparison of enhanced cognitive behaviour therapy (CBT-E) and interpersonal psychotherapy in the treatment of eating disorders. Behav Res Ther 70:64–71
Fardouly J, Vartanian LR (2015) Negative comparisons about one's appearance mediate the relationship between Facebook usage and body image concerns. Body Image 12:82–88
Field AE, Camargo CA, Taylor B, Berkey C, Frazier L, Gillman MW, Colditz GA (1999) Overweight, weight concerns, and bulimic behaviors among girls and boys. J Am Acad Child Adolesc Psychiatry 38:754–760
Fischer S, Peterson C (2015) Dialectical behavior therapy for adolescent binge eating, purging, suicidal behavior, and non-suicidal self-injury: a pilot study. Psychotherapy 52:78–92
Frisbey CM (2004) Does race matter? Effects of idealized images on African American women's perceptions of body esteem. J Black Stud 34:323–347
Galsworthy-Francis L, Allan S (2014) Cognitive behavioral therapy for anorexia nervosa: a systematic review. Clin Psychol Rev 34:54–72
Gilles LA (2001) Interpersonal psychotherapy for depression and other disorders. In: Barlow DH (ed) Clinical handbook of psychological disorders: a step-by-step treatment manual, 3rd edn. The Guilford Press, New York, pp 309–331
Godfrey KM, Gallo LC, Afari N (2015) Mindfulness-based interventions for binge eating: a systematic review and meta-analysis. J Behav Med 38:348–362
Gowers SG, Clark A, Roberts C, Griffiths A, Edwards V, Bryan C, Barrett B (2007) Clinical effectiveness of treatments for anorexia nervosa in adolescents: randomized controlled trial. Br J Psychiatry 191:427–435
Grabe S, Ward LM, Hyde JS (2008) The role of the media in body image concerns among women: a meta-analysis of experimental and correlational studies. Psychol Bull 134:460–476
Grilo CM (2006) Eating and weight disorders. Psychology Press, New York

Grilo CM, Crosby RD, Wilson GT, Masheb RM (2012) 12-month follow-up of fluoxetine and cognitive behavioral therapy for binge eating disorder. J Consult Clin Psychol 80:1108–1113
Halliwell E, Harvey M (2006) Examination of a sociocultural model of disordered eating among male and female adolescents. Br J Health Psychol 11:235–248
Hay PJ, Claudino AM (2012) Clinical psychopharmacology of eating disorders: a research update. Int J Neuropsychopharmacol 15:209–222
Heatherton TF, Polivy J (1992) Chronic dieting and eating disorders: a spiral model. In: Crowther J, Tennenbaum D, Hobfoll SE, Stephens MA (eds) The etiology of bulimia nervosa: the individual and family context. Hemisphere, Washington, DC, pp 133–155
Hoek HW, van Hoeken D (2006) Review of the prevalence and incidence of eating disorders. Int J Eat Disord 34:383–396
Horvath AO, Del Re AC, Fluckiger C, Symonds D (2011) Alliance in individual therapy. Psychotherapy 48:9–16
Hsu LKG, Holben B, West S (1992) Nutritional counseling in bulimia nervosa. Int J Eat Disord 11:55–62
Hudson JI, Hiripi E, Pope HG, Kessler RC (2007) The prevalence and correlates of eating disorders in the National Comorbidity Survey Replication. Biol Psychiatry 61:348–358
Johnson SM, Edwards KM, Gidycz CA (2015) Interpersonal weight-related pressure and disordered eating in college women: a test of an expanded tripartite influence model. Sex Roles 72:15–24
Jones A, Clausen L (2013) The efficacy of a brief group CBT program in treating patients diagnosed with bulimia nervosa: a brief report. Int J Eat Disord 46:560–562
Katter K (2010) New pathways: applying acceptance and commitment therapy to the treatment of eating disorders. In: Maine M, McGilley BH, Bunnell DW (eds) Treatment of eating disorders: bridging the research-practice gap. Academic, London, pp 163–180
Kaye W (2008) Neurobiology of anorexia and bulimia nervosa. Physiol Behav 94:121–135
Keery H, van den Berg P, Thompson JK (2004) An evaluation of the tripartite model of body dissatisfaction and eating disturbance with adolescent girls. Body Image 1:237–251
Keski-Rahkonen A, Hoek HW, Susser ES, Linna MS, Sihvola E, Raevuori A, Rissanen A (2007) Epidemiology and course of anorexia nervosa in the community. Am J Psychiatr 164:1259–1265
Keski-Rahkonen A, Hoek HW, Linna MS, Raevuori A, Sihvola E, Bulik CM, Kaprio J (2008) Incidence and outcomes of bulimia nervosa: a nationwide population-based study. Psychol Med 39:823–831
Kluck A (2010) Family influence on disordered eating: the role of body image dissatisfaction. Body Image 7:8–14
Klump KL (2013) Puberty as a critical risk period for eating disorders. A review of human and animal studies. Horm Behav 64:399–410
Knott S, Woodward D, Hoefkens A, Limbert C (2015) Cognitive behaviour therapy for bulimia nervosa and eating disorders not otherwise specified: translation from randomized controlled trial to a clinical setting. Behav Cogn Psychother 43:641–654
Labre MP (2005) The male body ideal: perspectives of readers and non-readers of fitness magazines. J Men's Health Gender 2:223–229
Le Grange D, Eisler I (2009) Family interventions in adolescent anorexia nervosa. Child Adolesc Psychiatr Clin N Am 18:159–173
Le Grange D, Crosby RD, Rathouz PJ, Leventhal BL (2007) A randomized controlled comparison of family-based treatment and supportive psychotherapy for adolescent bulimia nervosa. Arch Gen Psychiatry 64:1049–1056
Le Grange D, Swanson SA, Crow SJ, Merikangas KR (2012) Eating disorder not otherwise specified presentation in the US population. Int J Eat Disord 45:711–718
Le Grange D, Lock J, Agras WS, Bryson SW, Jo B (2015) Randomized controlled trial or family-based treatment and cognitive behavioral therapy for adolescent bulimia nervosa. J Am Acad Child Adolesc Psychiatry 54:886–894
Levine MP, Smolak L (1992) Toward a model of the developmental psychopathology of eating disorders: the example of early adolescence. In: Crowther J, Tennenbaum D, Hobfoll SE, Stephens MA (eds) The etiology of bulimia nervosa: the individual and family context. Hemisphere, Washington, pp 59–80

Lock J, Le Grange D, Agras WS, Moye A, Bryson SW, Jo B (2010) Randomized Clinical Trial Comparing Family-Based Treatment With Adolescent-Focused Individual Therapy for Adolescents With Anorexia Nervosa. Arch Gen Psychiatry 67(10):1025

MacFarlane K, Trottier K, Polivy J, Herman P, Arsenault J, Boivin M (2008) Eating disorders. In: Maddux J, Winstead B (eds) Psychopathology: foundations for a contemporary understanding, 3rd edn. Routledge, New York, pp 517–552

Machado PP, Machado BC, Goncalves S, Hoek HW (2007) The prevalence of eating disorders not otherwise specified. Int J Eat Disord 40:212–217

Madden S, Morris A, Zurynski YA, Kohn M, Elliot EJ (2009) Burden of eating disorders in 5-13-year-old children in Australia. Med J Aust 190:410–414

Maine M, Bunnell DW (2010) A perfect biopsychosocial storm: gender, culture, and eating disorders. In: Maine M, McGilley BH, Bunnell DW (eds) Treatment of eating disorders: bridging the research-practice gap. Academic, London, pp 3–16

Markowitz JC, Weissman MM (2012) Interpersonal psychotherapy: past, present and future. Clin Psychol Psychother 19:99–105

McIntosh VVW, Jordan J, Carter FA, Luty SE, McKenzie JM, Bulik CM, Joyce PR (2005) Three psychotherapies for anorexia nervosa: a randomized, controlled trial. Am J Psychiatr 162:741–747

Mehler PA, Anderson AE (2010) Eating disorders: a guide to medical care and complications, 2nd edn. Johns Hopkins University Press, Baltimore

Menzel JE, Schaefer LM, Burke NB, Mayhew LL, Brannick MT, Thompson JK (2010) Appearance-related teasing, body dissatisfaction, and disordered eating: a meta-analysis. Body Image 7:261–270

Minuchin S, Rosman BL, Baker L (1978) Psychosomatic families: anorexia nervosa in context. Harvard University Press, Cambridge

Mittnacht AM, Bulik CM (2015) Best nutrition counseling practices for the treatment of anorexia nervosa: a Delphi study. Int J Eat Disord 48:111–122

Molenaar EA, van Ameijden EJ, Vergouwe Y, Grobbee DE, Numans ME (2010) Effect of nutritional counselling and nutritional plus exercise counselling in overweight adults: a randomized trial in multidisciplinary primary care practice. Fam Pract 27:143–150

National Institute for Health and Clinical Excellence (2004) Eating disorders in over 8s management. NICE guideline (CG9). NICE, London. https://www.nice.org.uk/guidance/cg9/chapter/1-Guidance

Nouri M, Hill LG, Orrell-Valente JK (2011) Media exposure, internalization of the thin ideal, and body dissatisfaction: comparing Asian American and European American college females. Body Image 8:366–372

O'Connor M, Touyz S, Beumont P (1988) Nutritional management and dietary counseling in bulimia nervosa: some preliminary observations. Int J Eat Disord 7:657–662

Pike KM, Carter JC, Olmsted MP (2010) Cognitive-behavioral therapy for anorexia nervosa. In: Grilo CM, Mitchell JE (eds) The treatment of eating disorders: a clinical handbook. Guilford, New York, pp 83–107

Poulsen S, Lunn S, Daniel SIF, Folke S, Mathiesen BB, Katznelson H, Fairburn CG (2014) A randomized controlled trial of psychoanalytic psychotherapy or cognitive-behavioral therapy for bulimia nervosa. Am J Psychiatr 171:109–116

Preti A, Girolamo GD, Vilagut G, Alonso J, Graaf RD, Bruffaerts R, Demyttenaere K, Pinto-Meza A, Haro JM, Morosini P (2009) The epidemiology of eating disorders in six European countries: Results of the ESEMeD-WMH project. J Psychiatr Res 43(14):1125–1132

Rakhkovskaya LM, Warren CS (2014) Ethnic identity, thin-ideal internalization, and eating pathology in ethnically diverse college women. Body Image 11:438–445

Reas DL, Grilo CM (2008) Review and meta-analysis of pharmacotherapy for binge-eating disorder. Obesity 16:2024–2038

Roberts M, Lavender A, Tchanturia K (2011) Measuring self-report obsessionality in anorexia nervosa: Maudsley obsessive-compulsive inventory (MOCI) or obsessive-compulsive inventory-revised (OCI-R)? Eur Eat Disord Rev 19:501–508

Rogers RF, Paxton SJ, Chabrol H (2009) Effects of parental comments on body dissatisfaction and eating disturbance in young adults: a sociocultural model. Body Image 6:171–177

Schaefer LM, Thibodaux LK, Krenic D, Arnold E, Thompson KJ (2015) Physical appearance comparisons in ethnically diverse college women. Body Image 15:153–157
Smink FRE, van Hoeken D, Hoek HW (2006) Epidemiology of eating disorders: incidence, prevalence and mortality rates. Curr Opin Psychiatry 26:543–548
Smink FRE, van Hoeken D, Oldehinkel AJ, Hoek HW (2014) Prevalence of severity of DSM-5 eating disorders in a community cohort of adolescents. Int J Eat Disord 47:610–619
Stanton M (2013) The systemic epistemology of the specialty of family psychology. In: Bray JM, Stanton M (eds) The Wiley-Blackwell handbook of family psychology. Blackwell Publishing, West Sussex, pp 5–20
Stice E (1994) Review of the evidence for a sociocultural model of bulimia nervosa and an exploration of the mechanisms of action. Clin Psychol Rev 14:633–661
Stice E (2001a) A prospective test of the dual-pathway model of bulimic pathology: mediating effects of dieting and negative affect. J Abnorm Psychol 110:124–135
Stice E (2001b) Risk factors for eating pathology: recent advances and future directions. In: Striegel-Moore RH, Smolak L (eds) Eating disorders: innovative directions for research and practice. American Psychological Association, Washington, DC, pp 51–73
Stice E, Bearman SK (2001) Body image and eating disturbances prospectively predict increases in depressive symptoms in adolescent girls: a growth curve analysis. Dev Psychol 37:1–11
Stice E, Shaw HE (2002) Role of body dissatisfaction in the onset and maintenance of eating pathology: synthesis of research findings. J Psychosom Res 53:985–993
Stice E, Presnell K, Spangler D (2002) Risk factors for binge eating onset: a prospective investigation. Health Psychol 21:131–138
Stice E, Marti N, Spoor S, Presnell K, Shaw H (2008a) Dissonance and healthy weight eating disorder prevention programs: long-term effects from a randomized efficacy trial. J Consult Clin Psychol 76:329–340
Stice E, Shaw H, Becker CB, Rhode P (2008b) Dissonance-based interventions for the prevention of eating disorders: using persuasion principles to promote health. Soc Prev Res 9:114–128
Stice E, Shaw H, Becker C, Rohde P (2008c) Dissonance-based interventions for the prevention of eating disorders: using persuasion principles to promote health. Prev Sci 9:114–128
Stice E, South K, Shaw H (2012) Future directions in etiologic, prevention, and treatment research for eating disorders. J Clin Child Adolesc Psychol 41:845–855
Stice E, Becker CB, Yokum S (2013a) Eating disorder prevention: current evidence-base and future directions. Int J Eat Disord 46:478–485
Stice E, Burger K, Yokum S (2013b) Caloric deprivation increases responsively of attention and reward regions to intake, anticipated intake, and images of palatable foods. NeuroImage 67:322–330
Streigel-Moore RH, Silberstein LR, Rodin J (1986) Toward and understanding of risk factors for bulimia. Am Psychol 41:246–263
Striegel-Moore RH, Rosselli F, Perrin N, DeBar L, Wilson GT, May A, Kraemer HC (2009) Gender difference in the prevalence of eating disorder symptoms. Int J Eat Disord 42:471–474
Swanson SA, Crow SJ, Le Grange D, Swendsen J, Merikangas KR (2011) Prevalence and correlates of eating disorders in adolescents. Results from the national comorbidity survey replication adolescent supplement. Arch Gen Psychiatry 68:714–723
Tagay S, Schlottbohm E, Reyes-Rodriguez ML, Repic N, Senf W (2014) Eating disorders, trauma, PTSD, and psychosocial resources. Eat Disord 22:33–49
Thompson JK, Heinberg LJ, Altabe M, Tantleff-Dunn S (1999) Exacting beauty: theory, assessment, and treatment of body image disturbance. American Psychological Association, Washington, DC
Thompson KJ, Stice E (2001) Thin ideal internalization: mounting evidence for a new risk factor for body-image disturbance and eating pathology. Curr Dir Psychol Sci 10:181–183
Touyz S, Le Grange D, Lacey H, Hay P, Smith R, Maguire S, Bamford B, Pike KM, Crosby RD (2013) Treating severe and enduring anorexia nervosa: a randomized controlled trial. Psychol Med 43:2501–2511

van den Berg P, Thompson JK, Obremski-Brandon K, Coovert M (2002) The tripartite influence model of body image and eating disturbance: a covariance structure modeling investigation testing the meditational role of appearance comparison. J Psychosom Res 53:1007–1020

van Noort BM, Kraus MKA, Pfeiffer E, Lehmkuhl U, Kappel V (2016) Neuropsychological and behavioural short-term effects of cognitive remediation therapy in adolescent anorexia nervosa: a pilot study. Eur Eat Disord Rev 24:69–74

van Strien T, Engels RCME, Van Leeuwe J, Snoek HM (2005) The Stice model of overeating: tests in clinical and non-clinical samples. Appetite 45:205–213

Vocks S, Tuschen-Caffier B, Pietrowsky R, Rustenbach SJ, Kersting A, Herpertz S (2010) Meta-analysis of the effectiveness of psychological and pharmacological treatments for binge eating disorder. Int J Eat Disord 43:205–217

Vohs KD, Voelz ZR, Pettit JW, Bardone AM, Katz J, Abramson LY, Joiner TE (1999) Perfectionism, body dissatisfaction, and self-esteem: an interactive model of bulimic symptoms development. J Soc Clin Psychol 20:476–497

Wade TD, Hansell NK, Crosby RD, Bryant-Waugh R, Treasure J, Nixon M, N. G. (2013) A study of changes in genetic and environmental influences on weight and shape concern across adolescence. J Abnorm Psychol 122:199–130

Wade TD, Bergin JL, Tiggemann M, Bulik CM, Fairburn CG (2016) Prevalence and Long-Term Course of Lifetime Eating Disorders in an Adult Australian Twin Cohort. Aust N Z J Psychiatry 40(2):121–128

Wertheim EH, Martin G, Prior M, Sanson A, Smart D (2002) Parent influences in the transmission of eating and weight related values and behaviours. Eat Disord 10:321–334

Wildes JE, Emery RE, Simons AD (2001) The roles of ethnicity and culture in the development of eating disturbance and body dissatisfaction: a meta-analytic review. Clin Psychol Rev 21:521–551

Wilfley DE, Welch RR, Stein R, Spurrell EB, Cohen LR, Saelens BE, Matt GE (2002) A randomized comparison of group cognitive behavioral therapy and group interpersonal psychotherapy for treatment of overweight individuals with binge-eating disorder. Arch Gen Psychiatry 59:713–721

Wilson GT (1996) Treatment of bulimia nervosa: when treatment fails. Behav Res Ther 34:197–212

Wilson TG, Wilfley DE, Agras S, Bryson S (2010) Psychological treatments of binge eating disorder. Arch Gen Psychiatry 67:94–101

Wonderlich SA, Peterson CB, Crosby RD, Smith TL, Klein MH, Mitchell JE, Crow SJ (2014) A randomized controlled comparison of integrative cognitive-affective therapy (ICAT) and enhanced cognitive-behavioral therapy (CBT-E) for bulimia nervosa. Psychol Med 44:543–553

Suicide and Self-Harm

32

José Carlos Santos

32.1 Introduction

Suicidal behaviors are a major public health issue. The World Health Organization (WHO 2014a) estimates that more than 800,000 people per year, on average, die by suicide, representing an annual global age-standardized suicide rate of 11.4/100,000 population (15.0 for males and 8.0 for females). Worldwide, suicide is responsible for half (50%) of all violent deaths in men and 71% of violent deaths in women. Global averages indicate that suicide is more common among people over the age of 75 years yet all nations do not share this pattern. In some countries, suicide rates are highest among young people, and if we consider the 15–29 age group, suicide is the second leading cause of death worldwide. For every completed adult suicide, there are approximately 20 attempted suicides (WHO 2014a). Moreover, 48–500 million people experience suicide bereavement (bereavement as a result of losing a loved one to suicide) every year (Pitman et al. 2014).

WHO Member States have committed to fulfill the global target of reducing the suicide rate by 10% by 2020 (WHO 2013). The epidemiological characteristics of suicidal behaviors change between communities, in different demographic groups and over time. For this reason, an up-to-date surveillance of suicide and suicide attempts is always a key aspect of local and national prevention plans. Unfortunately, suicide is still stigmatized in many countries and even illegal in some (WHO 2014a), and, more importantly, these attitudes toward suicide can and do hamper help-seeking.

J.C. Santos
Escola Superior de Enfermagem de Coimbra, Nursing School of Coimbra, Coimbra, Portugal
e-mail: jcsantos@esenfc.pt

© Springer International Publishing Switzerland 2018

J.C. Santos, J.R. Cutcliffe (eds.), *European Psychiatric/Mental Health Nursing in the 21st Century*, Principles of Specialty Nursing,
https://doi.org/10.1007/978-3-319-31772-4_32

Underreporting of suicide is a reality, with a high rate of undetermined deaths in Europe, particularly in Estonia and Portugal (Värnik et al. 2010). This translates into a clear increase in the 2–20 benchmark for the ratio between the events of undetermined intent and suicide rates (Värnik et al. 2012). The same applies to data (when available) on self-harm episodes. For example, routine hospital data collected by the Hospital Episode Statistics may underestimate the overall rates of self-harm by up to 60% compared with data from the Multicentre Study of Self-harm in England (Clements et al. 2016). The person with suicidal behavior or suicidal ideation is perhaps the most challenging person in nursing-patient interventions, since suicide, despite all the advances, continues to be the most mysterious act of the human being. And thus the rest of this chapter focuses on suicide and self-harm, care of the suicidal person, and P/MH nursing response to people who engage in suicidal behavior and/or self-harm behavior.

32.2 Definitions

Research in this area is complex given the lack of agreement about suicidal behavior-related terminology and the differences in clinical and research practices (Edmondson et al. 2016). In this chapter, we use Shneidman's definition of suicide (Shneidman 1985, p. 3) as

> a conscious act of self-annihilation, best understood as a multidimensional malaise in a needful individual who defines an issue for which suicide is perceived as the best solution.

We also used Santa Mina and Gallop (1998, p. 794) definition of self-harm as

> an individual's intentional damage to a part of his or her own body, without a conscious intent to die, although the result may be fatal.

This includes nonfatal intentional self-poisoning/overdose and self-injury, which poses a major challenge in many countries and is associated with suicidal risk. Self-harm is distressing for both patients and their families and friends and places large demands on clinical services. It is therefore important to assess the evidence on treatments for patients who engage in self-harm (Hawton et al. 2016).

32.3 Suicide Prevention Policies

Although several suicide prevention programs have been implemented worldwide (Mann and Currier 2011), it has not been easy to assess the effectiveness of these programs due to the diversity of risk factors for suicidal behaviors which is still a rare epidemiological phenomenon. Thus, the WHO argues that countries with a comprehensive national response should focus on evaluation and improvement, updating their knowledge with new data and emphasizing effectiveness and efficiency. For this reason, suicide prevention activities should be carried out in conjunction with parallel and empirically robust evaluation activities. Even if a country is not yet ready to have a national prevention strategy, the process of consulting stakeholders usually generates interest and creates a favorable environment for making changes (WHO 2014a). However, suicide prevention efforts need to incorporate an ecological approach, a multilevel prevention network where health is only one among many other factors (Santos et al. 2014). Zalsman et al. (2016, p. 1) found that

> evidence for restricting access to lethal means in prevention of suicide has strengthened since 2005, especially with regard to control of analgesics and hot-spots for suicide by jumping. School-based awareness programs have been shown to reduce suicide attempts and suicidal ideation. The anti-suicidal effects of clozapine and lithium have been substantiated, but might be less specific than previously thought. Effective pharmacological and psychological treatments are important to prevent depression[1]. Insufficient evidence exists to assess the possible benefits for suicide prevention of screening in primary care, in general public education and media guidelines. However, in the quest for effective suicide prevention initiatives, no single strategy clearly stands above the others, which emphasizes the relevance of a global perspective on prevention in each country.

Nonetheless, suicide remains a major health problem: of the 20 countries with the highest global suicide rates, six are European countries. Young adults are particularly at risk, with suicide accounting for 17.6% of all deaths among people aged 15–29 years in high-income countries. It is ranked the second leading cause of death among this age group, both globally and in Europe, following road traffic accidents (WHO 2014b).

32.4 Assessment and Screening

Psychiatric and mental health (P/MH) nurses are highly likely to encounter people who present with an increased risk of suicide and/or self-harm. For this reason, the need for such nurses to be highly familiar with and competent in risk assessment of both suicide risk and risk of self-harm seems both obvious and logical (Cutcliffe and Santos 2012). However, the criterion reference for screening does not need to be suicidal behavior; rather, it can be clinical judgment that actionable risk is present. In contrast, the criterion reference for risk assessment should be suicidal behavior or other important outcomes (Boudreaux and Horowitz 2014).

For a better understanding, we need to distinguish between screening and assessment. According to Boudreaux and Horowitz, screening is performed to detect whether any actionable risk is present, requires easy administration by frontline staff, should be highly sensitive, and should have a strong ability to confidently rule out patients with no appreciable risk, whereas assessment is a more in-depth evaluation performed to further quantify the severity of risk to guide further clinical

[1] In our opinion, as Shneidman (1996, p. 6) said "the best route to understanding suicide is not through the study of mental diseases", however, in this context we respect the findings of these authors.

action (Boudreaux and Horowitz 2014). In this chapter, we elaborate on the notion of suicide risk assessment.

According to the New Zealand Guidelines Group (2003), the Registered Nurses Association of Ontario (2009), and Santos et al. (2012), the psychiatric/psychosocial assessment performed by P/MH nurses should have some guidelines.

Whenever possible, valid (and preferably user-friendly and expeditious) assessment instruments should be used. The Nurses' Global Assessment of Suicide Risk Instrument (NGASR), (Cutcliffe and Barker 2004; Cutcliffe and Santos 2012) which is a simple 15-item scoring scale, can be used to identify suicide risk. It was based on a review of relevant empirical literature which indicated that some variables have a greater effect on suicide risk than others. NGASR has been validated in several countries, namely, the United Kingdom, Canada, Australia, the United States, China, New Zealand, Portugal, the Netherlands, Germany, and Switzerland (Cutcliffe and Barker 2004; Façanha et al. 2016).

However, the nurses' approach should go beyond the assessment and consideration of the individual-level factors. According to Platt et al. (2005),

> individual-level health outcomes cannot be adequately studied by reference to the characteristics of individuals alone. It is also necessary to examine the characteristics of the social groups to which they belong, or the neighborhoods where they live and to acknowledge the interactions between individuals and contexts.

In addition to the use of instruments, an overall assessment should involve a systematic clinical assessment, including clinical interviews, and should also include the clinician's judgment.

32.5 Environment

P/MH nursing staff are primarily responsible for fostering and ultimately creating a therapeutic hospital environment to help decrease the suicide risk and prepare the patient for life outside the hospital setting (Mishara 2007). And this is a very

Box 1 Guidelines for psychiatric/psychosocial assessment performed by P/MH nurses

(a) Identify the acute and chronic psychiatric comorbidities.
(b) Assess the protective and risk factors associated with the behavior.
(c) Identify significant interpersonal problems and conflicts.
(d) Identify social stressors and concerns, such as unemployment and chronic illness.
(e) Identify dysfunctional thinking and behavior patterns.
(f) Consult with the family and friends, whenever possible.
(g) Assess the short-term risk of suicide.
(h) Assess the factors affecting long-term risk.
(i) Assess within a multidisciplinary team.
(j) Prescribe nursing care.

important issue, because patients sometimes die by suicide during hospitalization. In the United Kingdom, the National Confidential Inquiry (NCI) reported that 18,220 psychiatric patients, people who had contact with mental health services in the previous year, had taken their own lives, between 2003 and 2013. The NCI also reported a 73% increase in male patient suicides since 2006, particularly in male patients aged 45–54 years, and that the most common methods of suicide by patients were hanging, self-poisoning, and jumping/multiple injurious behaviors (National Confidential Inquiry into Suicide and Homicide by People with Mental Illness 2015a, b). Inpatient suicides accounted for 10% of psychiatric patient suicides and 2.5% of all suicides in the general population. In England, 20% of inpatient suicides (32 patients) occurred while the patients were absconding from the ward, and a slightly smaller percentage (17% of inpatient suicides) occurred while patients were involuntarily detained. Despite that, inpatient suicides continue to fall (across all countries), including in detained and absconding patients (National Confidential Inquiry into Suicide and Homicide by People with Mental Illness 2013). However, locked doors might not be able to prevent suicide and absconding (Huber et al. 2016). In fact, there were on average 18 suicides by inpatients under observation per year in the United Kingdom over a 7-year study period. Ninety-one percent of deaths under observation occurred under level 2 (intermittent) observation. A third of suicides under observation occurred off the ward. The commonest location for a death by suicide on the ward was the patient's bedroom, and the most frequently used method was hanging. Half of deaths occurred when observation was carried out by less experienced staff or staff who were likely to be unfamiliar with the patient (e.g., health care assistants or agency staff) (National Confidential Inquiry into Suicide and Homicide by People with Mental Illness 2015a, b). Despite the low inpatient suicide rates, nurses are negatively affected by suicide incidents. In a study conducted by Matandela and Matlakala (2016), nurses reported having experienced feelings of disbelief and hopelessness, blame and condemnation, guilt and inadequacy, emotional reactions, and fear of reprisal.

Suicides occur in general and psychiatric hospitals. However, Cheng et al. (2009) found that nonpsychiatric inpatients had less suicide communication, performed suicidal acts more rapidly after admission, and used more violent methods than psychiatric inpatients. This can be partly explained by the lack of experience of the general hospital team members, who are focused on the physical issues. According to Huang et al. (2014), the main reasons for suicide in general hospitals in their study were found to be a diagnosis of a (so-called) mental disorder, requiring money to meet medical expenses, lack of social support, and the hospital environment (Huang et al. 2014). Patients with (so-called) mental disorders appear to have an elevated risk of suicide. Having a serious disease, paying high medical expenses alone, the loss of social support, and unsafe hospital environments are also associated with an increased risk of suicide (Huang et al. 2014). Sakinofsky (2014, p. 131) found that

> the bulk of inpatient suicides actually occur not on the ward but off premises, when the patient was on leave or had absconded. Peaks occur shortly after admission and discharge.

Box 2 Measures associated with a safe environment

- Psychiatric wards with additional safety features (Tishler and Reiss 2009).
- Identify the most appropriate/safest wards and hospitalize suicidal patients accordingly (Lieberman et al. 2004).
- Install bars with breakaway capability, namely, shower curtain rods, closet rods, etc. (Lieberman et al. 2004).
- Redesign or enhance security strategies such as door-locking mechanisms, patient monitors, and alarms (Rose 2000).
- Find alternatives to plastic trash can liners (Rose 2000).
- Use blunt dining utensils and unbreakable plates and glasses (Lieberman et al. 2004).
- Place suicidal patients in rooms closest to the nursing station (Lieberman et al. 2004).
- Install unbreakable glass or plastic mirrors and windows (Lieberman et al. 2004).
- Conduct environmental rounds using active observation skills and a comprehensive checklist of potential environmental hazards (Mills and Bagian 2009).
- Update or establish procedures to educate hospital visitors about their role and patient suicide risks, particularly with regard to providing restricted items to patients (Lieberman et al. 2004).
- Update patient information transfer procedures (Wysocker 2000).
- Eliminate doors when not required by code (Mills and Bagian 2009).
- Install unlockable doors in patient bathrooms (Oregon Association of Hospitals and Health Systems 1999).
- Lock doors that may provide access to sharp objects (Oregon Association of Hospitals and Health Systems 1999).

> The most consistent predictor is a history of attempting suicide, but depressed mood (notably in people with schizophrenia), hopelessness, agitation, anxiety, and impulsivity also feature prominently. The timing of death is of concern, with peaks early on admission and shortly after discharge. It is possible to reduce suicide risk on the ward by having a safe environment, optimizing patient visibility, supervising patients appropriately, careful assessment, awareness of and respect for suicide risk, good teamwork and communication, and adequate clinical treatment.

However, health care teams, particularly P/MH nurses, cannot only focus on the environment, the disease, or risk management; they should rather focus on the patients, their singularity, specificity, and, above all, their ability to cope with the situation and on how nurses might be able to help (Cutcliffe and Santos 2012). Nurses often implement environment management strategies in an excessively defensive way so as to protect the patient's safety and well-being (Simões et al. 2014).

32.6 Evidence-Based Practice

As is well documented in the relevant literature, an important element within the evidenced-based practice movement is the assessment of the evidence for psychotherapeutic interventions; this is one necessary step in the process of achieving best practices. Focusing on the example of talking therapies rather than on

Box 3 Commonalities of effective psychotherapies

1. Being theoretically based and containing a language that is easy to understand.
2. High-risk cases with broad inclusion criteria.
3. Training clinicians well using manualized treatment and providing them with adequate supervision.
4. Treatment focus being specific to suicide rather than other associated symptoms or diagnoses.
5. Plan for compliance and continuity of care.
6. Interventions incorporating education on skill sets such as emotion regulation and problem solving.
7. Emphasis on internal locus of control and personal responsibility.
8. An element of crisis management.

pharmacology, commonalities in the various approaches to psychotherapy have been identified that appear to make psychotherapies effective (Leenaars 2011b). Rudd et al. (2009) and Rogers et al. (2011) (p. 134) identified eight commonalities across some studies.

In a recent Cochrane review on psychosocial interventions for self-harm in adults, Hawton et al. (2016) found that there was a significant treatment effect for cognitive-behavioral-based psychotherapy compared to treatment as usual at final follow-up since fewer participants repeated self-harm. For interventions typically delivered to individuals with a history of multiple episodes of self-harm/probable (so-called) personality disorder, group-based emotion-regulation psychotherapy and mentalization were associated with significantly reduced repetition when compared to treatment as usual. None of the following mixed interventions were associated with reduced repetition of self-harm compared to either alternative forms of psychological therapy: interpersonal problem-solving skills training, behavior therapy, home-based problem-solving therapy, and long-term psychotherapy.

Additionally, in a Cochrane review on the interventions for self-harm in children and adolescents, the same authors found that there are relatively few trials of interventions for children and adolescents who have engaged in self-harm, and only single trials contributed to all but two comparisons in this review. The quality of evidence was mostly very low. There is little support for the effectiveness of group-based psychotherapy for adolescents with multiple episodes of self-harm based on the results of three trials, the evidence from which was of very low quality. The results for therapeutic assessment, mentalization, and dialectical behavior therapy indicated that these approaches warrant further evaluation. Despite the scale of the problem of self-harm in children and adolescents, there is a paucity of evidence of effective interventions (Hawton et al. 2015).

In view of the above, the evidence is still scarce and involves some methodological issues. However, it is perhaps more important for therapists to understand that there are no universal formulations regarding suicide and that the search for a singular universal response is also a foolish and unrealistic fancy (Cutcliffe and Santos 2012). Health professionals must provide a person-centered care, and the patient-therapist relationship should be, in fact, an essential component in the effective psychotherapy with suicidal people (Leenaars 2011a). P/MH nurses should see this as an opportunity, in which interpersonal relationship and engagement are key concepts.

32.7 Core Practices: Latest Evidence

Gilje and Talseth (2014) conducted a meta-analysis on the psychiatric nurses' experiences with suicidal patients and identified four main themes: pondering humanistic and mechanistic views of suicide and suicidal patients, contemplating various responses to life and death encounters, discerning complex competencies while relating therapeutically, and, finally, needing informal and formal support. Care complexity remains an important issue within psychiatric nursing. It is necessary to strengthen interpersonal relationships and validate all interactions, taking into account a collaborative, respectful, and individualized approach, the belief in the person's value, and the practitioner's genuine care and concern (Gordon et al. 2014).

Therapeutic engagement and hope inspiration are key aspects in suicide prevention. Engagement seems to include several processes: forming a relationship (a human-human connection), conveying acceptance and tolerance, and hearing and understanding. Engaging with suicidal clients means to establish a relationship, a human-human connection, between client and nurse (Cutcliffe and Barker 2002), which is essential for an effective approach in this field (Cutcliffe and Santos 2012).

In turn, hope is perceived as a complex and multidimensional construct within the experience of illness and suffering. Regardless of their area of expertise, nurses must seek to inspire hope, exploring the patients' own resources and abilities. Hope has a therapeutic effect on health and well-being, which can be conveyed by reminding patients that, despite adversity or hardship, they can overcome difficulties and live a meaningful and goal-oriented life (Cutcliffe 2004). Despite the limited evidence on hope, Cutcliffe (2009) believes that there may well be formal or shared processes of hope inspiration and simultaneously particularized or nuanced processes of hope inspiration.

Cutcliffe and Stevenson (2007) put forward a three-stage model to reconnect the person with humanity. The first stage "reflecting an image of humanity" is divided into the following categories: experiencing intense, warm, care-based human-to-human contact and implicitly challenging suicidal constructs as a result of encountering contrary experiences. The second stage consists of "guiding the individual back toward humanity," with the following categories: nurturing insight and understanding, supporting and strengthening pre-suicidal beliefs, and encountering a novel interpersonal, helping relationship. Finally, the third stage is "learning to live": accommodating an existential crisis (past, present, and future) and going on in the context set by the existential relationship with suicide.

There are two other types of intervention: developing hope kits and borrowing hope. The hope kit is a tool that P/MH nurses can use as an intentional strategy to help patients identify meaningful images or representations of hope. It can contain items that represent hope to the patient, such as family photographs, music, objects or images with a particular symbolism or meaning, and shared personal experiences, among others. The development of personal hope kits will allow suicidal patients to access meaningful and available resources to help them regain hope and ease or mitigate their suffering and will to die (Moore 2005).

In turn, the strategy called "borrow hope" is based on the idea that hope can be borrowed or shared, without depending completely on the patient's own resources. The development of supportive relationships, the nurse's individual competences, and the inspiration of hope are key aspects that require the nurses' full commitment and self-knowledge. Encouraging patients to reflect on hope and its importance in the illness and recovery process and sharing obstacles that were overcome with and through hope are strategies that can help regain and improve hope (Edey and Jevne 2003).

Nonetheless, the health professional-patient relationship is essential in clinical practice. According to Michel (2011, pp. 9–10), when meeting a suicidal person "the goal for the clinician must be to reach, together with the patient, a shared understanding of the patient's suicidality." Health professionals must be aware that "most suicidal patients suffer from a state of mental pain or anguish and a total loss of self-respect." While interviewing patients, health professionals must adopt a non-judgmental and supportive attitude and "should encourage patients to deliver their self-narratives." Finally, "an approach that does not see patients as objects displaying pathology but as individuals that have their good reasons to perform an act of self-harm will help to strengthen the rapport" and "the ultimate goal should be to engage the patient in a therapeutic relationship, even in a first assessment interview."

According to Shneidman (1996, p. 133), suicidal people

> wish to die and they simultaneously wish to be rescued.

For this reason, the most important questions to be asked to a potentially suicidal person are "where do you hurt?" and "how can I help you?" This can be the first step for a person-centered approach. In addition to an individual approach, some studies reinforce the role played by the family in suicidal behaviors and promote the systemic approach, where the evaluation of the family environment, through expressed emotion, can help professionals to better understand suicidal behaviors and provide robust ideas for intervention (Santos 2014).

Conclusion

Suicide remains a complex behavior and one of the biggest challenges for mental health practitioners, mainly P/MH nurses. Including this issue in our daily lives, fighting against stigma and being person centered will help us improve our practices. A warm, confident, and supportive therapeutic relationship is a key ingredient. However, the question remains: "can we prevent the most mysterious act of the human being?" Successful cases of reducing suicide rates help us believe that it is possible to reduce the overall rates of this phenomenon.

However, to this end, greater political and social awareness, better access to health care services, and best practices are needed. Nurses, particularly P/MH nurses, have increased responsibilities (Santos 2015). Hence, an adequate training and knowledge, a less defensive practice, and more training in psychosocial skills may help suicidal people move from a death-oriented place to a life-orientated place (Cutcliffe and Santos 2012), i.e., make a difference between life and death.

References

Boudreaux E, Horowitz L (2014) Suicide risk screening and assessment. Designing instruments with dissemination in mind. Am J Prev Med 47(3S2):S163–S169

Cheng I, Hu F, Tseng M (2009) Inpatient suicide in a general hospital. Gen Hosp Psychiatry 31:110–115

Clements C, Turnbull P, Hawton K et al (2016) Rates of self-harm presenting to general hospitals: a comparison of data from the multicentre study of self-harm in England and hospital episode statistics. BMJ Open 6:e009749. doi:10.1136/bmjopen-2015-009749

Cutcliffe J (2004) The inspiration of hope in bereavement counselling. Jessica Kingsley Publisher, London

Cutcliffe J (2009) Hope: the eternal paradigm for psychiatric/mental health Nursing. J Psychiatr Ment Health Nurs 16:843–847

Cutcliffe JR, Barker P (2002) Considering the care of the suicidal client and the case for 'engagement and inspiring hope' or observations. J Psychiatr Ment Health Nurs 9(5):611–621

Cutcliffe JR, Barker P (2004) The nurses' global assessment of suicide risk (NGASR): developing a tool for clinical practice. J Psychiatr/Mental Health Nurs 11:393–400

Cutcliffe JR, Santos JC (2012) Suicide and self-harm: an evidence-informed approach. Quay Books, London

Cutcliffe JR, Stevenson C (2007) Care of suicidal person. Elsevier, London

Edey W, Jevne R (2003) Hope, illness, and counseling practice: making hope visible. Can J Couns 37:44–51

Edmondson A, Brennan C, House A (2016) Non-suicidal reasons for self-harm: a systematic review of self-reported accounts. J Affect Disord 191:109–117

Façanha J, Santos JC, Cutcliffe JR (2016) Assessment of suicide risk: validation of the nurses' global assessment of suicide risk index for the Portuguese population. Arch Psychiatr Nurs 30(4):470–475

Gilje F, Talseth A (2014) How psychiatric nurses experience suicidal patients: a qualitative meta-analysis. In: Cutcliffe JR, Santos J, Links PS, Zaheer J, Harder HG, Campbell F, McCormick R, Harder K, Bergmans Y, Eynan R (eds) Routledge international handbook of clinical suicide research. Routledge, Toronto

Gordon E, Stevenson C, Cutcliffe J (2014) Transcending suicidality: facilitating re-vitalizing worthiness. In: Cutcliffe JR, Santos J, Links PS, Zaheer J, Harder HG, Campbell F, McCormick R, Harder K, Bergmans Y, Eynan R (eds) Routledge international handbook of clinical suicide research. Routledge, Toronto

Hawton K, Witt KG, Taylor Salisbury TL, Arensman E, Gunnell D, Townsend E, van Heeringen K, Hazell P. (2015) Interventions for self-harm in children and adolescents. Cochrane Database Syst Rev 2015(12): CD012013. doi:10.1002/14651858.CD012013

Hawton K, Witt KG, Taylor Salisbury TL, Arensman E, Gunnell D, Hazell P, Townsend E, van Heeringen K. (2016) Psychosocial interventions for self-harm in adults. Cochrane Database Syst Rev 2016(5): CD012189. doi:10.1002/14651858.CD012189

Huang D, Hu D, Han Y, Lu C, Lu Y (2014) Five high-risk factors for inpatient suicide. Chin Nurs Res 1:14–16

Huber C, Schneebeerger A, Kowalinski E, Frohlich D, Felten S, Walter M, Zinkler M, Beine K, Heinz A, Borgwart S, Lang U (2016) The national confidential inquiry into suicide and homicide by people with mental illness. Lancet Psychiatry. http://www.thelancet.com/journals/lanpsy/article/PIIS2215-0366(16)30168-7/fulltext

Leenaars A (2011a) Psychotherapy with suicidal people: some common implications for response. In: Michel K, Jobes D (eds) Building a therapeutic alliance with the suicidal patient. American Psychological Association, Washington, DC, pp 231–254

Leenaars A (2011b) Evidence-based psychotherapy with suicidal people. A systematic review. In: Pompili M, Tatarelli R (eds) Evidence-based practice in suicidology. Hogrefe Publications, Toronto, pp 89–123

Lieberman D, Resnik H, Holder-Perkins V (2004) Environmental risk factors in hospital suicide. Suicide Life Threat Behav 34(4):448–453

Mann J, Currier D (2011) Evidence-based suicide prevention strategies: an overview. In: Pompili M, Tatarelli R (eds) Evidence-based practice in suicidology. Hogrefe Publishing, Toronto, pp 67–88

Matandela M, Matlakala M (2016) Nurses' experiences of inpatients suicides in a general hospital. Health SA Gesondheid 21:54–59

Michel K (2011) Introduction. In: Michel K, Jobes D (eds) Building a therapeutic alliance with the suicidal patient. American Psychological Association, Washington, DC, pp 3–10

Mills P, Bagian J (2009) Response to Tishler and Reiss' review of inpatient suicide. Gen Hosp Psychiatry 31:589

Mishara B (2007) Foreword. In: Cutcliffe J, Stevenson C (eds) Care of suicidal person. Elsevier, Edinburgh, pp xiii–xxiv

Moore S (2005) Hope makes a difference. J Psychiatr Ment Health Nurs 12(1):100–105

National Confidential Inquiry into Suicide and Homicide by People with Mental Illness (2013) Annual report 2013. University of Manchester, Manchester

National Confidential Inquiry into Suicide and Homicide by People with Mental Illness (2015a) In-patient suicide under observation. University of Manchester, Manchester

National Confidential Inquiry into Suicide and Homicide by People with Mental Illness (2015b) Annual Report 2015. University of Manchester, Manchester

New Zealand Guidelines Group (2003) The assessment and management of people at risk of suicide: best practice evidence-based guideline. New Zealand Guidelines Group and Ministry of Health, Wellington

Oregon Association of Hospitals and Health Systems (1999) Helpful hints on preventing inpatient suicide. Issues by Topic, December 1999

Pitman A, Osborn D, King M, Erlangsen A (2014) Effects of suicide bereavement on mental health and suicide risk. Lancet Psychiatry 1:86–94

Platt S, Davis S, Sharpe M, O'May F (2005) Contextual effects in suicidal behaviour: evidence explanation and implications. In: Hawton K (ed) Prevention and treatment of suicidal behaviour: from science to practice. Oxford University Press, Oxford, pp 53–70

Registered Nurses Association of Ontario (2009) Assessment and care of adults at risk for suicidal ideation and behaviour: nursing best practice guideline shaping the future of nursing. RNAO, Toronto, p 2009

Rogers J, Madura T, Hardy J (2011) Evidence-based psychosocial interventions for suicidal behavior. In: Pompili M, Tatarelli R (eds) Evidence-based practice in suicidology. Hogrefe Publishing, Toronto, pp 125–138

Rose N (2000) Six years' experience in Oxford: review of serious incidents. Psychiatr Bull 24:243–246

Rudd M, Joinier T, Trotter D, Williams B, Cordero L (2009) The psychosocial treatment of suicidal behavior: a critique of what we know (and don't know). In: Kleespies PM (ed) Behavioral emergencies. American Psychological Association, Washington, pp 339–350

Sakinofsky I (2014) Preventing suicide among inpatients. Can J Psychiatr 59(3):131–140

Santa Mina EE, Gallop R (1998) Childhood sexual and physical abuse and adult self-harm and suicidal behaviour: a literature review. Can J Psychiatr 43(8):793–800

Santos J (2014) Expressed emotion and suicidal behaviors. In: Cutcliffe JR, Santos J, Links PS, Zaheer J, Harder HG, Campbell F, McCormick R, Harder K, Bergmans Y, Eynan R (eds) Routledge international handbook of clinical suicide research. Routledge, Toronto, pp 63–76

Santos J (2015) Suicide: can we prevent the most mysterious act of the human being? Revista Portuguesa de Enfermagem de Saúde Mental, Número: Especial, 2, 1ª edn. ASPESM, Porto, pp 7–8

Santos J, Façanha J, Gonçalves M, Erse M, Cordeiro R, Simões R (2012) Guia Orientador de Boas Práticas Para a Prevenção de Sintomatologia Depressiva e Comportamentos da Esfera Suicidária, 1ª edn. Ordem dos Enfermeiros, Lisboa

Santos J, Erse M, Façanha J, Marques L, Simões R (2014) Contigo: promoção de saúde mental e prevenção de comportamentos suicidários na comunidade educativa – Número: 9, Série Monográfica, 1ª edn. Escola Superior de Enfermagem de Coimbra, Coimbra

Shneidman ES (1985) Definition of suicide. Wiley, New York

Shneidman E (1996) The suicidal mind. Oxford University Press, Oxford

Simões R, Erse M, Façanha J, Santos J (2014) Enfermagem em suicidologia – Suicídio e comportamentos autolesivos, 1ª edn. Lidel, Lisboa, pp 193–202. isbn:978-989-752-042-6, Depósito legal: 371456/14

Tishler C, Reiss N (2009) Inpatient suicide: preventing a common sentinel event. Gen Hosp Psychiatry 31:103–109

Värnik P, Sisask M, Värnik A, Laido Z, Meise U, Ibelshaüser A, van Audenhove C, Reynders A, Kocalevent R, Kopp M, Dosa A, Arensman E, Coffey C, van der Feltz-Cornelis C, Gusmão R, Hegerl U (2010) Suicide registration in eight European countries: a qualitative analysis of procedures and practices. Forensic Sci Int 202(2010):86–92

Värnik P, Sisask M, Värnik A, Arensman E, van Audenhove C, van der Feltz-Cornelis C, Hegerl U (2012) Validity of suicide statistics in Europe in relation to undetermined deaths: developing the 2-20 benchmark. Inj Prev 18(5):321–325

Wampold B (1997) Methodological problems in identifying efficacious psychotherapies. Psychother Res 7:21–43

WHO (2013) Mental health action plan 2013–2020. Switzerland, Geneva

WHO (2014a) Preventing suicide: a global imperative. Switzerland, Geneva

WHO (2014b) Data and statistics. In: WHO/Europe [website]. Copenhagen: WHO regional office for Europe; 2014. http://www.euro.who.int/en/health-topics/noncommunicable-diseases/mentalhealth/data-and-statistics. Accessed 09 Dec 2014

Wysocker A (2000) Suicide: risk management strategies. J Am Psychiatr Nurses Assoc 5(5):164–166

Zalsman G, Hawton K, Wasserman D, van Heeringen K, Arensman E, Sarchiapone M, Carli V, Höschl C, Barzilay R, Balazs J, Purebl G, Kahn J, Sáiz P, Lipsicas C, Bobes J, Cozman D, Hegerl U, Zohar J (2016) Suicide prevention strategies revisited: 10-year systematic review. Lancet Psychiatry 3:646–659

A Systematic Perspective of Violence and Aggression in Mental Health Care: Toward a More Comprehensive Understanding and Conceptualization

33

John R. Cutcliffe and Sanaz Riahi

33.1 Introduction and Background

Aggression and violence (A/V) in inpatient mental health care are an all too frequent occurrence with evidence indicating between 10% and 30% hospitalized psychiatric clients having engaged in violence prior to admission (Bjorkly 1995; Davison 2005). Similarly, the survey evidence, limitations notwithstanding, reveals that psychiatric/mental health (P/MH) nurses frequently encounter A/V incidents in their practice (UKCC 2001; Powell and Lloyd 2002; Whittington and Ritcher 2006a, b). The prevalence of A/V continues to rise internationally among healthcare professionals including nurses (UKCC 2001; Wells and Bowers 2002; Bourne 2003; Kynoch et al. 2009; Hahn et al. 2010). A/V have been linked with a number of documented outcomes: it places inpatient P/MH nurses at an increased risk for injury and/or low morale (Wykes 1994; Beech and Leather 2008; Nijman et al. 2005a); it leads to psychological and physical consequences (Foster et al. 2007; Hahn et al. 2010), increased absenteeism (Nijman et al. 2005a, b; Foster et al. 2007), increased staff turnover (Luckhoff et al. 2012), reduced job motivation (Arnetz and Arnetz 2001; Needham et al. 2005; Hahn et al. 2010), more 'fear-based' responses to clients who present with A/V issues (Duxbury 2002), and increased avoidance with, fewer interactions with clients (Michie and West 2004; Luckhoff et al. 2012);

J.R. Cutcliffe (✉)
Cutcliffe Consulting, Kingston, Canada

School of Nursing, Coimbra, Portugal
e-mail: jcutcliffe@outlook.com

S. Riahi
Director, Professional Practice, Clinical Information and Adolescent Services, Ontario Shores Mental Health, Ontario, Canada

© Springer International Publishing Switzerland 2018

J.C. Santos, J.R. Cutcliffe (eds.), *European Psychiatric/Mental Health Nursing in the 21st Century*, Principles of Specialty Nursing,
https://doi.org/10.1007/978-3-319-31772-4_33

it contributes to lower client satisfaction scores (Meehan et al. 2000; Abderhalden et al. 2006) and is very expensive (LeBel and Goldstein 2005).

While there appears to be a broad consensus as to the severity of this issue, there are conversely two areas where the absence of a consensus bedevils our efforts to tackle the problem, namely, (a) in definitions, conceptualizations, and the associated nomenclature of A/V in mental health care and (b) how we, as P/MH nurses and practitioners, should respond to and best manage A/V incidents (Lau et al. 2005; Riahi 2011). With regard to the first of these, even a cursory review of the extant literature illustrates that there is a great deal of ambiguity and inconsistency in definitions of A/V (Rippon 2000; Whittington 2000; Duxbury 2002; Bjorkly 2006), in what does/does not constitute a violent incident, let alone the well-documented difficulty in differentiating between incidents apparently motivated by so-called madness or badness (Cutcliffe 1999). A universally accepted definition of mental health-related A/V is therefore currently not available. And with regard to the second, the relevant theoretical and empirical literature in this area can be delineated into two broad positions (see also Bjorkdahl et al. 2010): One that emphasizes containment responses/measures posits the primacy of safety and security, maintaining order and enforcing rules/setting limits. The other approach is concerned with minimizing stress/demands/pressures made of clients; listening and understanding even when presented with angry, potentially violent clients; minimizing coercion; and perhaps ultimately moving toward the restraint-free mental health-care system(s) advocated for by the American Psychiatric Nurses Association (2007).

While there are encouraging signs within the literature that indicate that our understanding of A/V in inpatient mental health is clearly deepening and that there is a growing realization that the 'responsibility' for A/V incidents can rarely be attributed exclusively to the individual client (see, for instance, Nijman 2002; De Benedictis et al. 2011), there is also still an abundance of evidence that shows this position is still pervasive for some (NICE 2004; Davison 2005; Papadopoulos et al. 2012). P/MH nurses and other professionals frequently locate the causation, blame, and responsibility for the A/V with the client (Duxbury 1999; Duxbury 2002; Duxbury and Whittington 2005), while their own actions are seldom seen as contributing to causing A/V. Such a situation leads Stuart (Stuart 2003a, b, p. 122) to argue that:

"A serious limitation of clinical explanations of violent and disruptive behavior is their focus on the attributes of the mental illness and the mentally ill to the exclusion of social and contextual factors that interact to produce violence in clinical settings."

In response to these views, it needs to be acknowledged that there are a wide range of phenomena that linked to inpatient mental health A/V. As a result, what we intend to accomplish with this chapter is:

(a) Recognize and document the wide range of phenomena that have been found to have an association with A/V in inpatient mental health care and, in so doing, follow Meleis' (2007) and, more latterly, Cutcliffe et al.'s (2010) approach to model generation and development in nursing.
(b) Synthesize these propositions according to fit or congruence into a systemic model of A/V.

(c) Explore the empirical evidence pertaining to each of these propositions.
(d) Begin to consider application of this model to better inform our individual and/or organizational responses to A/V in mental health care.

In our discussion, the authors advance the argument that unless attention is paid to the associations and propositions that exist for A/V and all the identified phenomena, then efforts to reduce A/V will only have limited success.

33.2 Moving from Phenomena to Concepts to Propositions: A Summary of the Approach to Model Development

Meleis (2007) and more recently Cutcliffe et al. (2010) describe an approach to the development of models and theories in nursing which begins with noticing and naming phenomena. In the case of A/V in inpatient mental health care, numerous scholars, researchers, and clinicians have been engaging in this practice for many years, arguably beginning in the 1920s with Freud's psychoanalytical theories (Freud 1920). This has resulted in the proliferation of identified and named A/V--related concepts. Drawing on and refining the approach adopted in Nijman's (2002) work on advancing multifaceted models of A/V, the next step in Meleis' (2007) approach is to look for propositions wherein this refers to two or more concepts 'joined' together in some way. For example, the authors posited that there is a relationship between A/V in mental health care and (a) the physical environment in which the care is delivered; (b) the individual intrapersonal, client-related phenomena; and (c) the particular, more capacious mental health-care system and individual clinician-related phenomena. Meleis (2007) illustrates how propositions can be explored by asking the following questions: How does it happen? Why does it happen? When does it happen? Where does it happen? And who does it happen to? By answering these questions, the theoretician engages in the process of building a model or theory, because models and theories are simply a collection of propositions (Meleis 2007; Cutcliffe et al. 2010). In this instance, the authors applied such questions to the phenomena of A/V in inpatient mental health care and this allowed them to identify further propositions (e.g., the extent and nature of noise has a relationship with A/V in mental health care). Meleis (2007) explains how this enables propositions to be further developed, linked with other propositions, explained and/or depicted as a model, and, ultimately, tested. The authors then reference empirical work for each of the propositions they have included (Fig. 33.1).

33.3 Environmental-Related Phenomena

In this quadrant, the authors are referring to the physical setting/environment and structure of the care setting—not the interpersonal environment or 'milieu.' There There are a range of environmental phenomena that are linked with A/V in mental health care (Daffern et al. 2004; Chaplin et al. 2006; UKCC 2001; Whittington and

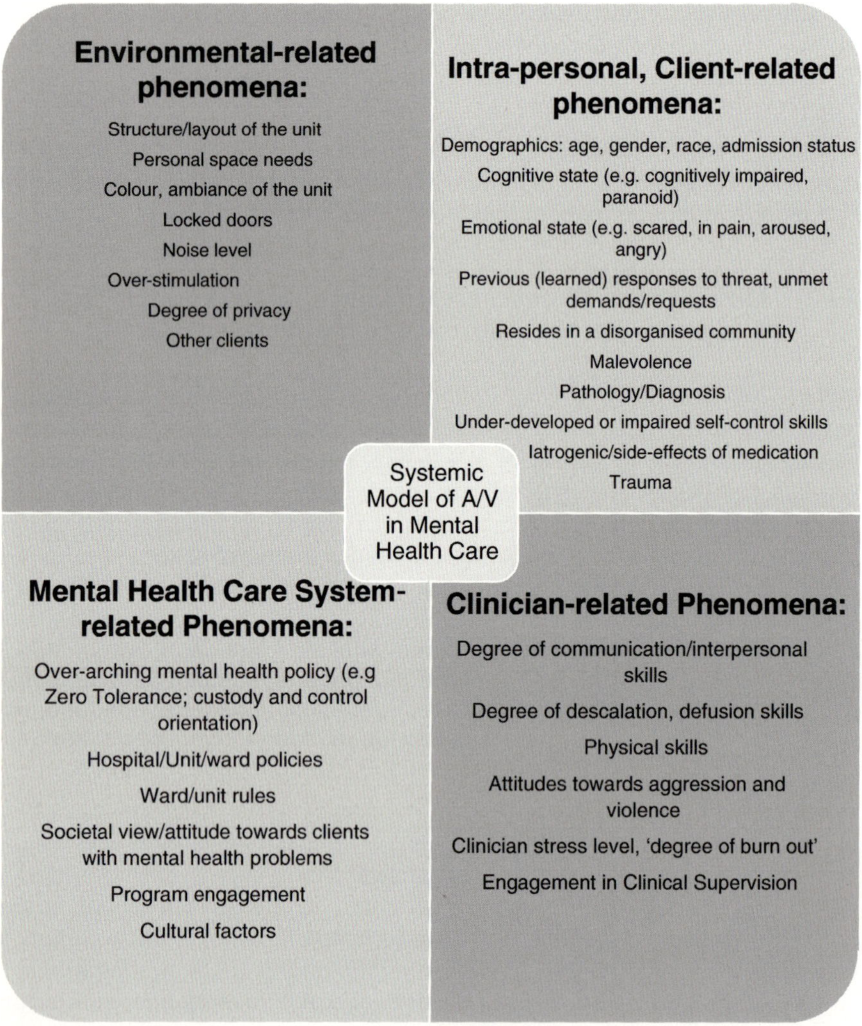

Fig. 33.1 Systemic model of phenomena that can contribute to A/V in mental health care

Ritcher 2006a, b), though the precise nature of these relationships remains uncertain. The knowledge base and associated body of work in this area has increased substantially over recent years and this is most welcome, especially when one considers the argument that environmental phenomena can be important determinants or contributing factors to A/V in psychiatric inpatient settings (Berkowitz 1993; Kayne et al. 1994; Duxbury et al. 2006).

A physical structure or ward design/layout that maximizes and provides for (personal) space, privacy, and freedom to move around and avoid overcrowding appears to be suggested by the limited evidence given that most A/V incidents have been reported to occur where the propensity for overcrowding and/or unrequited interpersonal contact is most likely, e.g., communal areas (see Ryden et al. 1991; Krakowski and Czobar 1994; Grassi et al. 2001; Ng et al. 2001). These earlier findings are corroborated in the more recent UK National Audit on Violence undertaken by the Royal College of Psychiatrists (Chaplin et al. 2006) who found that the design of many wards/units failed to meet many basic safety standards, that overcrowding and high bed occupancy figures are leading to increased numbers of A/V incidents, and/or that such incidents are not managed effectively when they occur. Similar findings have been discovered in correctional facilities (Southern Center for Human Rights 2012). However, as stated earlier, the precise nature of this relationship remains unclear; Nijman and Rector's (1999) study of crowding and aggression, for example, found only a modest correlation between the number of patients on the ward and number of aggressive incidents per patient, and that enlargement of the physical space available to patients midway through the study did not lead to a significant decline in incidents.

There appears to be little doubt that aversive stimulation can have a profound effect on A/V. Whittington and Ritcher (Whittington and Ritcher 2006a, b, p. 51) advance the view that:

> "Many aspects of the environment in which the ward-based patient finds himself or herself are unpleasant and much of the behavior of the patient in this setting is an understandable response to the aversive experience of being on the ward."

Sensory, 'Snoezelen rooms' (Champagne and Stromberg 2004; Champagne 2006; Champagne and Sayer 2012) and 'comfort rooms' (Cummings et al. 2010) as a means to help reduce aversive stimuli currently have limited empirical support, but the emerging evidence that does exist strongly supports the use of such rooms in inpatient mental health settings as a way to reduce A/V incidents, lower rates of seclusion, and restraint and improve client satisfaction (Champagne and Stromberg 2004; Champagne 2006; Champagne and Sayer 2012).

The environmental component of noise needs also to be considered. The previously referenced National Audit on Violence attempted to explore the possible relationship between noise and violent incidents. Service users and visitors were asked to describe anything that they felt 'triggered' violent incidents on their ward/unit and their answers indicated excessive noise: both expected noise, such as radios and people shouting, and unexpected noise, such as squeaking doors, doorbells ringing, and other service users being allowed to make noise late at night. In addition one also needs to acknowledge the limited evidence vis a vis noise and mental health problem per se. Berglund and Lindvall's (Berglund and Lindvall 1995) study published by the World Health Organization (WHO), for instance, declared that while environmental noise does not appear to cause mental health problems directly, there is evidence to suggest that it can accelerate and intensify the development of latent mental health problems. They conclude that 'community noise' may have adverse effects on mental health.

A further structural, environmental variable that appears to have a substantive relationship with rates of A/V is that of psychiatric units having locked doors. The limited literature is clear in highlighting an increasing widespread trend toward more locked doors. This is particularly evident in the United Kingdom (Adams 2000; Van Der Merwe et al. 2009) with more psychiatric facilities adopting 'locked door' practices that are already commonplace and widespread in North America. This is an interesting development given that, historically, the influence was moving in the opposite direction – with North American psychiatric facilities showing interest in the British-paradigm 'open door' policy (see Voineskos 1976), in addition to the view which Adams (2000, p. 327) reports, namely, that:

> "The 'wholesale unlocking' of mental hospital wards in the 1960s is described as being the most important single change in the milieu of the psychiatric hospital at that time."

There is a distinct paucity of literature in this area; the body of work that we do have is mostly descriptive, survey research and/or inconclusive (see Van Der Merwe et al. 2009). The large-scale 'City 128' (Bowers 2007) contained some qualitative and quantitative data pertaining to locked doors. Their qualitative, interview data indicated that locking the door made patients frustrated, angry, irritable, and more likely to be aggressive and refuse treatment. Their quantitative data showed the locked door was associated with an 11% increased risk of physical aggression to others, 25% elevated risk of aggression to objects, and was associated with more self-harm. Other surveys of views toward locked doors on inpatient wards, methodological limitations notwithstanding, are inconclusive. Haglund et al.'s (Haglund et al. 2006) qualitative study of 20 mental health nurses and 20 mental health nursing assistants revealed 8 categories of advantages and 18 categories of disadvantages. Nurses and mental health nurse assistants mentioned more disadvantages than advantages, and nurses mentioned more disadvantages than mental health nurse assistants. While the findings are inconclusive as to the relationship between locked doors and inpatient A/V, the nurses surveyed appeared to acknowledge the increased sense of confinement and emotional problems that can be experienced by clients when doors are locked (Haglund et al. 2006; see also Bowers et al. 2010). Accordingly, while there appears to be recognition of a possible causal relationship between locked doors, and the increased sense of confinement, loss of freedom etc., and the potential for an increase in violent incidents, we currently lack the data to support or refute this proposed connection.

A further environmental variable associated with increasing risk of violence and aggression is a lack of privacy (Davison 2005). The Royal College of Psychiatrists National Audit on Violence (Chaplin et al. 2006) and MIND (2004) highlighted the widespread problem with (lack of) privacy. The audit (Chaplin et al. 2006) asked the question of service users: can you think of anything that 'triggers' violent behavior on the ward/unit? The third most common response highlighted space, overcrowding, and lack of privacy.

For the authors the most disconcerting finding pertaining to environmental factors is that, despite the historical and contemporary evidence that illustrates the relationship between the physical environment of the psychiatric facility and incidents of A/V, the actual individuals who 'live' and work in these environments are seldom—if ever—consulted by the unit architects, designers, and hospital managers/administrators (Zborowsky et al. 2010; MIND 2006). Serious and comprehensive efforts and/or programs to help reduce A/V in mental health care must be mindful of the physical/structural environment and what can be done to produce an environment that is therapeutic, or at the very least produce an environment that minimizes aversive stimuli. This in part clearly requires consultation with the very people who live/work on the unit.

33.4 Client-Related (Intrapersonal) Phenomena

In this quadrant, the authors are referring to the range of phenomena associated with the client and/or 'within' the client. Whittington and Ritcher (Whittington and Ritcher 2006a, b) highlight how epidemiologically focused approaches to understanding A/V that situate demographic, clinical, and aggression phenomena 'within' the client or as 'intrapersonal' phenomena are commonplace. Numerous studies (see Johnson 2004; Davison 2005 for relatively recent and useful reviews of this extant work) have explored possible links between demographic phenomena and A/V such as age, gender, and race, and the findings are both equivocal and inconsistent. In many respects, the authors argue that these are entirely intuitively logical findings. Such models of A/V causality (e.g., males are more violent than females) fail to take into account any/all of the situational, contextual, historical, interpersonal, and cultural phenomena that can have a significant influence on rates of A/V. Studies have been undertaken regarding the possible link between admission status (i.e., admitted and/or detained against one's will) and A/V (Georgieva et al. 2012). Again, these findings are also intuitively logical in that higher rates of A/V are associated with involuntarily status (Kho et al. 1998; Nijman et al. 2002; Johnson 2004; Davison 2005). Whether this is a feature of or reaction to being detained against one's will per se or merely symptomatic of the type of individual and the clinical situation that he/she/they present, who most frequently require forced hospitalization, remains unclear.

The extant literature indicates a relationship between an individual's particular emotional state, mood, experience of pain, and resultant propensity for an A/V reaction(s) (Sweet and Mills 1997; Krakowski and Czobar 1999; Tang et al. 2008). Simplistically said, people in pain often have a "shorter fuse," less ability to tolerate stress and frustration, and thus have an increased risk of A/V reactions. There is also robust evidence that indicates how other "mental states" (e.g., feeling scared, experiencing paranoia, having a high degree of cognitive impairment) can have a significant influence on the increased risk of A/V. The presence and influence of certain psychotic delusions/hallucinations—especially if these are of a persecutory nature, contain content that leads to clients feeling threatened, and/or had a "command" element to their content – were repeatedly found in studies during the 1990s to indicate increased risk of A/V (Whittington and Ritcher 2006a, b). However interestingly, even in this area, more recent studies have produced equivocal results.

Numerous studies have demonstrated an association of A/V among individuals who have experienced some form of trauma (Felitti et al. 1998; Huckshorn 2004, 2006; LeBel and Goldstein 2005; LeBel 2011). Indeed, such is the significance of this emerging evidence that within the United States, the Substance Abuse and Mental Health Service Administration (recovered 2013) established a National Center for Trauma-Informed Care in 2005. Trauma has demonstrated neurological, biological, psychological, and social effects, as well as adoption of "risky" behaviors, such as A/V as a coping strategy (Felitti et al. 1998). The prevalence of trauma among mental health consumers has been reported to be as high as 90% (Champagne and Stromberg 2004; Rosenberg et al. 2001) and therefore integrating trauma-informed care practices are evidently significant in the preventative strategies of A/V. Although limited in number, the extant studies describing implementation of elements of trauma-informed care principles have reported reduced incidents of A/V and use of controlled interventions (such as restraints and seclusion) (Barton et al. 2009; Azeem et al. 2011; Chandler 2012; Goetz and Taylor-Trujillo 2012).

The 'fight or flight' response when an organism experiences a sense of threat—which can be real or imagined—is very well documented. Similarly, cognitive impairment whether organic and/or chronic in nature (e.g., learning disability, dementia) or temporary (e.g., acute confusional state, drug induced 'high', inebriated) has been linked repeatedly with increased risk of A/V (Powell et al. 1994; Owen et al. 1998a, b; Turnbull 1999; Stuart 2003a, b; Elbogen and Johnson 2009). There appears to be a particularly increased risk of A/V, when clients engage in substance/alcohol use/misuse (Douglas et al. 2009). Indeed, Hiday's (2006) critique of reported correlations between (so-called) severe mental illness and violence found that clients with a major mental disorder with no substance/alcohol use were three times less likely to be violent to those clients who did use drugs/alcohol. While this was a study of community—not inpatient populations – it is also noteworthy that clients who did not use alcohol/substances were not significantly more likely to be violent than the community "controls" and much less likely to be violent than community controls who did use drugs/alcohol. Tentative conclusions can be drawn from this work which clearly suggest that substance/drug use is significantly more of a risk factor for A/V than a so-called major mental health disorder. However, the risks posed by using drugs/alcohol when one has a history of major mental health problems should be acknowledged.

A significant portion of people who present to formal inpatient mental health facilities may have underdeveloped and/or incomplete developmental stages (and any associated 'tasks') and historical and experiential backgrounds that leave them with inadequate, ineffective, and/or inappropriate self-control, violence-moderating, abilities; this is likely to be the case when a client resides (currently or historically) in a "disorganized community" (Hiday 2006, p. 320/1). Indeed, a compelling case can be made that equipping or helping clients to develop these abilities or 'correct' whatever formative experiences/perceptions that contribute to an increased propensity for A/V could be regarded as one of the key functions of a mental health-care system. One only has to examine the vast array of interventions and programs that exist as attempts to modify, change, replace, alter, and reform the client's thoughts, perceptions, feelings, and resultant behavior to understand the legitimacy of this point. This key argument warrants further exploration. Firstly, one should acknowledge that the precise mechanism(s) of A/V are not comprehensively understood. Several theories, some more robust than others, have been advanced such as psychoanalytical theory (Freud 1920), drive theory (Dullard et al. 1939), and social learning theory (Bandura 1973). It is not within the scope of this paper to attempt to endorse one theory 'over' another, but examination of these theories shows they appear to have something in common. The theories posit that if certain tasks, functions, stages, etc. are not undertaken or completed, then this can give rise to problems with A/V in later life. For instance, Freud (1920) argued that if a person's aggressive impulses are not connected and intertwined with "love," then one could expect increased aggression and destructive behaviors from the individual. Alternatively, building on Freud's ideas, Bowlby (1989) advanced the idea that frustrated or unrequited early attachment needs in the child can and do lead to amplified and/or exaggerated distressed behavior, including A/V behavior, in the adult (see also Fonagy's 2003 work). Dullard et al.'s (1939) 'drive theory' similarly posits the causal relationship between A/V behavior and frustrated/unmet needs, goal-oriented activities. Interestingly, this theory alludes to the cumulative effect of repeated unmet needs/demands and increased risk for A/V, findings that have been reinforced/reiterated in recent studies (McDonnell and Gallon 2006). More recently, Bandura's work on the social learning theory of violence declares that A/V can be learned/acquired, vicariously, by observing and imitating the behaviors of others. Accordingly, if the person is not exposed to 'healthy' models of behavior, then this can and does give rise to acquired and reinforced models of A/V behavior. It may also be worthy of mention that learned responses and acquired behaviors vis a vis A/V can also occur within mental health facilities themselves.

Additional and compelling evidence of the potentially powerful effects of social learning and its effects of A/V can be seen in if one examines the client's socioeconomic background, whether or not the client has grown up or resides in what is termed a "disorganized community" (Hiday 2006, p. 320/1). Hiday's review found that:

"multiple empirical studies provide evidence that mental illness, substance abuse, violence and other deviant behaviors are more frequent in socially disadvantaged communities."

Hiday continues stating that:

> "Persons with severe mental illness who grow up and live in these communities learn to be violent just as everyone else."

And perhaps the most telling finding in this area is that reported by Silver (2000), Silver et al. (2002) and Swanson et al. (2002) who found that living in such socially disorganized communities/neighborhoods significantly raises the likelihood of violence above the likelihood predicted by individual risk factors.

A further intrapersonal variable that has a possible relationship with increased A/V is that of unwanted side effects of some/many psychotropic medications. It is well documented that many commonly used psychotropic drugs can give rise to unwanted iatrogenic effects including akathisia, increased agitation, and increased restlessness (Healy 2005; Kumar and Sachdev 2009). Any comprehensive model of A/V in mental health care then needs to be cognizant of these effects and their potential to contribute to increased risk. Interestingly, the service user literature reporting users' views, perceptions, and experiences of A/V is fairly consistent in highlighting this as a potential variable. Interestingly, findings related to these possible interactions rarely show up in the corresponding practitioner-focused findings and/or literature.

33.5 Mental Health-Care System-Related Phenomena

In this quadrant, the authors are referring to the factors that are related to the culture, customs, and practice of the particular mental health-care organization. Further, this quadrant also includes broader, cultural, societally based, and/or national mental health-care policies and positions. In contemporary occidental society, there is an almost automatic association between people experiencing mental health problems (or the so-called mentally ill) and violence per se (Cutcliffe and Hannigan 2001; Mullen 2001; Hannigan and Cutcliffe 2002; Stuart 2003a, b; Elbogen and Johnson 2009; Fazel et al. 2009). A recent nationwide study in the United Kingdom found that 34% of those surveyed expect the person with mental health problems to be violent (Department of Health 2007). Yet such perceptions are clearly at odds with the majority of the empirical evidence in this area. While methodological challenges and limitations in this area need to be acknowledged, studies tend to show either a decline in the rates of violence perpetrated by individuals with mental health problems or that findings are equivocal and inconclusive. Though some studies have found a clear statistical association between certain diagnoses and higher risk of A/V (see, e.g., Mullen 2001; Fazel and Grann 2006), other studies do not (see, e.g., the often cited study conducted by Bonta et al. 1998), and there remains a distinct lack of consistency across and between these findings (Steinert 2006). Schizophrenia, for example, has been found in some studies to indicate increased risk (Krakowski and Czobar 1999; Ehmann et al. 2001) and inversely to indicate no increase in risk in others (Walker and Seifert 1994; Grossman et al. 1995). Mania has been found to have an association with increased risk of A/V (Kho et al. 1998), but perhaps counterintuitively, depression has also been linked with increased risk of certain types of A/V.

The UK National Confidential Enquiry into Homicides and Suicides by Mentally Ill People (Appleby 1997) and Taylor and Gunn's (1999) critique indicated that contrary to the public misperceptions regarding violence and the (so-called) mentally ill, the percentage of homicides committed by mentally disordered people has declined over the last 40 years. Elbogen and Johnson's (2009) paper on the results from the National Epidemiological Survey on Alcohol and Related Conditions in the United States found very similar results. They discovered that so-called severe mental illness *IS NOT (our emphasis)* a robust predictor of future violence. People experiencing so-called severe mental illness report histories and environmental stressors associated with elevated risk of violence and that so-called severe mental illness alone *is not* (our emphasis) an independent contributor to explaining violence. They conclude that:

> "As severe mental illness was itself was not found shown to sequentially precede violent acts, the findings challenge perceptions that severe mental illness is a foremost cause of violence among society at large. The data shows it is simplistic as well as inaccurate to say the cause of violence among mentally ill individuals is the mental illness itself; instead, the current study finds that mental illness is clearly relevant to violence risk but that its causal roles are complex, indirect and embedded in a web of other relevant (arguably more) important individual and situational co-factors." (Elbogen and Johnson 2009, p. 159)

So, while prudence dictates that one acknowledges that mental pathology and/or certain diagnoses appear to be linked with some increased risk of A/V and that some of the evidence in this area does support a small association between mental health challenges and A/V (Stuart 2003a, b), there is an argument and a corresponding body of literature which indicates how we may have overexaggerated this risk and that there may be more important individual and situational phenomena (see also Hiday 2006).

One suggestion that is often advanced as a solution to inflated rates of A/V is to increase the number of nurses on the unit; to increase the ratio of clinical staff to clients, indeed Mason and Chandley (2002, p. 82) describe an:

"automatic call for an increase in staff as though quantity equates with safety."

Nevertheless, the existing, albeit limited, research evidence does not provide robust support for this response. Several reviews have reached the same conclusion, namely that the evidence in this area provides a mixed, confusing picture (Mason and Chandley 2002; Johnson 2004; Duxbury 2002). A handful of studies, both those of a noted vintage (Carmel and Hunter 1989) and more recently published (Chou et al. 2002), did find that higher ratios of clients to staff were related to more A/V incidents; however these papers 'cloud' this issue even more so as the findings can also be interpreted to indicate that that higher staffing levels are a response to rather than an antecedent of A/V. Other studies have found the opposite, that higher ratios of staff to clients were not related to higher rates of A/V (Morrison 1990; Owen et al. 1998a, b).

A more sophisticated analysis of this proposition seems to indicate that the relationship may have more to do with the *type of nurses rather than the number of nurses in proportion to the clients* (our emphasis). For instance, Owen et al. (1998a, b) indicate that three particular staff ratio-related phenomena have repeatedly been found to have a statistically significant positive correlation with increased rates of A/V incidents. These three phenomena are:

(a) Having a nursing staff compliment that includes more male nursing staff
(b) Having a staff compliment where more nurses do not have specialist psychiatric/mental health training or where nursing staff have not undergone specific education or training in dealing with/responding to A/V incidents
(c) Having wards that have higher rates of staff absenteeism

Inversely, wards with higher numbers of younger nursing staff and nurses with higher levels of specialist psychiatric expertise were found to have a statistically significant negative correlation with increased incidence of A/V incidents. Accordingly, while the degree of confounding findings in the limited literature in this area do not allow firm conclusions to be drawn regarding the "ideal" nursing staff to patient ratios, there is some evidence to indicate that having sufficient numbers of the "right" (e.g., much higher proportions of specialist P/MH nurses or nurses with specialist psychiatric education/training, higher numbers of younger staff) staff can make a difference.

There is a body of evidence pertaining to ward (and/or hospital) rules and incidents of A/V, and the evidence is currently insufficient to allow firm conclusions to be drawn. What can be stated, with a degree of empirical confidence, is that client reactions to rules or regimes have been frequently highlighted as a particular and significant antecedence to A/V incidents (Powell et al. 1994; Nijman et al. 1999; Duxbury 2002; Nijman 2002; Alexander and Bowers 2004; Davison 2005). Numerous authors have highlighted how mental health client A/V incidents are frequently triggered by unmet client requests/demands, power struggles, and/or controlling staff behavior (McDonnell and Gallon 2006; Papadopoulos et al. 2012). There is also ample anecdotal and narrative evidence that indicates how if there are cumulative incidents or episodes of unmet client requests/demands, power struggles, and/or controlling staff behavior, then the risk of A/V appears to increase. Whittington and Ritcher's (Whittington and Ritcher 2006a, b) work adds support to this view. There is also evidence indicating that inconsistency in the application of ward rules, or if the rules are communicated in a manner that conveys a sense of concern for the client's well-being, can have an influence on A/V incidents. It is important not to conflate ward/unit rules per se with ward structure, ward routine, and especially with structured, meaningful ward activities. High levels of boredom have been linked with increased rates of A/V in mental health units (UKCC 2001; Davison 2005; Duxbury 2002). Structured ward activities that have therapeutic value and involve meaningful and therapeutic interactions with staff appear to have a high degree of utility, not only in terms of their value regarding reducing rates of A/V. Frustration at the lack of activities can be one of the triggers for violence (National Institute for Clinical Excellence 2004; Chaplin et al. 2006).

In addition to ward or hospital level phenomena, are the broader, cultural, and/or federal (national) level policies to consider and their relationship with A/V in mental health care. By way of an example, the authors wish to highlight a policy purportedly designed to reduce and eradicate A/V: the policy of "zero tolerance" (UKCC 2001; Cowman 2006). The term "zero tolerance" can be traced back to the cities of New York and New Jersey on the east coast of the United States where it was inextricably tied to attempts to reduce or eradicate violence, vandalism, and public disorder offenses. It posits a largely untested model (and certainly untested model in inpatient mental health care) whereby if the relevant "authorities" do not respond harshly to the "minor offenses," then they are indirectly or inadvertently encouraging further (and usually escalating in severity) crimes. Leaving aside for the moment the absence of evidence in inpatient mental health care regarding the efficacy (or otherwise) of "zero tolerance" and the more broad criticism that "zero tolerance" is an ineffective response to violence in health-care settings (Holmes 2006), the idea of unthinkingly and unquestioningly transplanting this model into mental health care misses an axiomatic truth. "Zero tolerance" places all the responsibility for the A/V within or on the individual client and takes no account of the significant and wide range of other phenomena that can and do have more influence of rates of A/V. Not only is this inaccurate but the preponderance of evidence indicates that clients may have only a "minor" role. Whittington and Ritcher (Whittington and Ritcher 2006b, p. 49) offer similar remarks when they state:

> Actually, a patient's individual neurobiology and psychopathology are just additional features that probably only shape the speed and the extent of the patient's reaction. They are facilitators and inhibitors of aggression rather than originators.

As a result, efforts to reduce rates of A/V in mental health care need to include addressing (and replacing) any/all ill-thought-out policies such as "zero tolerance."

33.6 Clinician-Related Phenomena

Despite the existence of policies that ignore clinicians' possible contribution to A/V in mental health care (see, e.g., UKCC 2001), there is a growing body of literature that acknowledges how clinicians can and do have a significant influence. There are a range of clinician-related phenomena that are linked with A/V in inpatient mental health care (Johnson 2004; Chaplin et al. 2006; Whittington and Ritcher 2006a, b), though the precise nature of these relationships remains uncertain.

The degree or extent of training and/or preparation for dealing with A/V is one such phenomenon, and the literature in this area is inconclusive as to the possible efficacy of training. Johnson's (2010) review of 46 papers reporting on efforts to provide training to reduce incidents of A/V concluded that, due to methodological limitations and a lack of homogeneity between studies, no firm conclusions could be drawn. Similarly, Ritcher et al.'s (Richter et al. 2006) systematic review of 39 studies also found no clear trend regarding a reduction of violent incidents. Encouraging findings do exist in this body of work; the majority of studies found that trained employees tend to report increased confidence (in comparison to untrained) (see Richter et al. 2006; Bjorkdahl et al. 2012). Also, a few studies have found that enhanced use of de-escalation techniques and/or physical skills (defense skills) did result in a decrease of A/V incidents. As a result, while the findings should be interpreted with a degree of caution, there is some evidence to suggest that the "right" type(s) or kinds of training(s) may still bring positive results.

Related to degree of training/preparation for dealing with A/V incidents is the broader matter of competency in and degree of training/preparation in communication and interpersonal skills. Communication and interpersonal skills as a factor in potential A/V incidents becomes more clear when one becomes more aware of service user research findings regarding causes of A/V. Abderhalden et al. (2006, p. 74) summarize the findings of numerous studies and conclude that:

> among all research samples, **users consider staff behavior as a central cause of violence**, (emphasis added) describing it as provocative and disrespectful.

Accordingly, clinical staff who possess and are conversant with communication and interpersonal skills that convey a sense of respect (see Rogers 1951), that they are listening to and hearing the client's view and that lower the interpersonal "temperature" rather than "pouring fuel on the fire," would appear to be well placed to reduce the number of A/V incidents.

The literature pertaining to the relationship between level of qualification and A/V incidents is equivocal, and the authors of this paper would argue it is overly simplistic to posit a linear, causal relationship between these two phenomena. Mason and Chandley (2002) similarly contend that possessing professional qualifications is no guarantee of high-quality care. There is however widespread agreement within the literature that certain interpersonal styles (or idiosyncrasies) can be a significant contributing factor to A/V incidents, and moreover, these styles can affect the behavior one way or another (see, e.g., Mason and Chandley 2002). Bjorkdahl et al.'s (Bjorkdahl et al. 2010) recent work draws attention to the two different interpersonal styles for responding to A/V: the "bulldozer and the ballet dancer." The research underscores how certain interpersonal styles (and their associated approaches/interventions) are more likely to provoke or prevent the escalation of potentially violent incidents (see also Morrison's 1990 work). Practitioners who adopt an interpersonal approach that is characterized by attitudes and behaviors listed in Table 33.1 appear to be associated with a significantly higher incidence of A/V (Roper and Anderson 1991; Whittington and Wykes 1996). Whittington and Wykes' (1996) study, for example, found that 86% of assaults were immediately preceded by the assaulted nurse having delivered an aversive stimulus to the patient, e.g., frustration, activity demand, or physical contact.

It is documented that the most frequently reported effects of exposure to A/V incidents are anger, anxiety, fear, and guilt (Needham 2006). There is also evidence that exposure to A/V can lead to post-traumatic stress disorder (PTSD) or PTSD-like symptoms including one of the defining clinical features of PTSD, namely, avoidance of stimuli associated with the event, or which arouse recollection of the event (United States, Department of Veteran Affairs 2013). There is little, if any doubt, that exposure to A/V can leave residual physical and psychological difficulties for the "victim" (Riahi 2011), to the extent that in his review, Needham (2006) argues that post-incident care is necessary for both the perpetrators and victims of violence. This raises some key questions concerning the mental health and well-being of nurses and other mental health clinicians if no post-incident care is provided or received, particularly if the nurse is involved in repeated incidents, all of which go without post-incident support. This is regrettably another issue that is currently under-investigated though a small number of authors have advanced preliminary hypotheses and findings. Whittington and Wykes (1994a, b), for example,

Table 33.1 Clinician attitudes/behaviors that appear to be associated with a significantly higher incidence of A/V

Insistence of unbending adherence to ward/unit rules
Denial of requests
Denial of access to services
Impingements on personal liberty
Respond to/treat clients with a lack of respect
Unsolicited touch
Encroachment on personal space
Failure to acknowledge
Respond to/treat clients with a lack of "justice"
Provocation of clients (consciously and/or subconsciously)
Respond to/treat clients with a lack of respect
Use/abuse of power
Use of coercion/coercive measures
Lack of willingness to listen to the client (and his/her point of view) and negotiate
Insistence on retaining a sense of control
Paternalistic ("I know what's best for you") approach to mental health care

developed a cyclic model of exposure to violence; unresolved or unaddressed stress and/or trauma in the clinician that arises from exposure to violence can then result in specific behaviors which then, ironically, can lead to increased risk of further violent incidents (Luckhoff et al. 2012). Cutcliffe's (1999) study and, more recently, Ward's (2013) findings lend support to this model. Participants in Cutcliffe (1999) explained how their experience of A/V was influenced by how equipped and how supported they felt. Participants explained how if they had dealt with any previous incident, if they felt supported through that process, and if they had (via clinical supervision) deconstructed and learned from the previous experience, then they felt better prepared and better equipped to deal with the next incident. Inversely they also explained that if that had not dealt with the "aftermath" of an earlier incident, this can and did have a detrimental effect on their ability and willingness to deal with future violent incidents. It is also noteworthy that those clinicians who were able to engage with A/V repeatedly without suffering any apparent detriment were those who also actively engaged in restorative clinical supervision (see also Mason and Chandley 2002).

Clearly related to these factors is that of clinician "burnout." There is an intuitive logical, yet hitherto largely untested relationship between clinician degree of "burnout" (and/or elevated, unaddressed stress) and his/her response and attitude toward A/V. Identified clinical features of burnout include depleted physical energy, emotional exhaustion, less investment in interpersonal relationships, an increasingly pessimistic outlook, and increased absenteeism and inefficiency at work (Demerouti et al. 2000; Chang et al. 2006; Leiter and Maslach 2009). The authors will not belabor how each of these clinical features, on its own, can clearly influence a mental health nurse's ability to respond to and deal effectively with A/V incidents. The potential cumulative effects on a mental health nurse who experiences more than one of these features then become even more disconcerting, and regrettably, this remains an under-examined relationship.

Drawing these factors together, it becomes evident that a complex, multifactorial relationship appears to exist. Exposure to A/V incidents, stress response(s) to incidents, ability and opportunity to explore and deal with the intrapersonal responses resulting from dealing with (or exposure to) A/V incidents, and the degree of support, debriefing, clinical supervision, etc. all appear to be clinician-related phenomena that have a potential incidence on rates of A/V incidents. But also very encouraging are interrelated factors that are amenable to intervention(s); that is, there are a range of efficacious interventions that we know of that can a) reduce clinician stress levels; b) reduce impacts of PTSD-like symptoms; c) offer opportunities to debrief, deconstruct, and explore/learn from the incident; and d) help mental health nurses and other clinicians feel more supported.

33.7 Discussion and Conclusions

The authors of this chapter began with the premise that A/V in mental health care is a multidimensional, complex problem and that there are a wide range of phenomena that have an impact on rates of A/V in mental health care. In synthesizing these propositions into categories (or quadrants), according to shared commonality and patterns (e.g., several phenomena are related to the physical environment), and exploring empirical evidence pertaining to each of these, the authors can assert with a degree of empirical confidence that our original premise appears to be accurate. Each of the propositions (i.e., relationships between certain phenomena and A/V in inpatient mental health care) is supported, to a greater or lesser extent, by the empirical evidence. However, in certain cases the existing evidence is inconclusive. What this seems to suggest, is that while our systemic model may have some preliminary validity, there is a clear need for more focused empirical work, particularly to further test these proposed propositions. Moreover, as the existing propositions are subject to further empirical testing, and as new phenomena are discovered and explored, the findings could theoretically (a) be woven into the existing model, (b) indicate the need to edit or modify the quadrants, or (c) even, if there is sufficient evidence, signify the need to reject the model.

Despite the consensus that A/V in inpatient mental health care is a multidimensional, multifaceted, and complex problem, few attempts to reduce and/or minimize A/V have adopted a corresponding multidimensional, multifaceted approach, though the few studies that did have demonstrated positive outcomes (APA, APNA, and NAPHS 2003; Gaskin et al. 2007; Farrell et al. 2010; Scanlan 2010; Goetz and Taylor-Trujillo 2012). The significant majority of practice development initiatives and/or research studies focused on attempts to reduce rates of A/V adopted a single factor or single phenomenon approach. This is something of a disturbing disconnect for the authors and points to one of the most pressing issues in mental health care. As a result, there is a discernible need for our well-meaning efforts to reduce A/V to reflect this more comprehensive, more systemic conceptualization. Efforts and projects that adopt single factor (or phenomenon) approach rather than more comprehensive, systemic approaches have had, at best, only a minimal efficacy. These findings have an intuitive logic to them; changing only one component of a "broken" system and leaving the remainder of the system in a dysfunctional state are unlikely to produce significant and wide-scale improvements. The authors illustrate this problem by drawing an analogy of a car with four flat tires. If you are attempting to get the car functioning efficiently once more, inflating only one of the tires will not do it; the car merely goes round in circles. However, inflating each of the tires, even partially, produces a far more efficient performance from the car than having one fully inflated and three deflated tires.

A further implication arising out of exploring the various propositions within our systemic model is that of the need for mental health nurses to consider a more accurate reconceptualization of A/V in mental health care per se. In so doing, a more sophisticated understanding of the empirical evidence indicates the need to move away from views that disproportionately assign "responsibility" (or blame) to clients for causing A/V when the evidence indicates that the client-related phenomena may only account for a small portion of these incidents. For example, while Fazel and Grann (2006); Fazel et al. 2009 draw attention to the relationship between mental health problems and A/V, they qualify their remarks stating:

> "In many ways the most interesting aspect of our findings is that 19 out of 20 people committing violent crimes do so without having any severe mental health problems." (Fazel 2006)

A realistic appraisal of the evidence however does indicate that some A/V incidents in mental health care could be attributed to the individual client. Even in such cases, the propositions contained in this paper and the evidence associated with these seem to suggest that it may be inappropriate and unhelpful to expect the same (or even a higher) level of self-control, personal management abilities in some clients who (a) may have underdeveloped self-control mechanisms, systems, (b) have existed in and have personal experience of systems that 'teach' (and/or reinforce) clients to behave this way, and (c) have to live in conditions and environments which are well known to be replete with aversive stimulation.

Further, given that several experiential learning models posit the essential nature of experience (Kolb 1984; Lisko 2010), the questions needs to be asked: (a) How are clients supposed to engage in experiential learning and subsequent personal development, particularly around how they increase their control of their aggressive behavior, if they are denied the opportunity to become angry at all? (b) How are clients supposed to learn how to control their behaviors, to manage their emotions, and not 'hit out' when they feel angry, aggrieved, or frustrated, if an organization has a so-called 'Zero Tolerance' view of client frustration or anger?

Since 2001, the US National Association of State Mental Health Program Directors' (NASMHPD) stance has been that A/V in inpatient settings *is also caused by the characteristics of the institutional milieu* (emphasis added). They argue that institutions which focus on control, organizational rules, directions to staff to "keep order," and homogenized 'one-size-fits-all' treatment approaches and institutions that do not provide good staff supervision and training may trigger aggressive behaviors. While this may not be an easy 'truth' or position for some to digest, the evidence seems to suggest that there is more value in attempting to reduce A/V by focusing on the other three quadrants as well and adopting a more realistic perspective vis a vis responsibility for incidents. Accepting the cogency of this argument and acting accordingly will require integrity and a significant degree of bravery on the part of mental health clinicians and organizations and they will require support. Crucially, this also highlights the matter of adequate educational preparation and the necessity for better educated mental health nurses, both pre- and postgraduation, in the realm of how to minimize A/V incidents.

Interestingly, for the authors of this paper, how P/MH nurses and other mental health clinicians view and attempt to deal with A/V is actually symptomatic of a more pervasive philosophy, policy, and practice vis a vis mental health care per se. This pervasive view is effected if not actually driven by contemporary societal views and beliefs of mental health, so-called mental illness, and the individuals who experience mental health problems. Related research has repeatedly shown that nurses can be thought of as representative of the broader societal group and may well form their opinions about some mental health matters in the same way the general population does, via mass media, theological beliefs, political rhetoric and hyperbole, and other channels of (mis)information (Ogborne and Birchmore-Timney 1998; Forman et al. 2001; Ford 2010). Accordingly, given the overarching, media-perpetuated, societal views of 'the mentally ill' as violent per se (see Cutcliffe and Hannigan 2001; Edney 2004; Vermuelen 2008), given the clear and documented shift toward more coercive mental health policy in recent years (see Hannigan and Cutcliffe 2002), and given how some nurses apparently form their personal constructs, it may not be entirely surprising that some mental health nurses reportedly view clients as the principal cause of A/V in mental health care. Thus their emphasis on containment, the preponderance of ward and/or hospital rules and restrictions, and the almost automatic resistance to any practice development initiatives that suggests removing or reducing coercive measures. In keeping with this evidence and argument, one way that mental health facilities that wish to reduce or minimize A/V incidents might benefit would be to engage in a comprehensive examination and review of their hospital and ward rules and regimes. Searching and potentially difficult questions would then need to be asked: (a) Is this rule or restriction absolutely necessary? (b) Whose interests are being served by maintaining and enforcing the rule? (c) What is the therapeutic purpose (let alone the evidence) that underpins or drives this rule? And perhaps most importantly, (d) is there another, less coercive method that the unit could use in place of the rule/restriction?

By decreasing coercion and increasing choice, individuals involved at all levels of the system of care can help create a healing culture of hope and recovery and, ultimately, improve the quality of people's lives. Perhaps the mental health community can make progress in this area by reminding itself of the "core business" of mental health-care facilities, of remembering what drew us to the field of mental health care in the first instance. The authors posit that there may be merit in reminding ourselves of what the goals of mental health care are (and are not) and that contemporary mental health facilities are not and never have been intended to function as prisons or correctional facilities.

In conclusion, there is a robust body of evidence which shows that A/V in mental health care is a multidimensional, complex problem and that there are a wide range of phenomena that have an impact on rates of A/V in mental health care, and this has enabled the authors to synthesize these propositions into a systemic model of A/V. Despite the cogency of this body of evidence, the majority of projects aimed at reducing A/V in mental health care have not adopted a systemic, comprehensive view and have thus met with, at best, indifferent outcomes. As a result, the authors of this paper assert that organizations and mental health-care policy makers need to radically rethink their positions and show leadership regarding how to address the widespread problem of A/V in mental health care, most particularly, altering and broadening our understanding of the causes (antecedents) of such incidents. This has already happened in a number of facilities with encouraging results, for example, please refer to the well-documented success of the states, Massachusetts and Pennsylvania, USA (SAMSHA 2009). However, such an approach requires the rejection of client-focused causation models and the embracing of a systemic, more comprehensive understanding and conceptualization of A/V in mental health care.

Acknowledgment This chapter has been adapted and reproduced, with kind permission from the publisher, from the journal articles referenced: Cutcliffe JR, Riahi S (2013) A systemic perspective of violence and aggression in mental health care: towards a more comprehensive understanding and conceptualization – part one. Int J Ment Health Nurs 22(6):558–567 and Cutcliffe JR, Riahi S (2013) A systemic perspective of violence and aggression in mental health care: towards a more comprehensive understanding and conceptualization – part two. Int J Ment Health Nurs 22(6):568–578

References

Abderhalden C, Hahn S, Bonner YDB, Galeazzi GM (2006) Users' perceptions and views on violence and coercion in mental health care. In: Ritcher D, Whittington R (eds) Violence in mental health settings: causes, consequences and management. Springer, New York, pp psP69–psP92

Adams B (2000) Locked doors or sentinel nurses? Psychiatrist 24:327–328

Alexander J, Bowers L (2004) Acute psychiatric ward rules: a review of the literature. J Psychiatr Ment Health Nurs 11:623–631

American Psychiatric Nurses Association (2007) Seclusion and restraint standards of practice. http://www.apna.org/files/public/APNA_SR_Standards-Final.pdf (recovered July 2012)

American Psychiatric Association, American Psychiatric Nurses Association, and National Association of Psychiatric Health Systems (2003). Learning from each other: success stories and ideas for reducing restraint/seclusion in behavioural health. https://www.naphs.org/rscampaign/index

Appleby L (1997) National confidential enquiry into suicide and homicide by people with mental illness. Department of Health, HMOS, London

Arnetz JE, Arnetz BB (2001) Violence towards health care staff and possible effects on the quality of patient care. Soc Sci Med 52:417–427

Azeem MW, Aujla A, Rammerth M, Binsfeld G, Jones RB (2011) Effectiveness of six core strategies based on trauma informed care in reducing seclusions and restraints at a child and adolescent psychiatric hospital. J Child Adolesc Psychiatr Nurs 24:11–15

Bandura A (1973) Aggression: a social learning analysis. Prentice Hall, Englewood Cliffs, NJ

Barton SA, Johnson MR, Price LV (2009) Achieving restraint-free on an inpatient behavioural health unit. J Psychosoc Nurs 47(1):34–40
Beech I, Leather P (2008) Workplace violence in the healthcare sector: a review of staff training and integration of training evaluation models. Aggress Violent Behav 11:27–43
Berglund B, Lindvall T (eds) (1995) Community noise. Archives of the center for sensory research, vol 2, pp 1–195. http://www.who.int/docstore/peh/noise/guidelines2.html
Berkowitz L (1993) Aggression: causes, consequences and control. McGraw Hill, New York
Bjorkdahl A, Palmstinerna T, Hansebo G (2010) The bulldozer and the ballet dancer: aspects of nurses' caring approaches in acute psychiatric intensive care. J Psychiatr Ment Health Nurs 17:510–518
Bjorkdahl A, Hansebo G, Palmstinerna T (2012) The influence of staff training on the violence prevention and management climate in psychiatric inpatient units. J Psychiatr Ment Health Nurs 19:1–9
Bjorkly S (1995) Prediction of aggression in psychiatric patients: a review of prospective prediction studies *Clinical*. Psychol Rev 15:475–502
Bjorkly S (2006) Psychological theories of aggression: principles and application to practice. In: Ritcher D, Whittington R (eds) Violence in mental health settings: causes, consequences and management. Springer, New York, pp 27–46
Bonta J, Law M, Hanson K (1998) The prediction of criminal and violent recidivism among mentally disordered offenders: a meta-analysis. Psychol Bull 123:123–142
Bourne J (2003) A safer place to work: protecting NHS hospital and ambulance staff from violence and aggression. The National Audit Office, London
Bowers, L. (2007) The City-128 study of observation and outcomes. http://www.biomedcentral.com/1471-244X/7/S1/S122
Bowers L, Haglund K, Muir-Cochrane E, Nijman H, Simpson A, Van Der Merwe M (2010) Locked doors: a survey of patients, staff and visitors. J Psychiatr Ment Health Nurs 17(10):873–880
Bowlby J (1989) A secure base: parent-child attachment and healthy human development. Basic Books, New York
Carmel H, Hunter M (1989) Staff injuries from inpatient violence. Hospital Commun Psychiatry 40:41–46
Champagne T (2006) Creating sensory rooms: environmental enhancements for acute inpatient mental health settings. Ment Health Special Interest Section Quarterly 29(4):1–4
Champagne T, Stromberg N (2004) Sensory approaches in inpatient psychiatric settings: innovative alternatives to seclusion & restraint. J Psychosoc Nurs 42(9):35–44
Champagne, T., Sayer, E. (2012) The effects of the use of the sensory room in psychiatry. http://www.otinnovations.com/images/stories/PDF_Files/qi_study_sensory_room.pdf
Chandler GE (2012) Reducing use of restraints and seclusion to create a culture of safety. J Psychosoc Nurs 50(10):29–36
Chang EM, Daly J, Hancock KM, Bidewell JW, Johnson A, Lambert VA, Lambert CE (2006) The relationships among workplace stressors, coping methods, demographic characteristics, and health in Australian nurses. J Prof Nurs 22(1):30–38
Chaplin R, McGeorge M, Lelliott P (2006) The national audit of violence: in-patient care for adults of working age. Psychiatrist 30:444–446. https://doi.org/10.1192/pb.30.12.444
Chou KR, Lu RB, Mao WC (2002) Factors relevant to patient assaultive behavior and assault in acute in-patient psychiatric units in Taiwan. Arch Psychiatr Nurs 16:187–195
Cowman S (2006) Safety and security in psychiatric clinical environments. In: Ritcher D, Whittington R (eds) Violence in mental health settings: causes, consequences and management. Springer, New York, pp 253–271
Cummings KS, Grandfield SA, Coldwell CM (2010) Caring with comfort rooms: reducing seclusion and restraint use in psychiatric facilities. J Psychosoc Nurs 48(6):26–30
Cutcliffe JR (1999) Qualified nurses' lived experience of violence perpetrated by individuals suffering from enduring mental health problems: a hermeneutic study. Int J Nurs Stud 36:105–116

Cutcliffe JR, Hannigan B (2001) Mass media, monsters and mental health: a need for increased lobbying. J Psychiatr Ment Health Nurs 8(4):315–322
Cutcliffe JR, McKenna HP, Hyrkas K (2010) Nursing models: application to practice. Quay Books, London
Daffern M, Mayer MM, Martin T (2004) Environmental contributors to aggression in two forensic psychiatric hospitals. Int J Forensic Ment Health 3(1):105–114
Davison S (2005) The management of violence in general psychiatry. Adv Psychiatr Treat 11:362–370
De Benedictis L, Dumais A, Sieu N, Mailhot M-P, Létourneau G, Tran M, Stikarovska I, Bilodeau M, Brunelle S, Côté C, Lesage A (2011) Staff perceptions and organizational factors as predictors of seclusion and restraint on psychiatric wards. Psychiatr Serv 62(5):ps 484–ps 491
Demerouti E, Bakker AB, Nachreiner F, Schaufeli WB (2000) A model of burnout and life satisfaction amongst nurses. J Adv Nurs 32(2):454–464
Department of Health (2007) Survey of attitudes toward mental illness. Department of Health, HMSO, London
Douglas KS, Guy LS, Hart SD (2009) Psychosis as a risk factor for violence to others: a meta-analysis. Psychol Bull 135:679–706
Dullard J, Dobb L, Miller N, Mowrer OH, Sears RR (1939) Frustration and aggression. Yale University Press, New Haven
Duxbury J (1999) An exploratory account of registered nurses' experience of patient aggression in both mental health and general nursing settings. J Psychiatr Ment Health Nurs 6:107–114
Duxbury J (2002) An evaluation of staff and patient views of and strategies employed to manage inpatient aggression and violence on one mental health unit: a pluralistic design. J Psychiatr Ment Health Nurs 9:325–337
Duxbury J, Whittington R (2005). Causes and management of patient aggression and violence: staff and patient perspectives. J Adv Nurs 50:469–478
Duxbury JA, Bjorkdahl A, Johnson S (2006) Ward culture and atmosphere. In: Richter D & Whittington R (Eds). Violence in Mental Health Settings: Causes, Consequences, Management. New York: Springer Science–Business Media (pp. 273–291)
Edney DR (2004) Mass media and mental illness: a literature review. Canadian Mental Health Association, Toronto, ON. http://www.ontario.cmha.ca/about_mental_health.asp?cID=7601&Viewmode=print
Ehmann TS, Smith GN, Yamamoto A, McCarthy N, Ross D, Au T et al (2001) Violence in treatment resistant psychotic inpatients. J Nerv Ment Dis 189:716–721
Elbogen EB, Johnson SC (2009) The intricate link between violence and mental disorder: results from the national epidemiologic survey on alcohol and related conditions. Arch Gen Psychiatry 66(2):152–161. https://doi.org/10.1001/archgenpsychiatry.2008.537
Farrell GA, Shafiei T, Salmon P (2010) Facing up to 'challenging behaviour': a model for training in staff-client interaction. J Adv Nurs 66(7):1644–1655
Fazel S, Grann M (2006) The population impact of severe mental illness on violent crime. *Am J Psychiatr* 17:907–913
Fazel S, Grann M, Langstrom N (2009) Editorial: what is the role of epidemiology for forensic psychiatry. Crim Behav Ment Health 19:281–285
Felitti V, Anda R, Nordenberg D, Williamson D, Spitz A, Edwards V, Koss M, Marks J (1998) Relationship of childhood abuse and household dysfunction to many of the leading causes of death in adults: the adverse childhood experiences (ACE) study. Am J Preventive Med 14:245–258
Fonagy P (2003) Towards a developmental understanding of violence. Br J Psychiatry 183:190–192
Ford R (2010) An analysis of nurses' views of harm reduction measures and other treatments for the problems associated with illicit drug use. Aust J Adv Nurs 28(1):14–24
Forman RF, Bovasso G, Woody G (2001) Staff beliefs about addiction treatment. J Subst Abus Treat 21(1):1–9
Foster C, Bowers L, Nijman H (2007) Aggressive behavior on acute psychiatric wards: prevalence, severity and management. J Adv Nurs 58(2):140–149

Freud S (1920) Beyond the pleasure principle. Standard edition, vol 18. Hogarth Press, London
Gaskin CJ, Elsom SJ, Happell B (2007) Interventions for reducing the use of seclusion in psychiatric facilities: review of the literature. Br J Psychiatry J Ment Sci 191:298–303
Georgieva I, Vesselinov R, Mulder CL (2012) Early detection of risk factors for seclusion and restraint: a prospective study. Early Interv Psychiatry 6:415–422
Goetz SB, Taylor-Trujillo A (2012) A change in culture: violence prevention in an acute behavioural health setting. J Am Psychiatr Nurses Assoc 18(2):96–103
Grassi L, Peron L, Marangoni C, Zanchi P, Vanni A (2001) Characteristics of violent behavior in acute psychiatric inpatients: a five-year Italian study. Acta Psychiatrica Scandanavica 104:273–279
Grossman LS, Haywood TW, Cavanaugh JL, Davis JM et al (1995) State psychiatric hospital patients with past arrests for violent crimes. Psychiatr Serv 46:790–795
Haglund K, von Knorring L, von Essen L (2006) Psychiatric wards with locked doors—advantages and disadvantages to nurses and mental health nurse assistants. J Clin Nurs 15(4):387–394
Hahn S, Muller M, Needham I, Dassen T, Kok G, Halfens R (2010) Factors associated with patient and visitor violence experienced by nurses in general hospitals in Switzerland: a cross-sectional survey. J Clin Nurs 19(23–24):3535–3546
Hannigan B, Cutcliffe JR (2002) Challenging contemporary mental health policy: time to assuage the coercion? J Adv Nurs 35(5):477–484
Healy D (2005) Psychiatric drugs explained, 4th edn. Elsevier, Edinburgh
Hiday VA (2006) Putting community risk in perspective: a look at correlations, causes and controls. Int J Law Psychiatry 29:316–331
Holmes C (2006) Violence, zero tolerance and the subversion of professional practice. Contemp Nurse 21(2):212–227
Huckshorn KA (2004) Reducing seclusion and restraint use in mental health settings: core strategies for prevention. J Psychosoc Ment Health Serv 42(9):22–41
Huckshorn KA (2006) Reducing seclusion and restraint: deep change required. In: Module presentation for the National Executive Training Institutes. NASMHPD, Alexandria, VA
Johnson ME (2004) Violence on inpatient psychiatric units: state of the science. J Am Psychiatr Nurses Assoc 10:113–121
Johnson ME (2010) Violence and restraint reduction efforts on inpatient. Issues Ment Health Nurs 31:181–197
Kayne HL, Hicks C, Milner J (1994) Environmental characteristics related to patient assault. Issues Ment Health Nurs 15:319–335
Kho K, Sensky T, Mortimer A, Cross C (1998) Prospective study into factors associated with aggressive incidents in psychiatric acute admission wards. Br J Psychiatry 38:230–236
Kolb DA (1984) Experiential learning: experience as the source of learning and development. Prentice Hall, Englewood Cliffs, NJ
Krakowski MI, Czobar P (1994) Clinical symptoms, neurological impairment and prediction of violence in psychiatric inpatients. Hospital Commun 45(7):700–705
Krakowski MI, Czobar P (1999) Course of violence in patients with schizophrenia: relationship to clinical symptoms. Schizophr Bull 25:505–517
Kumar R, Sachdev PS (2009) Akathisia and second-generation antipsychotic drugs. Curr Opin Psychiatry 22(3):293–299
Kynoch K, Wu C, Chang A (2009) The effectiveness of interventions in the prevention and management of aggressive behaviours in patients admitted to an acute hospital setting: a systematic review. JBI Library Syst Rev 7(6):175–223
Lau J, Magarey J, McCutcheon H (2005) Violence in the emergency department: a literature review. Aust Emerg Nurs J 7(2):27–34
LeBel J, Goldstein R (2005) Special section on seclusion and restraint: the economic cost of using restraint and the value added by restraint reduction or elimination. Psychiatr Serv 56(9):ps 1109–ps 1114
LeBel J (2011) The business case for preventing and reducing restraint and seclusion use. HHS Publication No. (SMA) 11–4632. Substance Abuse and Mental Health Services Administration, Rockville, MD

Leiter MP, Maslach C (2009) Nurse turnover: the mediating role of burnout. J Nurs Manag 17:331–339

Lisko, S.A. (2010) Integration of theory and practice: experiential learning theory and nursing education nursing education perspectives. http://www.readperiodicals.com/201003/2021688841.html

Luckhoff M, Jordaan E, Swart Y, Cloete KJ, Koen L, Niehaus DJH (2012) Retrospective review of trends in assaults and seclusion at an acute psychiatric ward over a 5-year period. J Psychiatr Ment Health Nurs 20(8):687–695

McDonnell A, Gallon I (2006) Issues and concerns about 'control and restraint' training: moving the debate forward. In: Cutcliffe JR, Ward MW (eds) Key debates in psychiatric/mental health nursing. Churchill Livingstone, Elsevier, Edinburgh, pp 168–180

Mason T, Chandley M (2002) Managing violence and aggression: a manual for nurses and health care workers. Churchill Livingstone, Edinburgh

Meehan T, Vermeer C, Windsor C (2000) Patients' perceptions of seclusion: a qualitative investigation. J Adv Nurs 31:370–377

Meleis AI (2007) Theoretical nursing: development and progress, 4th edn. Lippincott Williams and Wilkins, Philadelphia, PA

Michie S, West MA (2004) Managing people and performance: an evidence based framework applied to health service organizations. Int J Manag Rev 5(6):91–111

MIND (2004) Ward watch report finds woeful conditions continue to prevail in many psychiatric hospitals. http://www.mind.org.uk/news/2046_ward_watch_report_finds_woeful_conditions_continue_to_prevail_in_many_psychiatric_hospitals

MIND (2006) Fit for their purpose—wards should be co-created by those who use them. http://www.mind.org.uk/campaigns_and_issues/report_and_resources/786_fit_for_their_purpose

Morrison EF (1990) The tradition of toughness: a study of nonprofessional nursing care in psychiatric settings. J Nurs Scholarsh 22(1):32–38

Mullen, P.E. (2001) Mental health and criminal justice: a review of the relationship between mental disorders and offending behaviours and on the management of mentally abnormal offenders in the health and criminal justice systems. http://www.criminologyresearchcouncil.gov.au/reports/mullen.pdf

National Institute for Clinical Excellence (2004) Short-term management of violent (disturbed) behavior in adult psychiatric inpatient and accident and emergency settings—second draft for consultation. NICE, London

Needham I (2006) Psychological responses following exposure to violence. In: Ritcher D, Whittington R (eds) Violence in mental health settings: causes, consequences and management. Springer, New York, pp 295–320

Needham I, Abderhalden C, Halfens RJ, Fischer JE, Dassen T (2005) Non-somatic effects of patient aggression on nurses: a systematic review. J Adv Nurs 49:283–296

Ng B, Kumar S, Ranclaud M, Robinson E (2001) Ward crowding and incidents of violence on an acute psychiatric inpatient unit. Psychiatr Serv 52(4):521–525

Nijman HLI (2002) A model of aggression in psychiatric hospitals. Acta Psychiatr Scand 106(2):142–143

Nijman HL, Rector G (1999) Crowding and aggression on inpatient psychiatric wards. Psychiatr Serv 50(6):830–831

Nijman H, Campo JLMG, Ravelli DP, Merckelbach HLGJ (1999) A tentative model of aggression on inpatient psychiatric wards. Psychiatr Serv 50(6):832–834

Nijman H, Merckelbach H, Evers C, Palmstierna T, Campo J (2002) Prediction of aggression on a locked psychiatric admission ward. Acta Psychiatrica Scandinavia 105:390–395

Nijman H, Bowers L, Oud N, Jansen G (2005a) Psychiatric nurses' experiences with inpatient aggression. Aggressive Behav 31:217–227

Nijman HL, Palmstierna T, Almvik R et al (2005b) Fifteen years of research with the staff observation aggression scale: a review. Acta Psychiatr Scand 111:12–21

Ogborne AC, Birchmore-Timney C (1998) Support for harm-reduction among staff of specialized addiction treatment services in Ontario, Canada. Drug Alcohol Rev 17:51–58

Owen C, Tarantello C, Jones M, Tennant C (1998a) Repetitively violent patients in psychiatric units. Psychiatr Serv 49:1458–1461

Owen C, Tarantello C, Jones M, Tennant C (1998b) Violence and aggression in psychiatric units. Psychiatr Serv 49(11):1452–1457
Papadopoulos C, Ross J, Stewart D, Dack C, James K, Bowers L (2012) The antecedents of violence and aggression within psychiatric in-patient settings. Acta Psychiatr Scand 125:425–439
Powell R, Lloyd K (2002) A national survey of violence experienced by community mental health researchers. Soc Psychiatr Psychiatr Epidemiol 36:158–163
Powell G, Caan W, Crowe M (1994) What events precede violent incidents in psychiatric hospitals? Br J Psychiatry 165:107–112
Riahi S (2011) Role stress amongst nurses at the workplace: concept analysis. J Nurs Manag 19:721–731
Richter D, Needham I, Kunz S (2006) The effects of aggression management training for mental health care and disability care staff: a systematic review. In: Ritcher D, Whittington R (eds) Violence in mental health settings: causes, consequences and management. Springer, New York, pp 211–227
Rippon TJ (2000) Aggression and violence in health care professions. J Adv Nurs 31:452–460
Rogers C (1951) Client-centered therapy: its current practice, implications and theory. Constable, London
Roper J, Anderson N (1991) The interactional dynamics of violence, part one: an acute psychiatric ward. Arch Psychiatr Nurs 4:209–215
Rosenberg SD, Mueser KT, Friedman MJ, Gorman PG, Drake RE, Vidaver RM, Torrey WC, Jankowski MK (2001) Developing effective treatments for posttraumatic disorders among people with severe mental illness. Psychiatr Serv 52:1453–1461
Ryden MB, Bossenmaier M, McLachlan C (1991) Aggressive behavior in cognitively impaired nursing home residents. Res Nurs Health 14:81–95
SAMSHA (2009) States in brief: Pennsylvania substance abuse and mental health issues At-A-Glance. SAMSHA, Washington, DC
Scanlan JN (2010) Interventions to reduce the use of seclusion and restraint in inpatient psychiatric settings: what we know so far a review of the literature. Int J Soc Psychiatry 56(4):412–423
Silver E (2000) Extending social disorganization theory: a multilevel approach to the study of violence among persons with mental illnesses. Criminology 38:1043–1074
Silver E, Mulvey EP, Monahan J (2002) Mental disorder and violent victimization: the mediating role of involvement in conflicted social relationships. Criminology 40:191–212
Southern Center for Human Rights (2012) Severe overcrowding creates chaos, violence, and corruption at donaldson correctional facility. http://www.schr.org/files/post/PR_Donaldson.pdf
Stuart H (2003a) Violence and mental illness: an overview. World Psychiatr 2(2):121–124
Steinert T (2006) Prediction of violence in inpatient settings. In: Ritcher D, Whittington R (eds) Violence in mental health settings: causes, consequences and management. Springer, New York, pp 47–68
Stuart H (2003b) Violence and mental illness: an overview. World Psychiatr 2(2):121–124
Swanson JW, Swartz M, Essock SM, Osher FC, Wagner HR et al (2002) The social-environmental context of violent behavior in persons with severe mental illness. Am J Public Health 92:1523–1531
Sweet C, Mills T (1997) Use of NOSIE to predict assaults among acute psychiatric patients. Psychiatr Serv 48:1177–1180
Tang NK, Salkovskis PM, Hodges A, Wright KJ, Hanna M, Hester J (2008) Effects of mood on pain responses and pain tolerance: an experimental study in chronic back pain patients. Pain 138(2):392–401
Taylor P, Gunn J (1999) Homicides by people with mental illness: myth and reality. Br J Psychiatry 174:9–14
Turnbull J (1999) Violence to staff—who is at risk. In: Turnbull J, Patterson B (eds) Aggression and violence: approaches to effective management. MacMillan, Basingstoke, pp 8–30
Vermuelen, M. (2008) An investigation into the representation of the mentally ill in popular film. http://nmmu.ac.za/documents/theses/M_Vermeulen%20Treatise.pdf

United Kingdom Central Council (2001) The recognition, prevention and therapeutic management of violence in mental health care a summary: an initiative supported by the government health departments and the statutory mental health bodies in the four countries of the United Kingdom. http://www.positive-options.com/news/downloads/UKCC_-_Therapeutic_Management_of_Violence_-_summary_-_2002.pdf

United States, Department of Veteran Affairs (2013) DSM criteria for PTSD. http://www.ptsd.va.gov/professional/pages/dsm-iv-tr-ptsd.asp

Van Der Merwe M, Bowers L, Jones J, Simpson A, Haglund K (2009) Locked doors in acute inpatient psychiatry: a literature review. J Psychiatr Ment Health Nurs 16(3):293–299

Voineskos G (1976) Locked wards in Canadian mental hospitals: the return to custodialism. CMA J 114:689–692

Walker Z, Seifert R (1994) Violent incidents in psychiatric emergency services and its effects on disposition decisions. Br J Psychiatry 164:826–828

Ward L (2013) Ready, aim fire! Mental health nurses under siege in acute inpatient facilities. Issues Ment Health Nurs 34(4):281–287

Wells J, Bowers L (2002) How prevalent is violence towards nurses working in general hospitals in the UK? J Adv Nurs 39:230–240

Whittington R (2000) Understanding the problem of violence in mental healthcare settings. NT Res 5:113–114

Whittington R, Wykes T (1994a) An observational study of associations between nurse behaviour and violence in psychiatric hospitals. J Psychiatr Ment Health Nurs 1(2):85–92

Whittington R., Wykes T. (1994b) Going in strong, confrontative

Whittington R, Ritcher D (2006a) Introduction. In: Ritcher D, Whittington R (eds) Violence in mental health settings: causes, consequences and management. Springer, New York, pp 1–7

Whittington R, Ritcher D (2006b) From the individual to the interpersonal: environment and interaction in the escalation of violence in mental health settings. In: Ritcher D, Whittington R (eds) Violence in mental health settings: causes, consequences and management. Springer, New York, pp 47–68

Whittington R, Wykes T (1996) An evaluation of staff training in psychological techniques for the management of patient aggression. J Clin Nurs 5:257–261

Wykes T (1994) Predicting symptomatic and behavioural outcomes of community care. Br J Psychiatry 165:486–492

Zborowsky T, Bunker-Hellmich L, Morel A, O'Niel M (2010) Centralized vs. decentralized nursing stations. Health Environ Res Des J Summer 3(4):19–42. 50–78

The Withdrawn or Recalcitrant Client

34

Richard Lakeman

34.1 Introduction

There are few groups who raise the anxiety of psychiatric/mental health nurses (P/MHNs) more than those who don't improve as expected, those who don't follow recommendations or those who fail to engage with P/MHNs in a cooperative way. Main (1957, p. 129) suggested that the sufferer who frustrates a keen therapist by failing to improve is always in danger of meeting primitive (retaliatory) human behaviour disguised as treatment. He observed that nurses would only give a sedative when they were unable to stand the patient's problems without experiencing anxiety, impatience, guilt, anger or despair, whatever their justification for the treatment. Today the reluctant, recalcitrant or a-motivated service user is at risk of coercion and increasingly desperate and frequently nonevidence-based treatment measures. An armoury of long-acting "depot" medications, other dangerous medications and electroconvulsive therapy (ECT) may be imposed on individuals who fail to improve at the pace expected of them, often perpetuating a cycle of further resistance and reluctance to engage with the mental health-care system. Accordingly, this chapter explores the nature of resistance and offers some interventions and principles of practice that might be helpful whatever the cause.

R. Lakeman
Adjunct Associate Professor, School of Health & Human Science,
Southern Cross University,
Lismore, NSW, Australia

Visiting Senior Lecturer, Faculty of Health,
University of Tasmania, Australia

Adolescent Mental Health Nurse Navigator/Clinical Nurse Consultant
Cairns & Hinterland Health Service District,
Queensland Health, Australia
e-mail: richard.lakeman@scu.edu.au

© Springer International Publishing Switzerland 2018

J.C. Santos, J.R. Cutcliffe (eds.), *European Psychiatric/Mental Health Nursing in the 21st Century*, Principles of Specialty Nursing,
https://doi.org/10.1007/978-3-319-31772-4_34

34.2 Understanding Resistance: Origins, Background and Overview

People who fail to follow health-care advice, who are seen to lack motivation or who actively resist caregivers are often labelled as resistant or reluctant. For the most part, resistance and social withdrawal are best understood as functions of the dynamics between people. People tend to resist what they fear, what they don't want and what is imposed on them. Yalom (1992, p. 220) tentatively proposed:

> perhaps symptoms are messengers of meaning and will vanish only when their message is comprehended.

P/MHNs need to consider what symptoms mean. As a first example, problems with drive and motivation may be part of recognised disorders, but this does not render those symptoms meaningless; often people diagnosed and treated for mental health problems have quite understandable reasons for resisting the well-meaning ministrations of treatment teams. It is worth familiarising oneself with some of the so-called disorders that are thought to impact on motivation and drive.

34.2.1 Neurological and Medical Conditions

Social withdrawal and a-motivation have long been considered part of a range of so-called disorders and syndromes including neurological conditions, the effects of traumatic injury, medical conditions and drug-induced states (see Marin and Wilkosz 2005). In neurology, a-motivation falls on a continuum from *apathy* or indifference at one end, *aboulia* or a lack of will or initiative in the middle and at the extreme pole, *akinetic mutism* (an absence of movement and speech). Treating the primary cause where possible, optimising the person's physical well-being, reducing medications that aggravate a-motivational symptoms, understanding and remediating cognitive deficits and creating an enriched positive environment are important treatment considerations. At the extreme end of the continuum, pharmacological treatments may be introduced as part of treatment, e.g. activating antidepressants, dopamine agonists and stimulants, in addition to specialist neuropsychological treatments (Marin and Wilkosz 2005).

34.2.2 Psychiatric Syndromes

In psychiatry degrees of a-motivation may be part of common syndromes such as (so-called) depression and psychosis and may be exacerbated by common pharmacological treatments (particularly the major tranquilisers). Bleuler who first coined the term schizophrenia suggested that the most prominent symptoms could be categorised as the "4 As", i.e. problems with *associations* between thoughts, *ambivalence*, *affect* and *autism*. Although debates continue about what were the more important symptoms of Bleuler's definition and in particular the importance of dissociation and splitting (see Moskowitz and Heim 2011), Bleuler recognised that some people with this complex syndrome of heterogeneous symptoms withdraw from the world and become preoccupied with their inner experience (*autism*). More recently distinctions have been made between (so-called) negative symptoms (an absence or diminishment of functioning), (so-called) positive symptoms (reflecting an excess) and cognitive symptoms (Marneros et al. 2012). Positive symptoms (which include delusions and hallucinations) are generally considered more amenable to treatment, and social withdrawal and cognitive problems are generally considered to be more disabling and resistant to pharmacological treatments. *A-volition* is the term used to describe a general decrease in the motivation to initiate and perform self-directed purposeful activities which is sometimes observed in people who may be diagnosed with schizophrenia.

Fusar-Poli et al. (2015) note the importance of distinguishing between symptoms which may be "secondary" to pharmacological treatments and those that appear persistent. Negative symptoms may be secondary to the use of neuroleptic drugs (which traditionally have been very tranquilising and induce states similar to Parkinson's disease). Negative symptoms may also be a response to unstimulating environments (a feature of impoverished community settings as well as traditional total institutions). More recently it has been noted that negative symptoms may not cluster together so neatly and unsurprisingly are inconsistently responsive to pharmacotherapy (Erhart et al. 2006). Regardless of cause however, apathy and a-motivation appear to be the most important predictor of poor functional outcomes in research involving people diagnosed with schizophrenia (Fervaha et al. 2013; Fusar-Poli et al. 2015).

What may be considered a contentious part of one syndrome may sometimes be considered an essential feature of others. *Anhedonia*, for example, is the loss of enjoyment in activities previously found enjoyable. This concept is central to notions of depression, although depression too is an amorphous syndrome with multiple possible causes. People diagnosed with schizophrenia often report anhedonia, but they have been found to enjoy activities "in the moment" as much as people without this diagnosis (Strauss 2013). Where they may differ is in the *anticipation* of pleasurable experiences (if people don't anticipate that an activity is likely to be pleasurable, their motivation to do it is reduced). There is some evidence that negative thoughts about one's ability to successfully perform goal-directed behaviour can prevent behaviour initiation, engagement and anticipatory pleasure (Campellone et al. 2016). Beck et al. (1979) famously observed that depression can be characterised as holding negative beliefs about oneself, the world and the future (known as the cognitive triad of depression). From this model the remedy is to assist the person to adopt more reasonable, realistic thoughts about themselves and the world and reduce ruminations and thinking which are predictive of bad outcomes. Finally fatigue or tiredness, chronic pain and indeed chronic stress can sap people's drive and motivation and can contribute to depression and hopelessness.

34.2.3 Resistance as a Psychological Concept

Resistance connotes a more active stance on the part of people to *not* move forward or do what is needed. In psychoanalytical traditions, resistance was first understood as an effort to repress anxiety-provoking insights and memories and later was ascribed to a reluctance to accept the interpretation of the therapist. In other words resistance is an attempt to control anxiety, and it is more or less functional and necessary for mental health. Resistance can be a function of people's stage of development. For example, it is a natural part of adolescence to resist the direction and control of adults and to identify more strongly with peer groups. This pushing against parental or adult authority assists in the process of identity formation and is arguably essential to enable the young person to leave the comfort of home. Resistance however can be reflected in distorted thinking, a failure to see the best way forwards, an unwillingness to change and sometimes in overt opposition to the P/MHN or the helping process. Generally speaking when engaging with a person in a therapeutic conversation, topics that appear to engender resistance and shifts in affect should be carefully noted and attended to. Sometimes the communication can be quite overt—"Don't go there", the subtext being that this topic is potentially too anxiety-provoking right now. The P/MHNs may use this moment to make an empathic comment, e.g. they can see or sense that this topic causes some discomfort and ask the person whether they would prefer to discuss it at a later time.

The notion of resistance as a feature of the psychology of the individual (whether unconscious or an actively chosen behaviour) can be useful. However, this view can obscure the more commonly encountered reasons for resistance, which are more to do with the *dynamics* or relationships between people. A view which considers interpersonal dynamics invites the nurse to consider how their own behaviour may influence the behaviour of the other(s) (see, e.g. Table 34.1). It can be empowering to "reframe" resistance as a P/MHNs issue: it is widely recognised that one cannot change clients, whereas one *can* change how one interacts with them.

Table 34.1 Resistance as a mental health-care professional (MHCP) problem

Resistance occurs when the MHCP
Fails to recognise that all clients are ambivalent about change
Wants more for clients than clients want for themselves
Goals clash with the client's
Is too intent on his/her own agenda
Is going too fast
Does not know what to do
Asks the wrong question or makes a poorly worded or unacceptable statement which to the client is unfathomable and unrealisable
Feels uncomfortable in response to the client's behaviour
Fails to cooperate with the client
Is resisting the client's position

Adapted with permission from Mitchell (2012, p. 8)

34.2.4 Trauma and Learned Helplessness

Childhood abuse, neglect and trauma have been found to play causal roles in depression, anxiety disorders, post-traumatic stress disorder, eating disorders, substance abuse, personality disorders, dissociative disorders and psychosis (Read et al. 2004). The greater the number of adverse childhood experiences a person is exposed to, the more likely they are to engage in risk-taking behaviour, have poor health maintenance behaviours, become ill from a range of often preventable diseases and die prematurely (Felitti et al. 1998). Not surprisingly people exposed to trauma early in their lives, particularly when they do not experience secure, warm and consistent attachment to a caregiver, subsequently have a great deal of difficulty trusting people and sustaining relationships with others (Pearlman and Courtois 2005). The relationships people have with P/MHNs may also be tenuous—why should people trust P/MHNs or other relative strangers when the person's experience of their primary caregivers or others in authority has been a failure to protect, inconsistency and sometimes abuse?

The person's experience of health and welfare systems may also exacerbate a sense of powerlessness and mistrust and a feeling that relationships with helpers are shallow, coercive and uncaring. Watkins (2001, p. 133) suggests that it is not surprising that people with "severe mental health problems" are unwilling to engage with mental health services, given there is sometimes a "legacy of distrust" founded on dealings with statutory agencies, traumatising experiences of past hospitalisations, enforced treatment and experiences of discrimination and racism in their past dealings with health professionals. The experience of having to tell a story multiple times or having to see multiple health professionals before engaging with a primary therapist can be psycho-noxious for someone with attachment trauma. Health professionals need to be alert to the impact of early attachment experiences, trauma and people's experience of engagement with the health-care system and anticipate that many people will not conform to a compliant or acquiescent patient role. Programmes such as 'Safe Wards' aim to reduce the potential for coercionon in hospital through encouraging P/MHNs to engage in respectful interactions and anticipating issues that may cause conflict and responding in a kind and empathic manner (Bowers, et al. 2015).

Health professionals may need to earn the trust of people they work with through demonstrating unconditional positive regard (Rogers 1957) and engaging in a certain kind of respectful, "containing" relationship which individuals may not expect or have experienced before. Indeed, purposefully doing the unexpected is a tool to deal with resistance. As Mitchell (2012, p. 37) notes, "… socially typical responses are, by and large ineffective in creating therapeutic movement. Typical responses beget typical reactions…". Responding to hostility, blaming, anger or expressions of hopelessness (which might ordinarily elicit rejection or defensive behaviour) with compassion, curiosity, empathy and hope may not only help build an alliance, they may also be inherently therapeutic.

Early research examining what happens to both animals and humans when exposed to repeated traumatic events over which they have little control elucidated the concept of "learned helplessness" (Seligman 1973, 1975; Mikulincer 2013).

Over time people in essence give up trying to change their situation or resist what they perceive as being beyond their control. They become apathetic and a-motivated. Resistance can be a highly adaptive response to situations of abuse or injustice, yet people often don't engage in health-affirming behaviour because they don't perceive that it will make a difference. This can in part explain highly institutionalised behaviour. The kind of resistance often seen in response to coercive care might also be considered a natural, if not healthy response.

34.3 The Coerced or Involuntary Client

All Western countries have legislation to enable such compulsory assessment and treatment. People who have committed crimes may also be compelled to submit to therapy including those who have committed sexual offences or who have been identified as having problems with illicit drugs or alcohol. Not surprisingly people tend to resist (often quite actively through anger and sometimes violence) the deprivation of their liberty and treatment or care imposed on them. Regardless of their legal status, people may perceive that they have little choice in their treatment or care or about important decisions in their lives. The *perception of coercion* and perception of choice are pivotal to the dynamics that may play out between the individual and MHCPs. Some people who are legally required to engage in treatment may have no perception of coercion at all, and others may welcome help and treatment regardless of perceived legal pressure. Others may not be subject to any legal order but fear that if they don't comply they will be compelled to go to hospital, lose entitlements (e.g. housing or pensions) or lose valued support. People's fears and perceptions around coercion need to be explored.

People may come to accept the need for coercion, particularly when they have been engaged in dangerous behaviour, but they often assert that coercive processes could have been undertaken in a more considerate manner (Sibitz et al. 2011). In many instances MHCPs have little choice but to work with people compelled to be involved with their service, and they may be required to enforce treatment plans in which they have little personal investment and with which they don't agree. This unique dynamic has rarely been explored. A useful strategy to build relationships and to minimise conflict around coercion is for MHCPs to acknowledge this shared position with the client, being honest about what aspects of care or treatment are non-negotiable and being clear about what choices are available. Honesty, transparency and maximising choice are critical ingredients of recovery-orientated practices (Lakeman 2010) as is wholeheartedly embracing and operationalising trauma-informed care (see Chap. 13).

34.4 Motivation and Readiness for Change

People may appear resistant or fail to adhere to treatment plans because they are not ready to change, or more particularly, MHCPs are not in step with their stage of readiness. *Motivational interviewing* (MI) encompasses a range of theories about change; it articulates ways to identify readiness and practices to assist in shifting people towards making positive changes in their life. It is based on an understanding that people are often *ambivalent* about change and may present with conflicting emotions and thoughts about taking a particular course of action. Ambivalent people met with highly directive or coercive demands for change from health professionals often "dig in" and resist change even further. Consider, for example, smoking cessation—most people are aware of the potential dangers of smoking, yet rarely does a health professional telling them they "should" stop lead to a commitment to changing behaviour. Resistance always arises when there is a mismatch between the MHCP's and the person's aspirations for behavioural change (ABCs)—most commonly when the MHCP's ABCs are high for change in particular area and the person's are low (e.g. the MHCP believes the person should exercise more and eat less junk food, whereas the person does not perceive this as important). The MHCP may ineffectually attempt to manipulate, persuade or cajole the person to change. Conversely the person may have a high ABC on one issue where the MHCP's is low (e.g. the person believes they need a medical intervention to reduce weight, whereas the MHCP believes they should make lifestyle changes). Such a clash of agendas needs to be worked through to prevent an unproductive struggle. The emphasise ought to be on negotiating mutually agreeable goals to progress.

People vary in their *desire* for change, perceived *ability* or confidence to make changes, specific *reasons* for making changes and perceptions of *need* for change (consider the acronym DARN). As illustrated in Table 34.2, the MHCP can ask

Table 34.2 Assessing motivation through listening and asking about change talk

Change talk	Statements about…	Questions to elicit change talk
Desire	Preference for change "I want to…" "I would like to…" "I wish…"	"Why would you want/like/wish/hope….?" How important is this to you?
Ability	Capability "I could…" "I can…" "I might be able to…"	"How would you do it, if you decided to?" "What are you able to do?" "What could you do?
Reasons	Arguments for change: "I would feel better if…" "I would have more… if…"	"What are your three best reasons for …?" "Why would you make this change?" "What would be some benefits of change?"
Need	Feeling obliged to change "I ought to…" "I have to…" "I should…"	"How important is it to you…?" "How much do you need to…?"
Commitment	The likelihood of change "I am going to…" "I will…" "I intend to…"	"What do you think you will do?" "What if anything do you intend to do?"
Taking steps	Action taken "I actually went out and…" "I cut down…"	"What have you done already?" "What would be a first step for you?"

Source: Adapted from Rollnick et al. (2008)

questions and listen for talk about change. Note that individuals will vary in the intensity of their desire, their confidence, how pressing their reasons and how compelling their perceived need for change. They may, for example, desire something greatly but have a low confidence in their capability to achieve it. Their ambivalence may be expressed in statements such as "I really want to give up smoking [desire], but I really don't think I can [ability]". Additionally, expressions of commitment to change suggest a greater *likelihood* of actually making change, and taking actual steps towards change may suggest that a person is *ready* to make change.

34.5 Responding to Resistance and Recalcitrant Behaviour

Just as numerous theoretical lenses can be employed for *understanding* resistant or difficult behaviour, so too many different approaches may considered in determining *how best to respond*. Mental health nurses who work with people with complex needs ought to develop and maintain a "toolbox"/set of useful psychotherapeutic skills. Education and supervised practice in solution-focused and strengths-based therapies (see, e.g. Ungar 2015), positive psychology and motivational interviewing (see, e.g. Rollnick et al. 2008; DiClemente and Prochaska 1998) will be particularly useful. The following are a precis of some general principles to consider when working with resistant clients.

34.5.1 Build an Alliance

The capacity to work productively with someone using any set of skills depends a great deal on the quality of the relationship that is formed between P/MHNs and person. Rogers (1957) famously observed that the necessary and sufficient conditions for personality growth of clients in therapy were congruence on the part of the therapist, communication to the client of the therapist's empathic understanding and unconditional positive regard. As has been noted, prior adverse experience (of the patient, the P/MHN or both), conflicting goals and resistant behaviour sometimes make it difficult to establish or sustain an ideal relationship. Trotter (2015) suggests that when working with involuntary clients (of all kinds), what has been emphatically demonstrated to work are role clarification, reinforcing and modelling prosocial values, collaborative problem solving, cognitive behavioural strategies and providing a service in an integrated way. Developing the relationship through appropriate use of empathy, humour, the communication of optimism, judicious use of self-disclosure, working with family and peers and employing principles of case management have all been found to be somewhat helpful. Clarifying with the person what the P/MHN's role is from the outset and revisiting that periodically are helpful in building a working alliance. This is particularly true when the P/MHN may have multiple roles in relation to the person. The P/MHN needs to be clear with what services or tasks they may be mandated to provide and which are negotiable.

Modelling unconditional positive regard and maintaining a friendly, concerned and professional countenance may be taken as a given. As important is modelling how to contain anxiety and strong emotions and to deal with inevitable ruptures that may occur in the relationship. Sometimes service users may express overt hostility or anger towards the P/MHN and be unable to regulate their emotions or arouse fear and anxiety in caregivers. The P/MHN needs to learn to contain these strong emotions in a similar way to that of a good-enough parent who calmly soothes an infant experiencing distress. This skill of emotional containment has recently been conceptualised as pivotal in the care and treatment of people with personality disorders (Goodwin 2005). It is now widely recognised that interpersonal environments characterised by high expressed emotion (i.e. over involvement, critical comments and hostility) contribute to a worsening of problematic behaviours in a wide range of mental health presentations (van Audenhove and Van Humbeeck 2003). P/MHNs need to learn to moderate and contain their own responses to distress and distressing behaviour (reduce expressed emotion) and model how to solve problems.

34.5.2 Be Motivational

Motivational interviewing involves some core skills that might be considered universally good practice in the helping field, e.g. resisting the righting reflex, understanding the person's motivation, listening and empowering (Rollnick et al. 2008). MI involves reaching agreement on a focus and setting an agenda and emphasises the "spirit" of the approach. Conversations exploring and building motivation to change progress through exchanging information, asking useful questions, listening reflectively and sometimes using structured approaches (e.g. eliciting the pros and cons about a particular behaviour). Summarising progress, returning to agenda setting and considering the next step are part of the iterative process.

People rarely benefit from being told that something is wrong with them, nor do they respond well to being told what to do. A first principle in motivational interviewing is "resisting the righting reflex", that is, to avoid correcting another's course, giving unsolicited advice or overusing direction. People have a natural tendency to resist persuasion (no matter how well motivated). If the P/MHNs or others argue for change (e.g. "You ought to do…"), then the person is likely to argue against change. Whilst there may be an occasional need to confront, inform or announce a different viewpoint, these strategies ought to be used the least and undertaken with great care and often with permission.

P/MHNs will be well acquainted with communicating empathically (e.g. "You feel… [identifying the correct emotion and intensity]… when or because… [identifying accurately the trigger]") (Egan 2013) or using selective reflection to enable deeper exploration about a topic of interest. A motivational form of reflection involves selectively reflecting the change talk (illustrated in Table 34.3) and/or the person's ambivalence. The goal (and natural tendency of the person) is for them to then argue *for* change or a different behaviour. Being motivational also means

Table 34.3 Twenty skills for ecological practice

Navigation skills
1. Make resources available—help the person identify internal and external resources
2. Make resources accessible—discuss how the person can access resources
3. Explore barriers to change—discuss the barriers to change and what resources are most likely to address which barriers
4. Build bridges to new services and supports—discuss supports that are available and build bridges to make new resources available and accessible
5. Ask what is meaningful—explore which resources are the most meaningful given the person's culture and context
6. Keep solutions as complex as the problems they solve—explore solutions that are as complex (multi-systemic) as the problems they address
7. Find allies—explore possible allies who can help the client access resources and put new ways of coping into practice
8. Ask whether coping strategies are adaptive or maladaptive—explore the solutions that the person is using to cope in challenging contexts and the consequences of the choices the person is making
9. Explore the person's level of motivation—discuss with the person their level of motivation to implement preferred solutions
10. Advocate—advocate with, or on the behalf of, the person, or show the person how to advocate independently to make resources more available and accessible
Negotiation skills
11. Thoughts and feelings—explore the person's thoughts and feelings about what brought the client into contact with the helping system
12. Context—explore the context in which problems occur and the conditions that sustain them
13. Responsibility—discuss who has responsibility to change patterns of coping that are causing problems for the person and/or for others in the person's life
14. Voice—help the person's voice be heard when they name the people and resources necessary to make life better
15. New names—when appropriate offer new names and descriptions for problems and explore the new meanings for the person
16. Fit—enable the person to choose one or more descriptions of the problem that fit with how they see the world
17. Resources—work together to find the internal and external resources to help the person put new solutions into practice
18. Possibilities—enable the person to experience possibilities for change that are more numerous than expected
19. Performance—identify times when the person is performing new ways of coping and discuss who will notice the changes
20. Perception—help the person find ways to communicate to others that they have changed or are doing better than expected

Adapted with permission from Ungar (2015)

understanding what motivates and drives specific individuals, their values and aspirations and whether they are motivated primarily by intrinsic or extrinsic rewards. Where people may appear high on desire but low on other aspects of motivation, then the MHCP may need to negotiate the provision of incentives. A long-standing and robust principle of behavioural psychology is that behaviour that is followed by positive consequences is likely to be repeated. Providing incentives or rewards for meeting specific behavioural goals (e.g. verified abstinence) has a strong evidence base in drug use (Carroll and Onken 2005), and increasingly direct incentives are proving to be useful to secure adherence to many health treatments of importance to public health. However, few things motivate individuals more than the praise, attention and approval of peers and trusted people. Therefore, praise people often and acknowledge their struggles and achievements.

34.5.3 Be Ecological/Solution Focused

A tradition and tendency of health and welfare services has been the focus on the identification of problems. Service users frequently develop or have reinforced a perception that they are at fault and need fixing. Often however, the person's problematic behaviour is a response to contexts beyond their control. As Ungar (2015, p. 66) notes "Individuals are not to blame for the strategies they use to cope in contexts that deny them choices". An ecological approach to problems emphasises the development and mobilisation of skills in navigation and negotiation (see Table 34.3) to identify and evaluate internal and external resources available to them and help people influence which resources they receive, by whom, how, when and where. Emphasising the idea of *resourcing* the person to deal with the world rather than fixing them goes a long way to avoiding conflict and positions the P/MHNs as an ally in coping. Giving people something they want or need is a shortcut to building a relationship. Indeed, whether or not people perceive they got something of value from their first encounter with a P/MHN may well influence the trajectory of the relationship from that time forward.

Being solution focused is in part a way of being as well as encompassing a set of techniques. An elegant and respectful way to demonstrate being solution focused is to judiciously attempt to reframe deficit and negative talk, statements about what people don't want into a desire for a solution, a more positive frame or a statement about what people want:

e.g. "I really hate that doctor… he never listens to me" [person]
"You would feel warmer towards your doctor if you had more opportunities to be heard" (P/MHN)
e.g. "I find it so hard to get out of bed right now" [person]
"You would like to have more energy in the mornings" (P/MHN)

The classic solution-focused question which can elicit aspirations for positive goal setting is the "miracle question". Have the person imagine or anticipate at some point in time in the future (the next day when they wake up or in a year's time) that their problems are resolved (and they don't need to know how it happened). Ask them to describe how it would be and what they would be doing. A variation of this approach (anticipatory open dialogue) can also be used with families or others in the network (Seikkula et al. 2006)—what they imagine things might be like and how they might help people get there.

34.5.4 Clarify and Set Meaningful Goals

People don't tend to resist what they really want. Often people may want something from the relationship but not always what is being offered. Early in the relationship, it is important to negotiate meaningful goals. Goal setting will proceed from an evolving understanding of the person, their context and the resources available to them. Where the individual's goals appear to be discordant with the health-care team, it is necessary to find some common ground. The aforementioned miracle question can be helpful to identify areas to aspire to. It is important to explore the person's motivation to attain a particular goal. Goal setting involves a commitment of one or more people to do something. As well as being specific, meaningful, action-orientated, realistic and with a clear time frame ("SMART"), the P/MHN may need to assist the person to determine who needs to do what and to identify motivational rewards or contingencies if the steps are not intrinsically motivating in themselves.

34.5.5 Engage Allies

An ecological approach acknowledges that people are part of a social system that is an integral part of a person's life and is a necessary resource for a person's well-being. P/MHNs are part of that system and whilst a fundamental goal is to be an ally to the person, the P/MHN also needs to mobilise other social resources. The P/MHN ought to negotiate who needs to be involved and what roles they need to assume. Consider, for example, someone who needs to lose weight. Some people may need information (and referral to a dietitian), some may need a coach (a referral to an exercise physiologist) or a companion to attend an exercise class with, whilst others might need a family intervention. All forms of family therapy and solution-focused therapy acknowledge that the solutions to problems or the resources to solve them are largely within the social group.

A sense that a team is working together to find solutions is a powerfully and reassuring idea. It is perhaps one of the critical ingredients of programmes such as assertive community treatment (the most evidenced-based programme for people with complex mental health needs) and is fundamental to innovative new programmes such as open dialogue (Lakeman 2014). Readers will note Ungar's (2015) list of negotiation skills (Table 34.3) ending with having the person's voice heard and their improvement witnessed by others. This involvement, witnessing and engagement with others are a powerful motivator of positive behaviour, and connectedness with others is perhaps the lynchpin of mental health. People need the opportunity to share their successes, help others and be needed by a social group. Engaging peer support and encouraging people to be peer supporters are a sound motivational strategy.

Lastly, P/MHNs need to remain engaged with allies themselves. When enmeshed in clinical roles, it is sometimes hard to see the forest (dynamics) for the trees (behaviours). Clinical supervision or at least open dialogue with others who are able to identify the dynamics involved in interactions, able to model the kind of containing presence that MHCPs need to model and able to enrich the P/MHN's toolbox of solution-focused strategies is essential to developing effective practice with the recalcitrant or highly resistant client.

References

Beck AT, Rush AJ, Shaw BF, Emery G (1979) Cognitive therapy of depression. Guilford, New York

Bowers L, James K, Quirk A, Simpson A, Stewart D, Hodsoll J (2015) Reducing conflict and containment rates on acute psychiatric wards: the safewards cluster randomised controlled trial. Int J Nurs Stud 52(9):1412–1422

Campellone TR, Sanchez AH, Kring AM (2016) Defeatist performance beliefs, negative symptoms, and functional outcome in schizophrenia: a meta-analytic review. Schizophr Bull 42(6):1343–1352

Carroll, K. M., & Onken, L. S. (2005). Behavioral therapies for drug abuse. American Journal of Psychiatry, 162(8), 1452–1460.

DiClemente CC, Prochaska JO (1998) Toward a comprehensive, transtheoretical model of change: stages of change and addictive behaviors. Plenum, New York

Egan G (2013) The skilled helper: a problem-management and opportunity-development approach to helping. Belmont, Cengage Learning

Erhart SM, Marder SR, Carpenter WT (2006) Treatment of schizophrenia negative symptoms: future prospects. Schizophr Bull 32(2):234–237

Felitti VJ, Anda RF, Nordenberg D, Williamson DF, Spitz AM, Edwards V, Marks JS (1998) Relationship of childhood abuse and household dysfunction too many of the leading causes of death in adults: the adverse childhood experiences (ACE) study. Am J Prev Med 14(4):245–258

Fervaha G, Foussias G, Agid O, Remington G (2013) A-motivation and functional outcomes in early schizophrenia. Psychiatry Res 210(2):665–668

Fusar-Poli P, Papanastasiou E, Stahl D, Rocchetti M, Carpenter W, Shergill S, McGuire P (2015) Treatments of negative symptoms in schizophrenia: meta-analysis of 168 randomized placebo-controlled trials. Schizophr Bull 41(4):892–899

Goodwin JM (2005) Redefining borderline syndromes as posttraumatic and rediscovering emotional containment as a first stage in treatment. J Interpers Violence 20(1):20–25

Lakeman R (2010) Mental health recovery competencies for mental health workers: a Delphi study. J Ment Health 19(1):62–74

Lakeman R (2014) The finnish open dialogue approach to crisis intervention in psychosis: a review. Psychother Austr 20(3):26–33

Main TF (1957) The ailment. Br J Med Psychol 30(3):129–145

Marin RS, Wilkosz PA (2005) Disorders of diminished motivation. J Head Trauma Rehabil 20(4):377–388

Marneros A, Andreasen NC, Tsuang MT (eds) (2012) Negative versus positive schizophrenia. Springer Science & Business Media, Berlin

Mikulincer M (2013) Human learned helplessness: a coping perspective. Springer Science & Business Media, New York

Mitchell CW (2012) Effective techniques for dealing with highly resistant clients, 2nd edn. Clifton W. Mitchell, Tennessee

Moskowitz A, Heim G (2011) Eugen Bleuler's dementia praecox or the group of schizophrenias (1911): a centenary appreciation and reconsideration. Schizophr Bull 37(3):471–479

Pearlman LA, Courtois CA (2005) Clinical applications of the attachment framework: relational treatment of complex trauma. J Trauma Stress 18(5):449–459

Read J, Mosher LR, Bentall RP (2004) Models of madness: Psychological, social and biological approaches to schizophrenia. Psychology Press, London
Rogers CR (1957) The necessary and sufficient conditions of therapeutic personality change. J Consult Psychol 21(2):95
Rollnick S, Miller WR, Butler CC (2008) Motivational interviewing in health care: helping patients change behaviour. Guilford, New York
Seikkula J, Arnkil TE, Hoffman L (2006) Dialogical meetings in social networks. Karnac Books, London
Seligman MEP (1973) Fall into helplessness. Psychol Today 7(1):43–48
Seligman MEP (1975) Helplessness. Freeman, San Francisco
Sibitz I, Scheutz A, Lakeman R, Schrank B, Schaffer M, Amering M (2011) Impact of coercive measures on life stories: qualitative study. Br J Psychiatry 199(3):239–244
Strauss GP (2013) The emotion paradox of anhedonia in schizophrenia: or is it? Schizophr Bull 39(2):247–250
Trotter C (2015) Working with involuntary clients, 3rd edn. Allen & Unwin, Sydney
Ungar M (2015) Working with children and youth with complex needs: 20 skills to build resilience. Routledge, New York
van Audenhove C, Van Humbeeck G (2003) Expressed emotion in professional relationships. Curr Opin Psychiatry 16(4):431–435
Watkins P (2001) Mental health nursing: the art of compassionate care. Butterworth-Heinemann Medical, Oxford
Yalom ID (1992) When nietzsche wept: a novel of obsession. Harper Collins, New York

35 Confronting Goffman: How Can Mental Health Nurses Effectively Challenge Stigma? A Critical View of the Literature

L. Bates and T. Stickley

35.1 Introduction

It is well documented that stigma has a significant impact upon the lives of people diagnosed with mental illnesses. Stigma is correlated with a number of social problems such as higher levels of poverty, poor physical and mental health, social isolation, deprivation and poor educational attainment as a consequence, leading in turn to a loss of social status (Crisp 2004; Elliot and Masters 2009; Jackson et al. 2009). In the UK, 56% of people with mental health problems have experienced stigma from their families and 52% from their friends (The Mental Health Foundation 2000; Healthcare Commission 2008). A question seldom addressed however is: how can mental health nurses effectively challenge stigma?

The methodology chosen to explore the question is a critical review, which allows the necessary freedom of exploration. As critical reviews do not follow any preordained structure, but rather seek to create discussion and critical reflection upon key issues arising from the literature, this introduction will demonstrate the path taken during the review and the reasons why the argument has developed into its current form (Cross and MacGregor 2010). We began by critically examining theories of stigma both to more clearly understand the concept and also to determine what mental health professionals could learn from these theories to assist them in reducing the impact of stigma upon those they work with. This led us to examine one particular aspect of Goffman's theory, which raised questions regarding the nature and causes of professional stigma amongst mental health professionals. The discussion then developed into a more wide-ranging critique of mental health policy and law and its contribution to the maintenance of stigmatizing attitudes.

L. Bates • T. Stickley (✉)
University of Nottingham, Nottingham, UK
e-mail: Theo.stickley@nottingham.ac.uk

© Springer International Publishing Switzerland 2018

J.C. Santos, J.R. Cutcliffe (eds.), *European Psychiatric/Mental Health Nursing in the 21st Century*, Principles of Specialty Nursing,
https://doi.org/10.1007/978-3-319-31772-4_35

35.2 Stigma and Its Theoretical Basis

The word 'stigma' retains its original sense of a person being marked or set apart; however, modern usage often implies invisible traits that result in a person being discriminated against by society (Thornicroft 2006; Hinshaw 2007). There are a number of theories which attempt to explain the mechanisms behind what causes and perpetuates stigma. One of the most prominent was put forward by Goffman (1963), who argued that individuals rely on stereotypes to interact effectively with strangers and categorize them. These categories carry a set of expectations about a person which form a 'virtual social identity'. The actual nature of the person, that is, reality and not the stereotype is referred to as their 'actual social identity'. Thus, according to Goffman, the roots of stigma lie in the perceived discrepancy between a person's virtual and actual social identities. Those who are part of a stigmatized group are treated by society in such a way that their life chances and prospects of realizing their own potential are significantly reduced. However, Goffman (1963) identifies certain types of people who are able to rise above stigmatizing others. 'The wise' do not share the stigma of a group or individual but are much closer to the stigmatized group than the general population, either as a result of working for organizations that cater for the stigmatized group or by being related to a stigmatized person. By assigning a position of privilege to those professionals who work closely with stigmatized groups, Goffman seems to assume that professionals have a superior level of insight and sympathy into the plight of the stigmatized group and therefore are above a point where they themselves would succumb to stigmatizing behaviour (Goffman 1963). The truth of this claim is of serious importance if nurses are to make significant contributions to reducing the impact of stigma on the lives of their clients. The professional, be that a doctor, a nurse, social worker or any other person whose job involves working with and supporting people with mental health problems, is clearly in a position of power and trust. However, there is increasing evidence that Goffman's claim is flawed. Many users of mental health services have identified encounters with health services as being amongst the most stigmatizing and distressing experiences of their illness (Thornicroft 2006; Sweeney et al. 2009). A study by Wahl (1999) in which service users were interviewed about their experiences of discrimination found that almost 25% reported some form of discrimination from those charged with their care. One of the most commonly reported complaints is of poor attitudes and intolerance towards people diagnosed with personality disorder (Ross and Goldner 2009; Westwood and Baker 2010). This complaint is supported by research which found that the chaotic interpersonal relationships and sometimes impulsive dangerous behaviour displayed by people with personality disorder meant nurses found it difficult to relate with these clients and believed they had more control over their own behaviour than did other clients (Munro and Baker 2007; Woollaston and Hixenbaugh 2008; Ross and Goldner 2009; Westwood and Baker 2010). However, professionals often state it is a personal priority to address the stigma faced by their clients but unknowingly reinforce it (Bertram and Stickley 2005). There has historically been a lack of literature which critically explores the underlying nature of discrimination against service users by mental health professionals. However, in the study by Wahl (1999) referred to earlier, most often this discrimination was passive rather than active and consisted of service users being discouraged from trying new and possibly challenging activities. This distinction between active and passive discrimination is important, as it hints at something wider than a straightforward cognitive process described in conventional models of stigma.

35.3 The Relationship Between Public and Professional Attitudes

The attitude of professionals towards mental illness as an incurable life-ruining event accompanied by a loss of or deficits in a person's ability to function is often quoted as the major factor driving stigmatizing behaviour (Repper and Perkins 2003). This belief becomes the basis for an approach to care which encourages superficial compliance and low-risk activities, with little or no responsibility being given to the service user (Amering and Schmolke 2009). However, mental health professionals, the mental health system and mental health law all operate against the backdrop of wider society and public concern. To fully understand the reasons for the stigma shown by professionals, it is essential to understand something of the public view of mental health and the policies and laws arising from this which govern mental health practice. In the UK, people's attitudes towards mental illness are becoming more positive, and acceptance is increasing. However, (1) 39% of people feel that those with mental illnesses are dangerous, (2) 67% of people stated asylums were still an appropriate method of treatment, (3) 19% and 15% of people, respectively, stated that those with mental illness appeared different to others and that weakness in personality was a significant factor in the development of mental illness (Office of National Statistics 2010). Attitudes such as these mean that people with mental health problems are at best isolated within their communities and at worst that others actively fear and avoid them. Most people's reactions appear to lie somewhere along the continuum between authoritarianism and benevolence (Green 2010). The general assumption by society is that people with mental health problems cannot be held responsible for their problems and should be treated compassionately (benevolence) but that if they object, then treatment should be carried out regardless as it is for their own good (authoritarianism). The media also has a role to play in creating and sustaining public attitudes; the recurring theme in the portrayal of mental health in the media is that of violence and dangerousness (Slopen et al. 2007; Rogers and Pilgrim 2010). The term 'moral panic' for such emphasis on violent or alarming aspects of a story, whilst diminishing the attention paid to other, less immediately interesting, facts is used to describe the effect created by the mass media in their reporting of violent incidents committed by those with mental health problems (Pearson 1999). The media's focus on the link between violent crimes and mental health problems is designed to reflect the preoccupations of the reader and serves to reinforce them, with the aim of increasing the circulation or rating of the particular newspaper or programme (Pearson 1999). The mechanisms of this process in action can be seen in the media response to the murders of Jonathan Zito and Isabel Schwartz in the mid-1990s. Both were ordinary members of the public who were attacked and murdered by people receiving treatment for mental health problems in the community (Paterson 2006). These murders became associated with the failure of community care and resulted in increased anxiety in society about the risk posed by people with mental health problems (Paterson and Stark 2001; Paterson 2006). Ultimately, these incidents and others like them resulted in a shift in policy away from the libertarian principles that had seen the closure of the asylums and the promotion of community care towards a more coercive and risk-averse mental health system (Paterson and Stark 2001, Paterson 2006).

35.4 Law and Policy in Mental Health: Does the System Create Stigma?

This 'moral panic' provides some understanding both of contemporary stigma and of the philosophy of control and coercion, which underpins much of the current legislation surrounding the treatment of those with mental health problems. The mental health system in the UK has undergone drastic changes over the previous 20 years, moving from a primarily hospital-based system of care towards a community-focused service. The physical change in the location has been accompanied by a philosophical shift in the values underpinning service delivery, reflected in the increasing emphasis on service user involvement and personal choice (Rogers and Pilgrim 2001; Ramon and Williams 2005).

Recent mental health policy has been heavily influenced by the current Recovery agenda that shifts emphasis from a biomedical model of mental health towards a more social and psychological understanding of mental well-being. This recovery approach arose out of a desire amongst users of mental health services to take back the self-hood which they felt the mental health system had deprived them of. Recovery does not mean an absence of symptoms but rather the ability of a person to integrate the experience of a mental health problem meaningfully into their life (Coleman 2004; Roberts and Wolfson 2004; Shepherd et al. 2008). Definition of terms is important here as the use of the term 'recovery' in this context refers to the ability and willingness of professionals to support people with mental health problems to direct and control their own lives in a way that allows them to live a life that is meaningful for them. This ethos has been recognized in a growing number of countries and has become mainstream in the UK policy agenda (Department of Health 2011), in spite of a paucity of research to support this (Stickley and Wright 2011a, b). Although there is widespread policy support for recovery and high-profile mental health awareness campaigns particularly within the NHS at trust level which have proved effective in reducing the degree of stigma (Schneider et al. 2011), stigma continues to cause a significant barrier to the ability of people with mental health problems to fully exercise their rights as citizens in the post-asylum era (Knapp 2007; Schneider et al. 2011).

The policies explored so far have all emphasized the need to develop inclusive, holistic and integrated services which aim to support the recovery and well-being of people with mental health problems. However, they are increasingly set against other mental health legislation, such as the recent amendments to the Mental Health Act (2007), which enshrine in law greater regulation and social control over people with mental health problems (Fawcett and Karban 2005). The tensions inherent between policy and legislation and a top-down risk-averse culture have an adverse effect upon the recovery of people with mental health problems. However, governmental responses to public anxiety were to increasingly emphasize the need to promote public safety within mental health policy at the expense of the rights of service users (Tidmarsh 2004; Barker 2010). Furthermore, as it is the lack of violent incidents which is seen by government as the most efficient means of measuring the efficacy of the law, Mental Health services have been placed under increased pressure to predict, manage and prevent violence committed by service users (Eastman and Peay 1999; Crisp 2004; Barker 2010).

In recent years, mental health legislation in the UK has become increasingly coercive; the implementation of Community Treatment Orders (CTOs) in 2007 is a primary example of this. Under a CTO, a person who has been detained under mental health law can be forcibly returned to hospital if there is concern that they are at risk of becoming unwell (Mental Health Act 2007). There was a marked discord between the expected and actual usage of CTOs. The government estimated that between 400 and 600 such orders would be made every year; however, the actual figures show that 4000 were implemented in the first year, indicating that coercive treatments were far more widely used than expected (Lawton-Smith 2010). Closer analysis of more general figures for involuntary inpatient admissions and community treatment orders shows a marked rise in the use both of forced detention and forced treatment in the community (National Health Service Information Centre 2010). Furthermore, Edgley et al. (2006) argue that the right to liberty is the most fundamental of human rights and that it is often breached by the execution of mental health law that favours protection of the public over individual liberty. The emphasis on preventing risk over promotion of the rights of individuals reflects a preoccupation with violence and dangerousness, which reinforces the media stereotypes of mental health problems. The impact of these policies upon the ability of a person to manage their own recovery and live a meaningful life is significant. The need for mental health professionals to practice in a risk-averse manner also has a negative impact upon their ability to support the recovery of service users (Berry et al. 2010). Through focusing on risk, professionals remove responsibility from the hands of service users and clients and place it in the hands of mental health services (Barker 2010). It is a combination of coercion, fear and separation which, its critics argue, gives mental health legislation the power to contribute to the stigmatization of those it was created to protect. Legislation which removes a person's rights coerces them into treatment and focuses extensively on diagnosis, and risk factors may perpetuate stigma and social exclusion by preventing a person from accessing schemes such as welfare to work or living independently because of fear of relapse (Fawcett and Karban 2005). Removing the right of a person to take responsibility through the use of the Mental Health Act also places a person in a situation where they have no direct power to change their circumstances and yet are pressured to take responsibility for their recovery (Beresford and Hopton 2003). As there is a direct link between the responsibilities a person has and the rights they are entitled to, practices which reduce those rights, such as the focus on risk, perpetuate the cycle of exclusion (Rogers and Pilgrim 2001; Fawcett and Karban 2005). Professionals are bound by a duty of care to protect not only those in their care but also the public from harm. Echoes of Foucault's (1967) assertion that modern societies fear madness in the guise of 'unreason' are clear in the newspaper headlines which report violent incidents committed by people with a history of mental health problems often accompanied by clear or implied statements that such people should be 'locked away'. Against this background of fear, mental health professionals are pressured through a combination of risk-averse legislation and their own fear of litigation to pursue avenues of compulsory treatment and detention that appear to be at odds with the increasing emphasis on recovery and social justice in the wider mental health arena (Fawcett 2007). The tension between care and control within psychiatry raises a number of further questions. First, does the law contribute to the stigmatization of those it seeks to protect? Second, what are the ethical implications of the law as it currently stands with regards to the autonomy of the individual and what does this mean for professionals seeking to promote the recovery and autonomy of their clients? Finally are there any realistic alternatives to the current system and if so what roles do professionals and nurses have in achieving change?

Campaigners for reform of mental health law have increasingly highlighted the potential of the law to contribute to stigmatization and discrimination, even when it seeks to support care and treatment. Some have even argued that the law creates more problems than it resolves (Sartorius 2002). The role of law as the framework for policy gives it the potential to exert the pressure needed to both influence and reform public opinion (Heginbotham and Elson 1999). The question of involuntary treatment is a good demonstration of the stigmatizing potential of mental health legislation. In physical medicine, a patient has the right to refuse treatment where they have capacity to understand the risks and benefits of potential treatment. This right exists even where failure to treat the condition would result in the patient's death (Matthews 1999; Szmukler 2010). Contrast this situation with the law governing involuntary treatment of mental health problems and a different picture emerges. This distinction between the physically ill and the mentally ill implies that the latter lack the competence or capacity to decide on their treatment. This assumed lack of competence means that society deems it necessary to create laws that coerce people into treatment against their wishes. The distinction between mental and physical health reflects a fear associated with the mental health problems which continues to affect politicians and lawmakers. As a result mental health law therefore becomes influenced by public attitudes towards mental illness (Eastman and Peay 1999).

The Mental Health Act alone is enough to indicate that as a society we feel it necessary to contain (so-called) mental illness as a separate entity and also that those who are mentally ill are qualitatively different in nature from those who are physically ill (Eastman and Peay 1999). It is for this reason that campaigners for reform of the mental health system have for many years targeted law and psychiatry's use of the law as stigmatizing and promoting discrimination against users of mental health services (Szmukler and Holloway 2000; Szasz 2004; Szmukler 2010). Szasz (2004) asserts that the foundation for mental health law is morally and medically unfounded and that it denies the rights of the individual against the rights of the system. The Mental Health Act (2007) is primarily designed to contain and manage risk and not to promote the rights of patients (Richardson 2010). It has been argued that the current system disempowers service users and makes an unjustifiable distinction between the rights of those with a physical illness and those with mental health problems (Matthews 1999; Dawson and Szmukler 2006; Ryan 2011). This view is supported by others critical of medical psychiatry who argue that what we perceive as mental illness and madness cannot be categorized as a disease in the medical sense of the word (Bentall 2003). However, the law can only be used as people wish it to be used (Eastman and Peay 1999). Law is a reflection of public concern, and politicians who enact laws such as the Mental Health Act do so in the belief that they are acting both for the good of the individual and for the safety of the public (Szmukler 2010). Indeed, the Mental Health Act (2007) was hailed as providing a landmark in the provision of rights for mental patients (Bean 1986). However, the discussion so far indicates that the actual reasons for the failure of professionals to combat stigma do not appear to lie exclusively in the personal beliefs and actions of individuals but in the fundamental tensions that underlie the policies which shape their practice (Berry et al. 2010). Many professionals are faced with a role confusion that permeates their entire practice. Their dilemma is whether their role is a caring one or whether they are agents of state control for mental illness. This tension prevents mental health services from being able to overcome the structural characteristics of the system. In other words, mental health services are suffering not from a crisis of attitude but a crisis of ideas (Bentall 2003).

35.5 Potential Solutions to the Current Situation

There are alternative options to the current laws that govern the mental health system which could improve the autonomy of service users and clients in choosing their treatment. The ethical basis of the law could arguably have the biggest effect upon reducing the stigma associated with the mental health system. Some of the potential future solutions, such as the capacity-based approach outlined within the Mental Capacity Act (2005), provide an example of what a more ethical mental health system could one day look like. A system of mental health law based upon capacity might eliminate some of the challenges and stigma by relocating the focus in the system from controlling risk to assessing capacity. This could achieve a complete and coherent ethical framework of practice over physical and psychological medicine (Dawson and Szmukler 2006). To achieve this, services would have to shift their focus away from control towards autonomy and social inclusion and promote involvement and recovery. A system which used capacity as a basis for judging the appropriateness of enforcing treatment would also have to consider the person's best interests and would also have to be flexible and open to the notion of fluctuating capacity (Barker 2010). Another fundamental part of any capacity-based system would be the introduction of advance directives (already enshrined in Scottish law), pre-existing declarations by a person before they become unwell concerning the forms of treatment they would wish to accept. Advance directives are not without problems; this may be seen in the ability of the Mental Health Act to override the contents of an advance directive and also over the definition of what constitutes 'treatment' within the mental health system (Barker 2010). The disability-inclusion model (Sayce 2000) highlights the potential of anti-discrimination law to be a tool in advocating for the rights and citizenship of people with disabilities on an equal footing to the rest of society. The ethos of this is present in the, although the Act fails to wholly protect the rights of those with mental health problems. The disability-inclusion model argues that exclusion results not from the inherent characteristics of an individual but the barriers society constructs against them. It calls upon service users not to accept a passive sick role but to fight for equal rights and responsibilities in law. It provides a significant challenge to the discriminating nature of current mental health law and paves the way forward for a more inclusive and more just mental health system (Sayce 2000). It also fits well with the capacity-based approach, basing its premise upon the promotion of autonomy, social inclusion and an emphasis on a recovery-orientated system of care.

Conclusion

The argument that has emerged through this review is that the mental health system creates an environment of almost institutionalized stigma. It is the requirement to be risk averse and to control and monitor behaviour which lies at the heart of the challenges facing nurses in reducing stigma. Such an approach denies the rights of the individual and compels professionals to restrict opportunities and challenges in favour of practice that effectively continues a cycle of exclusion (Beresford and Hopton 2003; Szmukler 2010). However, the causes of this are not entirely internal. The 'moral panic', created by media representation of violence committed by people with mental health problems, is reflected in the policies and laws which govern the mental health system (Paterson and Stark 2001; Paterson 2006). The degree to which this occurs lessens the ability of the mental health system to act independently to correct them. Yet the answer to the question of how nurses can challenge stigma hinges on their ability to effect meaningful change within the system and its laws. It must be acknowledged that a small minority of service users, such as those who have committed serious crimes, will inevitably attract significant stigma. However, this study has focused on the experiences of the majority, not minority, of service users within the NHS. Public attitudes alone cannot change institutional practices nor alter laws. Nurses alone cannot overturn a social phenomenon as embedded as stigma; however, by campaigning for changes in the law, it is possible that a change in the way mental health problems are perceived may occur and that this may lead to reduction in the degree of stigma attached to mental health problems. The education of nurses to equip them in this task should also form a fundamental part of any attempt to reduce public stigma. Mental health law contributes to the perpetuation of the stigma surrounding mental health problems. However, there are potential solutions to this problem such as the use of capacity-based law. Additionally, the law can also be used as a tool to fight for the rights of people with mental health problems and to create a system of laws against discrimination in housing and employment that would combat social exclusion and stigma.

References

Amering M, Schmolke M (2009) Recovery in mental health: reshaping scientific and clinical responsibilities. Wiley-Blackwell, Oxford

Barker P (2010) Mental health ethics: the human context. Routledge, London

Bean P (1986) Mental disorder and legal control. Cambridge University Press, Cambridge

Bentall RP (2003) Madness explained: psychosis and human nature. Penguin, London

Beresford P, Hopton J (2003) Recovery or independent living openmind. In: Barker P (ed) Mental health ethics: the human context. Routledge, London

Berry C, Gerry L, Hayward M et al (2010) Expectations and illusions: a position paper on the relationship between mental health practitioners and social exclusion. J Psychiatr Ment Health Nurs 17:411–421

Bertram G, Stickley T (2005) Mental health nurses, promoters of inclusion or perpetuators of exclusion? J Psychiatr Ment Health Nurs 12:387–395

Coleman R (2004) Recovery: an alien concept. P&P Press, Isle of Lewis

Crisp AH (2004) Every family in the land: understanding prejudice and discrimination against people with mental illness, Revised edn. London, Royal Society of Medicine Press

Cross J, MacGregor HN (2010) Knowledge, legitimacy and economic practice in informal markets for medicine: a critical review of research. Soc Sci Med 71:1593–1600

Dawson J, Szmukler G (2006) Fusion of mental health and incapacity legislation. Br J Psychiatry 188:504–509

Department of Health (2011) No health without mental health. Crown, London

Eastman N, Peay J (1999) Law without enforcement. Hart Publishing, Oxford

Edgley A, Stickley T, Masterson S (2006) Whose right? J Ment Health 15:35–42

Elliot L, Masters H (2009) Mental health inequalities and mental health nursing. J Psychiatr Ment Health Nurs 16:762–771

Fawcett B (2007) Consistencies and inconsistencies: mental health, compulsory treatment and community capacity building in England, Wales and Australia. Br J Soc Work 37:1027–1042

Fawcett B, Karban K (2005) Contemporary mental health: theory, policy and practice. Routledge, Oxford

Foucault M (1967) Madness and civilisation. Routledge Classics, London

Goffman E (1963) Stigma notes on the management of spoiled identity. Penguin, London

Green G (2010) The end of stigma? Changes in the social experience of long-term illness. Routledge, Oxford

Healthcare Commission (2008) Mental health service users' survey. Healthcare Commission, London

Heginbotham C, Elson T (1999) Public policy via law: practitioners sword and politicians shield. In: Eastman N, Peay J (eds) Law without enforcement. Hart Publishing, Oxford, pp 59–74

Hinshaw SP (2007) The mark of shame stigma and mental illness and an agenda for change. Oxford University Press, Oxford

Jackson L, Tudway JA, Giles D et al (2009) An exploration of the social identity of mental health inpatient service users. J Psychiatr Ment Health Nurs 2:167–176

Knapp M (2007) Mental health policy and practice across Europe: the future direction of mental health care. McGraw Hill International, Maidenhead
Lawton-Smith S (2010) Briefing paper 2 – supervised community treatment. http://www.mentalhealthalliance.org.uk. Accessed 18 Feb 2011
Matthews E (1999) Mental and physical illness: an unsustainable separation? In: Eastman N, Peay J (eds) Law without enforcement. Hart Publishing, Oxford, pp 47–58
Mental Capacity Act (2005) c.9. http://www.legislation.gov.uk. Accessed 31 Jan 2011
Mental Health Act (2007) c.12. http://www.legislation.gov.uk. Accessed 31 Jan 2011
Munro S, Baker JA (2007) Surveying the attitudes of acute mental health nurses. J Psychiatr Ment Health Nurs 14:196–202
National Health Service Information Centre (2010) In-patients formally detained in hospitals under the Mental Health Act 1983 and patients subject to supervised community treatment, annual figures, England 2009/10. http://www.ic.nhs.uk. Accessed 11 Feb 2011
Office of National Statistics (2010) Attitudes to mental illness 2010 research report. http://www.dh.gov.uk. Accessed 11 Feb 2011
Paterson B (2006) Newspaper representations of mental illness and the impact of the reporting of the 'events' on social policy: the 'framing' of Isabel Schwarz and Jonathan Zito. J Psychiatr Ment Health Nurs 13:294–300
Paterson B, Stark C (2001) Social policy and mental illness in England in the 1990s: violence, moral panic and critical discourse. J Psychiatr Ment Health Nurs 8:257–267
Pearson G (1999) Madness and moral panics. In: Eastman N, Peay J (eds) Law without enforcement. Hart Publishing, Oxford, pp 159–172
Ramon S, Williams JE (2005) Mental health at the crossroads: the promise of the psychosocial approach. Ashgate Publishing, Surrey
Repper J, Perkins R (2003) Social inclusion and recovery: a model for mental health practice. Elsevier Health Sciences, London
Richardson G (2010) Mental capacity at the margin: the interface between two acts. Med Law Rev 18:56–77
Roberts G, Wolfson P (2004) The rediscovery of recovery: open to all. Adv Psychiatr Treat 10:37–49
Rogers A, Pilgrim D (2001) Mental health policy in Britain, 2nd edn. Palgrave Macmillan, Basingstoke
Rogers A, Pilgrim D (2010) A sociology of mental health and illness, 4th edn. Open University Press/McGraw Hill, Maidenhead
Ross CA, Goldner EM (2009) Stigma, negative attitudes and discrimination towards mental illness within the nursing profession: a review of the literature. J Psychiatr Ment Health Nurs 16:558–567
Ryan CJ (2011) One flu over the cuckoo's nest: comparing legislated coercive treatment for mental illness with that for other illness. J Bioethical Inquiry 8:87–93
Sartorius N (2002) Iatrogenic stigma of mental illness: begins with behaviour and attitudes of medical professionals, especially psychiatrists. Br Med J 324:1470
Sayce L (2000) From psychiatric patient to citizen: overcoming discrimination and social exclusion. Macmillan Press, London
Schneider J, Beeley C, Repper J (2011) Campaign appears to influence subjective experience of stigma. J Ment Health 20:89–97
Shepherd G, Boardman J, Slade M (2008) Making recovery a reality. Sainsbury's Centre for Mental Health, London
Slopen NB, Watson AC, Gracia G et al (2007) Age analysis of newspaper coverage of mental illness. J Health Commun 12:3–15
Stickley T, Wright N (2011a) The British research evidence for recovery, papers published between 2006–2009 (inclusive). Part one: a review of the peer-reviewed literature using a systematic approach. J Psychiatr Ment Health Nurs 18:247–256
Stickley T, Wright N (2011b) The British research evidence for recovery, papers published between 2006–2009 (inclusive). Part two: a review of the grey literature including book chapters and policy documents. J Psychiatr Ment Health Nurs 8:297–307

Sweeney A, Beresford P, Faulkner A et al (2009) This is survivor research. PCCS Books, Ross-on-Wye

Szasz T (2004) Faith in freedom libertarian principles and psychiatric practices. Piscataway, Transaction Publishers

Szmukler G (2010) How mental health legislation discriminates unfairly against people with mental illness text of Gresham lecture. http://www.gresham.ac.uk. Accessed 6 Dec 2010

Szmukler G, Holloway F (2000) Mental Health Law: discrimination or protection London: South London & Maudsley NHS Trust. http://www.iop.kcl.ac.uk. Accessed 6 Dec 2010

The Mental Health Foundation (2000) Pull yourself together – a survey of stigma and discrimination faced by people who experience mental distress. http://www.mentalhealth.org.uk. Accessed 20 Jan 2010

Thornicroft G (2006) Shunned discrimination against people with mental illness. Oxford University Press, Oxford

Tidmarsh D (2004) The need for risk assessment: myth vs reality. In: Crisp AH (ed) Every family in the land: understanding prejudice and discrimination against people with mental illness. Royal Society of Medicine Press, London, pp 269–274

Wahl O (1999) Mental health consumers experiences of stigma. Schizophr Bull 25:467–478

Westwood L, Baker J (2010) Attitudes and perceptions of mental health nurses towards borderline personality disorder clients in acute mental health settings, a review of the literature. J Psychiatr Ment Health Nurs 17:657–662

Woollaston K, Hixenbaugh P (2008) Destructive Whirlwind: nurses perceptions of patients diagnosed with borderline personality disorder. J Psychiatr Ment Health Nurs 15:703–709

Part VI

Special Populations

Psychiatric/Mental Health Nursing Care of Children and Adolescents

36

António Jorge Soares Antunes Nabais, Lucília Rosa Mateus Nunes, John R. Cutcliffe, and José Carlos Santos

36.1 Introduction

The international epidemiological evidence, limitations notwithstanding, seems to suggest that the worldwide prevalence of mental health problems among children and adolescents is increasing (World Health Organisation 2017). In the European region, in some reports, one in five children was deemed to have evidence of mental health problems and this proportion appears to be increasing with more recent epidemiological studies demonstrating that mental health problems (or for some

During the 1970s and 1980s, the socio-emotional problems of children were not always understood and debated by health professionals as mental health problems, and parents or educators did not refer these children to mental health care. The justifications, given by parents when confronted with aggressive behavior or disobedience of their children, were related to the characteristics of children's own development or to parental anxiety, often mobilized as an argument by educators.

A.J.S.A. Nabais (✉)
Centro Hospitalar Lisboa Central, Hospital D. Estefânia,
Área Pedopsiquiatria: Rua Jacinta Marto, 1169-045 Lisboa, Portugal
e-mail: antunesnabais@gmail.com; antonio.nabais@chlc.min-saude.pt

L.R.M. Nunes
Nursing Department, Escola Superior de Saúde—Instituto Politécnico de Setúbal,
Campus do IPS, Estefanilha Edifício da ESCE, 2914-503 Setúbal, Portugal

J.R. Cutcliffe
Cutcliffe Consulting, Kingston, Canada

School of Nursing, Coimbra, Portugal
e-mail: jcutcliffe@outlook.com

J.C. Santos
Escola Superior de Enfermagem de Coimbra, Nursing School of Coimbra, Coimbra, Portugal
e-mail: jcsantos@esenfc.pt

© Springer International Publishing Switzerland 2018

J.C. Santos, J.R. Cutcliffe (eds.), *European Psychiatric/Mental Health Nursing in the 21st Century*, Principles of Specialty Nursing,
https://doi.org/10.1007/978-3-319-31772-4_36

psychiatric disorders) have become the main cause of disability and one of the major causes of morbidity in today's societies. According to this body of work, while some children/adolescents present with mental health problems that meet diagnostic criteria, many other children/adolescents report experiencing mental health problems that can be considered subliminal; they do not meet the diagnostic criteria for so-called "psychiatric disorders"; however, the child/adolescent still reports suffering and thus would likely benefit from specialized interventions and/or treatment. Contemporary thinking and some evidence suggest that emotional and behavioral problems in children might benefit from an early evaluation, with some research findings indicating that a later response from the professional mental health support services makes rehabilitation/recovery more difficult (Major and Seabra-Santos 2013).

Interestingly, key conceptualizations pertaining to mental health and child/adolescent have evolved in recent decades. Historically and traditionally, the age boundaries for the population of "children and adolescents" were determined to start before the child's birth and end at 18 years of age. However, more contemporary views have broadened such conceptualizations—increasing the upper age boundary to 25 years. And as such, these more contemporary views mirror the compelling evidence regarding human brain development and maturity (e.g., whereby the human brain is considered fully developed or fully mature/adult, until the person reaches their mid-twenties (Giedd et al. 1999; Sowell et al. 1999, 2001; Johnson et al. 2009). As a result, an argument can be constructed that suggests organizing care solely on the basis of age may not always be the most appropriate way to create responses in health and specifically in mental health.

36.2 Epidemiological Overview: Acknowledging the Nuanced View

Arriving at an undisputed and accurate epidemiological of mental health problems in children/adolescents in Europe and the rest of the world is no simple task. According to World Health Organization (WHO), 10–20% of children and adolescents worldwide experience mental health problems (for some—these are so-called psychiatric or mental disorders) (WHO 2017). Green et al. (2005) describing the problem in biomedical/diagnostic terms, indicate that the most common so-called "disorders" in childhood and adolescence include: "conduct disorder," "attention deficit hyperactivity disorder" (ADHD), "autistic spectrum disorders," "depression," and "anxiety disorders" (Green et al. 2005). Some recent studies have identified mental health problems, particularly depression, as the major cause of "disease" burden among young people (WHO 2017). However, according to a number of studies, the so-called ADHD is the most commonly experienced child/adolescent mental health problems with a worldwide prevalence estimate of 3.4% (Polanczyk et al. 2015), being more prevalent in the United States (8.7–10.6%) than in Europe (Visser et al. 2014). Interestingly, these varying patterns of diagnosis may very well reflect different medico-political, or/and cultural nuances in the practice (and accuracy) of diagnosis per se, rather than being accurate depictions of the scope of the problem in different countries (Office of the United States Surgeon General 2001). Not only do "classic" or "seminal" studies indicate that clients presenting with the same/very similar clinical "pictures" in the United States and the United Kingdom receive significantly different diagnoses (e.g., much broader conceptualization of schizophrenia in the USA leading to more diagnoses than the British psychiatrists, Kendell et al. 1971), but furthermore, studies indicate that cultural factors appear to have a significant affect and effect in shaping the form, course, response, and outcome of the mental health challenge (Jilek 2001).

> Pathoplastic effects of socio-cultural factors appear to shape the symptom profiles manifested by sufferers from schizophrenia differently in developed and developing countries. Schizophrenic patients in Western developed countries showed a higher frequency of depressive symptoms, primary delusions, thought insertion and thought broadcasting, while in non-Western developing countries visual and directed auditory hallucinations were more frequent" (Jilek 2001).

Establishing the precise epidemiology of mental health problems in children and adolescents and the efficacy of our responses to the same is further bedeviled by the fact that 42% of children with ADHD are followed up by a primary health care provider rather than a mental health practitioner. In addition to accurate identification of the mental health problem(s), this efficacy and therapeutic value of responses to these health challenges can be impeded and impacted negatively (Tatlow-Golden et al. 2016) (Table 36.1).

Establishing a precise epidemiology is also encumbered by the well-documented, related problems of: the over-medicalization of everyday life (Szasz 2007) and diagnostic inflation (Kudlow 2013). These questionable practices have led to a "diagnostic spiral" including the increasing (over) prescription of drugs, sometimes for life, even when such drugs have not been shown to have any substantial positive effect on any measure of "morbidity" for mental health problems (see Albarracin et al. 2015). According to the WHO Comprehensive Mental Health Action Plan 2013–2020 (2013, p. 13),

> children and adolescents with mental disorders should be provided with early intervention through evidence-based psychosocial and other non-pharmacological interventions based in the community, avoiding institutionalization and medicalization".

Further evidence of the creeping diagnostic inflation in child and adolescent psychiatric care is evident when one examines the data on rates of prescription of antidepressant and ADHD medication. From 2005 to 2012, the prevalence of antidepressant use increased by 26.1% in the United States, 54.4% in the United Kingdom, 60.5% in Denmark, and 17.6% in the Netherlands. Similarly, the prevalence of ADHD medication use has significantly increased by 111.9% in the Netherlands, 302.7% in Denmark, 62.4% in German, 56.6% in the United Kingdom, and 10.7% in the United States (Bachmann et al. 2016, 2017). Yet, these documented increases in prescriptions of psychotropic medication to children and adolescents are highly controversial (Connor 2011), especially given the ongoing and unresolved debate over its diagnostic validity, etiology, presentation, and treatment. Further, studies have found that cohorts treated for ADHD and subsequently followed up show poorer outcomes as adults than do participants in the control groups (see Zwi and York 2004). In summary, caution should be exercised when interpreting the figures on the epidemiology of mental health problems in children and adolescents, given the problems identified above. Though it can be stated with a degree of empirical confidence that mental health challenges and/or problems, especially those related to experiences of trauma and/or abuse, are a serious public health problem and require a substantive, serious response from the formal mental health services.

36.3 Assessment

A very useful and informative set of practice parameters for working with this client group has been advanced by the Association of Child and Adolescent Psychiatric Nurses (A Division of International Society of Psychiatric Nurses) (accessed May 16th 2017). According to these principles of care, the child/adolescent client and his/her family have a right to expect:

- A thorough assessment of current behavior, centered on issues that prompted admission.
- An opportunity to explain their perceptions of the behaviors and symptoms that prompted admission.
- A holistic assessment.
- The assessment should include examination of other factors integral to the child's functioning (e.g., client strengths, support system (or lack thereof), coping patterns, history or experience of trauma/abuse/neglect).
- An exploration of the child's experiences, relationships, and functioning within peer groups, family, school, and the neighborhood/community.
- An assessment of the child's thoughts, mood, and affect.
- A consideration of any verbal or non-verbal signs of danger to self or others,
- Review of evidence or history of any substance misuse: type, amount, frequency, context. Include legal, illegal, over-the-counter, and psychoactive substances.
- A review of achievement/non-achievement of developmental milestones.
- Review of medications: current, past years, side/adverse effects, dosage adjustments, and response.

As with assessment in adult mental health, the accuracy and validity of the assessment will be enhanced if this occurs within an emerging, trusting therapeutic relationship. A thorough assessment will draw upon a variety of sources of information in addition to that provided by the client him/herself; not least the information provided by the client's family.

36.4 Core Interventions

Regardless of the specific mental health issue(s) or problem(s) that the client presents with, a number of core practices that the P/MH should ensure are available. For mental health facilities that seek to use the "milieu" as a component of the care provided, then understandably the milieu needs to be managed in a way that creates opportunities for the client to feel heard and understood; to feel safe to explore his/her issues and problems; for the milieu itself to be calming or even soothing. Plus, this will create multiple opportunities for interactions with and observations of the child/adolescent in a variety of milieu settings with different people.

In one important way, the P/MH nursing care of the child/adolescent is no different from that of nursing the adult, older adult, or even family unit in that forming and maintaining a therapeutic interpersonal relationship is central to effective P/MH nursing care (Peplau 1988). Inextricably bound up with the development and maintenance of such relationships is therapeutic communication, or to paraphrase: using counselling skills or "working in a counselling way." Micro skills associated with such ways of working include:

- Be genuine.
- Be warm, friendly, affirming and supportive.
- Be respectful and communicate the same.
- Retain your own sense of hope and hopefulness, bring this into each counselling encounter and implicitly project this into the interpersonal dyad.
- Be non-judgmental, accepting, compassionate, and understanding.
- Listen—intently—to the person(s).
- Use full range of Heron's (1990) categories of therapeutic intervention: prescriptive, informative, confrontative, cathartic, catalytic, and supportive.
- Consider using full range of micro-skills to communicate empathy—such as: simple reflection, selective reflection, paraphrasing, empathic building, checking for understanding, clarifying, and appropriate self-disclosure.
- And consider thoughtful use of silence.

Invariably, working therapeutically with children and adolescents is very likely to require some work in the affective or "feeling" (emotional) domain. And while children and some adolescents may have difficulty identifying, exploring, discussing, and working with uncomfortable (often painful) emotions, this will need to be an area that the P/MH nurse feels confident and competent in. The P/MH nurse need not be afraid of emotion, even often raw and "messy" emotion, expressed with the interpersonal encounter as she/he needs to understand that such emotions will arise and be part of the encounter. Indeed, a core practice element is the "role modeling" that the P/MH nurse can engage in around the notion of acknowledging, accepting, expressing, exploring and finding meaning in the expression of emotion. The authors of this chapter deliberately eschew the term "managing" emotion as this has too many connotations of controlling, inhibiting, and discouraging emotion, and the research evidence in this area indicates that working with raw emotions remains an area of practice that many nurses are not comfortable with (Gray 2009; Hagen et al. 2017). Yet, literature in this area points out how strong, unresolved, or unaddressed emotions can interfere with effective change. Accordingly, the P/MH nurse can (should) demonstrate through her/his own actions how she/he can "hear" strong or raw emotion and not "run away" (literally or metaphorically) from such expressed emotion. The P/MH nurse can demonstrate how to bring such emotion (or and reactions to the emotion) more under control and help the child/adolescent learn to exercise more control over his/her emotions rather than the opposite.

Children and adolescents, arguably, need to learn and internalize that emotions and feelings are to be expected, especially if in response to challenging/traumatic experiences, and that such feelings need to be brought into the open and experienced (so-to-speak) rather than hidden or suppressed. In so doing, the P/MH nurse can help the child/adolescent begin to explore and learn about how to recognize his/her own emotions, how to give accurate names to them, how to differentiate between appropriate (and acceptable) and inappropriate (unacceptable) emotional expression. Such feeling orientated work can also occur in the form (or context) of: psychodrama, art therapy, or through "play exercises." Coupled with such work is exploring the meaning behind or underpinning the emotion. The child/adolescent should discover that the expression of emotion is still a form of communication.

36.5 Involving and Working with Families and Children/Adolescents

For the authors of this chapter, P/MH nursing in childhood and adolescence often needs the involvement of the family (Maybery and Reupert 2009). Research findings support the idea of family involvement in care; with family members of certain adolescent populations have identified several interventions that would fit their needs, including: multifamily groups, family therapy, and individual therapy (Oruche et al. 2014). Gaining a more comprehensive and deeper insight into and understanding of the child's challenges cannot be obtained solely from the client; the client's experiences do not occur in isolation because of their lack of autonomy and dependency care from extra uterine life and during the early years; it often falls to the parents the responsibility to organize the child's world.

It is important to know the set of "the priors" that parents have built on the performance they expect the child has, often in relation with their age, preventing the child stays in a pre-built and grounded restrictive context (Garnier 1995) nullifying their individuality. P/MH nurses might considering encouraging parents to engage in spontaneous interaction(s) with the child, stimulating creativity, originality and appropriateness to contexts. Spontaneity defines the degree of adequacy of the response that the individual presents in a new situation, or a measure of novelty in response to an old situation. It corresponds to a kind of intelligence that operates in the "here and now." Spontaneity manifests in word, in action, interaction, as well as in singing, dancing, or drawing. However we know that there are pathological spontaneity, distorting perceptions or dissociate the representation of roles, it is always important to assess the degree of adequacy of the response to the situation (Moreno 2013, 36).

36.6 Particular Psychiatric/Mental Health Nursing Challenges When Working with Children or Adolescents

36.6.1 Dealing with Aggression and Violence

Regrettably, both empirical and narrative evidence indicates that aggressive/violent behavior in children and adolescents who seek formal mental health care is common; though significant variation is to be found in the assorted studies that have attempted to estimate/measure the frequency of such incidents (see, for example, Baeza et al. 2013; Zahrt and Melzer-Lange 2011). However, the cause or antecedent for these behaviors is most often complicated, multi-factorial, convoluted and can involve many factors/experiences (see chapter—systemic model—Chap. 33). Thus a deeper and more comprehensive understanding of the range of factors and experiences that can contribute to development of aggressive/violent behavior is vital for P/MH nurses. Especially if these wish to avoid repeating the mistake of apportioning all responsibility (and blame) squarely on the shoulders of the client and his/her pathology (see chapter—systemic model—Chap. 33). It is critical for the P/MH nurse to be aware that acts of aggression are a form of communication in children/adolescents and similarly, rather than adopting an arbitrary response to aggression or violence, the P/MH nurse needs to try and understand the motivating factors, the client's background and history, the client's learned responses and behaviors and thus be able to respond appropriately to the aggression. For instance, understanding the profound differences between aggressive behaviors resulting from a fear/threat response and resulting from intimidation, malevolence, etc. should significantly inform the P/MH nurses' response to the behavior.

Our approach to responding to aggression/violence is embedded in a de-escalation framework and philosophy (see Chap. 25 Psychiatric/Mental Health Nursing Non-Physical Competencies for Managing Violence and Aggression: De-escalation and Defusion). The authors support and adopt the view regarding the use of physical restraint advanced by the APNA (2014) who regard all such uses as treatment failure and seek the elimination of seclusion and restraint. So while a mental health service that is free of physical restraint, seclusion, rooms, and mechanical restraint devices might be regarded as aspirational, it is particularly needed in cases where the child/adolescent has a history of trauma, abuse and/or neglect (see chap. 9). Further, a pro-active rather than reactionary response to aggression/violence is preferred. In this way, during a period of calm or/and receptivity in the client, the P/MH needs to explore and help the client recognize behaviors that indicate to staff that client's experience of arousal is increasing (or/and becoming upset), e.g. pacing, isolating in room, clipped speech, tense body posture. The P/MH nurse also needs to explore, consider, and learn new, alternate coping mechanisms that do not resort to aggressive or violent behaviors. Importantly, such explorations need the child/adolescent/family to participate collaboratively in the plan of care regarding episodes of aggression and extreme affect dysregulation. As pointed out in Chap. 33 (Riahi) P/MH nurses working with aggressive youth must recognize behaviors in themselves and during interactions with children that precede violent behavior. Recognition of such behaviors is the key to developing effective interventions (see chapter—systemic model—riahi). The authors of this chapter also recommend that responses to aggression/violence in should be discussed and negotiated in advance of any incidents and thus be a pro-active rather than reactive measure. The identification of triggers or antecedents to aggression and violence can help in the construction of a de-escalation plan. Plus, stress and anger management techniques should be explored and considered. For instance, distraction can be a useful technique that with practice can become very effective over time. Distraction, in this context, refers to anything the client/P/MH can do that will temporarily shift the client's focus or attention away from the noxious stimuli and strong negative emotion. Distraction ought to be personalized to the individual client, but as a rule, but this appears to be most effective as an intervention if the focus of your distraction is both absorbing and interesting to the client. There is some evidence that indicates how staying focused or even ruminating about the noxious stimuli/strong emotion can make it feel even stronger and even more difficult to control. Temporarily shifting the focus through distraction can then provide a little time and space for the client's emotions to decrease in intensity, making aggressive or violent behavior less likely. The P/MH nurse would be wise to remember that learning, practicing, and eventually becoming proficient in distraction—especially self-distraction—will take time. Clients are likely going to make mistakes and the P/MH nurse must be mindful of this. Lastly in this section is the need for formal debriefing sessions post-aggressive/violent incident. This is not an opportunity to pour on blame, but more an opportunity to—the child/adolescent will be able to process his/her feelings and perceptions with staff after an episode of aggression.

36.6.2 Dealing with Children and Adolescents with a History of Trauma, Abuse, Neglect, and/or Mistreatment

As detailed in Chap. 9 (Trauma-Informed Care: Progressive mental health care for the twenty-first century) there is no little or no major disagreement within the mental health workforce community that childhood experiences of trauma, abuse, or neglect are commonplace. Accordingly, the authors would argue that all child and adolescent formal mental health services should either incorporate the principles and practice of trauma-informed care, or at the very least weave these principles and practices into the unit philosophy. Given the restrictions in word space, the authors will not repeat all the relevant material from chapter nine, but rather review some of the principal interventions.

- Attempt to gain a history—children may be unwilling to share these experiences at first—without a trusting relationship established. However, if possible, explore occurrences or abuse, neglect, maltreatment, methods used and current status of perpetrator.
- Build trust, demonstrate unconditional acceptance and tolerance.
- Understand that the client's mental health problems are a manifestation of their attempt to deal with/live with/survive their traumatic past rather than manifestations of an "illness," "disease," or "disorder."
- Attempt to illicit details of family structure and dynamics, sociocultural issues/factors, behavioral patterns.
- Identify and explore any coping mechanisms that have been developed and employed by the child/adolescent subsequent to trauma experiences.

- Discuss and explore if the client has developed any coping methods that have been employed with success by the child/adolescent following experience of trauma.
- The identification, recovery and strengthening of personal inner resources.
- Emphasize the genuine possibility of "recovery."

36.6.3 Dealing with Children and Adolescents with a History of Self-Harm or/and Suicide Attempts

As detailed in Chap. 32 (suicide and self-harm), and the associated peer reviewed literature, the phenomena of self-harm and suicide are encountered fairly commonly in this population. While a precise epidemiology is very difficult to come by, given the problems in definition, concetptualization, reporting, and methodological limitations of studies, global estimates suggest the rate is increasing.

For the authors of this chapter, responses to adolescent self-harm are sometimes misinformed, overly-paternalistic. They fail to address the underlying psychological needs that causes the drive to self-harm and regrettably, are still conflated inappropriately with suicide and thus regarded as a failed suicide attempt. For example, some authors continue to conflate self-harm and suicide and depict the phenomena as one and the same; merely different points on a continuum of lethality (Anderson and Jenkins 2006; Claassen et al. 2006). This is unfortunate as the significant majority of the contemporary theoretical and empirical work clearly distinguishes self-harm from suicide and suicidal ideation. Perhaps these differences are most succinctly captured by Maris, Berman, Silverman, and Farberow (2000) when they state

> as a starting point, we must distinguish indirect self-destructive behaviors from behaviors more directly suicidal…In marked contrast, there are, however, a vast number of behaviors that are self-harmful, frequently injurious, self-negating, and self-defeating in which the individual engages but in which there may be no intention to die."

There are significant differences between suicide and self-harm, not only a difference in the outcome; self-harm is not necessarily a failed suicide attempt. Reduced to perhaps their simplest (most fundamental) differences, self-harm is a life orientated, coping-related act and suicide is a death-orientated act. As a result, it should therefore be no surprise that the responses to/interventions for self-harm and for genuine suicide attempts are not necessarily the same. While the findings around the reasons given for self-injurious acts are equivocal, a number of findings do occur with a noticeable frequency and degree of consistency. First is the finding that self-harm is complex. Second, the motive "to get relief from a terrible state of mind" was found to be the most commonly endorsed reason for self-harm (in boys and girls) (Rasmussen et al. 2016). Analogous findings are reported in Klonsky's work (see 2006 for example.) He studied the functions of non-suicidal self-injury in 39 young adults with a history of skin-cutting and other self-injurious behaviors including banging, burning, and severe scratching. Results indicate that self-injury is associated with improvements in affective valence and decreases in affective arousal. Specifically, participants tended to feel overwhelmed, sad, and frustrated before self-injury, and relieved and calm after self-injury.

The authors offer an important caveat here, by differentiating between suicide and self-harm, we are not suggesting that the issues are not linked and that any person who self-harms is, by the nature of the differences, not at risk of suicide. Indeed, methodological problems notwithstanding, numerous studies continue to highlight the significantly increased risk of eventual suicide for people, including adolescents, who engage in self-harm (Santa Mina and Gallop 1998; Cooper et al. 2005). However, there is a wealth of empirical evidence that shows that 95% and over of people who engage in self-harm do not go onto to take their own lives (Santa Mina and Gallop 1998; Anderson 2000; Welch 2001) (Table 36.1).

The second somewhat misinformed position that appears with conspicuous frequency in the associated literature is the automatic pathologizing of self-injurious acts. The Cornell Research Program on Self-Harm (2017) highlights the top 15 misconceptions regarding self-harm, these are listed in table one. These further underscore the major differences between self-harm and suicide but moreover, also illustrate that self-harm need not be pathologized. They stress how self-harm is a coping behavior that is not understandable to most of society. Indeed they go on to state

> "People who engage in repetitive self-injury have reported being diagnosed with depression, bipolar disorder, anorexia, bulimia, obsessive compulsive disorder, post-traumatic stress disorder, and/or anxiety and panic disorders. **Many who self-injure may not have any diagnosable disorder at all; a recent study found that almost half of college students with current self-injury behavior show no other identifiable mental illness**. (emphasis added)"

Table 36.1 15 top misconceptions regarding self-harm

1. Only females self-injure	9. People who self-injure only cut themselves
2. Self-injury is a suicide attempt or failed suicide attempt	10. Anyone who self-injures is part of the "Gothic" or "Emo" sub-culture
3. Only teenagers self-injure	11. People who self-injure enjoy the pain or can't feel it
4. Anyone who self-injures is crazy and should be locked up	12. There's nothing I (as a P/MH nurse) can do to help
5. Self-injury is not just attention seeking	13. All people who self-injure have been abused
6. Self-injury is untreatable	14. Someone who self-injures can stop if they really want to
7. People who self-injure are manipulative	15. Someone who self-injures is a danger to others
8. All people who self-injure have "Borderline Personality Disorder"	

Thirdly, is the understandable though often misinformed reactions of parents and care givers. Many parents and care givers sometimes react from a paternalistic, authoritarian position (see, for example, Holdsworth et al. 2001; McAllister et al. 2002), at least in part, because of the common reactions of shock, anger, sadness, or guilt. All of these are understandable reactions. However, even a cursory view of some of the narratives of their "care" experiences provided by hospitalized people who engage in self-harm makes for a harrowing listening[1]. The paternalistic and authoritarian interventions only serve to compound any feelings of low self-worth, reinforce misplaced perceptions about deserving to be treated in this way.

The P/MH nurses' role in part involves acknowledging and listening to the parents' feelings/reactions but steering them gently towards a more helpful conceptualization and resultant response(s). In place of authoritarian response, communicating understanding, compassion, non-judgment, and empathy will be more beneficial and therapeutic. Indeed, perhaps there is even a place for a discussion with the client/parents around how to de-stigmatize or even how commonplace (and thus not "abnormal") self-injurious behavior can be in adolescents. An argument can be constructed that some existential questioning should might even be expected during the tumultuous years of adolescence and young adulthood (Berman et al. 2006). Consider, for example, the many challenging situations that teenagers may well encounter: cyber and other forms of bullying; confusion and stigma regarding sexual orientation, exploration and choices, balancing emancipation from/retaining bond with parents, academic, sporting or artistic performance and expectations of success, peer group acceptance, family and parent dynamics/relationship, and by no means least, a past history of trauma, abuse, neglect, or mistreatment.

36.7 Concluding Remarks

The prevalence of mental health problems among children and adolescents appears to be on the increase. The number of people in the age group that are diagnosed with a so-called mental disorder and subsequently 'treated' with psychotropic medication appears to be on the increase. This is despite the existing, documented concerns about such "off label" medication use and the evidence pertaining to the limited efficacy of these medications. Nevertheless, the contemporary P/MH nurse is likely to encounter children and/or adolescents in the mental health care system and thus, after taking a nuanced view of the epidemiology, the chapter draws on the ACAPN practice parameters and uses these to inform our approach to assessment. Core interventions, which are drawn from and congruent with the principles and practices of trauma-informed-care

[1] see, for example, https://www.bing.com/videos/search?q=pateralistic+nursing+responses+to+people+who+self+harm&view=detail&mid=B463C02625B30DAAC99FB463C02625B30DAAC99F&FORM=VIRE;. https://www.bing.com/videos/search?q=pateralistic+nursing+responses+to+people+who+self+harm&&view=detail&mid=A1BF8F79917DB41FFE7AA1BF8F79917DB41FFE7A&rvsmid=4888B79E43DBB288B7DF4888B79E43DBB288B7DF&fsscr=0&FORM=VDFSRV.

are then explored, and P/MH nurses are then exhorted to involve and work collaboratively with clients and their families. The chapter then focuses on three particular challenges for the P/MH nursing care of children and adolescents. While these are by no means the only challenges that P/MH are likely to face, they are encountered frequently and show up with conspicuous regularity in the relevant extant literature. Namely: dealing with aggression and violence; dealing with children and adolescents with a history of trauma, abuse, neglect, and/or mistreatment and dealing with children and adolescents with a history of self-harm or/and suicide attempts.

References

Albarracin D, Ducousso-Lacaze A, Cohen D, Gonon F, Keller P, Minard M (2015) There is no cure for existence: on the medicalization of psychological distress. Ethical Hum Psychol Psychiatry 17(3):149–158

American Psychiatric Nurses Association Position on the Use of Seclusion and Restraint (2014) https://www.apna.org/i4a/pages/index.cfm?pageID=3728#PositionStatement. Accessed 19 May 2017

Anderson R (2000) Assessing the risk of self-harm in adolescents: a psychoanalytic perspective. Psychoanal Psychother 14(1):9–21

Anderson M, Jenkins R (2006) The national suicide prevention strategy for England: the reality of a national strategy for the nursing profession. J Psychiatr Ment Health Nurs 13(6):641–650

Bachmann J, Wijlaars L, Kalverdijk L, Burcu M, Glaeske G, Schuiling-Veninga C, Hoffmann F, Aagaard L, Zito J (2016) Trends and patterns of antidepressant use in children and adolescents from five western countries, 2005–2012. Eur Neuropsychopharamcol 26:411–419

Bachmann J, Wijlaars L, Kalverdijk L, Burcu M, Glaeske G, Schuiling-Veninga C, Hoffmann F, Aagaard L, Zito J (2017) Trends in ADHD medication use in children and adolescents in five western countries, 2005–2012. Eur Neuropsychopharamcol 2017(03):02

Baeza I, Correll CU, Saito E, Amanbekova D, Ramani M, Kapoor S, Chekuri R, De Hert M, Carbon M (2013) Frequency, characteristics and Management of Adolescent Inpatient Aggression. J Child Adolesc Psychopharmacol 23(4):271–281

Berman S, Weems CF, Stickle T (2006) Existential anxiety in adolescents: prevalence, structure, association with psychological symptoms and identity development. J Youth Adolesc 35(3):285–292

Center for Disease Control and Prevention (2013) Mental health surveillance among children — United States, 2005–2011. MMWR supplements 62(02):1–35. https://www.cdc.gov/mmwr/preview/mmwrhtml/su6202a1.htm

Claassen CA, Trivedi MH, Shimizu I, Stewart S, Larkin GL, Litovitz T (2006) Epidemiology of nonfatal deliberate self-harm in the United States as described in three medical databases. Suicide Life Threat Behav 36(2):192–212

Connor D (2011) Problems of over diagnosis and overprescribing in ADHD. Psychiatric times, Recovered May16th 2017 http://www.psychiatrictimes.com/adhd/problems-overdiagnosis-and-overprescribing-adhd/page/0/1

Cooper J, Kapur N, Webb R, Lawlor M, Guthrie E, Mackway-Jones K, Appleby L (2005) Suicide after deliberate self-harm: a four year cohort study. Am J Psychiatr 162(2):297–303

Cornell Research Program of Self-Harm Top 15 misconceptions of self-injury. http://www.selfinjury.bctr.cornell.edu/perch/resources/15-misconceptionsenglish-7.pdf. Accesed 19 May 2017

Garnier P (1995) Ce dont les enfants sont capables marcher, travailler, nager XVIII; XIX, XX siècles, Editions Métailié

Giedd J, Blumenthal J, Jeffries NO et al (1999) Brain development during childhood and adolescence: a longitudinal MRI study. Nat Neurosci 2:861–863

Gray B (2009) The emotional labour in nursing 1: exploring the concept. Nurs Times 105(8):26–29
Green H, McGinnity A, Meltzer H et al (2005) Mental health of children and young people in Britain, 2004. Palgrave MacMillan, New York
Hagen J, Knizek BL, Hiemeland H (2017) Mental health nurses' experiences of caring for suicidal patients in psychiatric wards: an emotional endeavor. Arch Psychiatr Nurs 31(1):31–37
Heron J (1990) Helping the client: a creative practical guide. Sage, Los Angeles
Holdsworth N, Belshaw D, Murray S (2001) Developing A&E nursing responses to people who deliberately self-harm: the provision and evaluation of a series of reflective workshop. J Psychiatr Ment Health Nurs 5:449–458
Jilek WG (2001) Cultural factors in psychiatric disorders. Paper presented at the 26th Congress of the World Federation for Mental Health, July 2001. http://mentalhealth.com/mag1/wolfgang.html
Johnson SB, Blum RW, Giedd JN (2009) Adolescent maturity and the brain: the promise and pitfalls of neuroscience research in adolescent health policy. J Adolesc Health 45(3):216–221
Kendell R, Cooper JE, Gourlay AJ et al (1971) Diagnostic criteria of American and British psychiatrists. Arch Gen Psychiatry 25:123–130
Klonsky DE (2006) The functions of self-injury in young adults who cut themselves: clarifying the evidence for affect regulation. Psychiatry Res 166(2–3):260–268
Kudlow P (2013) The perils of diagnostic inflation. CMAJ 185(1):25–26
Major S, Seabra-Santos MJ (2013) Uso de inventários comportamentais para a avaliação socio-emocional em idade pré-escolar. Avaliação Psicológica 12(1):101–107
McAllister M, Creedy D, Moyle W (2002) Nurses' attitudes towards clients who self-harm. J Adv Nurs 40(5):578–586
Maris R, Berman AL, Silverman MM (2000) Comprehensive textbook of suicidology. Guilford Press, New York
Maybery D, Reupert A (2009) Parental mental illness: a review of barriers and issues for working with families and children. J Psychiatr Ment Health Nurs 16:784–791
Oruche U, Draucker C, Alkhattab H, Knopf A, Mazurcyck J (2014) Interventions for family members of adolescents with disruptive behavior disorders. J Child Adolesc Psychiatr Nurs 27(2014):99–108
Peplau H (1998) Interpersonal relations in nursing: a conceptual frame of reference for psychodynamic nursing. Palgrave, New York
Polanczyk GV, Salum GA, Sugaya LS, Caye A, Rohde LA (2015) Annual research review: a meta-analysis of the worldwide prevalence of mental disorders in children and adolescents. J Child Psychol Psychiatry 56:345–365
Rasmussen S, Hawton K, Philpott-Morgan S, O'Connor R (2016) Why do adolescents self-harm? An investigation of motives in a community sample. Crisis 37:176–183
Santa Mina EE, Gallop R (1998) Childhood sexual and physical abuse and adult self-harm and suicidal behaviour: a literature review. Can J Psychiatr 43(8):793–800
Sowell ER, Thompson PM, Holmes CJ et al (1999) In vivo evidence for post-adolescent brain maturation in frontal and striatal regions. Nat Neurosci 2:859–861
Sowell ER, Thompson PM, Tessner KD et al (2001) Mapping continued brain growth and gray matter density reduction in dorsal frontal cortex: inverse relationships during postadolescent brain maturation. J Neurosci 21:8819–8829
Szasz T (2007) The medicalization of everyday life. Syracuse University Press, New York
Tatlow-Golden M, Prihodova L, Gavin B, Cullen W, McNicholas F (2016) What do general practitioners know about ADHD? Attitudes and knowledge among first-contact gatekeepers: systematic narrative review. BMC Fam Pract 17:129
The Association of Child and Adolescent Psychiatric Nurses A Division of International Society of Psychiatric Nurses (ISPN) (2017) Practice parameters child and adolescent inpatient psychiatric treatment: inpatient psychiatric treatment http://www.ispn-psych.org/docs/PracticeParameters.pdf. Accessed 18 May 2017
Visser SN, Danielson ML, Bitsko RH, Holbrook JR, Kogan MD, Ghandour RM, Perou R, Blumberg SJ (2014) Trends in the parent-report of health care provider-diagnosed and

medicated attention-deficit/hyperactivity disorder: United States, 2003–2011. J Am Acad Child Adolesc Psychiatry 53:34–46 (e32)

Welch SS (2001) A review of the literature on the epidemiology of parasuicide in the general population. Psychiatr Serv 52(3):368–375

WHO (2013) Comprehensive Mental Health Action Plan 2013–2020. WHO, Geneva

WHO (2017) Child and adolescent mental health. Available at: http://www.who.int/mental_health/maternal-child/child_adolescent/en/

Zahrt DM, Melzer-Lange MD (2011) Aggressive behavior in children and adolescents. Pediatr Rev 32(8):325–332

Zwi M, York A (2004) Attention-deficit hyperactivity disorder in adults: validity unknown. Adv Psychiatr Treat 10(4):248–256

António Jorge Soares Antunes Nabais Specialist Nurse in Mental Health and Psychiatry, Master in Sociology, Chief Nurse—Centro Hospitalar Lisboa Central—Hospital D. Estefânia—Área Pedopsiquiatria: Rua Jacinta Marto 1169-045 Lisboa: antonio.nabais@chlc.min-saude.pt; http://www.chlc.min-saude.pt/content.aspx?menuid=214&eid=2325&returnUrl=%2fcontentlist.aspx%3fmenuid%3d214. Professor Adjunto—Escola Superior Enfermagem Lisboa: Avenida Professor Egas Moniz, 1600–190 Lisboa: antonio.nabais@esel.pt http://www.esel.pt/ESEL/PT/ESEL/Docentes/antonionabais.htm

Lucília Rosa Mateus Nunes Specialist Nurse in Mental Health and Psychiatry, PhD Philosophy, Full Teacher, Head of Nursing Department, Escola Superior de Saúde—Instituto Politécnico de Setúbal, Campus do IPS, Estefanilha Edifício da ESCE 2914-503 Setúbal: lucilia.nunes@ess.ips.pt http://www.si.ips.pt/ess_si/FUNCIONARIOS_GERAL.FORMVIEW?P_CODIGO=8471

Psychiatric/Mental Health Nursing Care of the Older Adult: Mental Health in Old Age

37

Bengt Eriksson and Arild Granerud

37.1 Introduction

It is a well-documented fact that the European population is growing older (European Union (EU) 2015). Old age might bring increased risk of mental health problems in the later days of life, as a result of different changes related to, for example, social losses or physical ill health. Parallel to this, the power of resistance often decreases, not least as a result of reduced social networking. Therefore, old people's mental health should be addressed as an important field for research and improved practice. This chapter focuses on providing mental health care to and for older adults from a humanistic and holistic perspective. The view is psychosocial, resting on the conviction that both mental well-being and mental ill health are closely related to and dependent on one's social environment and personal story. The chapter deals with demographic developments in Europe and touches on different gerontological theories, but its main content is about mental ill health among old people, theories on mental health care and how they can take place, focusing on the local community perspective.

37.2 An Ageing Population

Next to Japan, Europe has the oldest population. The average length of life within the European Union (EU) is almost 80 years (European Union (EU) 2015); the average does vary greatly across the different countries of the EU. Examination of the epidemiological data indicate some general trends in that the average European lifespan is increasing and the differences in lifespan between men and women are

B. Eriksson (✉) • A. Granerud
Inland Norway University of Applied Science, Faculty of Public Health, Hedmark University College, Elverum, Norway
e-mail: bengt.eriksson@hihm.no; arild.granerud@hihm.no

© Springer International Publishing Switzerland 2018

J.C. Santos, J.R. Cutcliffe (eds.), *European Psychiatric/Mental Health Nursing in the 21st Century*, Principles of Specialty Nursing,
https://doi.org/10.1007/978-3-319-31772-4_37

decreasing. A study from a number of western European countries predicts that half the children born after the millennium will reach age 100 years (Christensen et al. 2009). Demographically, this means that an increasing part of the population will be constituted by older people and, by the year 2060, large parts of Europe will have twice as many older people (over 67 years) than today (Statistisk sentralbyrå (SSB) 2010). It is important to emphasize that this is a 'story of success', namely, that most people can look forward to living a 'full' (or entire) life, experiencing childhood, adolescence, adulthood, middle age and old age. The increasing average length of life has given rise to the concepts of 'the third age' and 'the fourth age' (Adams et al. 2011). The third age refers to the period when working (employed) life has past, but before health problems and the need for formal or informal support have put substantial limitations on everyday life. The third age can, therefore, be characterized by a high degree of freedom and self-realization but also has the potential for informal help and support to grown-up children, grandchildren, partners and society. The fourth age refers to the period of life around 80 years old and above and is more often coupled with health deficiencies and losses, causing a greater need for medical and social care. At the same time, this is the section of the population that is growing the fastest (European Union (EU) 2015). It is the post-war generation of 'baby boomers' who will, during the coming years, approach the age of 80 and beyond.

Despite the fact that older people do not constitute a united or homogenized group, they are often described as if they were. Rather, the opposite is more accurate. It is more relevant to regard older people as a group (or groups) that is as heterogenous (or composite) as other groups of people in earlier stages or phases of life. There are those who are extraordinarily positive, active and energetic and also those who struggle with diseases and functional deficiencies, social losses and a burdensome everyday life. However, in particular, in between there is a comprehensive group, mainly living a well-ordered and satisfying life, but not without obstacles and experiences of pain—in short, people living their lives like most other people in the population.

Accordingly, in our view, this is the most helpful, accurate and appropriate approach to how to view older people and their mental health status/challenges. Life as an old person, as for the entire lifespan, has risks for mental health problems. After becoming increasingly vulnerable and with physical health deficiencies, the risk of mental health problems can increase. However, it is not ageing itself that implies deteriorated mental health. Rather, the opposite, research on old people's quality of life shows that most have a positive view of life (Atchley 1999). Anyway, the ongoing demographic changes necessitate increased focus on health-care and social care services for old people, with the aim to prevent and cure ill health and maintain good health.

37.3 Theoretical Approaches to Ageing and Mental Health

Several theories have been advanced which seek to explain the psychosocial ageing process. Probably the most widely used, especially as a conceptual framework for research studies, is Erikson's theory (Erikson 1982). It has had a major impact on the view of old age and posited this as the last stage of psychosocial development. Erikson's theory tends to depict a positive view of old age. He describes the development of human beings in terms of evolution in eight stages, of which the last stage is old age; Erikson also describes the psychological challenges faced by people in the transition to this (and the other) phase. According to his theory, to avoid a psychosocial crisis, it is essential for individuals to know how to resolve the developmental and experiential challenges associated with this phase. At this stage, a meaningful whole can be created within the context of a person's entire life. To accept the life that is lived, with its events and experiences, can lead to the development of wisdom, which, according to Erikson, is closely related to acceptance of meeting death (Erikson 1982, 1995).

The theory about a lifespan focuses partly on another aspect of human life, namely, the close connection with, and dependence on, experiences during an entire life, from childhood, adolescence, working life and early old age to old age. The situation of life as an old person may be combined with experiences of mental ill health and takes place within the framework of the limitations and possibilities of the previous life. Experiences of, for example, mental health illness at a younger age follow the individual throughout his or her whole life, affecting interpretations and consequences of later life events. The lifespan can therefore be regarded as temporal (as a process or horizontal movement; Kohli 1985), but it can also be regarded vertically, i.e. in relation to other circumstances in the micro- or macro-environment. Focus is then directed towards the individual's personal biography in relation to important environmental events.

A theory of ageing that has gained increasing attention is that of gerotranscendence. Tornstam (1999, 2005) advanced the theory of gerotranscendence, and within that theory, gerotranscendence is viewed as the final stage in a natural process towards maturation and wisdom. It represents a shift in metaperspective, from a materialistic and rational view of the world, to a more cosmic and transcendent view (Hauge 1998). For Tornstam (1999, 2005), the theory of gerotranscendence is manifest (or has impacts) on different dimensions of the person. Changes in the so-called 'cosmic' dimension relate to an increasing sense of connection to earlier generations, a new understanding of life and death and acceptance of the mystery dimension of life. Self-confrontation, decrease of self-centredness, increased self-awareness and ego integrity are associated with the so-called dimension of 'self'. In old age, the individual with a transcendent perspective experiences a need to spend more time on meditation and less on material things and superficial social relationships (Hauge 1998; Tornstam 2005). With this theory, Tornstam offers a new way of understanding old age. His interpretation of withdrawal as another form of activity is special, and this activity is qualitatively different from the traditional form of social activity and engagement. Tornstam labels this form of activity transcendence and says that it helps to enhance the experience of a good life (Hauge 1998).

37.4 Mental Health Problems Among Older People

For most people old age means changes and adaptation, many of which are unwanted, such as the need to move to sheltered housing, physical diseases or functional impairments limiting everyday life, partner's diseases or death. These changes might be characterized as transitions connected to old age. Old people's health varies on the same continuum as everyone else's, from more or less normal stressors of everyday life, to serious illnesses that dominate the entire personality and the contexts of life. Various kinds of ill health, which can be more or less related to ageing, are often more frequently encountered as the person ages. They can, for example, be burdensome circumstances connected to experiences of losses in old age, or social losses that can lead to crises, but could also be more long-lasting experiences, such as anxiety and depression. On the other hand, serious mental health problems ('psychosis') do not often debut in old age. Older people with these forms of mental health problems have, in most cases, a long-lasting personal history of mental health problems. However, it is not unusual for transitions connected to old age, such as sudden disease and hospitalization, to give rise to states of mind such as delirium or acute confusion psychosis. Psychotic symptoms among elderly people present a challenge for medical and mental health-care professionals in inpatient, consultation/liaison and nursing home settings. Delirium is one of the most common causes of psychosis in elderly patients (Hassett et al. 2005).

37.5 Social Losses, Crisis and Transitions of Old Age

Transitions connected to old age are, for many people, expressed as crises, both acute traumatic crises and more long-lasting developmental crises. Age leads to increased risk of different experiences of loss, which could be loss of work, colleagues, friends and family but also loss of function due to reduced physical health (Haaning 2009). Similarly, Engedal (2008) found that factors such as poor health, limited social network, reduced flexibility on the basis of disability and existential feelings of meaninglessness reduce the ability to cope in old age. For many, this might lead to loneliness and depression (Thorsen and Clausen 2008; Kvaal et al. 2014). People who live alone tend to be lonelier than people who live with others. Widows and widowers are among the loneliest. According to Slagsvold and Daatland (2006), people with mental health problems have been found to be significantly lonelier than others, and physical health impairment also increases the risk of loneliness. Routasalo and Pitkala (2003) similarly reported that the experience of loneliness is a common feeling in old age, but there is a wide variation in prevalence in epidemiological studies from a few per cent to about 40% in some studies.

37.6 Grief and Depression

Emotional stress such as grief, related to loss of partner, friends or other relatives, is frequently reported in older adults (Borglin et al. 2005; Janlöv et al. 2005), but many older people also experience varying degrees of anxiety when life circumstances change for the worse (Janlöv et al. 2005, Brown and Harris, 1978). Depression is one of the dominant threats to public health in our time; studies have shown that around 12% of the population in western countries are affected (Kvaal et al. 2014). Depression is connected to the risk of suicide, with old people's risk of suicide being four times that of younger people. It has been argued that depression among old people is often connected to physical diseases, mainly cardiovascular diseases, and that these in turn involve a risk factor for the development of dementia (Kvaal et al. 2014). Depression is perceived as a severe multidimensional disorder that affects physical, mental, social and spiritual aspects of health and life. In its most severe form, it is perceived as unbearable (Hedelin and Strandmark 2001a).

37.7 Anxiety

Anxiety might be defined as a feeling of threat towards the entire personality, where the cause of this feeling of threat is unknown. Through its undefined character, anxiety becomes a self-reinforcing experience, making the affected person afraid of his or her anxiety. This means that anxiety is difficult to approach using the strategies normally available (Yochim et al. 2013). Existential anxiety is a kind of identity and developmental anxiety, connected to the fundamental conditions of our existence as human beings, coupled with, among other things, feelings of loneliness and isolation.

37.8 Dementia

Dementia is probably the kind of mental health suffering that most people connect with old age. It is a collective term for a group of interrelated states of deficiency, sharing their most loaded symptoms. Initially, the symptoms of dementia are memory difficulties, learning problems and, over time, the inability to routinely manage activities of daily life (Dahl 2004). The most common form of dementia is Alzheimer's disease (about 60% of cases), although vascular dementia represents about 25% of cases of dementia (Dahl 2004). These diseases are progressive, causing ever-increasing consequences for those who are affected. Relatives of people with dementia become strongly involved, so these diseases have been labelled 'the relative's disease'. Often, they imply a heavy emotional burden for the affected individual, shifting from moments of understanding one's situation to lack of understanding. Grief caused by the insight that intellectual capability disappears can give rise to depression. For relatives, it is often painful to experience how the intellectual and mental capacities of the affected loved one—his or her personality—disappear while, at the same time, the person's physical appearance is the same as it used to be.

37.9 Theoretical Approaches to Mental Health Care and Older Adults

Professional care for people with mental health problems, from mental health nurses and other helping professions, should always be based on the fundamental principles of humanistic caring and empathy. In addition, there are also particular theories, concepts and approaches that are applied to and operationalized in this field. The concepts of sense of coherence, coping and recovery are prominent.

37.9.1 Sense of Coherence

Various perspectives on ageing, such as knowledge of so-called mental disorders, start from a deficiency perspective that focuses mainly on negative factors. Antonovsky (1996) based his theory on health and developed the theory of 'salutogenesis' through studies of people who had experienced traumatic events but still managed to develop and maintain a positive basic attitude. Antonovsky identifies three characteristics that unite these people; they have a high degree of (1) comprehensibility, which means that they appear to understand the events in their environment and how their own situation is affected; (2) manageability, meaning that they make reasonable efforts to influence and control their situation and thus what will happen in life; and (3) meaningfulness, which means that they can put their own situation into a meaningful context, thereby giving life changes a direction and creating motivation to continue life. Antonovsky (1996) describes these three characteristics as sense of coherence. According to the salutogenic perspective, the nurse must contribute to the existence of elderly people, in which their own and ambient resources and factors promote health, and where the overall life situation is at the centre—rather than focusing on deficiencies, signs of (mental and physical) poor health and declining capabilities.

37.9.2 Coping

Mental health in elderly people, as in younger people, covers a wide range of emotions, situations and conditions. Coping is expending conscious effort to solve personal and interpersonal problems and seeking to master, minimize or tolerate stress or conflict (Weiten and Lloyd 2008). Various forms of coping can take different directions. They may involve dealing with different emotions, to preserve their self-esteem, to develop social interaction with other people or to solve different problems (Rønnmark 1999). To develop the structure and routines of everyday life can be a coping strategy—being out in nature or moving physically is another. Many different patterns of behaviour have been described as strategies for coping, but which strategies are used vary from person to person. There are also negative coping strategies, which attempt to deal with, for example, uneasiness and anxiety; this does not contribute to a positive solution but instead maintains the individual in a situation of health problems and dependence. For those who work in mental health with elderly people, it is important to know which coping strategies (positive or negative) they use, in order to connect their work to these and thereby reinforce an individual's resources.

37.9.3 Recovery from Mental Health Problems

Although there is consensus about the cornerstones of the concept of recovery from mental health problems, there is still no official and universally accepted definition of the concept (Davidson et al. 2005). One element that is common to all definitions of so-called mental illness is, however, that the process of recovery comprises a combination of collective social processes and individual intrapersonal changes. Currently, there are at least three different interpretations of the concept of recovery from so-called mental illness (Care Services Improvement Partnership, Royal College of Psychiatrists and Social Care Institute for Excellence 2007; Granerud and Eriksson 2014). First, recovery can be regarded as a process of improvement without treatment, powered by an individual's own resources and often supported by an informal network. Second, recovery can be seen as a result of effective clinical treatment, whereby recovery is defined by the absence of symptoms constituting a specific mental disease, in combination with the ability to function in daily life. In this regard, the focus is on an instrumental and behavioural definition of the concept. Third, recovery can be described as a personal process of change, in the sense that life is experienced as positive and meaningful, despite any remaining difficulties and shortcomings in everyday life. In this perspective, unique personal experiences play a larger role, and aspects such as hope, trust and security become important components on the road to recovery.

Adams and Partee (1998, p. 31) emphasize in particular the importance of hope in the recovery process stating:

> Hope is the anticipation of a desired event or condition – expectation of something good happening in the foreseeable future. Hope springs from a sense of 'the possible'.

Similarly, Anthony (1993, p. 15) defines personal recovery as:

> A deeply personal, unique process of changing one's attitudes, values, feelings, goals, skills, and/or roles.

The context in which we have searched for increased knowledge on recovery is primarily related to the last (i.e. the third) comprehension of the concept of recovery from mental illness. However, this process of personal change and development can be supported by professionals, such as mental health nurses, being sensitive to the individual's own pace, the need for time to reflect and growth 'from inside' as parts of the recovery process.

37.10 Psychiatric/Mental Health Nursing for Elderly People, Focusing on the Local Community Context

Most senior citizens will sooner or later need services from the public. Having reached the fourth stage of life, many experience a greater need for assistance. In most European countries, municipalities commonly provide the services necessary for older adults in their daily lives. Social and medical care and support for older adults is aimed mainly at physical health problems. Most senior citizens with impaired physical health have several physical health challenges. In addition, sometimes accidents occur, such as fractures that may be difficult to heal. Furthermore, older adults are heavy consumers of different drugs (Westlund and Sjøberg 2005), which often interact with each other and produce different effects. Senior citizens often define health based on the ability to be active and participate in social activities/contexts (Nilsson et al. 1998). Participation in or performance of various activities help provide a sense of independence (Borglin et al. 2005). For many older people with disabilities, there are fewer opportunities to fill their days with meaningful activities, which can lead to a feeling of emptiness and a sense of a monotonous life (Tollén et al. 2008). Relationships with other people are perceived as the mainstay of good mental health (Hedelin and Strandmark 2001b). Through verification of themselves and their values in relation to others, the person's mental health has been found to improve (Hedelin and Jonsson 2003). Mental health challenges have been found to, in some cases, be harder to overcome (or cope with) than physical changes (Nilsson et al. 2000). Sensory loss, such as reduced vision and hearing, has also been found to lead many senior citizens to participate less in social interactions and therefore contributes to a greater sense of loneliness (Graneheim and Lundman 2010).

P/MH nursing with older people usually involves personal and prolonged contact. The relationship between the caregiver and the older adult is therefore crucial to the quality of services and service user experiences of mental health care. Where there is a specific relief effort in the form of practical chores, combined with a human presence and insight that we all as humans share fundamental living conditions, there is an improvement in the prospects of achieving and maintaining good mental health. A good relationship is characterized by physical and mental presence and continuity, with opportunities for the helper to be able to spend time, show empathetic understanding and convey hope, trust and confidence. To develop the possibility of such relationships within psychiatric/mental health (P/MH) nursing requires an organization and leadership that support and facilitate the work. Aspects of P/MH nursing must be expanded and, above all, local community 'actors' must create a common strategy to support older adults with mental health problems, who often exhibit more diffuse symptoms than younger people and whose symptoms often coincide with changes in their life situation. We believe that P/MH nursing for elderly people should be based on the following four key concepts:

1. *Everyday life*: the overall objective is to help create an everyday life that is as good as possible. Special measures may be required from time to time, but the important thing is everyday life, with the familiar environment and the 'near and dear things' all around.
2. *Social support*: human beings are social beings. Positive and supportive contacts with others in personal and informal networks are important. Support from volunteers in the community, including more casual contact from health and social workers in the public sector, is the major constituent of good mental health. Four different forms of social support can be described: emotional, cognitive, social affiliation/network and practical. All these forms belong in the arena of mental health care for older people.

3. *Knowledge*: knowledge about older adults and ageing is important, similar to knowledge about mental health and appropriate responses. Particularly in the public sector, social- and health-promoting institutions can increase knowledge about mental health and so-called mental health disorders in older people and provide better help and support. In addition, volunteers, non-profit organizations and consumer organizations should engage in the interface between older adults and mental health.
4. *Communication and cooperation: P/MH nursing* for older adults is an under-focused area. The solution is cooperation and communication across all levels, and between professional groups in municipal health services, based on the understanding that all have important knowledge and resources to supply—but also a shared responsibility—and that the people concerned are at the interface.

37.11 Concluding Remarks

A more multidimensional vision must be developed in which both ageing and expression of mental health problems can be considered, but in which factors such as personal stories, social class, gender, ethnicity and religion must also be reflected as well. Variations among older adults are large so one cannot talk about this population as a unified group. Mental health problems may be related to physical illnesses, social losses of ageing transitions or psychiatric/mental health problems in earlier life. They can express themselves as crisis reactions, anxiety, grief and depression, or severe psychiatric symptoms. The risk of developing dementia increases with age. P/MH nurses and other helping professions can play a major role in strengthening older people with various mental health problems, by supporting their personal recovery and coping ability. Contribution to the establishment and maintenance of an everyday life of the best possible quality could be the overarching goal, guided by a wish to enhance the old person's sense of coherence.

This text is based on previous publications in Norwegian by the authors.

References

Adams SM, Partee DJ (1998) Hope. The critical factor in recovery. J Psychosoc Nurs Ment Health Serv 36:29–32

Adams KB, Roberts AR, Cole MB (2011) Changes in activity and interest in the third and fourth age: associations with health, functioning and depressive symptoms. Occup Ther Int 18:4

Anthony WA (1993) Recovery from mental illness: the guiding vision of the mental health service system in the 1990's. Psychosoc Rehabil J 16:11–23

Antonovsky A (1996) The salutogenic model as a theory to guide health promotion. Health Promot Int 11:11–18

Atchley RC (1999) Continuity and adaption in aging. Creating positive experiences. John Hopkins University Press, Baltimore

Borglin GE, Hallberg AK, Rahm I (2005) The experiences of quality of life among older people. J Aging Stud 19:201–220

Brown GW, Harris T (1978) Social origins of depression. The Free Press, New York

Care Services Improvement Partnership, Royal College of Psychiatrists and Social Care Institute for Excellence (2007) A common purpose: recovery in future mental health services. Social Care Institute for Excellence, London

Christensen K, Doblhammer G, Rau R et al (2009) Ageing populations: the challenges ahead. Lancet 374:1196–1208

Dahl TE (2004) To meet people with loss of memory. In: Hummelvoll JK (ed) Not only the parts – but the whole. Psychiatric nursing and mental health. Gyldendal Akademisk, Oslo

Davidson L, O'Connell MJ, Tondora J et al (2005) Recovery in serious mental illness: a new wine or just a new bottle? Prof Psychol Res Pract 36:480–487

Engedal K (2008) Old age psychiatry in practice. Forlaget Aldring og helse, Tønsberg

Erikson EH (1982) The life cycle completed: a review. Norton, New York

Erikson EH (1995) Childhood and society. Vintage, London

European Union (EU) (2015) The 2015 ageing report. European economy 3|2015. Publications Office of the European Union, Luxembourg. http://europa.eu/epc/pdf/ageing_report_2015_en.pdf

Graneheim UH, Lundman B (2010) Experiences of loneliness among the very old: the Umeå 85 + project. Aging Ment Health 14:433–438

Granerud A, Eriksson B (2014) Mental health problems, recovery and the impact of Green Care Services – a qualitative, participant focused approach. Occup Ther Mental Health 30:317–336

Haaning MG (2009) Mastering ageing. In: Glasdam S, Appel Esbensen B, Andersen-Ranberg K (eds) Gerontology: life as elderly in modern society. Copenhagen, Nyt Nordisk Forlag Arnold Busck/Dansk sygeplejeråd

Hassett A, Ames D, Chiu E (eds) (2005) Psychosis in the elderly. Taylor & Francis, London

Hauge S (1998) An analysis and critique of the theory of gerotranscendence. Report 4/98. Vestfold College, Tønsberg

Hedelin B, Jonsson I (2003) Mutuality as background music in women's lived experience of mental health and depression. J Psychiatr Ment Health Nurs 10:317–322

Hedelin B, Strandmark M (2001a) The meaning of depression from the life – world perspective of elderly women. Issues Ment Health Nurs 22:401–420

Hedelin B, Strandmark M (2001b) The meaning of mental health form elderly women's perspectives: a basis for health promotion. Perspect Psychiatr Care 37:7–14

Janlöv AC, Hallberg IR, Petersson K (2005) The experience of older people of entering into the phase of asking for public home help – a qualitative study. Int J Soc Welf 14:326–336

Kohli M (1985) Die Institutionalisierung des Lebenslaufs. Historische befunde und theoretische argumente. Kølner Z Soziol Sozialpsychol 37:1–29

Kvaal K, Halding AG, Kvigne K (2014) Social provision and loneliness among older people suffering from chronic physical illness. A mixed-methods approach. Scand J Caring Sci 28:104–111

Nilsson M, Sarvimäki A, Ekman SL (1998) Ageing with joy or resigning to old age: older people's experiences of the quality of life in old age. Health Care Later Life 3:94–110

Nilsson M, Sarvimäki A, Ekman SL (2000) Feeling old: being in a phase of transition in later life. Nurs Inq 7:41–49

Rønnmark L (1999) Fallen leafs. On coping when loss of children. Institutionen før Socialt Arbete, Gøteborgs Universitet, Gøteborg

Routasalo P, Pitkala KH (2003) Loneliness among older people. Rev Clin Gerontol 13:303–311

Slagsvold B, Daatland SO (2006) Ageing, local variations: results from the Norwegian study of life course, ageing and generation – runde 1 (report 15/06). Norsk Institutt for Forskning om Oppvekst, Velferd og Aldring, Oslo

Statistisk Sentralbyrå (SSB) (2010) Population projections. National and regional figures, 2012–2100, Oslo. http://www.ssb.no/english/subjects/02/03/folkfram_en/. Accessed 03 May 2016

Thorsen K, Clausen S (2008) Disability, loneliness and depression: what does solitude mean for how persons with disabilities experience depression? Tidsskr Norsk Psykologforening 1:19–27

Tollén A, Fredriksson C, Kamwendo K (2008) Elderly persons with disabilities in Sweden: their experiences of everyday life. Occup Ther Int 15:133–149

Tornstam L (1999) Transcendence in later life. Generations 23:10–15

Tornstam L (2005) Gerotranscendence. A developmental theory of positive aging. Springer Publishing Co., Inc., New York

Weiten W, Lloyd MA (2008) Psychology applied to modern life, 9th edn. Wadsworth Cengage Learning, Boston

Westlund P, Sjøberg A (2005) Antonowsky not Maslow – salutogenic care and nursing. Fortbildningsførlaget, Solna

Yochim BP, Mueller AE, Segal DL (2013) Late life anxiety is associated with decreased memory and executive functioning in community dwelling older adults (Report). J Anxiety Disord 27:567

38 Psychiatric/Mental Health Nurses Care of the Client Who Presents with Both Mental Health and Substance Misuse Problems

John R. Cutcliffe, Rodger Travale, and T. Green

38.1 Introduction: The Shift in Substance Misuse Policy (Decriminalisation, Legalisation and the Move to Treatment-Driven Responses)

If one examines the relevant theoretical, empirical and practice-based literature, it would be difficult to overlook or ignore the sweeping and significant shifts in global drug policy that have occurred in the last 5 years. The quantum shift in such policy can be characterised as the need to move away from a criminal justice-based response to a treatment-based response; to those people who present with substance misuse problems. Coupled with this shift is the underpinning philosophical position (and resultant legislative-legal positions) regarding a person's right to imbibe certain substances. This is perhaps best exemplified by the efforts during the last two decades, to decriminalise/legalise marijuana (see Cutcliffe and Saadeh 2014a, b). For the authors of this chapter, it is not possible or practicable to have a meaningful dialogue around what might be the best or most appropriate care responses to this population without first acknowledging and applying the contemporary global policy shift

J.R. Cutcliffe (✉)
Cutcliffe Consulting, Kingston, Canada

School of Nursing, Coimbra, Portugal
e-mail: jcutcliffe@outlook.com

R. Travale
Healthcare Manager, Chiron Health Services, Prince George Regional Correctional Centre, British Columbia, Canada

T. Green
Clinical Instructor and Psychiatric Nurse Practitioner, Wright State University Ohio, New York, NY, USA

© Springer International Publishing Switzerland 2018

J.C. Santos, J.R. Cutcliffe (eds.), *European Psychiatric/Mental Health Nursing in the 21st Century*, Principles of Specialty Nursing,
https://doi.org/10.1007/978-3-319-31772-4_38

vis-à-vis substance (mis)use. Accordingly, it is necessary to review the key aspects of this policy shift.

Many European and occidental countries have historically had, and in some cases still have, a 'hard line' drug policy, one that champions the criminalization of substance use (possession, distribution, etc.) Interestingly, the published evidence does not offer robust support for this policy, nor does it indicate that countries that enact the most 'hard line' policies have the lowest rates of consumption and usage. For instance, despite the enactment of the 'Nixonesque' so-called 'War on drugs', absolutist policy over the last 40 years or so, it is interesting to note that the USA currently has the highest rates of marijuana and cocaine use in the world (see, e.g. GCDP 2011; Cutcliffe and Saadeh 2014a, b). Countries with more so-called 'liberal' substance use policies and laws (e.g. Canada, some countries in the European Union) have lower rates of substance use. Indeed, the most compelling case example of the efficacy and value of more liberal, treatment-driven policies over draconian, criminalization policies can be found in Portugal, who decriminalised all personal substance possession offences in 2001.

Empirical evaluation of the impacts of this policy 'U-turn' continues to this day, and while the authors are cautious about reaching premature conclusions, the evidence produced so far is both consistent and convincing (see EMCSSA 2013). Five years subsequent to the new policy, substance use among teenagers was found to have declined, the number of people who actively sought treatment for substance use-related problems doubled, and rates of new secondary infections, most notably HIV infections, dropped (Greenwald 2009; Hughes and Stevens 2007, 2010). It is also noteworthy that the chorus of protestations prior to Portugal's new policy being implemented, such as that Portugal would be a 'magnet for dug users', that their beaches would be 'littered with discarded, used needles', that this would lead to 'substance tourism' and that the decriminalisation would result in a vast, surge-like increase in the number of hard line substance users all turned out to be inaccurate (O'Neil 2013). Portugal is by no means the only European country that has shifted its policy on substance misuse and/or relaxed/replaced its criminal justice response. The Netherlands and its iconoclastic 'coffee shops' have long been very visible examples of a more relaxed attitude towards substance use, even though, technically, marijuana isn't legal in the Netherlands. Similarly trends are evident in Spain, where possession and/or the use of marijuana is illegal, but not a criminal offence if it is for personal use. Some German parliamentarians champion progress towards legalisation (see Sabine Bätzing, member of Germany's Bundestag for the Social Democratic Party). As a result, the general trend in the European drug policy is a shift to prevention and decriminalisation rather than punishment.

38.2 What Is 'Dual Diagnosis' and What Are 'Concurrent Disorders'?

At the outset, it needs to be recognised that there is a considerable and unresolved debate concerning the terms/definitions used to depict or capture this population (Hryb et al. 2007). Moreover, whether or not one of these terms can be used as the name of the category for a heterogeneous group of individuals with complex needs is also a contested issue. Most commonly, the term 'dual diagnosis' (DD) is conferred onto individuals who simultaneously experience a mental health problem and substance misuse problem. The National Institute for Mental Health (recovered 2016) in the USA offers little more depth in their definition, stating as they do that:

> Dual diagnosis (also called co-occurring disorders, COD) is the condition of suffering from a mental illness and a comorbid substance abuse problem.

Interestingly, the Substance Abuse and Mental Health Services Administration (SAMSHA) uses the term *co-occurring disorders* (COD) rather than dual diagnosis, when referring to this population, and states that co-occurring disorders refer to the population of clients who experience co-occurring substance-related and mental disorders. Patients said to have (so-called) co-occurring disorders have one or more substance-related disorders as well as one or more mental disorders (Hryb et al. 2007). Other definitions are slightly more broad; Segen's medical dictionary (recovered 2016), for instance, defines DD as:

> The simultaneous presence of two mental health related conditions—e.g., a developmental and a mental disorder, learning disability and substance abuse, depression and substance abuse, etc.

This lack of a widely agreed upon conceptualisation, let alone definition, for this population is one of the most pressing issues bedevilling efforts to advance our knowledge, understanding and resultant practice. In order to obtain meaningful findings with regard to the efficacy (or otherwise) of treatment responses to this population, it is perhaps tautological to point out P/MH nurses/researchers need to be clear that they are comparing 'like WITH like'. Without some standardised definition of what counts as or constitutes a case that warrants the term 'dual diagnosis' and what does not, comparisons of outcomes between (or across) clients become largely meaningless (Proctor et al. 2011; Velentgas et al. 2013).

38.3 Assessment

According to SAMHSA (2006), a vast literature exists on screening and assessment in substance abuse care and a similarly large body of work in assessment in mental healthcare settings. What is less proliferate is the literature on assessment/treatment that specifically addresses persons with (or suspected of having) co-occurring problems. However, in order for such an assessment to be clinically meaningful and useful, it will necessarily include procedures, practices and tools drawn from both the substance abuse and mental health fields (SASMHA 2006). Indeed, Munro and Edward (2008) advance the point that improved education to enhance the assessment and diagnosis of this client group is also considered essential for P/MH nurses. A number of instruments/assessment scales and clinical interview assessment guides have been produced to gauge the severity of the person's substance misuse/mental health problems, and a selection of these are listed in Table 38.1.

Table 38.1 Dual diagnosis/co-occurring disorders assessment instruments

Authors	Instrument	Available at
Rosenberg et al. (1998)	Dartmouth Assessment of Lifestyle Instrument (DALI)	Rosenberg, S.D., Drake, R.E., Wolford, G.L., Mueser, K.T., Oxman, T.E., Vidaver, R.M., Carrieri, K.L. & Luckoor, R. (1998) Dartmouth Assessment of Lifestyle Instrument (DALI): A substance use disorder screen for people with severe mental illness (1998) *American Journal of Psychiatry*, 155(2), 232–8
Matson and Bamburg (1998)	Assessment for Dual Diagnosis (ADD)	http://www.sciencedirect.com/science/article/pii/S0891422297000310
K. W. Wanberg	Adolescent Self-Assessment Profile II (ASAP II)	http://aodassess.com/software_applications/AMS/AMS_Sample_Profile.pdf
Stallvik and Nordahl (2014)	American Society of Addiction Medicine (ASAM) second edition-revised	Stallvik, Marianne; Nordahl, Hans M. (2014) Convergent Validity of the ASAM Criteria in Co-Occurring Disorders. *Journal of Dual Diagnosis*, 10(2), 68–78
World Health Organisation (2010)	The Alcohol, Smoking and Substance Involvement Screening Test (ASSIST): manual for use in primary care	http://apps.who.int/iris/bitstream/10665/44320/1/9789241599382_eng.pdf

38.4 The Clinical Assessment Interview: Fundamentals and Rudiments

As with any mental health assessment, the accuracy and validity of assessment in this population are enhanced when the P/MH nurse has established a trusting, therapeutic interpersonal relationship with the client/survivor. The clinical assessment interview needs to be comprehensive and holistic and should consider physical, psychological and social issues/needs. Specific attention in the assessment needs to include questions pertaining to the individual's history and patterns of behaviour regarding substance misuse and mental health histories. The Saskatoon Regional Health Authority—Mental Health and Addiction Services Concurrent Model Working Group (MHASCMWG) (2007)—published a comprehensive assessment guide for this population. Here the authors summarise the main areas for assessment and include some examples. Readers are referred to the original documents for more comprehensive and detailed assessment questions.

1. Emotional and Psychological Well-Being

Areas to consider: physical appearance, behaviour, speech/thought (form and content), appetite, sleep, affect/mood, cognition, memory, insight, psychiatric history, medical history, social and family history, suicidal thoughts, plans, etc.

2. Substance Use and Problem Gambling

Areas to consider: the reason(s) client is presenting to services, patterns of substance use (types, quantities, frequency), method(s) used, any history of substance use, problems/consequences experienced due to current or past substance use, history of admissions/detoxification due to substance use, details of previous recovery attempts, memory impairment, lack of concentration, difficulty retaining new information, insomnia, anxiety, depressed feelings and restlessness/agitation.

3. Danger to Self or Others/Personal Safety

Areas to consider: history of intentional self-harm, history of driving while impaired, engaging in high-risk sexual activity (e.g. unprotected sex), wandering/absconding, risk of suicide (thoughts, plans, attempts), risk of violence towards others (thoughts, plans, history), history of being harmed/exploited by others and safety of immediate physical and emotional environment.

4. Spirituality

Areas to consider: sense of purpose, sense of meaning in life, feeling of connection to others, society, culture, belief in a higher power, cultural practices and religious affiliation.

5. Stressful Life Events/Trauma

Areas to consider: what are the significant sources of stress in the present and normal coping strategies, recent untoward stressful events, unresolved trauma that contributes to current stress or limits coping strategies and willingness to engage in problem-solving and to reach out for support.

6. Physical Health

Areas to consider: overview of physical health status assessment will be required, chronic health problems, disability, chronic pain, acute/short-term physical health problems, commitment/motivation to pursue a healthy lifestyle or aspire to self-care, nutritional status, recent significant weight loss/gain, housing and symptoms of withdrawal.

7. Daily Living Skills

Areas to consider: ability/confidence/concern level about performance of daily living skills, presence/absence of relevant skill sets, willingness/capacity/opportunity to learn daily living skills, motivation/strengths/limitations and availability of formal/informal supports to counter deficits.

8. Personal Response to Illness, Substance Use, Abuse and Dependency

Areas to consider: willingness to accept and take responsibility for own problems; degree of distress related to loss of function/aspirations; degree of discomfort with consequences of choices made/substance; estrangement from friends/family; financial losses; disruption of employment and social connections; sense of self-worth, self-esteem and self-motivation; willingness to assume responsibility; strive for independence/self-sufficiency; willingness and ability to engage in problem-solving; and utilise available support.

9. Family and Caregiver Concerns

Areas to consider: explore family's attitudes to and understanding of client's illness/problems/substance use, explore impact of client's symptoms/behaviour on client's parents/spouse/children and degree of connection/estrangement with family and explore patterns of guilt/blame and of taking/avoiding responsibility and willingness to remain connected.

10. Friendships/Social Relationships

Areas to consider: size/extent and quality of friendship/social network, level of satisfaction and reliance on social relationships/activities, willingness to severe contacts with 'substance'-related contacts and comfort and ability to maintain social and significant relationships.

11. Recreation/Leisure

Areas to consider: explore client's awareness of recreation and leisure/education activities, what is the client's level of participation in meaningful recreational activity, identify areas of social and coping skill development required and assess what is the client's current reliance on/importance of his/her structure/routine, what barriers prevent engagement/participation in social activities.

12. Work/Education

Areas to consider: what are the client's personal interests, motivation and current skills and what is the client's capacity for new learning/problem-solving skills/abilities, employment situation, continuing education/training situation, ambition/goals rework/education, past work and education history.

13. Financial Status

Areas to consider: employment status/prospects, income sources, financial comfort level (e.g. sufficient to cover basic day-to-day living expenses, pay the bills), ability to manage finances and budget, helpful and unhelpful spending patterns (e.g. during a manic phase) and need for advocacy/trusteeship.

14. Housing/Accommodation

Areas to consider: current housing/accommodation status, congruence between current housing and the client's needs/preference/income, ability to manage and 'run' a home and any special housing/environmental needs.

15. Legal/Advocacy Issues

Areas to consider: existence of unresolved criminal or civil legal matters, need for a formal advocate or guardian, existence of Community Treatment Order and how informed/aware is the client of his/her rights in relation to healthcare and rights in relation to certification or determination of capacity.

16. Medication Management

Areas to consider: awareness of prescribed medication regime, comfort/satisfaction with medication regime, does the client fully understand the rationale for the medication prescribed, is the client adhering to the prescribed medication regime, risk for future non-compliance, what is the extent of the client's understanding of how the medication allegedly works and incidence, frequency and severity of side effects and iatrogenic effects (Box 38.1).

Box 38.1 Additional questions to consider asking during admission and assessment processes—adapted from Saskatoon Regional Health Authority—Mental Health and Addiction Services Concurrent Model Working Group (MHASCMWG 2007) and SAMSHA (2006)

1. What brought you (the client) here today?
2. What, if any problems, have you experienced with: housing/accommodation instability, difficulty budgeting resources, social problems, legal problems, employment difficulties, cognitive impairments, violence, suicide ideation and/or attempts?
3. What do you hope to achieve by engaging in treatment? What are your goals and expectations?
4. How are you hoping that we can we help you?
5. Have you tried previously to address this concern/problem/issue and if so, what happened?
6. Have you ever talked to others about emotional/mental health/alcohol or drug problems?
7. Have these problems ever resulted in you being hospitalised or required you to see treatment in some form of residential facility (inpatient, detox.)?
8. What are your current living circumstances?
9. How do you feel about these living arrangements?
10. What kind of supports do you have?
11. How often do you use them?
12. Have you had any contact with mental health and/or addiction services in the past?

38.5 Guiding Principles for Working with This Population

Cleary et al. (2008a, b), who have made significant and pioneering contributions to this area of P/MH nursing care, advanced a number of principles for guiding the care of the client who presents with mental health and substance misuse problems. Interestingly, as with the chapter on Trauma-Informed Care (Chapter 9), an argument can be constructed which suggests that many of these principles merely represent high-quality, empowering P/MH nursing practice and are not necessarily specific to the treatment of clients experiencing mental health and substance misuse problems. Significant support for this position can be found in the relevant body of literature; further support for the position is also clearly evident in the large body of work concerned with service user views, experiences and evaluations of mental healthcare services (See Cutcliffe et al., 2015). For example, in an examination of mental health service evaluations for the UK, Portugal, Canada, Germany, Switzerland and Australia, the findings indicated that, in many cases, service users encounter a mental healthcare inpatient experience that is often devoid of warm therapeutic relationships, respectful interactions, information or choice about treatment and any kind of formal/informal 'talk therapy'. Instead such care experiences are personified by: coercion, disinterest, inhumane practices, custodial and controlling practitioners and a gross over use of pharmacological 'treatments'. As a result, one could argue that it is of even greater import to (re)familiarise ourselves with the principles, especially if we wish to nudge our services closer to being truly trauma informed.

1. Engagement

Successful treatment is predicated on engagement with the client and not a cursory, 'lip service' engagement. There is a well-developed body of work, both contemporary and that of a more recognised vintage that focuses on engagement in P/MH nursing (e.g. Sainsbury Centre for Mental Health 1998; Jeynes and Minett 1999; Cutcliffe and Barker 2002; MacKay et al. 2004; Cooper 2009; Polacek et al. 2015), and readers should refer to this for the specific interventions and micro-skills that can be used to facilitate and promote engagement. Without first working to establish the trusting therapeutic relationship, the engagement and treatment efficacy is likely to be reduced (Collins and Cutcliffe 2003; Kreyenbuhl et al. 2009). When seeking to engage with such clients, the P/MH nurse ought to communicate empathy and adopt a non-judgemental approach.[1] Successful engagement is further predicated on the P/MH nurse's ability and willingness to listen, provide opportunities for the client to tell his/her story and hear concerns and provide reassurance. The P/MH nurse is also responsible for injecting hope into the clinical encounter (Koehn and Cutcliffe 2012). As the tentative therapeutic relationship is formed, the

[1] Adopting a non-judgement approach for working with this population requires the P/MH nurse to become aware of his/her own prejudices and misinformed beliefs vis-à-vis drug use and drug users.

P/MH nurse will need to discuss boundaries around confidentiality, choice, proactive discussion of potential iatrogenic and side effects. Lastly, where possible, the P/MH nurse might consider involving appropriate care givers/significant others.

2. Treatment Aims

Cleary et al. (2008a, b) assert that the next principle involves having awareness of how treatment and/or care can have several aims rather than only one. There are well-documented problems that arise when there is little or no philosophical/policy congruence between the mental health and the substance misuse services (see, e.g. Swinden and Barrett 2008). This is arguably, expressly the case, when the particular values, philosophy and policy endorsed by mental health/substance misuse services are not contemporary and do not take account of the recent, major shift(s) in drug policy—globally. So, even as such services move towards and adopt/embrace a *harm reduction* approach, individual client treatment aims are not necessarily the same. The Commission for Healthcare Audit and Inspection (2008) offers similar remarks when they report how harm reduction interventions were not provided broadly enough across the treatment system or sufficiently integrated into it. Lessening or minimising the harms associated with substance use, not necessarily having abstinence as the goal, is a much more in keeping with recent shifts in substance misuse policy (ISPC 2009; LACDD 2009; GCDP 2011). Accordingly, treatment aims should be negotiated (ala Peplau 1988); complete and total abstinence may not always be the most helpful treatment aim, especially if such aims are coupled to termination of mental health services if the service user is found to be using substances. Other treatment aims could/should include physiological stabilisation and management of any substance withdrawal symptoms, addressing the specific needs/problems that are associated with the mental health problems and minimising chance of recidivism or/and lengthening the period of time of sobriety.

3. Assessment

It seems somewhat redundant to include the guiding principle of the need for accurate and comprehensive assessment, of both the mental health issues and the substance misuse issues; however, Cleary et al. (2008b) do include this. The author recommends the use of established and reliable assessment instruments to help data collection; this is in addition to comprehensive clinical interviewing. (*Please refer to the section in this chapter on assessment.*)

4. Care Plans

For some, utilising the nursing process and with that producing written care plans may not be considered to be engaging in evidence-based practice (given the lack of evidence that links engaging in care planning with better outcomes for clients—see Moloney and Maggs 1999). For others, care planning is inextricably linked to critical thinking and problem-solving and thus would seem highly appropriate to include as a principle for working with this client group (Sinatra-Wilhelm 2012; Yildrim and Özkkahraman 2011). Care plans should be negotiated and co-constructed with the client—thus maximising the possibility of completing the programme of care and achieving treatment goals. Goals need to be clear and above all realistic. And here the problem of low success rate for substance misuse and concurrent disorder programmes should be acknowledged. Consider aiming for short-term and achievable targets. Assessments and evaluations ought, where possible, to use the same instruments to enhance consistency and accuracy. Cleary et al. (2008) match client needs with resources.

5. Cycle of Change

Numerous theoretical models of addiction have been advanced over recent decades (see EMCDDA 2013 for a recent review), some which have gained more traction than others. One such theoretical model which appears to have 'stood the test of time' is Prochaska et al. (1992) and their 'transtheoretical model of behaviour change' model. Cleary et al. (2008) argue that P/MH nurses who work with this population need to be aware of the fluid or changing nature of people's intention to change their behaviour. This readiness to change, and moreover the cyclic nature of this contemplative process, is captured in the 'transtheoretical model of behaviour change'. In utilising this model in practice, the P/MH nurse assesses the client's readiness and willingness to act on acquiring/refining new healthier behaviour and provides strategies or processes of change to guide the individual through the stages of change to action and maintenance (Prochaska et al. 1992). Their model describes five stages: (1) Precontemplative: according to Prochaska et al. (1992), people at this stage do not intend to start the healthy behaviour in their foreseeable near future. In this stage the client can learn more about healthy behaviour, weigh up the benefits and drawbacks of changing their behaviour and begin to consider the effects their negative behaviours have on others. And Prochaska et al. (1992) declare that one of the most effective steps that others (e.g. the P/MH nurse) can help with at this stage is to encourage clients to become more mindful of their decision making and more conscious of the multiple benefits of changing an unhealthy behaviour. (2) Contemplative: according to Prochaska et al. (1992), people at this stage intend to start the healthy behaviour within the foreseeable future (i.e. within the next 6 months). This stage is also associated with ambivalence in the client as though they have become more aware of the benefits of changing their behaviour; these are still 'offset' by the drawbacks and thus create a sense of ambivalence. This ambivalence invariably can impede the client in changing, causing them to keep putting off taking action. This stage also sees clients exploring and learning about the kind of person they could be if they changed their behaviour. P/MH nurses can influence and help effectively during this stage by encouraging clients to work at reducing the drawbacks associated with changing their behaviour. (3) Preparation: according to Prochaska et al. (1992), clients at this stage are ready to start taking action within the immediate short-term future, commonly depicted as within the next 30 days. This step also may contain evidence of the client taking the first 'small steps', such as, clients may share with their friends and family that they want to change their behaviour. In this stage, the P/MH nurse should encourage the client to seek support from friends they trust, to share their plan to change with people and begin to think about how they would feel if they behaved in a healthier way. (4) Action: according to Prochaska et al. (1992), this stage is characterised by clients who have recently (within recent months) changed their (problematic) behaviour and need to continue to work hard to keep making progress and staying sober. This will typically involve a process of learning how to strengthen their conviction/commitment to change and learning how to better resist urges to imbibe. For example, clients may well be taught 'substitution techniques' where healthy/positive behaviours are substituted for and thus replace harmful and/or problematic behaviours, positive reinforcement for and recognition of taking steps forwards and/or avoiding people and situations that tempt them to behave in unhealthy ways (Prochaska et al. 1992). (5) Maintenance (monitoring): according to Prochaska et al. (1992), clients in this stage have changed their problematic behaviour over 6 months ago. The key task then in this stage is restructuring of one's contacts, interactions and where one spends time—as continued progress is predicated on clients being aware of situations that may tempt them to return to the unhealthy behaviour. Prochaska et al. (1992) assert that clients should seek out support from and talk with people whom they trust (i.e. not those acquaintances associated with one's substance use past), spend time with people who behave in healthy ways and remember to engage in healthy activities to cope with stress instead of relying on unhealthy behaviour.

6. Motivational Interviewing

One of the interventions that appears to be garnering a robust evidence base pertaining to its efficacy is that of motivational interviewing (MI) (Miller and Rollnick 1991). Indeed, in their systematic review of psychosocial treatments for this population, Cleary et al. (2008b) conclude that MI is a key component of the P/MH nurse's therapeutic tool kit for this population. The aim of such an intervention is to stimulate, encourage and support the client's commitment to making positive, healthy behavioural changes. It is not uncommon for there to be disconnected between what the client says are his/her goals/aims and what actual behaviours he/she engage in, and thus an aspect of MI is helping the client have goals/aims and behaviour that are congruous with one another. Working in partnership with the client, the P/MH nurse can help identify the benefits/drawbacks of continuing to use the substance(s) and compare this to the identified benefits/drawbacks of discontinuing to use the substance(s) (Laker 2007). According to Chanut et al. (2005), MI includes providing the client with factual, contemporary and accurate information on the potential harms associated with continued use of the substance and should explore with the client the possible/likely repercussions and/or consequences of continued use—particularly impacts on family/significant other relationships and employment status.

7. Traps to Avoid

Many traps and disappointments can be avoided when working with this population by the P/MH nurse adopting an appropriate degree of expectation of success. Holding onto somewhat crude expectations of prompt and/or continued abstinence, especially given the published evidence in this area, would be unhelpful and counter-productive. For example, the evidence for an abstinence-only approach has poor efficacy. A review of 12 studies of the long-term effectiveness of abstinence-only TC found that, while substance abuse decreased during treatment, relapse was frequent after leaving the community (Malivert et al. 2012). The most predictive factor for abstinence at follow-up was treatment retention; relapse rates varied between 34% and 100% in the studies reviewed. It is inevitable that working with this client population can evoke a variety of emotional responses in the P/MH nurse (Cleary et al. 2008a, b). And thus the P/MH nurse will need to monitor themselves for unhelpful (but understandable) emotional responses.

8. Active Treatment

According to Cleary et al. (2008a, b) treatment for this population, treatment should be active not passive. In this way, for instance, the P/MH nurse does not wait for cravings to occur before responding but rather will anticipate such reactions and together with the client and develop strategies to deal with these. Similarly, the physical environment should be considered and 'managed'—actively.

9. Relapse Prevention

While P/MH nurses need to be mindful of the limited success rate for substance misuse programmes, (see Cutcliffe et al. 2016) they should work from the premise that the client wishes to avoid relapse or recidivism. That is not to suggest the P/MH bludgeon his/her way forwards, ignorant of the distinct possibility that the treatment episode may not result in prolonged abstinence; it is more the case that he/she remains hopeful, he/she should work from the premise that lasting change is possible, and importantly, he/she is aware that there are a range of P/MH nursing activities that appear to be linked, empirically, to improved outcomes. For example, the P/MH nurse should work at encouraging completion of the programme, given that programme completion is one of the best predictors of treatment success (Cutcliffe et al. 2016). Creating/providing structure and staying busy and occupying the client's time with meaningful activity appear to be evidence-based interventions. An awareness of and perpetual vigilance for early warning signs of potential cravings/relapse, in addition to, an awareness of and recognition of early warning signs of potential mental health deterioration, seem to be valuable relapse prevention interventions (Warren 2007). The P/MH nurse is encouraged to consider creating a plan of contingency actions: a 'Mental Health Advance Directive' (see, e.g. Washington State Hospital Association Mental Health Advance Directives 2017), a negotiated plan of how the formal mental healthcare team and P/MH nurse will respond if the client deteriorates. Importantly, relapse prevention mindfulness and planning do not 'stop at the door' to speak metaphorically; the planning has to include post-discharge actions. Such planning for post-discharge should include, though this may not be easy for the client, plans for how to stay away from 'high-risk' people and high-risk areas and how and where to develop (new?) relationships with abstinent friends in order to help reduce the social and peer pressure. Plus, peer group support and post-discharge support groups should also be explored.

10. Treatment Diversity

Cleary et al. (2008a, b) advance the view that to speak of 'the' population of clients who experience mental health problems simultaneously to substance misuse challenges is not to speak of a single, homogenous group. A more careful and detailed examination of this population indicates that they are a heterogeneous group, and therefore personalised and individualised programmes that take account of the client's gender, age, culture, ethnicity, spirituality, background and history will be required. Moreover, given the compelling body of evidence regarding the possibility (note: statistical likelihood) that client's from this population will be trauma victims/survivors (i.e. have a history of abuse/neglect), the principles and practices of trauma-informed care need to be enacted.

38.6 Conclusion: Psychiatric/Mental Health Nursing Responses

Providing effective P/MH nursing care to clients who present with both mental health and substance misuse-related problems makes a number of demands on such nurses. Arguments have been advanced regarding the need for P/MH nurses to come to terms with (and resolve) their own often misinformed and prejudicial views regarding this population. Indeed, given the global and hugely significant shift in policy regarding drugs/substances, it is incumbent for P/MH nurses to adopt attitudes that are congruent with rather than antagonistic too such policy (see also Moore 2013). P/MH nursing responses to this population will invariably need to include interventions aimed to address the substance misuse issues/needs/challenges and other interventions aimed to address or help with the client's mental health problems. Additional P/MH nursing responses to clients experiencing substance misuse issues have been covered in Chap. 30. Combining approaches and interventions with P/MH nursing responses to other mental health problems appears to hold the most potential for providing efficacious interventions, though it should be borne in mind that programmes aimed to minimise recidivism do not have a high success rate.

References

Chanut F, Brown TG, Dongier M (2005) Motivational interviewing and clinical psychiatry. Can J Psychiatr 50(11):715–721

Cleary M, Walter G, Hunt GE, Clancy R, Horsfall J (2008b) Promoting dual diagnosis awareness in everyday clinical practice. J Psychosocial Nurs 46(12):43–49

Cleary M, Hunt GE, Matheson S, Walter G (2008a) Psychosocial treatments for people with co-occurring severe mental illness and substance misuse: a systematic review. J Adv Nurs 65(2):238–258

Collins S, Cutcliffe JR (2003) Addressing hopelessness in people with depression and suicidal ideation: building upon the therapeutic relationship utilising a cognitive behavioural approach. J Psychiatr Ment Health Nurs 10(2):175–186

Commission for Healthcare Audit and Inspection (2008) Improving services for substance misuse: commissioning drug treatment and harm reduction services. National Treatment Agency for Substance Misuse, London

Cooper PD (2009) The person who experiences mental health and substance use problems. In: Barker P (ed) Psychiatric and mental health nursing: the craft of caring, 2nd edn. Edward Arnold, London, pp 252–261

Cutcliffe JR, Barker P (2002) Considering the care of the suicidal client and the case for 'engagement and inspiring hope' or observations. J Psychiatr Ment Health Nurs 9(5): 611–621

Cutcliffe JR, Saadeh B (2014a) Grounded in evidence or a puritanical legacy: a critique of United States of America 21st century drug policy. Subst Use Ment Health 7(3):195–206. https://doi.org/10.1080/17523281.2013.826271

Cutcliffe JR, Saadeh B (2014b) Time to get serious? Psychiatric/mental health nurses and an evidence-informed drug policy for the United States of America. Subst Use Ment Health 7(4):473–486. https://doi.org/10.1080/17523281.2014.924550

Cutcliffe JR, Santos JC, Kozel B, Taylor P, Lees D (2015) Raiders of the lost art: have psychiatric/mental health nurses lost, forgotten or abandoned the therapeutic use of self? The case of acute psychiatric settings in the United Kingdom, Portugal, Canada, Switzerland, Germany and Australia. Int J Ment Health Nurs 24:375–385

Cutcliffe JR, Travale RT, Richmond M, Green T (2016) Considering the contemporary issues and unresolved challenges of therapeutic communities for clients with alcohol and substance use problems. Issues Ment Health Nurs 37(9):642–650. https://doi.org/10.3109/01612840.2016.1169465

Edward K-L, Munro I (2009) Nursing considerations for dual diagnosis in mental health. Int J Nurs Pract 15:74–79

European Monitoring Centre for Drugs and Drug Addiction (EMCDDA) (2013) Insight: models of addiction. Publication Office of the EU, Luxembourg. http://www.emcdda.europa.eu/attachements.cfm/att_213861_EN_TDXD13014ENN.pdf

Global Commission on Drug Policy (2011) War on drugs: the report of the global commission on drug policy. United Nations, New York

Greenwald G (2009) Drug decriminalization in Portugal: lessons for creating fair and successful drug policies. Cato Institute, Washington, DC. Retrieved from http://www.cato.org/publications/white-paper/drug-decriminalization-portugal-lessons-creating-fair-successful-drug-policies

Hryb K, Kirkhart R, Talbert R (2007) A call for standardized definition of dual diagnosis. Psychiatry 4(9):15–16

Hughes C, Stevens A (2007) The effects of decriminalization of drug use in Portugal, Briefing Paper 14. The Beckley Foundation Drug Policy Programme, London

Hughes CE, Stevens A (2010) What can we learn from the Portuguese decriminalization of illicit substances? Br J Criminol 50:999–1022

International Substance Policy Consortia (ISPC) (2009) Press release United Nations substance policy review: out of ideas and out of touch. Available at http://www.governanceanddevelopment.com/2012/03/global-substance-policy-roundup-ii-budding.html

Jeynes P, Minett R (1999) Engagement in people with mental health problems: a case study. Br J Ther Rehabil 6(10):487–491

Koehn C, Cutcliffe JR (2012) The inspiration of hope in substance abuse counselling. J Humanistic Counseling 51:78–98. Education and Development Journal of Humanistic Couseling

Kreyenbuhl J, Nossel IR, Dixon LB (2009) Disengagement from mental health treatment among individuals with schizophrenia and strategies for facilitating connections to care: a review of the literature. Schizophr Bull 35(4):696–703

Laker CJ (2007) How reliable is the current evidence looking at the efficacy of harm reduction and motivational interviewing interventions in the treatment of patients with a dual diagnosis? J Psychiatr/Ment Health Nurs 14(8):720–726
Latin American Commission on Drugs and Democracy (LACDD) (2009) Drugs and democracy: towards a paradigm shift: a statement by the Latin American commission on drugs and democracy. Available at: http://www.drogasedemocracia.org/Arquivos/declaracao_ingles_site.pdf
MacKay MM, Hibbert R, Hoagwood K, Rodriguez J, Murray L, Legerski J, Fernandez D (2004) Integrating evidence-based engagement interventions into "real world" child mental health settings. Brief Treat Crisis Intervention 4:177–186
Malivert M, Fatséas M, Denis C, Langlois E, Auriacombe M (2012) Effectiveness of therapeutic communities: a systematic review. Eur Addict Res 18(1):1–11
Matson JL, Bamburg JW (1998) Reliability of the assessment of dual diagnosis (ADD). Res Dev Disabil 19(1):89–95
Mental Health and Addiction Services Concurrent Model Working Group (MHASCMWG): Saskatoon Regional Health Authority (2007) Integrated screening and assessment for mental health and addiction services concurrent disorders. https://www.saskatoonhealthregion.ca/locations_services/Services/mhas/Documents/Resources%20for%20Professionals/CompleteScreeningDocumentJanuary2007_2_.pdf
Miller WR, Rollnick S (1991) Motivational interviewing: preparing people for change. Guilford Press, New York
Moloney R, Maggs C (1999) A systematic review of the relationships between written manual nursing care planning, record keeping and patient outcomes. J Adv Nurs 30(1):51–57
Moore J (2013) Dual diagnosis: training needs and attitudes of nursing staff. Ment Health Pract 16(6):27–31
Munro I, Edward K-L (2008) Mental illness and substance use: an Australian perspective. Int J Ment Health Nurs 17:255–260
National Institute for Mental Health (2016) Glossary. http://www.nimh.nih.gov/health/topics/schizophrenia/raise/glossary.shtml
O'Neil T (2013) Ten years ago Portugal legalized all substances – what happened next? Retrieved from http://www.alternet.org/story/151635/ten_years_ago_portugal_legalized_all_substances_DOUBLEHYPHENwhat_happened_next
Peplau HE (1988) Interpersonal relations in nursing, 2nd edn. MacMilian, London
Polacek MJ, Allen DE, Damin-Moss RS, Schwartz AJA, Sharp D, Shattell M, Souther J, Delaney KR (2015) White paper: engagement as an element of safe inpatient psychiatric environments. J Am Psychiatr Nurses Assoc 21:181–190
Prochaska JO, DiClemente CC, Norcross JC (1992) In search of how people change: applications to addictive behaviors. Am Psychol 47:1102–1114
Proctor E, Silmere H, Raghavan R, Peter Hovmand P, Greg Aarons G, Bunger A, Griffey R, Hensley M (2011) Outcomes for implementation research: conceptual distinctions, measurement challenges, and research agenda. Admin Pol Ment Health 38(2):65–76
Rosenberg SD, Drake RE, Wolford GL, Mueser KT, Oxman TE, Vidaver RM, Carrieri KL, Luckoor R (1998) Dartmouth assessment of lifestyle instrument: (DALI) a substance use disorder screen for people with severe mental illness. Am J Psychiatr 155(2):232–238
(The) Sainsbury Centre for Mental Health (1998) Keys to engagement: review of care for people with severe mental illness who are hard to engage with services. The Sainsbury Centre for Mental Health, London
Sinatra-Wilhelm T (2012) Nursing care plans versus concept maps in the enhancement of critical thinking skills in nursing students enrolled in a baccalaureate nursing program. Creat Nurs 18(2):78–84
Stallvik M, Nordahl HM (2014) Convergent validity of the ASAM criteria in co-occurring disorders. J Dual Diagn 10(2):68–78
Substance Abuse and Mental Health Services Administration: Co-occurring Center for excellence (2006) OCE overview paper #2: screening, assessment, and treatment planning for persons with co-occurring disorders, Rockville, MD. http://store.samhsa.gov/shin/content//PHD1131/PHD1131.pdf

Swinden D, Barrett M (2008) Developing a dual diagnosis role in mental health. Nurs Times 104(19):26–27

Velentgas P, Dreyer NA, Wu AW (2013) Outcome definition and measurement. In: Velentgas P, Dreyer NA, Nourjah P, Smith SR, Torchia MM (eds) Developing a protocol for observational comparative effectiveness research: a user's guide. Agency for Healthcare Research and Quality, Rockville, MD

Wanberg KW (2007) Adolescent Self-Assessment Profile II – (ASAP II). http://aodassess.com/software_applications/AMS/AMS_Sample_Profile.pdf. Accessed 15 Mar 2017

Warren RK (2007) Evidence-based practice to reduce recidivism: implications for state judiciaries. National Center for State Courts for the Crime and Justice Institute and the National Institute of Corrections. http://static.nicic.gov/Library/023358.pdf

Washington State Hospital Association Mental Health Advance Directives (2017). Association of Washington Public Hospital Districts. http://www.nrc-pad.org/images/stories/PDFs/mentalhealthadvancedirectiveinfo_washstate.pdf. Accessed 13 Mar 2017

World Health Organisation (2010) The alcohol smoking and substance involvement screening test (ASSIST): manual for use in primary care. http://apps.who.int/iris/bitstream/10665/44320/1/9789241599382_eng.pdf

Yildrim B, Özkkahraman S (2011) Critical thinking in nursing process and education. Int J Humanities Soc Sci 1(13):257–261

Non-European and European Migrants in Acute Adult Inpatient Mental Healthcare: Dissociation and Identity

39

Yasmine Souiah-Benchorab, Stephen Adshead, and Jean-Manuel Morvillers

39.1 Introduction

Since time immemorial, all countries have been subject to the phenomenon of migration (Otte 2008). When it takes place in groups, as among nomadic populations, migration can be organised and regular. Inversely, migration can also involve rather more isolated and aimless individual homeless people. Among this group of migrants, we assume that there were, and still are, those who could be classed as political refugees or asylum seekers and people presenting with varying degrees of mental health problem (Foucault 1964; Castel 1995; Wagniart 1999). Medicine, especially psychiatry, has been interested in this latter population, at least since the nineteenth century (Arveiller 1996). At the beginning of the twentieth century, sociologists became especially interested in the repercussions of mass migration, particularly for the United States, with its reputation for being the 'great melting pot'.

Y. Souiah-Benchorab (✉)
EPS Maison Blanche, Paris, France
e-mail: Yasmine.Souiah-Benchorab@ch-maison-blanche.fr

S. Adshead
School Of Health and Human Sciences, University of Essex (Southend on Sea), Colchester, UK

J.-M. Morvillers
EPS Maison Blanche, Paris, France

Université Paris 13, Sorbonne Paris Cité, Chaire Recherche Sciences Infirmières, Laboratoire Educations et Pratiques de Santé (LEPS), (EA 3412), UFR SMBH, F-93017 Bobigny, France

© Springer International Publishing Switzerland 2018

J.C. Santos, J.R. Cutcliffe (eds.), *European Psychiatric/Mental Health Nursing in the 21st Century*, Principles of Specialty Nursing,
https://doi.org/10.1007/978-3-319-31772-4_39

These sociologists also developed a focus on the link possible relationship migration and mental health (Wirth 1956; Zorbaugh 1976). The history of patterns of migration in Europe reflects that migrant populations most often voyaged from neighbouring countries and/or provinces; today migrants are more likely to originate from more distant, poorer countries, who are beset with armed conflicts or economic crises, beyond the borders to the South and East of the European Union (EU) (Bhugra et al. 2014).

It is well known that migration to the European Union (EU) has grown considerably in recent years (Breteau 2015). According to Eurostat, in 2009, at least 4% of the total EU population was made up of citizens of countries outside the EU, but this figure does not account for naturalised citizens, so the actual number of migrants could be considerably more (Rechel et al. 2011). People may choose to migrate for economic reasons, hoping for a better life, or for political reasons, to flee war and famine (ibid.; p. 169–171); thus, migrants can be considered as a heterogeneous class of displaced people with each individual facing very different 'problems of living' (e.g. Barker and Buchannan-Barker 2005). The importance of the language that psychiatric/mental health nurses and other mental healthcare professionals use to describe displaced people should not be underestimated. It is indeed significant that the 'welcome' which historically was extended to immigrants across Europe has altered significantly in recent years, along with a change in the political rhetoric about them (*op. cit,* p. 7).

Some authors have suggested that, from the point of view of the migrant, migration first and foremost represents the loss of and mourning for one's country, friends and culture, and this can sometimes appear unacceptable to the indigenous population (Grinberg et al. 1986). But whether or not the experience of migration in itself can provoke psychotic disorders in a vulnerable displaced population remains unclear. Grinberg et al. (*op. cit*) had no hesitation in talking about trauma, in the psychoanalytic sense, as the prime motive for migration. Although the unfavourable social conditions of starting life in a new culture can be considered an aggravating factor (*op. cit. p. 51*), it may also be protective, relative to the horror of a war zone at home (see, e.g. Frissa et al. 2013). Even so, most of the relevant literature is concordant, advancing the view that having experienced or engaged in migration can be an important risk factor for the development of serious mental health problems (Cantor-Graae and Selten 2005) for both the first *and* second generations of an immigrant family (Bourque et al. 2011).

It is then perhaps not surprising that both the Commission of the European Communities (2005) and the World Health Organization (WHO-IOM 2010) have published major reports in recent years, recognising that migrants are particularly at risk of mental health problems and making the case that we need to prioritise their needs (see also Lindert, Schinina, *in* Rechel, 2011 Chap. 11 p. 169). However, given the heterogeneous nature of the 'migrant' population and the limited theoretical, empirical and clinical data available on the mental health needs of this population(s), the question should be asked: How can we, as psychiatric/mental health (P/MH) nurses, use our knowledge and skills to provide help to the migrant who is experiencing emotional/psychological distress?

> People who are hostile, belligerent or violent are, quite rightly, identified as presenting a threat to others. However, this threat may be a displacement of the threat, which the person feels, rightly or wrongly, is directed at her or his own Self.

Gradually, as he became more stable, the prefect of the city of Paris granted him an accompanied outing (or 'escorted leave' in the UK). This outing was to be carried out as part of the therapeutic group we had convened. During the group's coffee break, he confided: 'There is progress in my file. You will find me a home'. He went on: 'I would be better off at home in Morocco, to eat my bread and drink my water'. During the excursion, the patient did not attempt to run away. As our therapeutic alliance with him strengthened, it became possible to ask him what had caused him to assault a passer-by. He replied, 'It is the evil eye. I have no luck; so I did not need the evil eye'.

Faced with the OQTF measure and the impossibility of appealing, we prepared a care plan to prepare him for his return to his home country. Contact was made with the Consulate of Morocco, and based on the photographs we had obtained, we were able to find the real identity of this patient. The records attest to the fact that the famous name, Michael, was in the end his real name. It turned out that his passport had been out of date for several years and that his last travel documents had been issued in Barcelona. It was only at this point in our engagement with him that Michael authorised us to contact his family. His family thought he was dead because they had not heard from him for at least 5 years. This is not uncommon in this type of case. His brother, who lives in Morocco, sent us his birth certificate in order to establish his true identity and apply for a new passport so that he could return to his country. For this it is necessary for him to leave the hospital and be accompanied on a visit to the civil service. He was so eager to leave that at one time he said to the nurse investigator: 'It is today that I must go to the consulate'. But it wasn't the right day. He had to be detained further because of reasons associated with processing his documents. Even so, he was very disappointed saying, 'You lied to me; you said you would come'. When the day arrived to be taken to the consulate, the patient was smiling and thanking the team. The social worker who accompanied him reported that: 'He seemed happy and sure of his choice, despite my explanations on the progress of his file, and the disappointment of his family'. His brother, having heard the news, said: 'I must come to Paris to try to find him'.

39.4 Results 2: Mr. SD's Story

39.4.1 Mr. SD or 'Male Beauty' (16 Months of Hospitalisation)

This client has given himself a nickname synonymous with masculine beauty. He is rather tall, with a poorly maintained beard, half-length, blond hair with blue glacial eyes, and presented with a body odour that was hardly tolerable. He has a slight Anglo-Saxon accent. He had been admitted to the SDRE for punching a woman in the ear who, according to him, 'took a picture'. Having hit her to the floor, he kicked her face while she was on the ground. Two knives and a knuckle punch were found on him. This patient was described in the medical reports as dissonant, with fixed, tense, worried and rather reluctant eyes. He appeared to be experiencing some degree of paranoid persecutory ideation, aggravated by his vulnerable situation of homelessness, without papers or means of support. Upon arrival, the patient was calm and was placed in an ordinary reception room. The contact with him was minimal. He seemed very suspicious. He justified the carrying of weapons with the statement that: 'Four strangers have been threatening me on the stairs where I usually sleep'. A few days after the introduction of the neuroleptic treatment, he recounted the day of his arrest and said, discordantly, 'a group that had a bomb wanted to photograph it'. At the medical nurse interview, he avoided making eye contact and engaged in a form of dialogue and inaudible lip movements that were incomprehensible to anyone else but him. Thus, he chose to express himself through drawing diagrams, to try and explain where he wanted to go, and refused to verbalise his requests.

At some point, his condition got worse and this was accompanied by various somatic complications. A fall and aggravation of his vital signs made his transfer to the emergency department necessary. We note that before the transfer, he was agitated, slapping and scratching his caregiver. Despite receiving care, his condition continued to worsen. He had to be intubated in resuscitation to the point of having to be fed by a gastric tube. The diagnosis of thyrotoxicosis by Graves' disease was then made. The team would visit him regularly over this time. During stabilisation, he refused the endocrinologist permission for an operation, with an unshakeable will, but did accept other forms of treatment. He refused a proposal to see another doctor. He gave no reason for this but said, 'No! No! Dr. Xendocrinologist'. Upon his return to our care, he displayed a disorder of swallowing. His dental condition was catastrophic. An appointment with a stomatologist was made. The verdict was without question: All his teeth had to be extracted and a total prosthesis was necessary. Again, the patient was opposed to his treatment. Upon leaving the hospital, he gave a few more details to his psychiatrist of the CMP. What did not change however was the fact that he felt assaulted by the person who took the picture, but he recognised his responsibility for his physical aggression. However, he thought that his behaviour was related to his somatic pathology.

During our various interviews, he always insisted that he had never had a family and that he remembered having grown up in institutions and being moved around a lot. He purported to have studied at a high school in Switzerland and worked as a removal man. According to him, he had a passport from the European Union. He came to France for a holiday and after 3 weeks an armed gang assaulted him. He said he had confidence in the care team because he understood that, in his words, 'they are not part of the gang'. Throughout his hospitalisation, P/MH nurses helped him take care of his hygiene, and we offered him baths as a therapeutic intervention. He would show his displeasure by refusing to speak to us. As his hospitalisation continued, some hours of leave were granted. At first, we had no information on how he used to occupy his time or how his leave might benefit him. Then, little by little, he opened up to us and told us that he would sleep in front of the same supermarket every time. Once he returned with 90 euros and asked us to redo his ID for him. At the announcement of his discharge by the administrative authorities, he refused to leave the hospital. He argued this refusal by saying, 'I'm sick'. Then one day he agreed to leave the ward and continue his care at the CMP. He kept all his appointments with the psychiatrist. An action was taken out with a lawyer so that he would be recognised as a ward of the French state. Eventually he was admitted to a home, and he agreed to stay there because life outside was becoming more and more unbearable for him.

39.5 Results 3: Mr. L.Y.Z's Story

39.5.1 L.Y.Z: 6 Months of Hospitalisation

This client was originally from China, specifically Qingdao, in the far east of the country; he was physically very tall and thin and had medium-length hair at first presentation. The patient had also displayed hetero-aggressive acts. He had a rather cold, hermetic disposition and was particularly reluctant to engage in any dialogue. He had three episodes of hospitalisation and now found himself in the SDRE context. The first two hospitalisations were very complicated. He often protested against hospitalisation under duress by fasting and refusing any treatment, leading to the point where the healthcare team had to physically restrain him to inject medication. Through the intermediary of the interpreter, he said, 'I just defended myself against the gentleman who bothered me'. He added, 'He insults me'. When asked, 'In what language?', he retorted, 'I understood this by telepathy'. At the time of his first hospitalisation, after treatment, this patient, who had agreed to return to China, then ran away from the service. His second hospitalisation took place at another medical centre because his name was misspelt, either by the police or by the patient himself. An identical clinical picture was drawn up there, and the same protests and refusals were recorded in his notes. At the arrival of the interpreter, he specified that he ultimately refused to return to China because his parents were deceased and his siblings were too old. His siblings included seven children, of whom he was the youngest.

As a result of the hospitalisations, a therapeutic alliance could be established with this patient. This allowed us to go a step further in the analysis of his clinical presentation. In his migratory journey, it will be noted that he travelled to France with a visa. He was able to join a Chinese community, work in a restaurant and stay with other Chinese people. But in 2004, the restaurant boss returned to China. As a result, the patient had no more work and so soon he had no more housing. He found himself on the street, no longer able to send money to China for his wife and son. They then broke off their relations with him. At first he just wanted to find odd jobs, but after a while he did nothing—maybe because his psychic disorders became too intrusive. This behaviour seemed to change from his first to his last admission, but he never gave an explanation for this. Our team, however, was able to start to play scrabble with him and then he started to converse with them in French.

39.6 Discussion

Yassine or 'Michael' was an economic migrant whose identity remained largely intact, despite the loss of his home culture, probably because its formation had already been completed within his childhood. However, his identity had been put under threat by his migration to a new culture. His particular 'problem of living' therefore appeared to be the construction of a new identity within a foreign culture (see, e.g. Schrauf and Rubin 2003). The loss of his paperwork, as the physical manifestation of his identity, left him exposed to a hostile world which he could not defend himself against; in theory, this was because he was simultaneously excluded from the foreign culture by his inability to speak the French language. Thus, while reverting to his childhood identity, 'Michael', appeared to offer him some resilience, it also meant his best chance of making a full recovery was returning to his family and place of birth.

SD or Male Beauty, on the other hand, was an economic migrant who appeared to lose his identity completely; his psychotic symptoms and history of violence made him a very vulnerable person. Barker (2005; Barker and Buchanon, 2005, p. 62) has noted and uses the mathematical metaphor of 'chaos' to refer to extreme states of undifferentiated arousal like this. Barker describes it as a 'psychic storm that often threatens to engulf, overwhelm and ultimately drown the person' (ibid. p. 202). Unlike Yassine, SD did not have a stable identity in his childhood that would have helped his identity remain resilient to stress. Furthermore, as an adult he became an economic migrant who travelled around Europe in search of a better life; so SD lacked an extended family or any form of nurturing relationships in the form of a social support structure. Thus, it is perhaps not surprising that his recovery involved a protracted period of dependence upon the state reflecting his initial reports of spending his childhood in residential care.

The last case, L.Y.Z., could also be classed as an economic migrant. He seems to have had a traumatic separation from his wife and children in China and from the Chinese community in France because of economic reasons, or so we are informed. As a result he seems to have suffered from quite a severe form of emotional detachment. Higher rates of unresolved attachments, like his, have been found in migrant populations in the past (Van Ecke et al. 2005); but it is unclear whether such unresolved attachments could be associated with the sort of splitting, of mind from emotions, that has become the defining feature of schizophrenia, since Blueler first diagnosed the disorder in 1911 (see, e.g. Park and Thakkar 2010). However, it does appear that L.Y.Z.'s recovery was made possible by his ability to engage in the French language. According to Schrauf and Rubin (2003), it is possible that an identity that is constructed in a non-native language can replace an identity that is constructed in a native language, for instance, in a first-generation immigrant. However, in theory, this phenomenon could also contribute to the identity of second-generation bilingual immigrants becoming split between their native and non-native communities.

At the time of writing, two out of the three clients have recovered enough to leave the hospital, although in all cases the therapeutic alliance with the nursing team has been an important part of their recovery. Yassine eventually recovered the life he had had in his home country, while for L.Y.Z, it is less clear that he will be able to return to his home country very soon. As for 'masculine beauty', it is certain that he came from another country, but he decided to stay and continue working with us, and it is hoped he may one day find employment. This means that while all three of these patients could be counted among 'those who cannot come back' (Grinberg et al. 1986), each one of them has recovered something of an identity from receiving ethnonursing care.

It is true that in each case the building of a therapeutic alliance was made difficult because of a refusal to engage and that this situation was made worse by the language barrier. Moreover, the core identity of these patients was often concealed by their behaviour, which suggested that they were using their behaviour as some kind of defence mechanism against, what they perceived to be, a hostile world. Thus, the symbolic role played by the body and/or its image was highlighted for us and, in the circumstances, eventually came to replace the verbal constructions of the self usually developed with a language. For instance, Yassine believed he was envied by other people. When asked the question, 'What do people envy about you?', he used to answer, 'My hair and my look'. His proof was that they cast the evil eye on him. The evil eye, in Arabic 'ayn', is a malevolent glare from someone or something that will injure the person or the thing glared at, with or without intention. Thus, the 'evil eye' represents a culturally appropriate non-verbal signal for danger or threat, but it is not necessarily a signal perceived by anyone else other than the recipient.

For the patient who defined his identity as a 'masculine beauty', the non-verbal link to others in his community was marked by him physically distancing himself from them. This was because of his persistent poor personal hygiene, and his reference to the 'group', a word that he used to define most others, was also used to refer to its opposite, to the individuality of the individual and *ultimately* to the social isolation of himself as the migrant-vagrant. In all three cases, then, there appears to have been an issue regarding identity that was attributable to their migrant status, which made them more or less vulnerable to stress. The greatest distress seemed to appear as the result of an absence of identity, but more importantly, the amount of distress appeared to vary in proportion to the ability to maintain an existing identity within the context of a home culture or the ability to construct a new identity within the context of an adopted culture.

However, a note of caution is advised regarding this interpretation. According to Devereux (2009), the renunciation of an identity in the context of migration could also represent a defence against a past which, in itself, poses a threat of psychic destruction. 'To be understood' in this context means being recognised and thus identified in a bad way, which carries with it a threat of destruction. Thus, the refusal to be understood, to be predictable, would support the thesis that certain, of our patients, who present these identity conflicts, are trying to protect themselves against being known and against absolute destruction by becoming incomprehensible to others; remaining unidentifiable, unknown, means escaping the danger they are to themselves. As Devereux adds, the identity is thus made incomprehensible even to the patients themselves. Having said that, it is true that not all first-generation migrants who display psychotic disorders and commit serious hetero-aggressive acts may present with the sort of identity issues we have described here. We share the analysis of Baubet and Moro (2003) when they affirm that 'there is no specific pathology linked to migration: Migration constrains individual development through the encountering of obstacles, and this will be expressed through psychopathology, the clinical expression of which is conditioned by a whole set of individual and cultural factors in specific social contexts. Migration reduces the question of identity to a number of essential dimensions: historical continuity, the sense of self (*op. cit.*, p. 147) and our relationship to others'.

Finally, we are required to note that, in two other cases we have dealt with, the presence of social links, with family or the ethnic community, proved to be a protective factor against the development of the most severe forms of mental illness, through the sharing of an ethnic identity (Veling et al. 2008). We note this not to make claims regarding the aetiology of identity problems in the context of mental illness but rather to highlight the way in which they occur and how we might treat the symptoms when we find ourselves providing care to people with this presentation.

39.7 Implications for Psychiatric/Mental Health Nurses

The approach to care adopted by the nurse in these situations, where the question of identity is central, demanded an approach based on patience and a willingness/ability to question the particular meaning(s) the client gave to his suffering. As Leininger (1979) declared, to be able to offer genuine humanistic nursing care, the nurse needs openness to the other person's experience of their world. However, the cases indicate that mental health needs for such clients extend beyond those that can be situated in their experiences of migration and transcultural adaptation. Today, every nurse must acquire cultural skills and be aware of the impact of migration on mental health. These skills will allow the nurse to construct a good therapeutic alliance, which may be long and difficult, especially in the context of foreign languages, but not impossible. The nurse should still try and help the client to reintegrate with his/her social groups as soon as possible, as this can take time. Reintegration in a supportive community can also be achieved using ethnopsychiatric consultations based on a similar model to therapeutic groups. The groups we held consisted of a number of co-therapists, managed by a main therapist, which the client would attend, along with his/her family and a translator, if needed. In this way, the therapeutic group was able to help reconstruct the client's identity within a cultural frame of reference, along with their wider belief systems and values.

Conclusion

Besides the act of migration in itself and the psychic trauma caused by leaving one's country, family, etc., studies have shown that migrants can be confronted with social adversity and feelings of social defeat. These psychosocial factors can promote psychological breakdowns, and even psychotic disorders, that result in more or less enduring illnesses, especially if these promoting factors persist.

Nurses and their healthcare institutions must ensure a benevolent approach to greeting these patients as it is rare that they are well received in their new environments. This is why the focus on building a therapeutic alliance is so important, enabling individuals to avoid feelings of constraint, or risk of them experiencing feelings of persecution, which we have found in the delirious cases. Additional to individual care, group therapies (ethnopsychiatry), in which the nurse can often be a co-therapist, are also of great help to the patient.

References

Arveiller J (1996) Le voyage automatique. Fugues, vagabondage et psychiatrie. Evol Psychiatr 61(3):579–612

Barker P, Buchannan-Barker P (2005) The tidal model: a guide for mental health professionals. Routledge, Hove

Baubet T, Moro MR, Congrès de psychiatrie et de neurologie de langue française (éd) (2003) Psychiatrie et migrations [rapport de psychiatrie], Masson, Paris, p 62

Bhugra D, Gupta S, Schouler-Ocak M, Graeff-Calliess I, Deakin NA, Qureshi A, Carta M (2014) EPA guidance mental health care of migrants. Eur Psychiatry 29(2):107–115

Bourque F, van der Ven E, Malla A (2011) A meta-analysis of the risk for psychotic disorders among first- and second-generation immigrants. Psychol Med 41(5):897–910

Breteau AP (2015) Le nombre de migrants et de réfugiés a explosé au XXIe siècle. *Le Monde.fr*. Consulté à l'adresse http://www.lemonde.fr/les-decodeurs/article/2015/09/03/le-nombre-de-migrants-et-refugies-a-explose-au-xxie-siecle-dans-le-monde_4744977_4355770.html

Cantor-Graae E, Selten J-P (2005) Schizophrenia and migration: a meta-analysis and review. Am J Psychiatr 162(1)

Castel R (1995) Les métamorphoses de la question sociale. Fayard, Paris

Commission of the European Communities (2005) Green paper improving the mental health of the population: towards a strategy on mental health for the European Union. Office for Official Publications of the European Communities, Luxembourg. http://ec.europa.eu/health/ph_determinants/life_style/mental/green_paper/mental_gp_en.pdf

Devereux G, Bastide R, Gobard H, Jolas T (1983) Essais d'ethnopsychiatrie générale. Gallimard, Paris

Devereux G (2009) La renonciation à l'identité défense contre l'anéantissement. Payot & Rivages, Paris

Foucault M (1964) Histoire de la folie à l'âge classique. Union générale d'éditions, Paris

Frissa S, Hatch SL, Gazard B, Fear NT, Hotopf M, SELCoH study team (2013) Trauma and current symptoms of PTSD in a south East London community. Soc Psychiatry Psychiatr Epidemiol 48(8):1199–1209

Grinberg L, Grinberg R, Ba MN, Legrand Y, Legrand C (1986) Psychanalyse du migrant et de l'éxilé. Césura Lyon éditions, Lyon

Leininger M (1997) Overview of the theory of culture care with the Ethnonursing research method. J Transcult Nurs 8(2):32–52

Leininger MM (1979) Transcultural nursing. MASSON International Nursing Publications, New York

Marcel G (1948) The philosophy of existence (trans: Harari M). London: The Harvill Press

Morvillers JM, Lobrot M (2013) *L'impact de l'implication: importance de l'engagement de soi dans l'exercice soignant et le développement de la personne* (Vol. 1–1). Paris: De Boeck-Otte, M. (2008). *Cro Magnon*. Perrin, Paris

Otte M (2008) Cro Magnon. Perrin, Paris
Park S, Thakkar KN (2010) "splitting of the mind" revisited: recent neuroimaging evidence for functional Dysconnection in schizophrenia and its relation to symptoms. Am J Psychiatry 167(4):366–368
Rechel B, Mladovsky P, Devillé W, Rijks B, Petrova-Benedict R, McKee M (éds) (2011) Migration and health in European Union, McGraw Hill/Open University Press, Maidenhead
Rubin DC, Schrauf RW, Greenberg DL (2003) Belief and recollection of autobiographical memories. Mem Cogn 31:887–901
Van Ecke Y, Chope RC, Emmelkamp PMG (2005) Immigrants and attachment status: research findings with Dutch and Belgian immigrants in California. Soc Behav Personal Int J 33(7):657–674
Veling W, Susser E, Van Os J, Mackenbach JP, Selten JP, Hoek HW (2008) Ethnic density of neighbourhoods and incidence of psychotic disorders among immigrants. Am J Psychiatr 165(1):66–73
Wagniart JF (1999) *Le vagabond à la fin du XIXème siècle* (Belin)
Wirth L (1956) The ghetto. University of Chicago Press, Chicago
WHO/IOM (2010) Health of migrants—the way forward. Report of a global consultation Madrid, Spain, 3–5 March 2010. http://www.who.int/hac/events/consultation_report_health_migrants_colour_web.pdf
Yin RK (2014) Case study research: design and methods. Sage, London
Zorbaugh HW (1976) The gold coast and the slum: a sociological study of Chicago's near north side. University of Chicago Press, Chicago

Working with Individuals Who Are Homeless

40

Cheryl Forchuk

40.1 Introduction

The purpose of this chapter is to give psychiatric/mental health nurses an overview of some of the issues they may need to consider when providing care for people who are homeless. Working with people who are homeless is an example of a specialty area of nursing. Homelessness has been found to be a problem that is increasing in many communities and countries. For example, recent studies have found increases in the homeless population in Canada (Collins 2010; City of Vancouver 2016), Australia (Australian Bureau of Statistics 2011), New Zealand (Collins 2010), United States (The US Department of Housing and Urban Development 2016), and the United Kingdom (Department for Communities and Local Government 2016). People with mental illnesses, including addiction, are overrepresented among the homeless population (Fazel et al. 2008), and people who are homeless have an increased use of emergency medical services (Hwang et al. 2010, 2011) and suffer early mortality (Hwang et al. 2009). Nurses who work with the homeless population may be employed in primary care facilities, emergency medical services, mental health organizations, or community nursing agencies including outreach programs and "street nursing" programs. The focus may vary depending on the goals of the agency overall. However, understanding some of the contextual issues regarding working with this population is important regardless of clinical agency.

C. Forchuk
Western University, London, ON, Canada
e-mail: cforchuk@uwo.ca

© Springer International Publishing Switzerland 2018

J.C. Santos, J.R. Cutcliffe (eds.), *European Psychiatric/Mental Health Nursing in the 21st Century*, Principles of Specialty Nursing,
https://doi.org/10.1007/978-3-319-31772-4_40

40.2 Mental Health and Housing

Consistently, people with mental illness, including substance abuse, are overrepresented in the homeless population (Aubry et al. 2016; Fazel et al. 2008; Goering et al. 2002; Iaquinta 2016; Mental Health Commission of Canada 2013). This phenomenon has been seen in a number of countries, including Spain (Marquez and Urraza 2016), Denmark (Benjaminsen 2016), Switzerland (Jaeger et al. 2015), Japan (Okamura et al. 2015), and China (Yim et al. 2015). Deinstitutionalization of individuals with mental illness has been a worldwide trend that was often not accompanied by an increase in community mental health services and appropriate community housing policies (Forchuk et al. 2007a, b). The issues related to mental health and housing are varied and complex. Research has shown that people with severe mental illness are at risk of losing their housing, living in substandard housing that is not aligned with their preferences, or being placed in inappropriate housing (Nelson et al. 2011). In obtaining housing in the private market, people with (so-called) mental illness may experience discrimination from landlords (Forchuk et al. 2006). A common myth is that people are homeless because that is how they would like to live. In a study of housing preference (Nelson et al. 2011), less than 1% stated they actually preferred to be homeless. People described themselves as homeless because they had run out of other choices (Forchuk et al. 2011). Through a Community-University Research Alliance (CURA) on mental health and housing, we were able to conduct focus groups and interviews with psychiatric survivors who have experienced homelessness. Our objective of the study was to understand the two questions: What issues of concern do psychiatric survivors have about their current housing situation? What preferences do they have related to housing?

40.3 Concerns

When asked to identify problems or concerns in accessing housing, survivors identified a few different issues. Many survivors identified a concern of homelessness and precarious housing situations which could lead to frequent moving. They also identified the lack of affordable and/or desirable housing available to them. They described most housing as being in poor quality, being too small, being in poor neighborhoods, having lack of privacy, or having restrictive rules. The survivors identified an overall lack of choice in housing (Forchuk et al. 2011).

40.3.1 Gender Issues

Interestingly, women survivors identified some specific sex and gender concerns with regard to housing. The issues included access to child care, rate of subsidy, and safety for the woman and/or her children. One woman said "She was in there [hospital] because she was sexually abused. She was placed in a home with two guys. When she complains, they tell her that she is lucky to be out of hospital." Another woman said "Being on the 3rd floor of a complex with no elevator which is not practical with two infants and the presence of a child molester in the same building." As a solution one woman added that "...there should be one house with all women, one man, and two that are mixed."

40.3.2 Safety Issues

Safety was a general concern for many participants, especially among female survivors. Survivors cited concerns over victimization (break-ins, stealing, sexual abuse, etc.) and proximity to the drug and sex trade.

40.3.3 Preferences

Women survivors listed a few preferences for their housing needs, which included a choice over the gender of living companions and a safe place for their children.

To further combat safety concerns, some survivors identified a preference for security at their housing, which included an effective lock on their door.

40.3.4 Supports

In addition to concerns and preferences over housing, survivors also described necessary supports to being housed. Some of the items that survivors identified were access to transportation (83%), access to a telephone (81.7%), money for rent deposit (78%), and assistance from others to help them access preferred housing (64%) (Nelson et al. 2011).

40.4 Selected Findings from Homelessness and Diversity Study

The author served as the principal investigator on a study that explored the intersecting vulnerabilities in individuals who are homeless and have psychiatric challenges. Current literature on intersectionality suggests that when people experience more than one type of disadvantage, the combination is essentially greater than the sum of individual issues (Cairney et al. 2014; Crenshaw 1995; Davy 2011; Dhamoon and Hankivsky 2011). The study also examined some of the issues related to diversity issuers among people who are homeless (Forchuk et al. 2007a, b). The main goal of the Homelessness and Diversity Issues in Canada initiative is to support policy-relevant research on homelessness and its diversity. The rationale for this study was to dispel the common perceived notion that psychiatric survivors are a homogeneous group with similar needs. However, there are far more additional disadvantages experienced by this group. People further marginalized by visible/

Table 40.1 Disabilities of community mental health sample vs homeless sample

Disability	Community mental health sample $n = 318$ (100%)	Homeless sample $n = 132$ (100%)
Visually impaired	125 (39.3%)	56 (42.4%)
Physically disabled	126 (39.6%)	61 (46.2%)
Hearing disabled	61 (19.2%)	27 (20.5%)
Learning disabled	116 (36.5%)	51 (38.6%)
Psychiatrically disabled	219 (68.9%)	89 (67.4%)
Other disability	15 (3.1%)	5 (3.8%)

cultural minority group status, sexual orientation, and/or disabilities were studied to understand its relation to housing and homelessness.

The findings in this study were consistent with other research: We found the majority of people were unpartnered at the time of the interviews. Only four people (3% of the sample) were in a married/common law relationship at the time of the interview, and over half of those interviewed had never been married. We also found that homelessness and poverty are integrally related, and less than half of individuals who were sampled had completed high school. In comparison with the general Canadian population in 2006, over 87% of individuals aged 25–29 had completed high school (Statistics Canada 2010). One of the interesting things we found in the study on diversity was the layers of disadvantage related to multiple health challenges and disabilities. Table 40.1 compares the homeless population to a community sample of people with mental health problems in the same community and conducted in the same time period. All conditions are self-reported.

To indicate sources of disability as illustrated in Table 40.1, people checked all disabilities that applied to them personally. The results show many people had more than one disability. Two fifths of these people report being visually impaired. One of the issues for those experiencing homelessness, as well as others in extreme poverty, is that they may not be able to afford and maintain/replace eyeglasses that would correct the problem. A similar number report being physically disabled, while over one third stated they experienced a learning disability. Although every individual in the community sample reported having a history of mental illness, two thirds of these individuals disclosed having a psychiatric disability. Interestingly, the reports of disability among the community sample were almost identical to the incidents among the homeless sample. These numbers indicate that a significant health burden is being borne by this population.

40.4.1 Individual or Systems Issues as Cause?

It is important to understand that homelessness is generally a systemic issue rather than simply the fault of individuals. Changes in housing, income support, and mental health policies have led to a dramatic increase in homelessness in Canada (Forchuk et al. 2007a, b). In a randomized intervention study, Forchuk and colleagues found that the prompt provision of income and housing supports upon discharge from psychiatric wards made a significant difference in housing outcomes (Forchuk et al. 2008). A total of 14 individuals who had no prior history of homelessness, but had lost their housing upon admission to the psychiatric hospital, were randomly assigned to the intervention group ($n = 7$; income support and housing assistance) or to the usual care group ($n = 7$). While all seven individuals in the intervention group maintained their housing at the 6 month follow-up, this pilot study had to be stopped when six of the seven individuals in the usual care group were still homeless. The only "successful" participant in this group had been recruited for the first time into the sex trade to avoid homelessness; 6 months later, she was still in the sex trade. The intervention then became usual care, and discharge to homelessness dropped by over 92.5% (Forchuk et al. 2013).

40.5 Psychiatric/Mental Health Nursing Issues to Consider

Understanding that homelessness is a multifaceted issue is crucial. This section will talk about issues to consider in the nursing field. As healthcare professionals, we have an obligation to understand the depth of the issues concerning our community. Discussions related to why the person is currently homeless often lead to strategies to address the homelessness. For example, homeless youth have often discussed sexuality identity crises, while others may identify substance abuse. Obviously different types of strategies would help for very different issues.

40.5.1 The Experience of Homelessness

Homelessness means living in the moment. It is extremely difficult to implement a strategy or plan when homeless, since the individual usually ends up essentially living in the moment. The focus ends up on the following: Where is my next meal coming from? Where will I sleep tonight? How can I be safe, right now? This focus on immediacy is very much a survival tactic. However, such a focus runs counter to the view of the future needed for most plans. Housing First is a strategy to first focus on getting the person housed, and the supports to remain housed, before expecting any progress on other goals (Gaetz et al. 2013). Housing First means there is low (or no) barrier to housing. People do not need to be sober, compliant with treatment/in treatment or meet any other conditions to be housed. With this approach, housing is considered a basic human right (Tsemberis and Asmussen 1999).

40.5.2 Mental Health

Mental health, including addiction issues, is very common. People with such issues have been found to be consistently overrepresented in the homeless population (Aubry et al. 2016; Fazel et al. 2008; Goering et al. 2002; Iaquinta 2016; Mental Health Commission of Canada 2013). There are multiple issues that related to this including systemic issues such as the "deinstitution" of psychiatric treatment without adequate investment in community mental health services, income, and housing supports (Forchuk et al. 2007a, b). People may be discharged directly from hospitals to homelessness if adequate supports are not in place (Forchuk et al. 2008, 2013). Although housing is a well-known social determinant of health, healthcare providers such as nurses often forget to ask questions related to housing. Substance use, depression, and anxiety can also be seen as responses to the difficult situation of being homeless.

40.5.3 Peer Support

Peer relationships are often important to people who are homeless as a source of strength and to give hope for recovery. Such relationships can also keep people drawn to the streets. While on the street, people often describe having a "street family" that has replaced blood relatives. They often rely on each other for finding temporary accommodation as well as providing safety. Peer relationships can draw people, particularly young people, into the drug and/or sex trade as a source of needed income. On the other hand, a relationship with someone who has successfully transitioned from homelessness to being housed can provide powerful peer support and hope. Drop-in programs for people who are homeless can be structured to accommodate groups and support formal or informal peer support (Haldenby et al. 2011).

40.5.4 Family Support

Family relationships can be strained. For youth in particular, there may be a history of domestic violence or major family conflict that contributed to the decision to leave home. However, even with strained family relationships, individuals may be able to identify specific people in the family that they could reach out to. Building health supports is an important strategy to rebuilding stability (Haldenby et al. 2011).

40.5.5 Food

Food is often a concern. People who are homeless are often hungry. They generally have few funds for food and no place to store or prepare food. They may take advantage of meal programs offered through social or religious organizations. Nurses should be aware of when and where such programs operate in case they need to direct people to such programs. If a person who is homeless has had to wait for a long period, for example, in the emergency room of a hospital, it should be assumed that the person is hungry. Such hunger can interfere with assessment and with the establishment of rapport. Providing some food prior to assessment can often help both with the hunger and the assessment/rapport.

40.5.6 Sexuality

Sexuality issues can become very complex when homeless. People who identify as LGBTQ (lesbian, gay, bisexual, transgendered, queer or questioning) are often overrepresented in the homeless population (Ray 2006; Rosario et al. 2012). Lack of family acceptance of one's sexuality could have contributed to the current situation of homelessness (Cray et al. 2013; McLaughlin et al. 2012). To add to the complexity, once on the street, young people in particular may be recruited into the sex trade. This can begin with the offering of entry level sex jobs such as massage parlors or dancing. Youth may be offered "a job" and "a place to stay" which sounds very appealing. People on the street may engage in "survival sex" to have a space to stay for the night (Reid et al. 2005). While on the street, they may also be at risk for sexual assault. Some of the women expressed a fear of being assaulted, physically and sexually, and implemented their own survival strategies to prevent this from occurring and to minimize harm. For some, they aligned themselves with other males in a variety of ways as a means of negotiating their safety in what they perceived to be a hostile and dangerous environment (Reid et al. 2005). Some women will wear multiple layers of clothing to hide their sexuality in an attempt to reduce the risk of sexual assault.

40.5.7 Illness

Communicable illnesses and infestations are a constant issue on the street. It is easy to become physically ill when on the street or in a homeless shelter. Both constant exposure to the elements (such as cold, wet, heat) and the crowding of shelters can contribute to this problem. Simple things, like difficulty washing or doing laundry can add to the spread of communicable illness or problems such as head or body lice.

40.5.8 Income

Income is almost always an issue when one is homeless. Lack of income is a common cause of homelessness. Once homeless finding gainful employment is very difficult without an address or phone number.

Conclusion

Nurses may encounter people living with homelessness in almost any practice area. It is important to understand the broader context of homelessness. It is also important to ask appropriate questions to discover vulnerable housing situations as well as to help plan strategies. The best practice standard is to address "Housing First" since other problems are almost impossible to address while still homeless.

References

Aubry T, Goering P, Veldhuizen S, Adair CE, Bourque J, Distasio J, Latimer E, Stergiopoulos V, Somers J, Streiner DL, Tsemberis S (2016) A multiple-city RCT of housing first with assertive community treatment for homeless Canadians with serious mental illness. Psychiatr Serv 67(3):275–281. doi:10.1176/appi.ps.201400587

Australian Bureau of Statistics (2011) Census of population and housing: estimating homelessness in Australia. (2049.0). Retrieved from Australian Burau of Statistics http://www.ausstats.abs.gov.au/Ausstats/subscriber.nsf/0/EB59F237159F7102CA257AB100170B61/%24File/20490_2011.pdf

Benjaminsen L (2016) Homelessness in a Scandinavian welfare state: the risk of shelter use in the Danish adult population. Urban Stud 53(10):2041–2063. doi:10.1177/0042098015587818

Cairney J, Velhuizen S, Vigod S, Streiner DL, Wade TJ, Kurdyak P (2014) Exploring the social determinants of mental health service using Intersectionality theory and CART analysis. J Epidemiol Community Health 68:145–150. https://doi.org/10.1136/jech-2013-203120

City of Vancouver (2016) City releases 2016 homeless count results and updates on low-income housing. Retrieved from http://vancouver.ca/news-calendar/city-releases-2016-homeless-count-results-updates-low-income-housing.aspx

Collins D (2010) Homelessness in Canada and New Zealand: a comparative perspective on numbers and policy responses. Urban Geogr 31(7):932–952

Cray A, Miller K, Durso LE (2013) Seeking shelter: the experiences and unmet needs of LGBT homeless youth. Center for American Progress, Washington, DC

Crenshaw K (1995) Mapping the margins: intersectionality, identity, politics and violence against women of color. In: Crenshaw K, Gotanda N, Peller G, Thomas K (eds) Critical race theory. The New Press, New York, pp 357–383

Davy Z (2011) The promise of intersectionality theory in primary care. Qual Prim Care 19(5):279–281. http://search.ebscohost.com/login.aspx?direct=true&db=cin20&AN=2011365254&site=ehost-live

Department for Communities and Local Government (2016) Rough sleeping statistics autumn 2015, England. Homelessness. Retrieved from https://www.gov.uk/government/uploads/system/uploads/attachment_data/file/503015/Rough_Sleeping_Autumn_2015_statistical_release.pdf

Dhamoon K, Hankivsky O (2011) Why the theory and practice of intersectionality matter to health research and policy. In: Hankivsky O (ed) Health inequalities in Canada: intersectional frameworks and practices. UBC Press, Vancouver, BC, pp 16–50

Fazel S, Khosla V, Doll H, Geddes J (2008) The prevalence of mental disorders among the homeless in Western countries: systematic review and meta-regression analysis. PLoS Med 5(12):1670–1681. doi:10.1371/journal.pmed.0050225

Forchuk C, Ward-Griffin C, Csiernik R, Turner K (2006) Surviving the tornado of mental illness: psychiatric survivors' experiences of getting, losing, and keeping housing. Psychiatr Serv 57(4):558–562. doi:10.1176/appi.ps.57.4.558

Forchuk C, Jensen E, Csiernik R, Gorlick C, Ray SL, Berman H, Joplin L (2007a) Diversity and homelessness: minorities and psychiatric survivors. Can J Nurs Res 39(3):191–193

Forchuk C, Joplin L, Schofield R, Csiernik R, Gorlick C, Turner K (2007b) Housing, income support and mental health: points of disconnection. Health Res Policy Syst 5:14. doi:10.1186/1478-4505-5-14

Forchuk C, Kingston-MacClure S, Van Beers M, Smith C, Csiernik R, Hoch J, Jensen E (2008) Developing and testing an intervention to prevent homelessness among individuals discharged from psychiatric wards to shelters and 'No Fixed Address'. J Psychiatr Ment Health Nurs 15(7):569–575. doi:10.1111/j.1365-2850.2008.01266.x

Forchuk C, Nelson G, Hall GB (2011) It's important to be proud of the place you live in: housing preferences of Mental Health Consumer-Survivors. In: Forchuk C, Csiernik R, Jensen E (eds) Homelessness, housing, and mental health finding truths-creating change. Canadian Scholar's Press, Toronto, pp 91–105

Forchuk C, Godin M, Hoch JS, Kingston-MacClure S, Jeng MS, Puddy L, Jensen E (2013) Preventing psychiatric discharge to homelessness. Can J Commun Ment Health 32(3):17–28. doi:10.7870/cjcmh-2013-028

Gaetz S, Scott F, Gulliver T (eds) (2013) Housing first in Canada: supporting communities to end homelessness. Canadian Homelessness Research Network Press, Toronto

Goering P, Tolomiczenko G, Sheldon T, Boydell K, Wasylenki D (2002) Characteristics of persons who are homeless for the first time. Psychiatr Serv 53(11):1472–1474

Haldenby A, Berman H, Forchuk C (2011) Homelessness and health in adolescents. In: Forchuk C, Csiernik R, Jensen E (eds) Homelessness, housing, and mental health finding truths-creating change. Canadian Scholar's Press, Toronto, pp 91–105

Hwang SW, Wilkins R, Tjepkema M, O'Campo PJ, Dunn JR (2009) Mortality among residents of shelters, rooming houses, and hotels in Canada: 11 year follow-up study. Br Med J 339:1068–1070

Hwang SW, Ueng JJ, Chiu S, Kiss A, Tolomiczenko G, Cowan L, Levinson W, Redelmeier DA (2010) Universal health insurance and health care access for homeless persons. Am J Public Health 100(8):1454–1461

Hwang S, Gogosis E, Chambers C, Dunn J, Hoch J, Aubry T (2011) Health status, quality of life, residential stability, substance use, and health care utilization among adults applying to a supportive housing program. J Urban Health 88(6):1076–1090

Iaquinta MS (2016) A systemic review of the transition from homelessness to finding a home. J Community Health Nurs 33(1):20–41. doi:10.1080/07370016.2016.1120593

Jaeger M, Briner D, Kawohl W, Seifritz E, Baumgartner-Nietlisbach G (2015) Psychosocial functioning of individuals with schizophrenia in community housing facilities and the psychiatric hospital in Zurich. Psychiatry Res 230(2):413–418. doi:10.1016/j.psychres.2015.09.029

Marquez GM, Urraza XA (2016) The impact of the crisis on homelessness in Spain: social intervention in a context of greater need and fewer resources. Eur J Soc Work 19(1):31–45. doi:10.1080/13691457.2015.1022712

McLaughlin KA, Hatzenbuehler ML, Xuan Z, Conron KJ (2012) Disproportionate exposure to early-life adversity and sexual orientation disparities in psychiatric morbidity. Child Abuse Negl 36(9):645–655. doi:10.1016/j.chiabu.2012.07.004

Mental Health Commission of Canada (2013) Turning the key: assessing housing and related supports for persons living with mental health problems and illness. Author, Ottawa. http://www.mentalhealthcommission.ca/sites/default/files/PrimaryCare_Turning_the_Key_Full_ENG_0_1.pdf

Nelson G, Hall GB, Forchuk C (2011) Current and preferred Housing of Mental Health Consumer-Survivors. In: Forchuk C, Csiernik R, Jensen E (eds) Homelessness, housing, and mental health finding truths-creating change. Canadian Scholar's Press, Toronto, pp 107–121

Okamura T, Takeshima T, Tachimori H, Takiwaki K, Matoba Y, Awata S (2015) Characteristics of individuals with mental illness in Tokyo homeless shelters. Psychiatr Serv 66(12):1290–1295. doi:10.1176/appi.ps.201400517

Ray N (2006) Lesbian, gay, bisexual and transgender youth: an epidemic of homelessness. National Gay and Lesbian Task Force Policy Institute and the National Coalition for the Homeless, New York

Reid S, Berman H, Forchuk C (2005) Living on the streets in Canada: a feminist narrative study of girls and young women. Issues Compr Pediatr Nurs 28:237–256

Rosario M, Schrimshaw EW, Hunter J (2012) Risk factors for homelessness among lesbian, gay, and bisexual youths: a developmental milestones approach. Child Youth Serv Rev 34(10):186–193. doi:10.1016/j.childyouth.2011.09.016

Statistics Canada (2010) Healthy people, healthy places (Cat. No. 82–229-X2009001). Minister of Industry, Ottawa. http://www5.statcan.gc.ca/olc-cel/olc.action?objId=82-229-X&objType=2&lang=en&limit=0

Tsemberis S, Asmussen S (1999) From streets to homes: an innovative approach to supported housing for homeless adults with psychiatric disabilities. J Community Psychol 27(2):225–241

The US Department of Housing and Urban Development (2016) The 2016 Annual Homeless Assessment Report (AHAR) to Congress. Retrieved from https://www.hudexchange.info/resources/documents/2016-AHAR-Part-1.pdf

Yim LC-L, Leung HC-M, Chan WC, Lam MH-B, Lim VW-M (2015) Prevalence of mental illness among homeless people in Hong Kong. PLoS ONE 10(10):e0140940. doi:10.1371/journal.pone.014094

Mental Health Problems and Risks in Refugees During Migration Processes and Experiences: Literature Overview and Interventions

41

Cossu Giulia, Maura Galletta, and Carta Mauro Giovanni

41.1 Introduction and Background

According to the United Nations High Commissioner for Refugees, the number of refugees and internally displaced people has reached its highest point since World War II; it could be over 65 million, and this figure is still rising (UNHCR's annual Global Trends Report, 2015). The figure is up from 37.5 millions 10 years ago. About 22 millions of these are asylum seekers. In the last year, 1 million asylum seekers came to Europe, and almost 4000 have died in the Mediterranean Sea (UNHCR's annual Global Trends Report 2015; Carta et al. 2015). Refugees are people fleeing conflict or persecution. They are defined and protected by international law and must not be expelled or returned to situations where their life and freedom are at risk (UNHCR's 2015). Such international legal protection started back in 1951, when the United Nations Convention relating to the status of refugees defined a refugee as someone who fears being persecuted for reasons of race, religion, nationality, membership of a particular social group, or political opinion. A refugee lives outside his/her country of origin and is unable or unwilling to be protected by that country. The term refugee is sometimes used to indicate persons forced to flee from their own countries. Actually a distinction should be made between those who have received official hospitality in the country of arrival and whose rights are guaranteed by the Geneva Convention and those who have not. Today most of the people who escape atrocities prefer to remain underground – i.e.,

C. Giulia • M. Galletta • C.M. Giovanni (✉)
Department of Medical Science and Public Health, University of Cagliari, Cagliari, Italy
e-mail: mgcarta@tiscali.it

© Springer International Publishing Switzerland 2018

J.C. Santos, J.R. Cutcliffe (eds.), *European Psychiatric/Mental Health Nursing in the 21st Century*, Principles of Specialty Nursing,
https://doi.org/10.1007/978-3-319-31772-4_41

without official recognition – since an application for asylum might cause their exposure to the risk of retaliation by their country of origin. According to the rules of the European Union, if a person receives the status of refugee in one country, she/he cannot leave it for another EU country. Most refugees arrive in Italy but have relatives in other countries, particularly in Northern Europe. For this reason nobody wants to be recognized as a refugee upon their arrival.

Refugees have been often subjected to a range of traumatic experiences: human rights violations, persecution, war trauma, gender-based violence, significant family losses, and dangerous travels. Lack of information about immigration status, potential hostility, and undignified and protracted detention are all potential traumatic and stressful events. Not surprisingly, asylum seekers and refugees might have been exposed to events that have influenced their mental health (WHO/Europe 2015). According to the fifth edition of the Diagnostic and Statistical Manual of Mental Disorders (5th ed.; *DSM-5*), the so-called trauma- and stressor-related disorder includes so-called disorders that arise from exposure to a traumatic or stressful events. These include so-called reactive attachment disorder, disinhibited social engagement disorder, post-traumatic stress disorder (PTSD), adjustment disorders, and acute stress disorder. Many individuals who have been exposed to a traumatic or stressful event exhibit anxiety, fear-based symptoms, and most prominent clinical characteristics as anhedonic and dysphoric symptoms, externalizing angry and aggressive symptoms, or dissociative symptoms (DSM-5); most of these symptoms evolve into a so-called structured disorder. Other frequent mental health problems and challenges among asylum seekers are depression and anxiety "disorders" (Naja et al. 2016). Two comprehensive systematic reviews and meta-analyses showed that these subjects are about ten times more likely than the general population to have post-traumatic stress disorder (PTSD), with a higher incidence rate in younger people (Fazel et al. 2005; Bogic et al. 2015). Similarly, a study on Bosnian refugees showed that after 3 years, 45% of the people suffering from post-traumatic stress disorder still presented significant symptoms; symptoms remained even after over 10 years since exposure to traumatic events (Mollica et al. 1999; Mollica et al. 2007). The Lebanese population has shown a high risk of psychiatric disorders documented 20 years after the Lebanese war, particularly among those who were children at that time (Karam et al. 2008). The results of a study made on Syrian refugees in Turkey are quite similar to the findings of the cited studies in Lebanon (Acarturk et al. 2015), thus supporting the need to consider the long-term consequences on these populations.

As a result, subsequent to a review of the relevant theoretical and empirical literature, the chapter highlights concepts, phenomena, and propositions that could serve as the basis for a theoretical framework of risk factors, mediation, and protective factors involved in the possible onset and development of mental health problems among refugee populations during their migration experience. The review will also take into account the risk factors attributable to the three phases (e.g., premigration, migration, post-migration) of the migration process according to a conventional time perspective. The potential protective factors on refugees' mental health will be identified on different levels: the personal level (i.e., skills, strategies, demographic characteristics), the community level (i.e., support from the community or from family members on the territory), and the cultural level (i.e., cultural meaning systems and beliefs). We are assuming that this is a purely explicative distinction of dimensions that may depend one upon the others. Also clinical practices will be put in question as well as their probable ethnocentrism trend. Interventions treating symptoms of mental disorders among refugees population will be reviewed, and preventive measures will be discussed. The goal is to support and strengthen clinical knowledge on existing responses and treatments that could actually prove to be useful and effective response to the emergency to provide adequate care to a risk population as that of refugees and asylum seekers.

41.2 Risk Factors

Population movements expose migrants to a range of risk factors that may impact on various health issues: the reproductive system, drug and alcohol abuse, higher newborn mortality, and mental disease (Fazel et al. 2005; Bogic et al. 2015). Migration process can be conventionally explained in three stages, which can expose migrants to specific ranges of traumatic experiences. The first stage is called "premigration": it can be characterized by human rights violations, persecution, economic hardship, war trauma, and disruption of social support and of family and community networks. The second stage is called "migration," namely, physical relocation of individuals from one place to another which can be characterized by extremely dangerous journeys with an uncertain migration outcome, violent separation from the loved ones, and extremely precarious living conditions. Finally the "post-migration" stage may expose migrants to such factors as undignified and protracted detention, hostility, uncertainty about the outcome of the application for political asylum, difficulties in language learning, acculturation and adaptation, concern about family members left behind, and possibility of reunification (Bhugra 2004; Bhugra and Gupta 2011). Moreover once a mental health problem has become manifest, post-migration factors become critical in the process of development and potential chronicity of the problem (Carta et al. 2013; Mollica et al. 1999, Mollica et al. 2007; Lindert et al. 2009; Bogic et al. 2003, Bogic et al. 2015; Ginzburg 2010).

41.3 Resilience, Sense of Coherence, Coping Strategies, and Community Network Support as Mediating Factors

Overall the acculturation process can be mediated by economic, educational, social, psychological, physical, and cultural factors. Individual factors such as gender, age, language proficiency, and economic educational status contribute to the inclusion process, too, albeit in different ways (Hadgkiss and Renzaho 2014). Porter and Haslam (2005) in their meta-analysis found that individuals with higher levels of education who experienced significant decrease in their socioeconomic and professional status after migration had worse post-migration outcomes. The individual coping strategies generate a response to stressors, influence the acculturation process outcome, and may therefore become a potential protection factor. The coping strategies developed after traumatic events are commonly described as a way to manage adverse or problematic conditions (Aldwin and Tracey 1987; Carver et al. 1989; Taylor and Stanton 2007). Action-oriented and intrapsychic efforts to manage stressful events can include:

- The cognitive ability to *process* and restore past and present stressful *events*
- Reframe the situation
- Focus on future wishes
- Relaxation and meditation
- Avoid any exposure to conditions that might recall the traumatic event

These strategies were discussed in different studies on refugee populations, showing their potential role in mediating the psychological burden following exposure to stressful events (Halcón et al. 2004; Goodman 2004; Khaawaja et al. 2008).

An individual's ability to recover quickly from "illness" and drastic changes and successfully adapt to adversity, trauma, tragedy, threats, or stressor – known as resilience (Davydov et al. 2010) – has emerged as a potential predictor of mental health outcomes among refugees (Schweitzer et al. 2007). Sense of coherence (SOC) (Antonovsky 1979) refers to an internal psychological mechanism that mediates the effects of external stressors. SOC refers how people see life and, in stressful situations, identify and use their resources to maintain and develop their health. SOC is a tripartite construct consisting in three dimensions: comprehensibility (the ability to understand processes and events), manageability (the ability to manage stressful events), and meaningfulness (the ability to assign and process meanings). Some studies have shown SOC can be an extremely powerful predictor of psychological coping and mediate the effects of external stressors among Southeast Asian refugees (Ying et al. 1997; Ying and Akutsu 1997).

Hofstede (2011) attempted to identify macrocultural dimensions in order to better define the acculturation phenomenon. He described cultural dimensions in terms of collectivism/individualism, feminine/masculine, orientation to power, and avoidance of uncertainty. Nevertheless not all the cultures have the same dimensions; furthermore, these characteristics may interact generating similar or different cultural outcomes than those of the host country (Bhugra 2014). In fact in some cultural contexts, religion, gender role expectations, and attitude toward the institutions and medical services can modulate the relationship between stressful events and mental health outcomes (Kamperman et al. 2007). A recent qualitative study of attributions in war survivors has underlined social attachment and support, coping strategies, personality hardiness, community involvement, and normalization of everyday life as the main helpful factors in recovery from post-traumatic symptoms (Ajdukovic et al. 2013). Lack of awareness and knowledge about mental health problems and medical care opportunities may ultimately increase the attribution ambiguity and foster more stigmatizing dynamics (Schomerus et al. 2012).

The post-migration process, and the procedure to be granted legal asylum in particular (in Italy) which lasts about 1 year, can expose refugees to a vast number of social stressors such as difficulty in participating in society, stigmatization, exclusion from welfare benefits and work, discrimination, racism, and stereotyping by the host community. Potential community intervention to protect from the overall burden of migration psychological distress includes family and community cohesion, support, and collective identity (Siriwardhana et al. 2014). Community approaches aim to achieve a strong social impact and social inclusion (Williams and Thompson 2011; Bolton et al. 2014); more specifically, some of these interventions are oriented to engage and empower local community groups to take an active part and true participation in diagnosing and solving their own health problems (Morgan 2001; Harpham and Few 2002). Resilience, SOC, and coping strategies, but also individual qualities, religious beliefs and culture, knowledge, social community, and family support, can all modulate the relationship between events, acculturation outcomes, and mental health. These dimensions can become potential protective factors reducing the overall burden of mental illnesses and levels of psychological distress (Siriwardhana et al. 2014). The interaction between these elements can have a decisive influence on the ability to seek help and support, use institutional and social resources, and access to health services.

41.4 From Ethnocentrism to Culturally Sensitive Practices

Modern medicine and health care, including mental health care, have been developed thanks to the contribution of scientists of different cultures. For example, despite the contemporary anti-Islamic sentiment that proliferates certain groups (see, e.g., many of the remarks and policies advance by candidate Donald Trump during the recent presidential elections in the USA or comments made during the "Brexit" campaign), Carta and Moro (2014) pointed out that:

> The great Greek and Roman medical tradition was saved thanks to the contribution of the doctors of the Arabic courts, who transcribed the Greek classics into Arab when Christian fundamentalism denied the science such as Ibn Rusd and Moshe ben Maimon.

On the one hand, it is necessary to underline that modern medicine and mental health care are the products of the contribution of different cultures, whose merits and paternity ought to be acknowledged; on the other hand, many psychiatric clinical practices tend to ethnocentrism (REF). Ethnocentrism is the attitude to use practices and standards that are strongly related to mental health conceptions influenced only by western symbols and meanings (REF). Not surprisingly, the most recent edition of the DSM emphasizes the need to assess mental health needs and problems in a more interpretive culture framework:

> Diagnostic assessment must therefore consider whether an individual's experiences, symptoms, and behaviors differ from sociocultural norms and lead to difficulties in adaptation in the cultures of origin and in specific social or familial contexts. (DSM-5, p?)

In particular, as regards to the spectrum of trauma-related problems, DSM-5 specifies that:

> Cultural syndromes and idioms of distress influence the expression of PTSD and the range of comorbid disorders in different cultures by providing behavioral and cognitive templates that link traumatic exposures to specific symptoms. For example, panic attack symptoms may be salient in PTSD among Cambodians and Latin Americans because of the association of traumatic exposure with panic-like *khyâl* attacks and *ataque de nervios*. Comprehensive evaluation of local expressions of PTSD should include assessment of cultural concepts of distress.

The overall trend seems indeed to perceive refugees like a homogeneous population linked by traumatic experiences of human rights violations and physical abuse; accordingly it becomes necessary to consider the complexity of the cultural differences involved in a massive population movement. The limitations imposed by ethnocentricity are now recognized by many scientists and professionals, who underline how some aspects of trauma-related mental disorders are shaped by cultural determinants (Marsella 2010; Drožđek and Bolwerk 2010; Drozdek and Wilson 2007; Wilson and So-Kum Tang 2007).

The bias of imposing treatment without cultural appropriateness could generate a distorted picture of psychosocial disabilities and functioning, poor outcome, and ineffective treatment; it may as well increase distrust of nontraditional practices. Several efforts have been made to adapt clinical practices, as much as possible, to a more culturally sensitive approach. Tool validations in different languages (Mollica et al. 1999, 2007; Dinh et al. 2009), or support by a native language consultant or lay counselor (Neuner et al. 2008), have been implemented in the clinical practice, although the approach of mere linguistic adaptation of PTSD measurement and treatment was criticized (Myers 2011). Culturally sensitive approaches and treatments that pay higher attention to the varying social context have been explored and applied. In the case of Congolese and Somali men and women refugee groups in the USA, mental health concerns were often dealt in their community first, with the help of families or friends. The role of mental health professionals seems to be not well understood by all refugees, and this could have a strong effect on hesitancy to access medical services, thus in turn worsening the stigma dynamics (Piwowarczyk et al. 2014).

An analysis of the recorded and transcribed statements, beliefs, and knowledge about post-traumatic stress disorder among older Iranian refugees in the USA has shown a holistic approach to health care that views the mind, the body, and the spirit as inseparable (REF). These three elements are indicated with a unique word: *salamati*. This holistic view could contribute to their difficulties in describing symptoms that conform to western biomedical standards (Martin 2009). More culture-sensitive programs could favor the effective work with refugees within a social justice framework, but it requires potential modification of empirically supported screening and treatments and overall flexibility of clinicians.

41.5 Treating Mental Health Problems Among Refugee Populations

Some approaches and types of treatment of trauma among refugee populations have obtained more specific attention. Some of the major approaches will be illustrated, to provide an overview of what the scientific literature has underlined. Psychological, social, physical, biofeedback, and complementary and alternative medicine treatments shall be herein described. Some treatments use group techniques including community, family members, or individual session's therapy; in some cases these have been integrated and used in a multidisciplinary way (Slobodin and de Jong 2015).

41.5.1 Community-Based Interventions

The goal of community-based interventions is to involve communities and families as real healing agents through cohesion, support, and collective identity identification. This approach might also act as a potential protective factor that effectively reduces the overall burden of mental health problems (Siriwardhana et al. 2014). The local community has been empowered to take an active part and true participation in the diagnosis and care process (Morgan 2001; Harpham and Few 2002). Participation in health outcomes can be implemented in some steps of the process, e.g., the planning or implementation intervention phases. Community-based interventions mainly focus on outreach, workshops, train-the-trainer models, employment of refugees, and mentoring programs. All activities are generally aimed at achieving a strong social impact and social inclusion (Stone 1992; Williams and Thompson 2011; Bolton et al. 2014).

41.5.2 Complementary and Alternative Medicine

The National Center for Complementary and Alternative Medicine (NCCAM) divides complementary and alternative medicine (CAM) into four domains: mind/body medicine, biologically based practices, manipulative and body-based practices, and energy medicine (Pearson and Chesney 2007). Some of these promising approaches are emerging in the physical rehabilitation of torture survivors and include physical therapy; others focus on meditation, specific diet and exercise, and acupuncture (Mollica 2011). Several studies and reviews have documented the use of CAM among refugees, finding evidence of the use of CAM in combination with or without standard medicine on refugee populations (MacDuff et al. 2011). The conclusions were limited by some methodological problems in the included studies, namely, poor documentation of intervention methods and lack of randomized control trials. More evidence-based approaches and further investigation would be appropriate.

41.5.3 Trauma-Focused Cognitive Behavioral Therapy

As an adapted form of cognitive behavioral therapy, trauma-focused cognitive behavioral therapy (TF-CBT) is a component-based psychosocial treatment model that integrates also attachment, humanistic, empowerment, and caregiver therapy elements. In the first part of the therapy, psychoeducation is provided to patients and their caregivers concerning the impact of trauma and common reactions. With the aim of helping identify and cope with a range of emotions and behavioral adjustments, relaxation and stress training skills are provided. Cognitive processing is enhanced by illustrating the relationships among thoughts, behaviors, and feelings, while the trauma is gone through narration, with patients' describing their personal traumatic experiences (Buhmann et al. 2015; Lambert and Alhassoon 2015).

41.5.4 Narrative Exposure Therapy

NET (Narrative Exposure Therapy) is a narrative approach, a short, pragmatic, and cross-cultural application mainly used as PTSD treatment (REF). It can be applied across cultures and easily fits into the social and setting backgrounds (Gwozdziewycz and Mehl-Madrona 2013). In NET the patient constructs a narrative of his whole life, from birth to present day, recording a new biography with the therapist support instead of defining a single traumatic event as the only target of therapy. Patients are encouraged to reconstruct a narration of their lives and contextualize their experiences in a more social justice and emotionally aware framework (Gwozdziewycz and Mehl-Madrona 2013; Buhmann 2014).

41.5.5 Interpersonal Psychotherapy (IPT)

Interpersonal psychotherapy (IPT) is a short psychotherapy focus on interpersonal issues, which are considered fundamental in the genesis and maintenance of psychological distress. The targets of IPT are symptom resolution, improving interpersonal functioning, and increasing social support. Social functioning is assessed and discussed with consequent benefits on the quality of life and mood symptom experience. The patient's interpersonal functioning problems are previously analyzed and structured in four areas, interpersonal disputes, role transitions, grief, and interpersonal deficits (Stuart and Robertson 2012), in order to generate the interpersonal inventory assessment that is an important starting point of therapy. Therapy works by identifying dispute, role transition, or grief and linking them with emotional and interpersonal accomplishments occurring during the final part of the treatment. Despite the growing body of evidence concerning the effectiveness of this therapy (Swartz et al. 2014), few studies have addressed its effectiveness among refugees (Meffert et al. 2014).

41.5.6 Basic Body Awareness Therapy

Basic Body Awareness Therapy (BBAT) is a recommended form of physiotherapy that combines a number of different movements from the Western and Eastern traditions. The Body Awareness Therapy was developed and taken from Swedish physiotherapy and implemented in the treatment of psychiatric disorders. BBAT has somatic, biological, physiotherapy bases and includes other professional practices, such as psychiatry and psychotherapy. Since the spectrum of trauma disorders often includes a strong psychosomatic base as an important part of the pathology, therapy is focused on body awareness exercises aimed at total coordination and nonverbal therapeutic process. The therapist guides the patient's movements to empower confidence in their own resources (Gyllenstcn et al. 2009). Chronic pain is very common among traumatized refugees, and it is believed to maintain the mental symptoms of trauma. The literature reports only a very limited amount of scientific trials about physical activity as part of the treatment of traumatized refugee populations (Stade et al. 2015; Gyllensten et al. 2009).

41.5.7 Biofeedback Treatments

Biofeedback has already been performed in a few preliminary studies on traumatized refugees (Muller et al. 2009) in combination with cognitive behavioral intervention treatment and physical activity for pain management. The intervention is performed by integrating various biofeedback technologies and physical activity tasks to make specific body movements (Schwartz and Andrasik 2015). While the patient performs tasks that stimulate images of a stressful situation or relaxation, the biofeedback technology can detect the patient's internal bodily functions with far greater precision than a person alone could. This information is evaluated by the patient and the therapist, in order to direct the progress of treatment. Trauma-related symptoms such as muscle tension due to hyperarousal can produce pain and more stress (Vlaeyen and Linton 2000). In this sense, movement task activity with biofeedback can help patients become more aware and learn new coping strategies to manage their physiological reactivity and somatic and psychological symptoms.

41.5.8 Physical Activity

Physical activity has already been performed within a cognitive behavior therapy (CBT) intervention with the aim of helping traumatized refugees cope with pain. This has suggested that physical activity adds value to pain management intervention outcomes (Liedl et al. 2011). The effectiveness of interventions that use physical activity – with or without integration of conventional therapies – has already been amply demonstrated in a wide range of mental disorders, including depression, anxiety, and PTSD (Manger and Motta 2005; Carta et al. 2008; Mura and Carta 2013).

41.5.9 Mindfulness

The definition of mindfulness is based on Buddhist and psychological literature, and it refers to a set of meditation and awareness practices, defined "mindful," to the focus on present-oriented experience with a certain emotional attitude, and to mind-sets designed to achieve body-set acceptance perceptions. The patient doing meditation is instructed to watch thoughts and feelings come and go on their own, without judging them. Mindfulness focuses on relaxation and gentleness and leads the person to watch thoughts and emotional reactions from a completely different perspective. Some trial has already illustrated how to utilize acceptance and mindfulness techniques in integrated treatments (culturally adapted CBT, or CA-CBT) for traumatized refugees and ethnic minority populations (Hinton et al. 2013).

41.5.9.1 Eye Movement Desensitization and Reprocessing

Eye movement desensitization and reprocessing (EMDR) is known particularly for treating PTSD after traumatic experiences. EMDR aims to alleviate the distress associated with traumatic memories, by facilitating the access to and the processing of traumatic experience in order to get to an adaptive resolution. The therapeutic goal is to relieve distress, reformulate negative beliefs, and reduce physiological arousal. During EMDR therapy, the patient remembers emotionally disturbing materials while simultaneously focusing on an external stimulus – like hand tapping or audio stimulation – and performing lateral eye movements. Information processing is enhanced through new associations forged between the traumatic memory and more adaptive emotions and information (Shapiro and Maxfield 2002). Since EMDR seems to be an easily implementable technique in specific contexts, among Traumatized Refugees, it is receiving a lot of attention (Bower et al. 2004; Regel and Berliner 2007; Jackie June ter Heide et al. 2011).

41.5.9.2 The Effectiveness of Cultural Sensitivity Practices and the Role of Community Support

Some kinds of treatment are receiving more attention than others. Narrative Exposure Therapy seems to be the most implemented and evaluated approach among refugees (Robjant and Fazel 2010). A recent meta-analysis concerning RCT of NET revealed that it shows a total average effect size of 0.53 (Cohen's d). The effect size found in a trial that actively involved refugees in the care process as counselors was of 1.02 (Gwozdziewycz and Mehl-Madrona 2013). This may suggest that NET can be actually more effective on refugee clinical populations. The common cultural background between counselors and treated refugees could be the key. If it were true, then a culturally sensitive approach could really serve as a key component in the therapeutic process among refugee populations. So far a limited number of studies have included a refugee community member as a therapist or a counselor (Neuner et al. 2008; Meffert et al. 2014). Other studies have included a native speaker or a certified translator in the NET therapeutic process, but these were not from the same refugees' cultural community (Stenmark et al. 2013; Hijazi et al. 2014). Family support is often recognized as a key context for refugees and their mental health, serving as a resource for adjustment and coping (Voulgaridou et al. 2006). Multiple-family group intervention can be effective in increasing access to mental health services, while family support can mediate the intervention effect in depression symptoms among refugees (Weine et al. 2008).

41.6 Preventing Mental Health Problems Among Refugees

Refugees' exposition may span generations with significant negative impacts on public health and socioeconomic development (World Health Organization 2015). Despite this, few studies have verified the effectiveness of prevention programs on refugees' well-being (Kirmayer et al. 2011). Preventive efforts to reduce the onset of mental disorders among migrants should focus on mental health education and on emotional, social, and economic support; and they should address the barriers against traditional western mental health services and human rights (Porter 2007). Considering the factors that have proved crucial for refugees' quality of life, post-migration interventions should provide an integrated approach including trauma therapy, work orientation, language training, and support for bureaucratic and political awareness, while facilitating the creation of a supportive refugees' network in the host community. Preventive activities aimed at facilitating and speeding up the integration process have already proved a protective factor against experiences of discrimination and mental disease, in a perspective of long-term health benefits (Beiser 2006). Community-oriented intervention in the early stages of refugee resettlement has been performed among young refugees in the USA, with the aim to prevent or detect the initial stages of mental illness. Results showed how community-based mental health services seem more effective than the traditional primary care model (Weine et al. 2006; Weine 2008; Weine 2011; Dura-Vila et al. 2013). Community collaboration opposes the feeling of being isolated, alone, and discriminated; it is also a great facilitator in the access to information and resources by refugee community members, especially by the younger ones, thus supporting the successful adaptation to host countries (Birman et al. 2008; Tyrer and Fazel 2014). Preventive interventions have often been conducted with minimum methodological quality standards; therefore, more studies are required on its application and on the effect it might have on public health.

References

Acarturk C, Konuk E, Cetinkaya M, Senay I, Sijbrandij M, Cuijpers P, Aker T (2015) EMDR for Syrian refugees with posttraumatic stress disorder symptoms: results of a pilot randomized controlled trial. Eur J Psychotraumatol 18(6):27414

Ajdukovic D, Ajdukovic D, Bogic M, Franciskovic T, Galeazzi GM, Kucukalic A, Lecic-Tosevski D, Schützwohl M, Priebe S (2013) Recovery from posttraumatic stress symptoms: a qualitative study of attributions in survivors of war. PLoS One 8(8):e70579

Aldwin CM, Tracey R (1987) Does coping help? A re-examination of the relation between coping and mental health. J Pers Soc Psychol 53(2):337–348

Antonovsky A (1979) Health, stress and coping. Jossey-Bass, San Francisco
Beiser M (2006) Longitudinal research to promote effective refugee resettlement. Transcult Psychiatry 43(1):56–71
Bhugra D (2004) Migration and mental health. Acta Psychiatr Scand 109(4):243–258
Bhugra D (2014) All medicine is social. J R Soc Med 107(5):183–186
Bhugra D, Gupta S (2011) Migration in mental health. Cambridge University Press, Cambridge
Birman D, Beehler S, Harris EM, Everson ML, Batia K, Liautaud J, Frazier S, Atkins M, Blanton S, Buwalda J, Fogg L, Cappella E (2008) International family, adult, and child enhancement services (FACES): a community-based comprehensive services model for refugee children in resettlement. Am J Orthopsychiatry 78(1):121–132
Bogic M, Ajdukovic D, Bremner S, Franciskovic T, Galeazzi GM, Kucukalic A, Lecic-Tosevski D, Morina N, Popovski M, Schützwohl M, Wang D, Priebe S (2003) Factors associated with mental disorders in long-settled war refugees: refugees from the former Yugoslavia in Germany, Italy and the UK. Br J Psychiatry 200(3):216–223
Bogic M, Njoku A, Priebe S (2015) Long-term mental health of war-refugees: a systematic literature review. BMC 15:29
Bolton P, Lee C, Haroz EE, Murray L, Dorsey S, Robinson C, Ugueto AM, Bass J (2014) A transdiagnostic community-based mental health treatment for comorbid disorders: development and outcomes of a randomized controlled trial among Burmese refugees in Thailand. PLoS Med 11(11):e1001757
Bower RD, Pahl L, Bernstein MA (2004) Case presentation of a tattoo-mutilated, Bosnian torture survivor. Torture 14(1):16–24
Buhmann CB (2014) Traumatized refugees: morbidity, treatment and predictors of outcome. Dan Med J 61(8):B4871
Buhmann C, Andersen I, Mortensen EL, Ryberg J, Nordentoft M, Ekstrøm M (2015) Cognitive behavioral psychotherapeutic treatment at a psychiatric trauma clinic for refugees: description and evaluation. Torture 25(1):17–32
Carta, M.G. & Moro, M.F. (2014) Conflicts and mental health in the Mediterranean, Conference: XVI World Congress of Psychiatry. Madrid 2014, At Madrid, Volume 2. Abstracts Regular Symposia, Conference Paper January 2014
Carta MG, Hardoy MC, Pilu A, Sorba M, Floris AL, Mannu FA, Baum A, Cappai A, Velluti C, Salvi M (2008) Improving physical quality of life with group physical activity in the adjunctive treatment of major depressive disorder. Clin Pract Epidemiol Ment Health 26(4):1
Carta MG, Wallet Oumar F, Moro MF, Moro D, Preti A, Mereu A, Bhugra D (2013) Trauma and stressor related disorders in the tuareg refugees of a camp in Burkina Faso. Clin Pract EpidemiolMental Health 9:189–195
Carta MG, Moro MF, Bass J (2015) War traumas in the Mediterranean area. Int J Soc Psychiatry 61(1):33–38
Carver CS, Scheier MF, Weintraub JK (1989) Assessing coping strategies: a theoretically based approach. J Pers Soc Psychol 56(2):267–283
Davydov DM, Stewart R, Ritchie K, Chaudieu I (2010) Resilience and mental health. Clin Psychol Rev 30(5):479–495
Dinh TQ, Yamada AM, Yee BW (2009) A culturally relevant conceptualization of depression: an empirical examination of the factorial structure of the Vietnamese depression scale. Int J Soc Psychiatry 55(6):496–505
Drožđek B, Bolwerk N (2010) Group therapy with traumatized asylum seekers and refugees: for whom it works and for whom it does not? Traumatology 16(4):160–167
Drozdek B, Wilson JP (2007) Voices of trauma: treating psychological across cultures. Springer
Dura-Vila G, Klasen H, Makatini Z, Rahimi Z, Hodes M (2013) Mental health problems of young refugees: duration of settlement, risk factors and community-based interventions. Clin Child Psychol Psychiatry 18:604–623
Fazel M, Wheeler J, Danesh J (2005) Prevalence of serious mental disorder in 7000 refugees resettled in western countries: a systematic review. Lancet 365:1309–1314

Ginzburg ES (2010) Comorbidity of posttraumatic stress disorder, anxiety and depression: a 20-years longitudinal study of war veterans. J Affect Disord 123(1-3):249–257
Goodman JH (2004) Coping with trauma and hardship among unaccompanied refugee youths from Sudan. Quant Health Res 14(9):1177–1196
Gwozdziewycz N, Mehl-Madrona L (2013) Meta-analysis of the use of narrative exposure therapy for the effects of trauma among refugee populations. Perm J 17(1):70–76
Gyllensten AL, Ekdahl C, Hansson L (2009) Long-term effectiveness of basic body awareness therapy in psychiatric outpatient care. A randomized controlled study. Adv Physiother 11(1):2–12
Hadgkiss EJ, Renzaho AM (2014) The physical health status, service utilisation and barriers to accessing care for asylum seekers residing in the community: a systematic review of the literature. Aust Health Rev 38(2):142–159
Halcón LL, Robertson CL, Savik K, Johnson DR, Spring MA, Butcher JN, Westermeyer JJ, Jaranson JM (2004) Trauma and coping in Somali and Oromo refugee youth. J Adolesc Health 35(1):17–25
Harpham T, Few R (2002) The Dar Es Salaam urban health project, Tanzania: a multi-dimensional evaluation. J Public Health Med 24(2):112–119
Hijazi AM, Lumley MA, Ziadni MS, Haddad L, Rapport LJ, Arnetz BB (2014) Brief narrative exposure therapy for post-traumatic stress in Iraqi refugees: a preliminary randomized clinical trial. J Trauam Stress 27(3):314–322
Hinton DE, Pich VH, Stefan G, Otto MW (2013) Acceptance and mindfulness techniques as applied to refugee and ethnic minority populations with PTSD: examples from "culturally adapted CBT". Cogn Behav Pract 20(1):33–46
Hofstede G (2011) Dimensionalizing cultures: the hofstede model in context. Online Read Psychol Culture 2(1):8
Jackie June ter Heide F, Mooren GTM, Kleijn W, de Jongh A, Kleber RJ (2011) EMDR versus stabilisation in traumatised asylum seekers and refugees: results of a pilot RCT. Eur J Psychotraumatol 2:5881
Kamperman AM, Komproe IH, de Jong JT (2007) Migrant mental health: a model for indicators of mental health and health care consumption. Health Psychol 26(1):96–104
Karam EG, Fayyad J, Nasser Karam A, Cordahi TC, Melhem N, Mneimneh Z, Dimassi H (2008) Effectiveness and specificity of a classroom-based group intervention in children and adolescents exposed to war in Lebanon. World Psychiatry 7:103–109
Khaawaja NG, White KM, Schweiter R, Greenslade J (2008) Difficulties and coping strategies of Sudanese refugees: a qualitative approach. Transcult Psychaitry 45(3):489–512
Kirmayer LJ, Narasiah L, Munoz M, Rashid M, Ryder AG, Guzder J, Hassan G, Rousseau C, Pottie K (2011) Canadian collaboration for immigrant and refugee health (CCIRH): common mental health problems in immigrants and refugees: general approach in primary care. CMAJ 183(12):E959–E967
Lambert JE, Alhassoon OM (2015) Trauma-focused therapy for refugees: meta-analytic findings. J Couns Psychol 62(1):28–37
Liedl A, Müller J, Morina N, Karl A, Denke C, Knaevelsrud C (2011) Physical activity within a CBT intervention improves coping with pain in traumatized refugees: results of a randomized controlled design. Pain Med 12(2):234–245
Lindert J, Ehrenstein OS, Priebe S, Mielck A, Brähler E (2009) Depression and anxiety in labor migrants and refugees--a systematic review and meta-analysis. Soc Sci Med 69(2):246–257
MacDuff S, Grodin MA, Gardiner P (2011) The use of complementary and alternative medicine among refugees: a systematic review. J Immigr Minor Health 13(3):585–599
Manger TA, Motta RW (2005) The impact of an exercise program on posttraumatic stress disorder, anxiety, and depression. Int J Emerg Ment Health 7(1):49–57
Marsella AJ (2010) Ethnocultural aspects of PTSD: an overview of concepts, issues, and treatments. Traumatology 16(4):17–26
Martin SS (2009) Illness of the mind or illness of the spirit? Mental health-related conceptualization and practices of older Iranian immigrants. Health Soc Work 34(2):17–26

Meffert SM, Abdo AO, Alla OA, Elmakki YO, Omer AA, Yousif S, Metzler TJ, Marmar CR (2014) Pilot randomized controlled trial of interpersonal psychotherapy for Sudanese refugees in Cairo, Egypt. Psychol Trauma 6(3):240–249

Mollica RF (2011) Medical best practices for the treatment of torture survivors. Torture 21(1):8–17

Mollica RF, McInnes K, Sarajlic N, Lavelle J, Sarajlic I, Massagli MP (1999) Disability associated with psychiatric comorbidity and health status in Bosnian refugees living in Croatia. JAMA 282(5):433–439

Mollica RF, Caridad KR, Massagli MP (2007) Longitudinal study of posttraumatic stress disorder, depression, and changes in traumatic memories over time in Bosnian refugees. J Nerv Ment Dis 195(7):572–579

Morgan LM (2001) Community participation in health: perpetual allure, persistent challenge. Health Policy Plan 16(3):221–230

Muller J, Karl A, Denke C, Mathier F, Dittmann J, Rohleder N, Knaevelsrud C (2009) Biofeedback for pain management in traumatised refugees. Cogn Behav Ther 38(3):184–190

Mura G, Carta MG (2013) Physical activity in depressed elderly. A systematic review. Clin Pract Epidemiol Ment Health 12(9):125–135

Myers SJ (2011) Cross-cultural measurement of posttraumatic stress disorder in post-conflict settings. Am J Public Health 101(4):581–582

Naja WJ, Aoun MP, El Khoury EL, Abdallah FJ, Haddad RS (2016) Prevalence of depression in Syrian refugees and the influence of religiosity. Compr Psychiatry 68:78–85

Neuner F, Onyut PL, Ertl V, Odenwald M, Schauer E, Elbert T (2008) Treatment of post-traumatic stress disorder by trained lay counselors in an African refugee settlement: a randomized controlled trial. J Consult Clin Psychol 76(4):868–694

Pearson NJ, Chesney MA (2007) The national center for complementary and alternative medicine. Acad Med 82(10):967

Piwowarczyk L, Bishop H, Yusuf A, Mudymba F, Raj A (2014) Congolese and Somali beliefs about mental health services. J Nerv Ment Dis 202(3):209–216

Porter M (2007) Global evidence for a biopsychosocial understanding of refugee adaptation. Transcult Psychiatry 44(3):418–439

Porter M, Haslam N (2005) Predisplacement and postdisplacement factors associated with mental health of refugees and internally displaced persons: a meta-analysis. JAMA 294(5):602–612

Regel S, Berliner P (2007) Current perspectives on assessment and therapy with survivors of torture: the use of a cognitive behavioural approach. Eur J Psychother Counsel 9(3):289–299

Robjant K, Fazel M (2010) The emerging evidence for narrative exposure therapy: a review. Clin Psychol Rev 30(8):1030–1039

Schomerus G, Auer C, Rhode D, Luppa M, Freyberger HJ, Schmidt S (2012) Personal stigma, problem appraisal and perceived need for professional help in currently untreated depressed persons. J Affect Disord 139(1):94–97

Schwartz MS, Andrasik F (2015) Biofeedback: a practitioner's guide, 4th edn. The Guilford press, London

Schweitzer R, Greenslade J, Kagee A (2007) Coping and resilience in refugees from the Sudan: a narrative account. Aust N Z J Psychiatry 41(3):282–288

Shapiro F, Maxfield L (2002) Eye movement desensitization and reprocessing (EMDR): information processing in the treatment of trauma. J Clin Psychol 58(8):933–946

Siriwardhana C, Shirwa SA, Roberts B, Stewart R (2014) A systematic review of resilience and mental health outcomes of conflict-driven adult forced migrants. Confl Heal 8:13

Slobodin O, de Jong JT (2015) Mental health interventions for traumatized asylum seekers and refugees: what do we know about their efficacy? Int J Soc Psychiatry 61(1):17–26

Stade K, Skammeritz S, Hjortkjær C, Carlsson J (2015) "after all the traumas my body has been through, I feel good that it is still working."--basic body awareness therapy for traumatised refugees. Torture 25(1):33–50

Stenmark H, Catani C, Neuner F, Elbert T, Holen A (2013) Treating PTSD in refugees and asylum seekers within the general health care system: a randomized controlled multi-center study. Beh Res Ther 51(10):641–647

Stone L (1992) Cultural influences in community participation in health. Soc Sci Med 35(4):409–417
Stuart S, Robertson M (2012) Interpersonal psychotherapy: a clinician's guide, 2nd edn. Edward Arnold, London
Swartz HA, Grote NK, Graham P (2014) Brief interpersonal psychotherapy (IPT-B): overview and review of evidence. Am J Psychother 68(4):443–462
Taylor SE, Stanton AL (2007) Coping resources, coping processes and mental health. Annu Rev. Clin Psychol 3:377–401
Tyrer RA, Fazel M (2014) School and community-based interventions for refugee and asylum seeking children: a systematic review. PLoS One 9(2):e89359
UNHCR's annual Global Trends Report (2015), 20 JUNE 2016
Vlaeyen JW, Linton SJ (2000) Fear-avoidance and its consequences in chronic musculoskeletal pain: a state of the art. Pain 85(3):317–332
Voulgaridou M, Papadopoulos R, Tomaras V (2006) Working with refugee families in Greece: systemic considerations. J Fam Ther 28:200–220
Weine S (2008) Family roles in refugee youth resettlement from a prevention perspective. Child Adolesc Psychiatr Clin N Am 17(3):515–518
Weine S (2011) Developing preventive mental health interventions for refugee families in resettlement. Fam Process 50(3):410–430
Weine SM, Kulauzovic Y, Besic S, Lezic A, Mujagic A, Muzurovic J et al (2006) A family beliefs framework for developing socially and culturally specific preventive interventions for refugee families and youth. Am J Orthopsychiatry 76:1–9
Weine S, Kulauzovic Y, Klebic A, Besic S, Mujagic A, Muzurovic J, Spahovic D, Sclove S, Pavkovic I, Feetham S, Rolland J (2008) Evaluating a multiple-family group access intervention for refugees with PTSD. J Marital Fam Ther 34(2):149–164
WHO/Europe (2015) Mental health and psychological support for refugees, asylum seekers and migrants on the move in Europe: a multi-agency guidance note
Williams ME, Thompson SC (2011) The use of community-based interventions in reducing morbidity from the psychological impact of conflict-related trauma among refugee populations: a systematic review of the literature. J Immigr Minor Health 13(4):780–794
Wilson JP, So-Kum Tang C (2007) Cross-cultural assessment of psychological trauma and PTSD. Springer, New York
World Health Organization (2015) Policy brief on migration and health: mental health care for refugees. http://www.euro.who.int/__data/assets/pdf_file/0006/293271/Policy-Brief-Migration-Health-Mental-Health-Care-Refugees.pdf?4a=1
Ying YW, Akutsu PD (1997) Psychological adjustment of southeast Asian refugees: the contribution of sense of coherence. J Commun Phychol 25(2):125–139
Ying YW, Akutsu PD, Zhang X et al (1997) Psychological dysfunction in southeast Asian refugees as mediated by sense of coherence. Am J Community Psychol 25:839

Printed by Printforce, the Netherlands